Memorable Neurology

Second Edition

Jonathan Heldt, M.D.

Also available from the same author:
Memorable Psychopharmacology
Memorable Psychiatry

The content of this book is not intended to be a replacement for proper medical training, nor is it intended to substitute for professional medical advice, diagnosis, or treatment. Always seek the advice of your physician or other qualified health provider with any questions you may have regarding a medical condition.

Editing and behavioral consultation provided by **Juliane Heldt, BCBA (Board Certified Behavior Analyst)**.

Revision 2.0. Last revised August 10, 2021.

ISBN: 1737210825
ISBN-13: 978-1737210825

DEDICATION

To **Dr. William Hemmerlin**. Thank you for showing me that anything is teachable with the right combination of passion for the learner, dedication to the craft, and ample servings of liquid nitrogen ice cream.

CONTENTS

Introduction

Neuroanatomy

Clinical Neurology

ACKNOWLEDGMENTS

To **Nick** for keeping me happy, warm, and well fed while working on this book.

1 INTRODUCTION

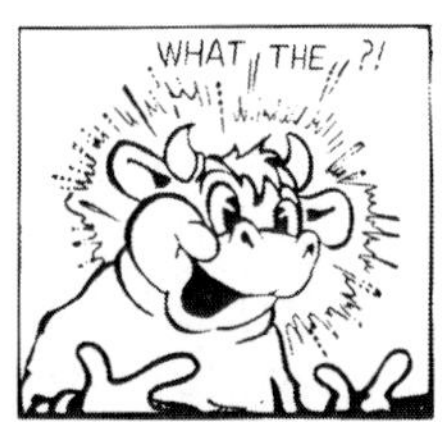

Before we begin, your author has something that he needs to disclose: he is not a neurologist. More than that, he doesn't even *like* neurology. Even on his best days, he finds the subject dense, tedious, and technical in a way that resists easy memorization and understanding. So what exactly makes him feel qualified to write a book on the subject when there are plenty of *actual* neurologists from whom you could learn?

In short, this book is written for people who feel the same way! Because learning neurology can be painful at times, this book liberally uses mnemonics, visual aids, practice questions, and a few spoonfuls of sugar to help everything go down. It also focuses on the highest yield information (the things that are most likely to show up on tests and in clinical settings) rather than trying to present a comprehensive listing of every possible disease and disorder. With that in mind, this book will be helpful mostly for people who need a core understanding of neurology, including medical students, nurse practitioners, physician assistants, and doctors in various other specialties like psychiatry and internal medicine.

This book is roughly divided into two halves. The first half covers the **anatomical foundations** upon which neurology rests, as learning the basic neuroanatomy of both the central and peripheral nervous system is essential for understanding the diseases that you will see in clinical practice. The second half of the book will take everything that you've learned about neuroanatomy and show what can go *wrong* at each step along the way which forms of the basis of **clinical neurology**.

As you go through the book, you will realize that, when it comes to classifying neurologic disorders, there is often **more than one way to slice the bread**, as many diseases will not fit neatly into a single category but are classifiable in several ways. For example, Guillain–Barré syndrome is a disease in which someone's immune system attacks their own nerves by removing the protective sheath around them following an infection, leading to dysfunctional nerve transmission in the peripheral nervous system. Does that make Guillain–Barré syndrome an autoimmune disease? A demyelinating disease? A post-infectious disease? A peripheral neuropathy? In short: all of the above! Because nature does not always carve neatly, it is often impossible to categorize its disorders into mutually exclusive categories. However, rest assured that we will cover all the important major diseases in due time.

As you read, look for boxes like the one below to highlight the **most clinically relevant information**. If you are short on time, you can rapidly review the information by only looking at the boxes. Each box will also contain a memory aid to help you to get the information to stick. The most high-yield information has been collected together in a few pages at the end of this book which you can refer to as you progress throughout the text. You may even consider snapping a photo to take with you for future reference!

By design, some of the mnemonics and analogies in this book may be silly, amusing, or even slightly risqué. This is done in order to make the information more accessible, as provoking an emotional response is a good way of getting information to stick. Nothing in this book is intended to stigmatize, trivialize, or humiliate anyone struggling with any of the diseases mentioned. Instead, the goal is to make the necessary clinical information more accessible to their healthcare providers.

Concepts in boxes are particularly **high-yield**!

*An **easy way** to remember them will be in **italics** below.*

Before we begin, it's worth pointing out that this book assumes that the reader is familiar with **basic concepts from anatomy, physiology, and cell biology**. Make sure that you have an introductory understanding of things such as action potentials, neurotransmitters, and hormones as well as a background in how various organ systems work, including the circulatory, respiratory, gastrointestinal, genitourinary, immune, endocrine, and musculoskeletal systems. If you feel rusty on any of these subjects, now is a good time to go back and do some reviewing on your own.

Now, let's get started…

2 THE NERVOUS SYSTEM

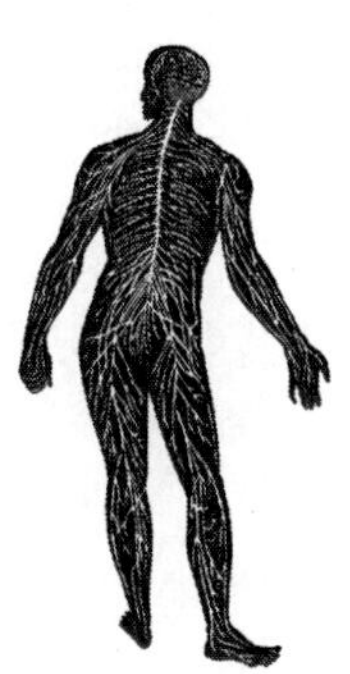

Neurology is the study of the **nervous system** or the organ system consisting of all the **neurons** (or nerve cells) in the human body. Neurons are the building blocks of the nervous system in the same way that bricks are the building blocks of a house. Just as one brick isn't really useful for much, a single neuron on its own is kind of pointless. This is because the primary function of a neuron is to **communicate** with other cells, including not only other neurons but also muscle cells (to tell them to contract) and endocrine cells (to tell them to release a specific hormone at a specific time). Knowing how an individual neuron works will be crucial to understanding the nervous system as a whole, so let's start there.

Like most cells in the human body, a neuron has a **cell body** (also known as a soma) where the nucleus, mitochondria, endoplasmic reticulum, and other organelles are housed. The entirety of a neuron's anatomy relates back to its primary function: to communicate. Like an antenna, the neuron needs an apparatus to both **receive and transmit signals**. Neurons communicate by passing along an electrical signal known as an **action potential**. A neuron *receives* signals by way of its **dendrites** or spiny processes that shoot off from the soma like the branches of a tree to receive signals from other neurons or from the environment. The neuron then *transmits* signals by way of its **axon**, a long slender "tail" that passes along action potentials to other cells. Many axons are wrapped in a fatty substance known as **myelin** which acts to protect the nerve (like tape wrapped around an electrical wire) and to increase the speed of the action potential.

A drawing of a typical neuron is found in the following image:

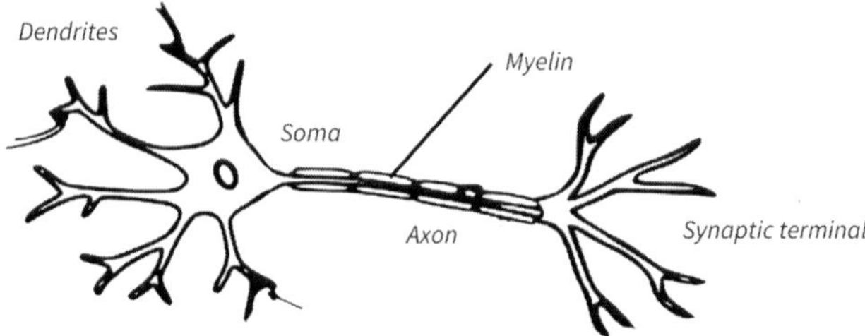

When the signal reaches the **terminal** end of the axon, it causes the release of **neurotransmitters** which then diffuse across the space between cells (known as a **synapse**) and bind to receptors on the dendrites of nearby neurons. By activating these receptors, a new action potential is generated, thereby passing the signal from the **pre-synaptic neuron** to the **post-synaptic neuron** and beginning the cycle anew.

A visual depiction of a synapse is found in the following image:

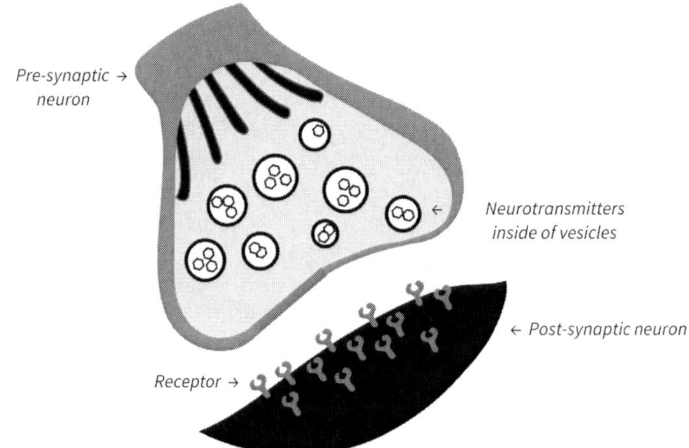

The process of releasing neurotransmitters into the synaptic cleft is found in the following image, going from left to right:

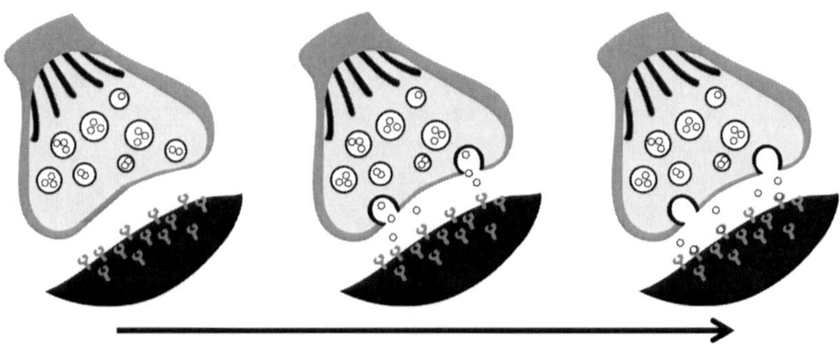

Neurotransmitters are not made on demand when an action potential arrives at a synapse, as manufacturing these chemicals takes time which would slow down the near-instantaneous speed that allows the nervous system to operate as quickly and efficiently as it does. Instead, prior to their release, neurotransmitters are stored in lipid bubbles known as **synaptic vesicles**. When an action potential arrives at a synaptic terminal, it causes an influx of **calcium** ions into the pre-synaptic neuron. Calcium then stimulates a group of protein complexes known as **SNARE proteins** that help guide the vesicles to the cell membrane. Once there, they fuse with the membrane and release their contents into the synapse in a process known as **exocytosis**. You can remember the steps leading to neurotransmitter release by thinking of them being like a group of soldiers marching into battle. **Call**-cium is the battle **call**, and **SNARE** proteins are the battle **drums** marching the neurotransmitters into the synapse.

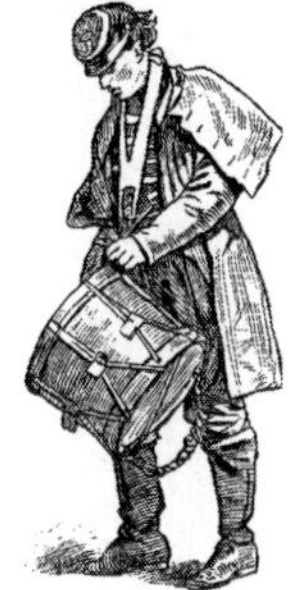

Neurotransmitter release relies upon an influx of **calcium** into the **pre-synaptic nerve terminal**, which then activates **SNARE proteins** to mediate **vesicle fusion** with the cell membrane.

***Call**-cium is the battle **call**, while **SNARE** proteins march neurotransmitters into the synapse.*

While a single neuron is so small you need a microscope to see it, a bunch of neurons grouped together can be visible to the naked eye. A group of neurons running together like this is known as a **nerve**. Together, all of the neurons in the human body make up the **nervous system** which takes in information from the environment and then uses it to coordinate the actions of the entire organism.

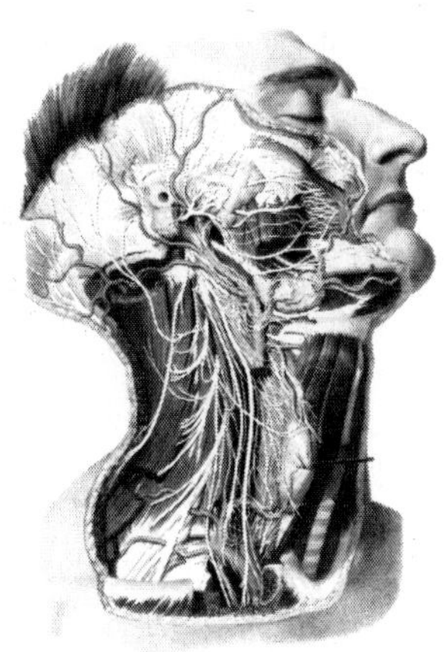

The nervous system is divided into two parts: the **central nervous system**, which includes the brain and spinal cord, and the **peripheral nervous system**, which consists of all the neurons outside of the central nervous system. The peripheral nervous system is further divided into the **somatic nervous system**, which consists of both **sensory** and **motor** nerves carrying information and making movements about which we are consciously aware, as well as the **autonomic nervous system**, which regulates vital functions such as one's heartbeat, breathing, digestion, urination, and other processes that we are often controlling *un*consciously. The autonomic nervous system is itself split into two systems: the **sympathetic nervous system**, which has an *activating* effect on the body (also known as the "fight or flight" response), and the **parasympathetic nervous system**, which promotes homeostatic processes such as eating and digesting (the so-called "feed and breed, then rest and digest" response). We'll now go over each of these systems in more detail.

THE CENTRAL NERVOUS SYSTEM

The **central nervous system** (sometimes abbreviated CNS) is divided into two main parts: the brain and the spinal cord. The **brain** is the "capital city" of the nervous system and acts as the primary organ that coordinates activity among all the different parts of the body. The brain is divided into three parts: the **cerebrum**, the **cerebellum**, and the **brainstem**. From there, the central nervous system continues on as the **spinal cord**, as seen in the following image:

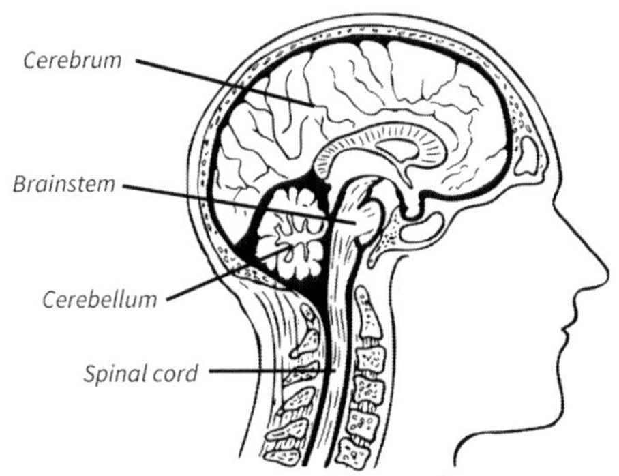

*Components of the **central nervous system**.*

THE CEREBRUM

The cerebrum is the largest part of the brain and is responsible for **higher order functions** such as learning, memory, communication, sensation, and movement. The outermost layer of the cerebrum, known as the **cerebral cortex**, is made up of neuronal cell bodies. Because the cell bodies themselves are not covered in myelin like the axons are, they have a greyish appearance to the naked eye, so someone thought to give them the (super imaginative) name of "**grey matter**." Underneath the grey matter lie the myelinated axons connecting these neurons to one another. Myelin is a fatty substance that appears white, so (naturally) these axons were called "**white matter**." The cerebrum is split into left and right hemispheres by a deep "canyon" known as the **longitudinal fissure** that runs down the middle of the brain. However, a white matter tract known as the **corpus callosum** exists that connects these two halves of the brain together and allows them to communicate. (You can think of this as the cor-**plus** callo-**sum** to remember that it **adds** the two halves of your brain together.)

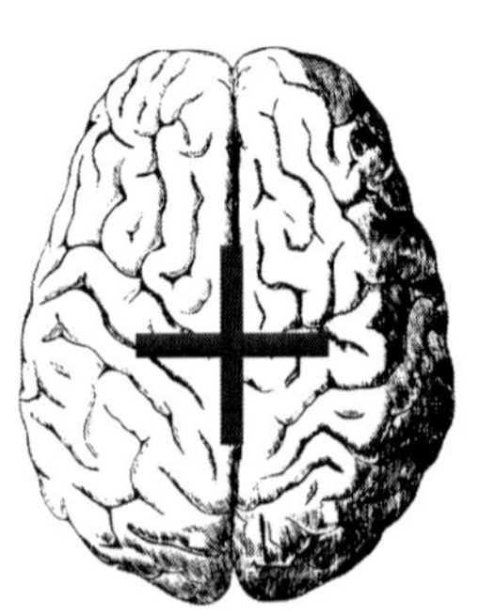

The **corpus callosum** connects the **right and left hemispheres** which are separated by the **longitudinal fissure**.

*The cor-**plus** callo-**sum adds** the two halves of the brain together.*

When talking about the different halves of the brain, neurologists will often make reference to a **dominant hemisphere** and a **non-dominant hemisphere**. The dominant hemisphere is the one that controls your dominant hand (for most people, the right hand). However, because neurons controlling voluntary muscles cross over from left-to-right and right-to-left on their way down to the peripheral nervous system (as we will talk about further in Chapter 7), the dominant hemisphere ends up being on the *opposite* side as the dominant hand (so a right-handed person has a left-dominant hemisphere and vice versa). Besides controlling the dominant hand, the dominant hemisphere has a few other jobs to perform, most notably understanding and producing **language**. Up to 99% of right-handed individuals have their language centers in their left cerebral hemisphere, while only around 70% of left-handed individuals do. This makes handedness an important consideration when discussing an individual patient's clinical presentation. (This is why neurologists will often begin talking about a patient by saying, "This is a 76-year-old *right-handed* male..." The fact that he is right-handed means that it is exceedingly likely that his language centers will be located on the left side of his brain, as opposed to a left-handed individual where this is less likely.)

Below the cerebral cortex is the **cerebral subcortex**. The subcortex contains many key structures that each perform a variety of functions, including fine-tuning movement, directing sensory information to the correct part of the brain, and taking care of such vital processes as eating, drinking, and social bonding.

THE CEREBELLUM

Tucked away in a little space behind the cerebrum is the **cerebellum**, a "little brain" that helps to coordinate complex movements, balance, and posture. (If you're not falling out of your chair as you read this, it's because your cerebellum is working!) In contrast, someone with a dysfunctional cerebellum will have imprecise, erratic, and uncoordinated movements. So don't let it's "little" status fool you: the cerebellum plays a big role in movement despite its diminutive size!

THE BRAINSTEM

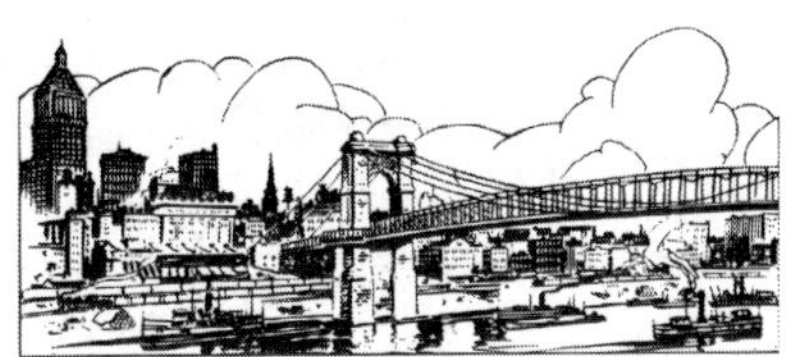

If the brain is the capital city, then the **brainstem** is the "bridge" connecting the brain to the "highway" of the spinal cord. While learning to associate the brainstem with the word "bridge" early on is helpful, it threatens to obscure the fact that the brainstem is so much more than *just* a bridge. Indeed, the brainstem is not just an inert lump of tissue over which other more important neurons cross. Instead, the three parts of the brainstem (the **midbrain**, **pons**, and **medulla oblongata**) each perform a variety of functions on their own, with many of these being among the most vital and basic to survival such as breathing, sleeping, and maintaining a heartbeat. The brainstem is so essential for survival that most medical practitioners will only consider someone "brain dead" once it is clear that the brainstem has stopped functioning. (Compare this to someone who has suffered a widespread loss of cerebral tissue, who may technically still be considered "alive" because their heartbeat and respiration are continuing on their own due to an intact brainstem.)

THE SPINAL CORD

The **spinal cord** is the final part of the central nervous system. It acts as a "highway" connecting neurons traveling between the brain and the organs in the rest of the body. Like the brain, the spinal cord is made up of both grey matter and white matter. However, the pattern here is reversed, with the grey matter on the *inside* and the white matter on the *outside*.

Like any highway, the spinal cord travels in a central location. When it comes time to go to their final destinations in the muscles, skin, and organs scattered throughout the body, these nerves form "exits" from the central highway around the level at which their target organ lies. Like a real highway exit, these nerves have both an "on-ramp" and an "off-ramp," with motor nerves getting *off* the highway exiting on the *anterior* side of the spinal cord while sensory nerves getting *on* the highway enter on the *posterior* side. These **nerve roots** join together to form two-way "side streets" known as **spinal nerves** that go on to innervate the target organs directly. (Some nerves exit directly from the brain rather than first traveling in the spinal cord. These are known as **cranial nerves**.) Together, cranial nerves and spinal nerves collectively form the peripheral nervous system, which is where we will now turn our attention.

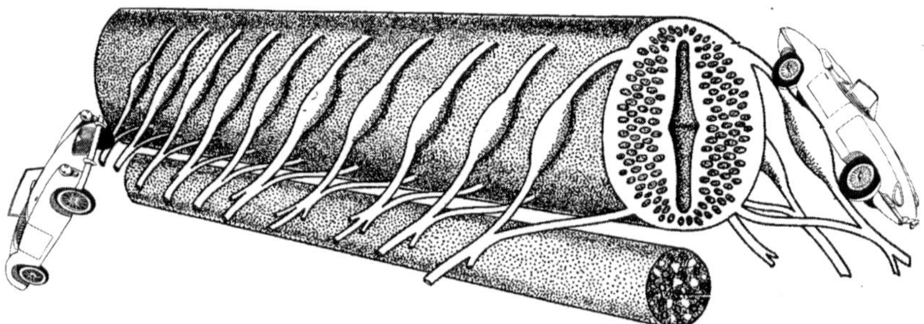

Spinal nerves *connecting to* ***the spinal cord****. Note the resemblance to highway* ***on-ramps*** *and* ***off-ramps****!*

Nerves from the brain cross the **brainstem** and travel via the **spinal cord** to the level of their target organ. They then exit the spinal cord as **peripheral nerves**.

Associate these words!
Brain *= Capital city*
Brainstem *= Bridge*
Spinal cord *= Highway*
Peripheral nerves *= Side streets*

THE PERIPHERAL NERVOUS SYSTEM

The **peripheral nervous system** is made up of all the nerves connecting target organs to the central nervous system. These nerves have one of two functions: either they are **sensory nerves** transmitting information about the environment *up to* the central nervous system or they are **motor nerves** carrying instructions *down from* the central nervous system to make something happen. Nerves carrying sensory information are also known as **afferent** nerves while those carrying motor signals are called **efferent** nerves. You can remember the difference between afferent and efferent nerves by thinking that **A**fferent nerves **A**scend to **A**lert the brain while e**F**ferent nerves **F**low down to e**F**fect change. The afferent division is the simpler of the two, and it is where we will head next.

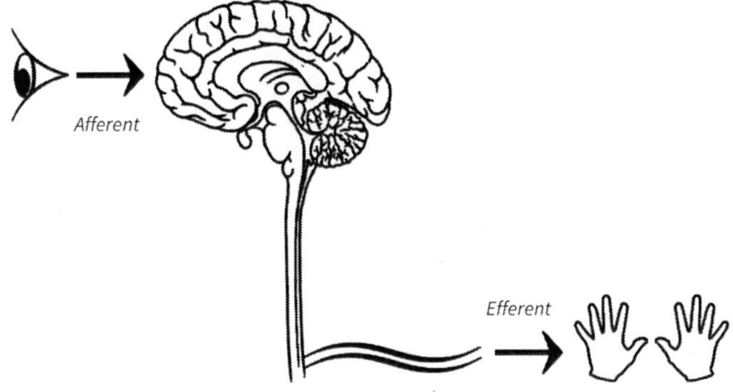

Afferent nerves carry **sensory information** up to the central nervous system, while **efferent nerves** carry **motor signals** down from the central nervous system.

*Afferent nerves **A**scend to **A**lert the brain,*
*while e**F**ferent nerves **F**low down to e**F**fect change.*

THE AFFERENT DIVISION

The **afferent division** acts to relay information about the environment to the central nervous system so that someone can respond appropriately to their situation. Sensory information comes in a few different varieties including **touch**, **pain**, **temperature**, **vibration**, and **proprioception** (with proprioception being one's sense of the position of their body parts in space, as in your ability to tell if someone has lifted your arm up or down even if your eyes are closed). We also have other senses that instead come from specialized **sense organs**, like the eyes and ears, that are specifically structured to provide unique forms of information about the environment. These **special senses** are **vision**, **hearing**, **balance**, **smell**, and **taste** (each of which we will cover in more detail in Chapters 10 and 11).

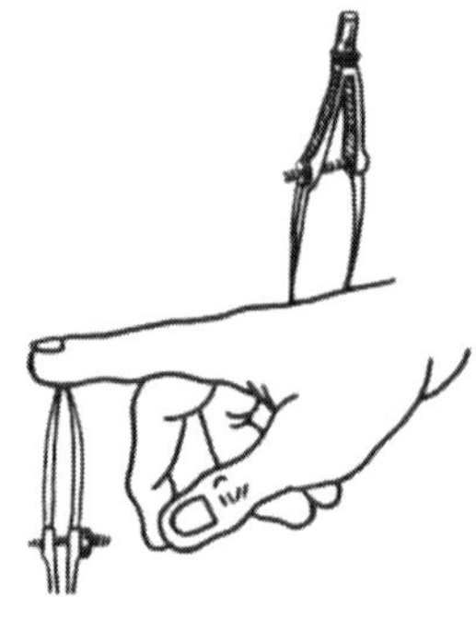

While seemingly a simple concept, the sense of touch requires some additional explanation. It turns out that touch is really *two* senses: **crude touch** (also known as non-discriminative touch) and **fine touch** (also called discriminative touch). Crude touch can only tell you whether or not you are being touched, while fine touch is sensitive enough to distinguish between two contact points in the same area. You can test this on yourself using two pin points both on the tip of your finger and on the back of your hand. With your eyes closed, you will be able to tell the difference between two points with your finger much better than with the back of your hand, as your fingertips are the better of the two at fine touch.

There are two types of neurons that carry sensory information from the skin: **protopathic** neurons (which carry **crude touch**, **pain**, and **temperature**) and **epicritic** neurons (which carry **fine touch**, **vibration**, and **proprioception**). Protopathic and epicritic neurons have a few key differences. First, they travel in different parts of the spinal cord (which will become important when we talk about various forms of spinal cord injury in Chapter 7). In addition, epicritic neurons are **myelinated** (meaning they have that insulating sheath wrapped around them to enable action potentials to travel more quickly down axons) while protopathic neurons are **unmyelinated** and carry action potentials much more slowly (this will come into play clinically when talking about demyelinating diseases in Chapter 25). For now, just remember the distinction between the two by thinking of **proto**pathic nerves as carrying the "lower" or "baser" senses like crude touch that likely developed first (which makes sense as "proto-" means "primitive") while epi**critic** should make you think of a snobby **critic** who thinks he is better than everyone else with his "finer" or "more sophisticated" senses.

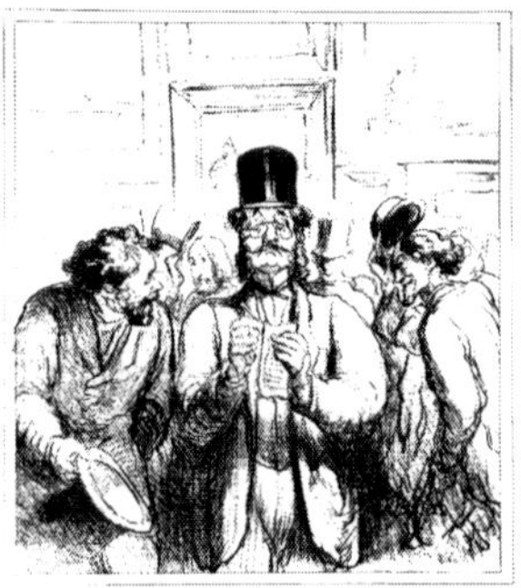

Protopathic neurons convey **crude touch**, **pain**, and **temperature**, while **epicritic neurons** convey **fine touch**, **vibration**, and **proprioception**.

***Proto** means "**primitive**" so the **proto**pathic senses are more **basic**, while a snobby epi**critic** thinks he has **more sophisticated senses** than everyone else.*

While these different sensory modalities travel *separately* in the spinal cord, they travel *together* in the peripheral nervous system as cranial and spinal nerves. Specific spinal nerves (and some cranial nerves) are responsible for innervating specific areas known as their **dermatomes**. (For example, the spinal nerve that exits from the spinal column below the tenth thoracic vertebra innervates the area around the belly button.) We'll go over dermatomes in more detail in Chapter 9.

THE EFFERENT DIVISION

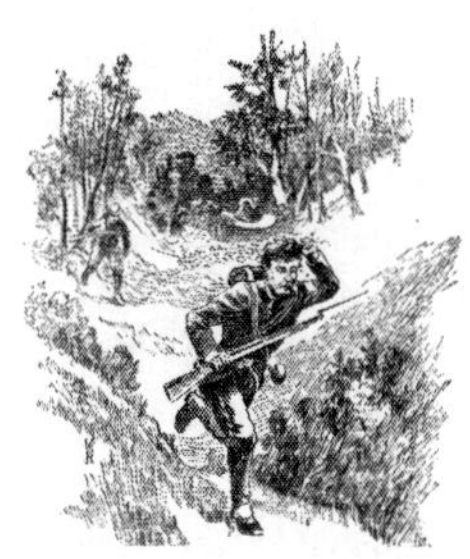

While the afferent division helps to bring information about the environment *into* the central nervous system, the **efferent division** enables an organism to not just be *aware* of its environment but to *respond* to it as well. After all, it would be pointless to know about something without being able to do something about it! For example, just being able to see a swarm of bees flying towards you doesn't really help that much. It is only if you are able to act on this information by running away that it confers any advantage.

The efferent division acts in two distinct ways that form the basis for a *further* subdivision of the nervous system. The **somatic nervous system** involves sending signals to muscles throughout the body to enable **voluntary movements** such as walking, eating, stretching, and working with our hands. In contrast, the **autonomic nervous system** effects changes in **unconscious bodily processes** that we do *not* have as much awareness of or control over, including our heart rate, blood pressure, and release of certain hormones. We'll talk about the somatic nervous system first.

THE SOMATIC NERVOUS SYSTEM

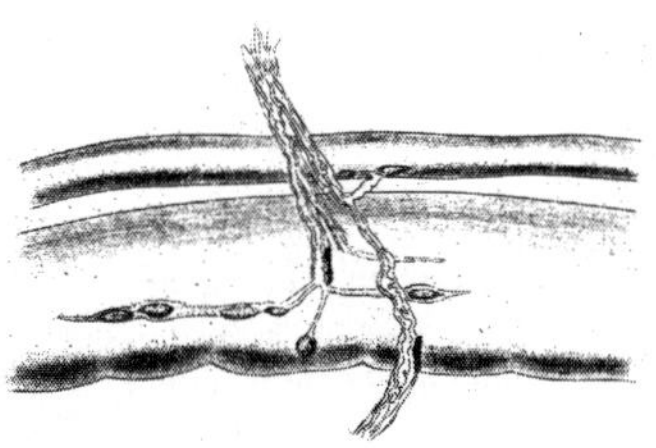

The somatic nervous system involves all of the skeletal muscles over which we have direct voluntary control. (It's worth pointing out that some muscles can involve *both* voluntary and involuntary control. For example, the muscles we use to breathe or blink will contract without conscious effort most of the time, though if we choose to we can hold our breath or shut our eyes.)

Similar to the afferent division and its dermatomes, different muscles in the body are innervated by specific cranial and spinal nerves, with the muscle groups that a particular motor nerve innervates known as its **myotome**. Efferent nerves carry signals down from the brain to the muscles and meet them at the **neuromuscular junction** or the point at which the axon of a motor neuron terminates onto the muscle. When an action potential arrives at the neuromuscular junction, it triggers an influx of **calcium** ions into the neuron. The neuron then releases a neurotransmitter known as **acetylcholine** (ACh) into the synapse between the neuron and the muscle. Acetylcholine binds to a specific type of acetylcholine receptor known as a **nicotinic receptor** on the muscle itself which causes the muscle to depolarize and contract. (The process is overall quite similar to what happens at most synapses except that the post-synaptic cell is a muscle cell rather than another neuron.) We will talk about diseases specific to the neuromuscular junction in more detail in Chapter 17.

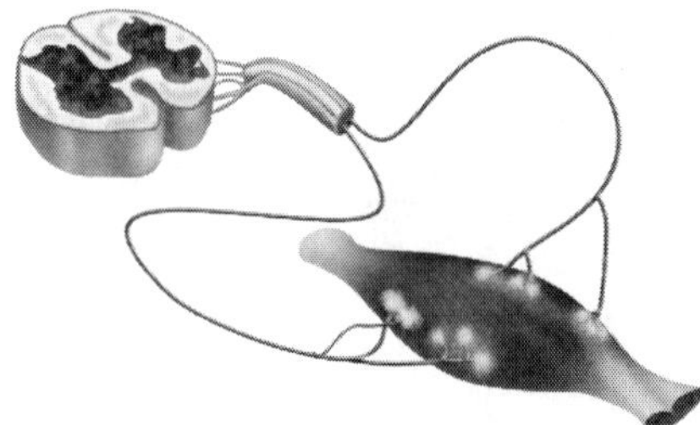

THE AUTONOMIC NERVOUS SYSTEM

In contrast to the somatic nervous system (where there is some degree of conscious control over the impulses that are sent down), the effects of the **autonomic nervous system** are not things that we can control directly and, in some cases, are not even visible to us. (For example, can you tell whether your stomach is secreting acid at this exact moment?) For this reason, the autonomic nervous system can initially be harder to understand. It is best thought of as our body's attempt to take care of the basics (like digesting food and circulating blood) so that our conscious awareness can be reserved for more complicated things like cooking dinner or doing math.

The autonomic nervous system is itself divided into two opposing forces: the **sympathetic nervous system** and the **parasympathetic nervous system**. These systems should be familiar to you if you've studied physiology, but we'll briefly review them here, starting with the parasympathetic nervous system.

PARASYMPATHETIC NERVOUS SYSTEM

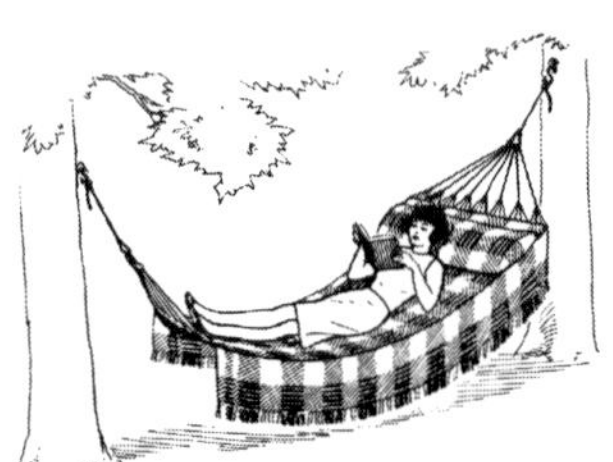

The **parasympathetic nervous system** is activated when the body doesn't have any immediate stresses to face down and is able to focus on **homeostatic activities** like resting, eating, urinating, defecating, and reproducing ("**feed and breed**, then **rest and digest**"). The parasympathetic nervous system largely arises from nerves coming directly from the brain as well as the spinal nerves coming out of the sacral vertebrae, so it is said to have **craniosacral** outflow.

The **parasympathetic nervous system** is activated in the **absence of immediate stressors** and promotes **homeostatic functions** such as feeding and reproducing.

*Think "**feed and breed,** then **rest and digest.**"*

The parasympathetic nervous system uses the neurotransmitter **acetylcholine** at all of its synapses (both the one near the spinal cord and the one closer to the target organ). However, despite the same *neurotransmitter* being found at both synapse types, different *receptors* are found in each. At the first synapse acetylcholine binds to a **nicotinic receptor**, while at the target organ it binds to a different kind of receptor known as a **muscarinic receptor**. This becomes clinically important because certain drugs and diseases affect one type of acetylcholine receptor but not the other, leading to different presentations depending on which are involved.

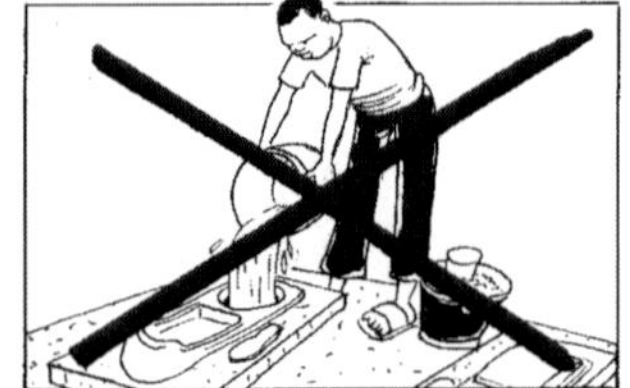

You can remember the effects of *muscarinic* receptor activation using the mnemonic **SLUDG-E BM**, with BM being a common medical abbreviation for a bowel movement (making this mnemonic an unpleasant but highly relevant mental image). SLUDG-E BM stands for **S**alivation, **L**acrimation (excessive tear production), **U**rination, **D**iaphoresis (excessive sweating), **G**astrointestinal hypermotility, **E**mesis, **B**radycardia (slow heart rate), and **M**iosis (constricted pupils).

Muscarinic acetylcholine receptors are responsible for most of the **efferent effects** of the **parasympathetic nervous system**.

SLUDG-E BM:
S*alivation*
L*acrimation*
U*rination*
D*iaphoresis*
G*astrointestinal hypermotility*
E*mesis*
B*radycardia*
M*iosis*

In contrast, the effects of nicotinic receptors largely involve the **motor system** (remember that nicotinic receptors are the ones at the neuromuscular junction!) and the higher processes of the brain like **memory** and **behavior**. For this reason, drugs that affect acetylcholine can be used to treat conditions like Alzheimer's disease where the patient's memory is impacted. You can remember both of these functions by thinking of the phrase "**Nic's muscle memory**" to correlate **nic**otinic receptors, **muscle** contraction, and **memory** formation.

Nicotinic acetylcholine receptors are found at the **neuromuscular junction** as well as in the brain where they are involved in **memory and behavior**.

Think of ***Nic's muscle memory****.*

THE SYMPATHETIC NERVOUS SYSTEM

In contrast to the parasympathetic nervous system and its "feed and breed, then rest and digest" functions, the **sympathetic nervous system** instead generates a "**fight or flight**" state in response to a threat (whether that is a physical threat like a swarm of bees or a more social one like giving a speech in public). In response to a perceived threat, the sympathetic nervous system kicks into high gear and makes the heart beat faster, the airway open wider, and the pupils dilate (among many other things) to enable us to either fight the threat or run away from it. In contrast to the *para*sympathetic nervous system and its craniosacral outflow, the sympathetic nervous system instead largely arises from nerves coming off of the spinal cord in the thoracic and lumbar regions and is therefore said to have **thoracolumbar** outflow.

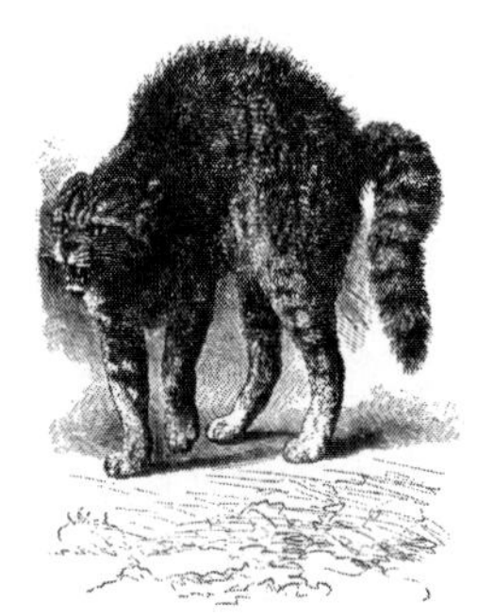

The **sympathetic nervous system** is activated in the **presence of immediate stressors** to enable a **physiologic response to the threat**.

*Think "**fight or flight.**"*

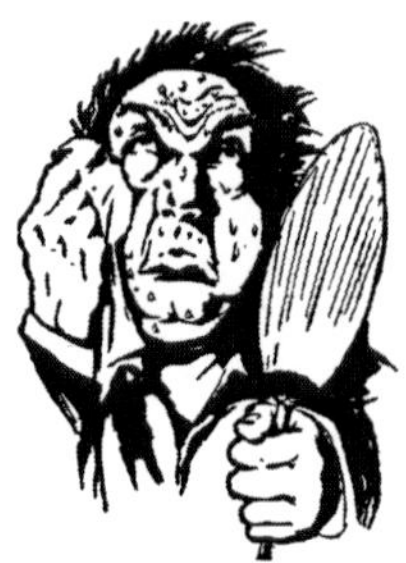

In contrast to the parasympathetic nervous system (which uses the same neurotransmitter at both synapses, even if the *receptor* differs between the two), the sympathetic nervous system uses a different neurotransmitter at each synapse. At the synapse near the spinal cord, acetylcholine binds to a *nicotinic* receptor. However, at the synapse near the target organ, a different neurotransmitter known as **norepinephrine** is used. This is true across all organs in the body that respond to the sympathetic nervous system with the sole exception of **sweat glands**! At sweat glands, acetylcholine is used again, with a *muscarinic* receptor. (This explains why **D**iaphoresis is the **D** in SLU**D**G-E BM. While sweating is normally a *sympathetic* function, because it involves the muscarinic acetylcholine receptor, widespread activation of muscarinic receptors will include sweating in addition to the other *para*sympathetic effects.)

For future reference, a quick review of the neurotransmitters and receptors used in the parasympathetic, sympathetic, and somatic nervous systems is found below, with N standing for nicotinic receptors, M standing for muscarinic receptors, and NE standing for norepinephrine. (We haven't talked about anterior horn cells yet, but we'll go over them in Chapter 8 when we discuss the spinal cord.)

The Parasympathetic Nervous System

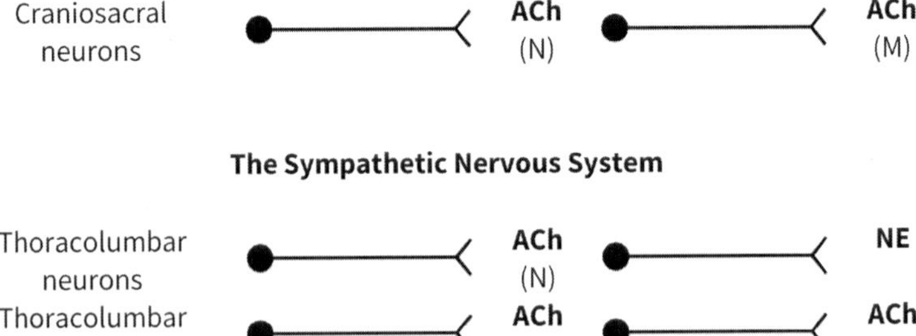

The Somatic Nervous System

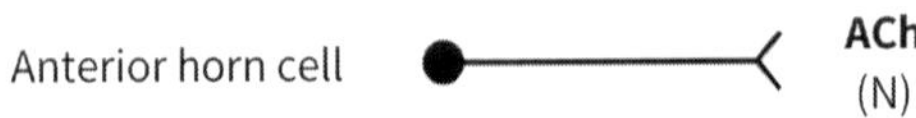

GLIAL CELLS

We first learned about the nervous system at the level of the neuron, then we zoomed out to look at the nervous system on the scale of the whole person. To finish off, we're going to jump back to the microscopic level to talk about other cells belonging to the nervous system that are *not* neurons but are still essential for neuronal functioning. Just as you need more than just bricks to make a house (with additional materials like mortar and rebar being required to support the structure of the building), neurons rely on a variety of support cells to function. These support cells are collectively known as **glial cells** (from the Greek word for "glue") and come in a few varieties.

OLIGODENDROGLIA AND SCHWANN CELLS

Myelin is not made by the neuron itself. Instead, it is created by two types of glial cells: **oligodendroglia** (which live in the *central* nervous system and myelinate *multiple* neurons each) and **Schwann cells** (which instead live in the *peripheral* nervous system and myelinate only a *single* neuron each). Diseases of these myelin-producing cells can result in poor signal transmission and nerve dysfunction. One fact that will become important when we talk about nervous system tumors is that oligodendroglia have a characteristic "fried egg" appearance under the microscope as seen below. File this away as a bit of trivia for now, but it will come into play later!

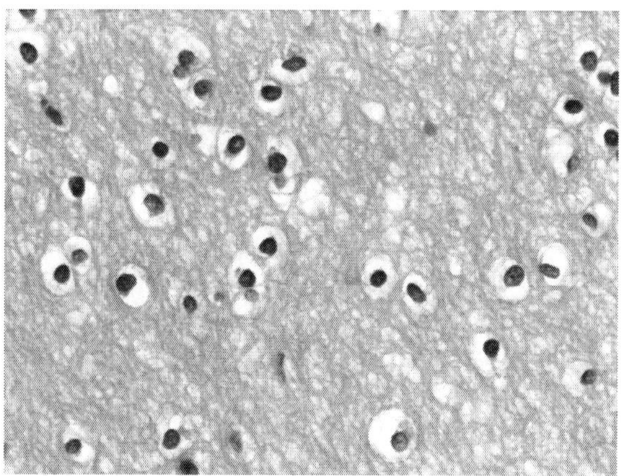

*Microscopic view of the brain showing **oligodendrocytes** with their characteristic fried-egg appearance.*

Oligodendrocytes myelinate multiple neurons in the **central nervous system** and have a **fried egg** appearance when examined under a microscope.

*Think of them as ol-**egg**-odendrocytes.*

Schwann cells myelinate a **single neuron** in the **peripheral nervous system**.

***Sch-wann** cells can myelinate only **wann** (one) **cell at a time**.*

ASTROCYTES AND SATELLITE CELLS

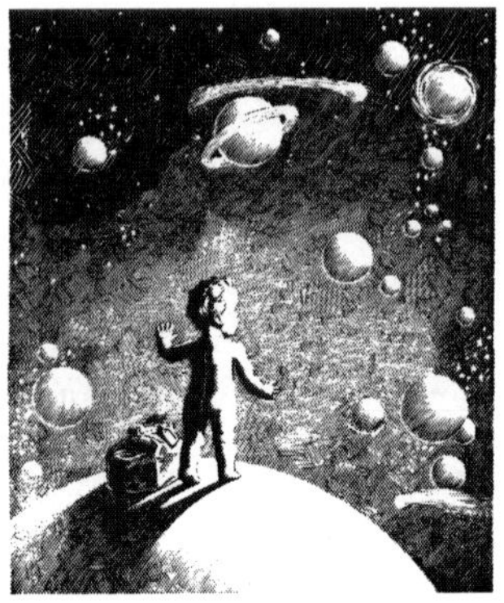

Astrocytes and **satellite cells** are the **support staff** of the nervous system. They provide nutrients to neurons, maintain a clean environment, regulate blood flow, and repair damage following an injury. They differ between the two halves of the nervous system, with astrocytes being found exclusively in the *central* nervous system while satellite cells are found only in the *peripheral* nervous system. To remember the location and function of astrocytes and satellite cells, connect **astros** (stars) and **satellites** with the mental image of **space**. This will help you think of these cells as being located in the *space* around the neuron!

Astrocytes and **satellite cells** help to **support neurons** in a variety of ways.

***Astro**-cytes and **satellite** cells are found in the **space** between neurons.*

EPENDYMAL CELLS

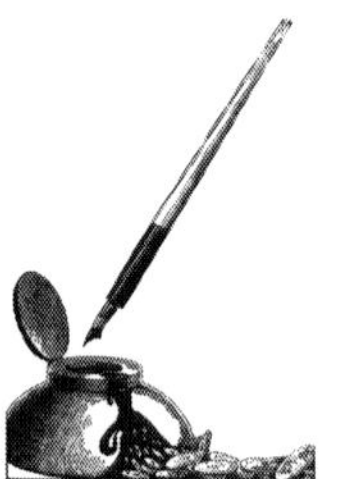

The **ependyma** is a layer of cells lining the **ventricular system**. (We will talk about the ventricular system more in Chapter 12, but it is a series of cavities inside the brain and spinal cord through which a liquid known as **cerebrospinal fluid** flows.) Ependymal cells are involved not only in producing the cerebrospinal fluid but also in circulating it and absorbing it back into the system. To link the ependyma to its role regulating cerebrospinal fluid, try to imagine dipping an e-**pen**-dyma in (cerebrospinal) **fluid** to write.

Ependymal cells line the ventricular system where they produce, circulate, and absorb **cerebrospinal fluid.**

*Visualize dipping an e-**pen**-dyma in (cerebrospinal) **fluid**.*

MICROGLIA

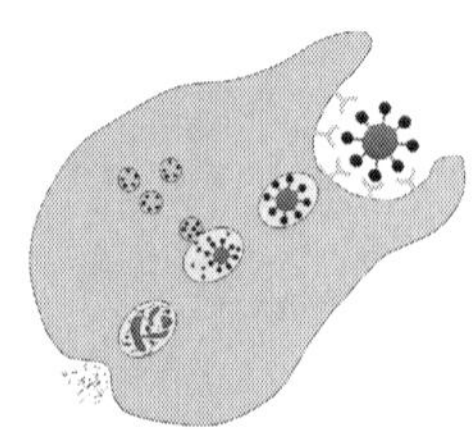

Microglial cells are found in the central nervous system where they help to protect the brain and spinal cord from infectious diseases by, well, eating them! In this way, microglial cells are part of both the nervous system and the immune system. Microglia also help to remove debris from injured or defective neurons which prevents the damage from spreading to nearby healthy neurons.

PUTTING IT ALL TOGETHER

Let's recap what we've learned! The nervous system is made up of specialized cells known as **neurons** whose main function is to communicate. It does this by sending electrical signals known as **action potentials** to muscles, glands, and other nerves. Neurons receive assistance from a variety of supporting cells known as **glial cells**.

The nervous system is divided between the **central nervous system** (consisting of the brain and spinal cord) and the **peripheral nervous system** (everything else, including cranial and spinal nerves). The peripheral nervous system itself is divided between the **afferent division** (sensory information) and the **efferent division** (motor signals). The efferent division is divided into the **somatic nervous system** (which innervates skeletal muscles over which we have voluntary control) and the **autonomic nervous system** (which innervates internal organs over which we have little conscious awareness). Finally, the autonomic nervous system is itself further subdivided into the **sympathetic nervous system** (which does "fight or flight") and the **parasympathetic nervous system** (which does "feed and breed, then rest and digest"). Whew! A visual summary of the organization of the nervous system is found in the following chart:

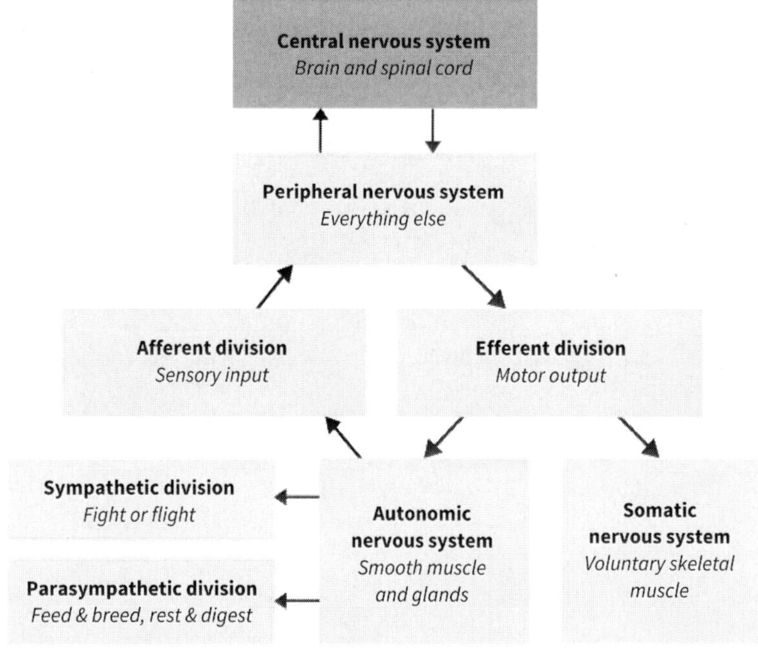

We've covered a lot of ground here, and the truth is that most of it is not going to be *immediately* relevant in a clinical sense. Nevertheless, it is important to absorb all of the concepts here because they will come back to haunt us in later chapters! Don't feel like you need to have complete understanding yet, as learning more about the anatomy and pathology of the nervous system in the rest of the book will reinforce and deepen your comprehension of these concepts as we continue our journey through the nervous system.

REVIEW QUESTIONS

1. A 43 y/o F who works on a farm accidentally ingests an unknown quantity of an insecticide. Upon arrival to the hospital, she is suffering from severe nausea with copious vomiting, diarrhea with fecal incontinence, excessive tear and saliva production, and diffuse sweating across her entire body. On examination, her pupils are narrow and non-reactive to light as seen in the following image:

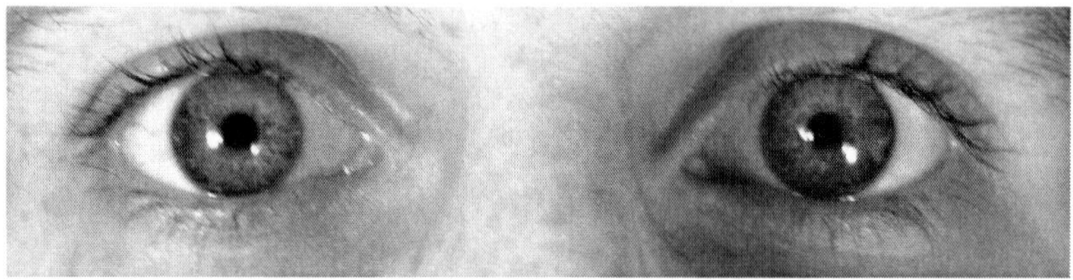

Which of the following signs and symptoms seen in insecticide poisoning is *not* related to parasympathetic nervous system activation?

- A. Nausea and vomiting
- B. Diarrhea
- C. Lacrimation
- D. Salivation
- E. Diaphoresis
- F. Miosis

2. A 46 y/o F is diagnosed with Guillain–Barré syndrome, a disease in which the immune system attacks the myelin sheath of peripheral nerves. Which of the following actions or processes is *least* likely to be affected by this disease?

- A. Feeling her cell phone vibrating in her pocket
- B. Sensing the position of her hand in space with her eyes closed
- C. Noticing that her arm is too close to a hot stove
- D. Being able to tell whether she is being poked by one needle or two
- E. Taking a kickboxing class

3. An 8 y/o M is hospitalized due to a *Streptococcus pneumoniae* infection of the meninges, or the membranes covering the central nervous system. During the course of the infection, he sustains widespread damage to his ependymal cells. Abnormalities in which of the following would be most directly attributable to ependymal cell injury?
    - A. Nervous tissue of the brain
    - B. Nervous tissue of the spinal cord
    - C. Peripheral nerves
    - D. Arterial blood
    - E. Venous blood
    - F. Cerebrospinal fluid
    - G. None of the above

4. A 53 y/o F begins taking amitriptyline, a potent antidepressant with strong anticholinergic effects at muscarinic receptors. Which of the following side effects is she *least* likely to experience?
    - A. Blurred vision
    - B. Dry mouth
    - C. Constipation
    - D. Rapid heart rate
    - E. Excessive urination

1. **The best answer is E.** Some insecticides contain organophosphates, a poison that causes acetylcholine to build up in synapses across the body. This leads to the characteristic SLUDG-E BM signs and symptoms due to hyperactivation of muscarinic receptors. Because acetylcholine is the neurotransmitter found in synapses across the parasympathetic nervous system, signs and symptoms of organophosphate poisoning often resemble a state of parasympathetic nervous system excitation (answers A–D, F). One exception to this is sweating which is instead related to the sympathetic nervous system. While the sympathetic nervous system generally uses norepinephrine (rather than acetylcholine) as its primary neurotransmitter, in the case of sweating the neurotransmitter at both of the synapses involved is acetylcholine.

2. **The best answer is C.** A demyelinating disease will primarily affect functions that involve myelinated, rather than unmyelinated, neurons. This means that vibration (answer A), proprioception (answer B), and discriminative touch (answer D) are all likely to be impaired. Neurons controlling voluntary movement are also myelinated, so some degree of motor weakness is likely to be observed as well (answer E). The primary processes that would not be affected are non-discriminative touch, heat sensation, and pain sensation, as these signals travel on unmyelinated neurons.

3. **The best answer is F.** Ependymal cells can be found lining the ventricular system which is the series of cavities through which cerebrospinal fluid flows. Because of this, damage to ependymal cells can cause dysfunction in cerebrospinal fluid, including an excessive build-up of fluid in the ventricular system known as hydrocephalus. While dysregulation of cerebrospinal fluid may have downstream effects on nervous tissues and/or the blood vessels traveling through them (answers A through E), the most direct effect of ependymal damage will be on cerebrospinal fluid itself.

4. **The best answer is E.** Another question on acetylcholine! This time, we are looking at what happens when acetylcholine's effects are blocked rather than increased. To understand what is happening here, assume that anticholinergic effects will be the exact opposite of what is seen in the SLUDG-E BM mnemonic, with constricted pupils turning into dilated ones (answer A), salivation turning into mouth dryness (answer B), gastrointestinal hypermotility turning into constipation (answer C), and bradycardia turning into tachycardia (answer D). Excessive urination is unlikely to be seen with use of anticholinergic drugs, with urinary *retention* being more common.

3 THE CEREBRAL CORTEX

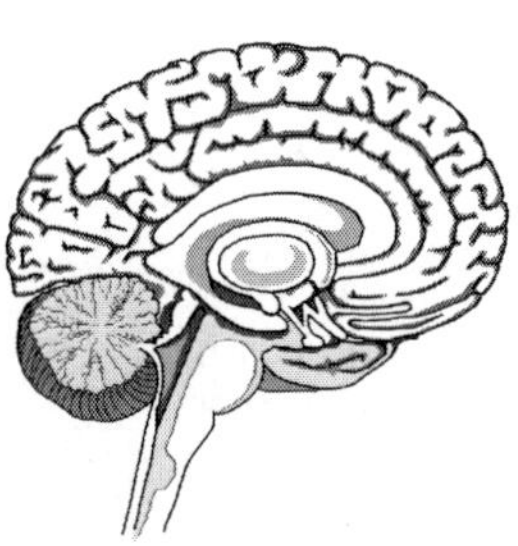

Now that we have talked about the organization of the nervous system as a whole, it's time to talk about its individual components in more detail. We will first begin with the **central nervous system** before moving onto the peripheral nervous system. Our first stop will be the **brain** which is the "capital city" of the entire nervous system, as it is the organ where most sensory information is sent up *to* as well as where most motor impulses come down *from*.

At first glance, the brain can seem like a giant amorphous blob, especially given that it has a physical consistency not unlike Jell-O or uncooked tofu. Yet within this lump of nervous tissue lies a surprisingly high degree of structure and organization. This is because neurons that serve similar purposes tend to cluster together, and for this reason the brain can be described in terms of **distinct anatomical regions** that each have a specific function or set of functions. This organization forms the basis for the field of **neuroanatomy** which will be our focus for the first half of this book.

To begin our study of neuroanatomy, we will look first at the cerebrum. Because the cerebrum is the largest part of the brain by size, it is easier to break it down further rather than covering it as a single entity. The first thing to know about the cerebrum is that it isn't simply a lump. Instead, the cerebrum has an outer portion known as the **cortex** as well as an underlying region known as the **subcortex**. We will start first with the cortex before discussing the deeper underlying structures of the subcortex in the next two chapters, essentially working our way from the outside in (like eating an apple).

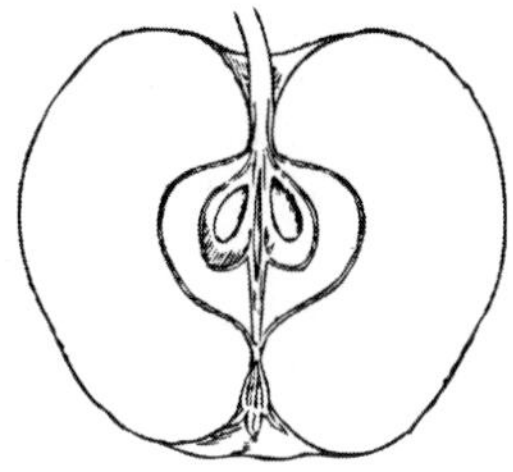

THE FOUR LOBES OF THE BRAIN

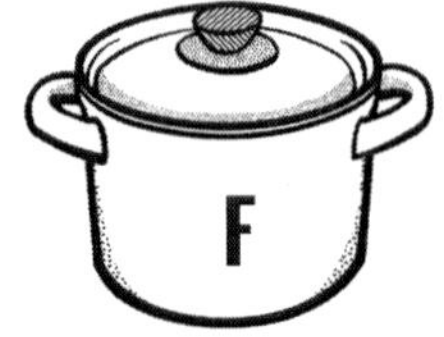

The cerebral cortex is largely made up of **grey matter** (which, as you'll recall from the previous chapter, consists of neuronal cell *bodies*, as compared to white matter which consists of myelinated axons). The cell bodies contained in the grey matter of the cerebral cortex play key roles in many of the "higher functions" that make us human, including creating plans, performing actions, learning information, sensing our environment, and feeling emotions. (This contrasts with many of the structures in the subcortex which perform functions that are more basic to survival such as hunger, thirst, and sleep.)

The cerebral cortex is itself divided into four lobes known as the **frontal lobe**, the **parietal lobe**, the **occipital lobe**, and the **temporal lobe**. Each of these carries out distinct functions, as we will discover next. You can remember the order of the four lobes from front-to-back and top-to-bottom with the acronym **FPOT**.

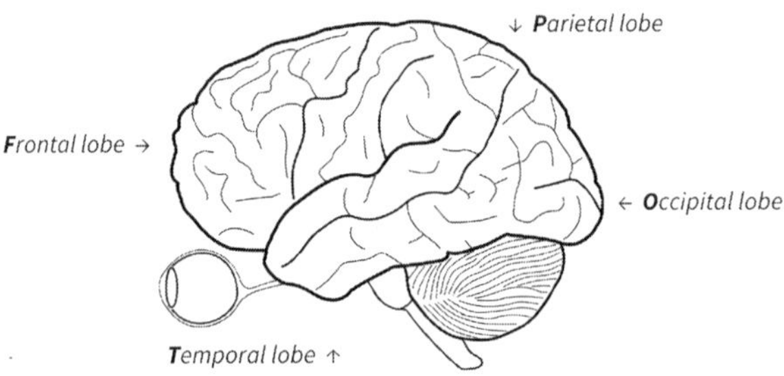

The **cerebral cortex** is responsible for **higher cognitive functions** and is divided into **four lobes**, each of which has unique functions.

From front-to-back and top-to-bottom, the lobes are ***FPOT****:*
Frontal, Parietal, Occipital, and Temporal.

THE FRONTAL CORTEX

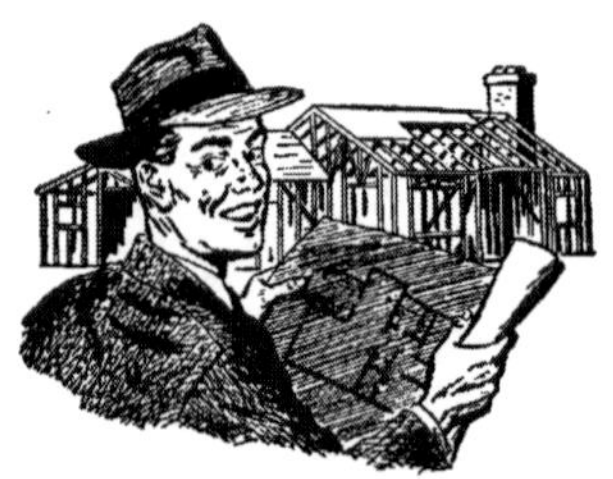

The **frontal cortex** is found just behind the forehead and is the "brainiest" part of the brain. In particular, a region known as the **prefrontal cortex** is involved in **executive functions** such as decision-making and planning. For example, when you are making a complex decision, you may try to weigh the potential benefits ("This job has a much higher salary…") as well as the downsides ("…but the commute would be so much longer."). When doing this, you are primarily using your prefrontal cortex. The frontal cortex is also involved in planning complex tasks that require multiple thoughts and ideas to be held in mind at once, such as a chef keeping track of multiple dishes or an architect drawing up plans for a new house.

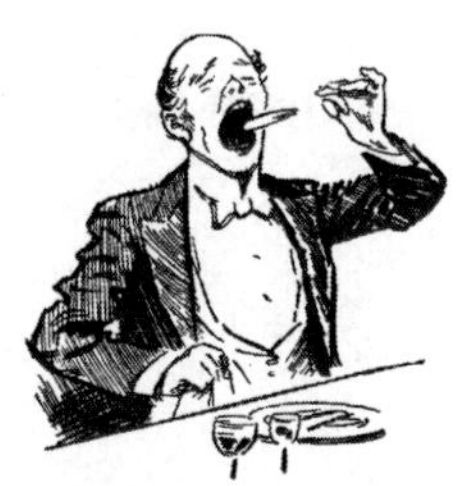

Another important task of the prefrontal cortex is to **say "no" to other parts of the brain** which tend to act more reflexively or instinctually. For example, if you sit down to a meal with friends while you are hungry, one part of your brain (the hypothalamus, which we will learn about in the next chapter) will give off hunger signals, tempting you to immediately start eating all the food around you. However, when you notice that not everyone's food has arrived yet, your prefrontal cortex steps in to inhibit this initial impulse, bringing your behavior in line with social norms and allowing you to avoid the social embarrassment of bad manners. In contrast, people who have sustained damage to their frontal cortex often become unable to override their baser instincts, leading to impulsive, inappropriate, and even aggressive behavior.

Finally, the back of the frontal lobe contains the **primary motor cortex** which generates signals controlling **voluntary movements** such as giving someone a high-five or hitting a ball. (To be clear, these motor signals are not sent directly to your muscles but are first altered and refined in the basal ganglia, which we will talk about in Chapter 5.) To remember that the motor cortex lies in the front part of the brain, think of the brain as being like a standard car with the engine or **motor in the front**.

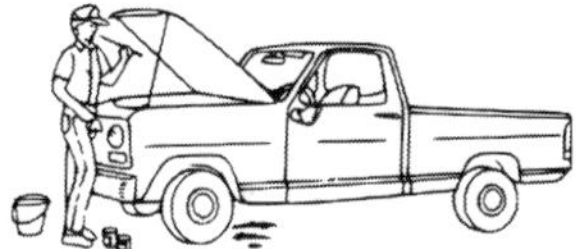

The **primary motor cortex** lies in the **frontal lobe**.

*It's **like a car**: the **motor** is in the **front**.*

Various parts of the body are mapped to specific places in the motor cortex in a predictable way, with the lower extremities being controlled from the *medial* part of the brain (closer to the longitudinal fissure) while the upper extremities and facial muscles are controlled from the *lateral* part, as seen in the following image. This is clinically relevant because the medial part of the motor cortex is supplied by a different artery than the lateral part, so you can often figure out the location of a stroke based on which muscle groups have become unresponsive (with weakness of the face suggesting a different artery than weakness of the feet).

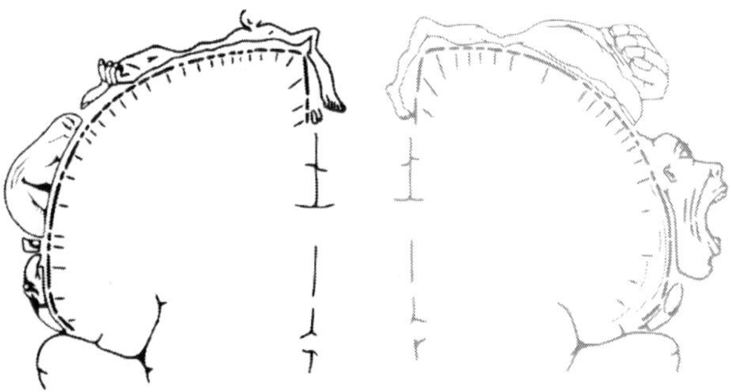

*The **primary motor cortex** (with the somatosensory cortex on the right).*

THE PARIETAL CORTEX

The **parietal lobe** lies just behind the frontal lobe and is separated from it by the **central sulcus**, a deep groove making a "canyon" between the two lobes. The parietal cortex is involved in processing **sensory information** from different parts of the body. Neurons carrying sensory information travel from the body to the **somatosensory cortex** which lies just behind the central sulcus.

The somatosensory cortex is similar to the motor cortex in that specific parts of the body are mapped to specific areas of the brain, with the same overall pattern (lower parts more medial, upper parts more lateral) as seen in the following image. When looking at the drawing, you'll notice that some parts of the body are bigger than others. This is because the number of sensory neurons does *not* necessarily correlate with the physical size of the organ! For example, while the hand is smaller than the leg, it is more densely innervated and sensitive to stimuli (especially fine touch) so it takes up more real estate in the parietal cortex.

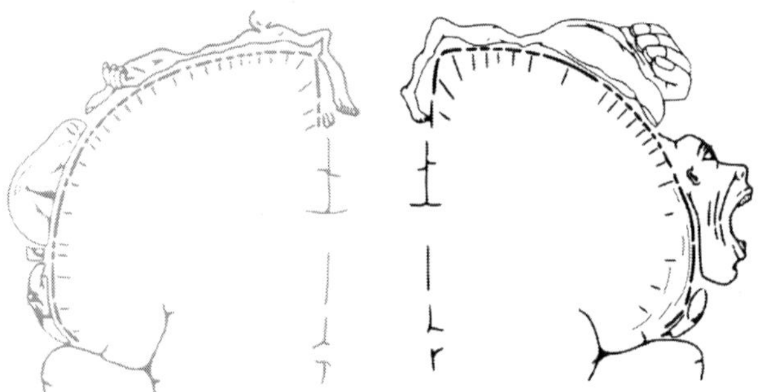

*The **somatosensory cortex** (with the primary motor cortex on the left).*

More than just receiving each of the senses individually, the parietal cortex is also involved in maintaining an **overall awareness of one's environment**. This can be seen in people who suffer damage to their non-dominant parietal lobe, as they often show signs of **hemispatial neglect** or an ignorance of sensory information coming from one side. For example, if you ask them to draw a clock, they may draw the numbers entirely on the one side only. This is not because the nerves carrying this sensory information are damaged but rather because the part of the brain set up to gather them (the parietal cortex) cannot receive them properly.

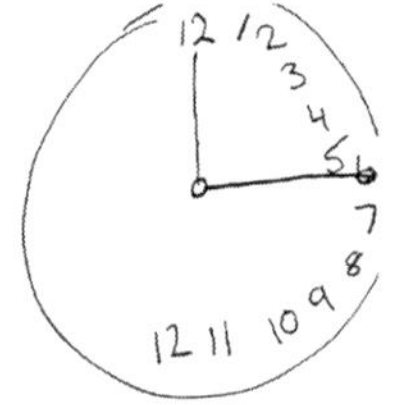

To remember the association of the parietal cortex to sensation and awareness, think of it as the **pariah**-tal cortex. A **pariah** is an outcast who could be quite **sensitive** to criticism, just as the pariah-tal cortex is quite sensitive to sensory information coming from the body.

The **parietal lobe** is the site of the **primary somatosensory cortex.**

*The **pariah**-tal cortex is quite **sens**itive (**sens**ory).*

THE OCCIPITAL CORTEX

The **occipital lobe** is the smallest of the four lobes and is found at the back of the brain. It primarily serves as the site of the **visual cortex**. In contrast to sensory information from the body (which goes to the parietal cortex), sensory information from the **eyes** travels to the occipital cortex where it is processed into the picture that we actually "see." You can remember that the occipital lobe is the site of the visual cortex by thinking that what you see through bin**oc**ulars goes back from the eyes to the **oc**cipital lobe.

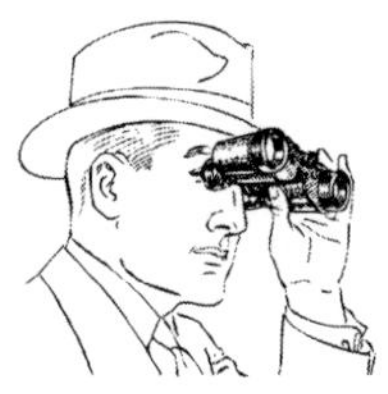

The **occipital lobe** is the site of the **visual cortex**.

*Sensory information from bin**oc**ulars goes to the **oc**cipital cortex.*

When bilateral damage to the occipital lobe occurs, it can result in a rare but fascinating disorder known as **Anton's syndrome**. Someone with Anton's syndrome is completely blind, but they will adamantly deny that they are blind (even when presented with clear evidence) and will make up answers to any questions requiring sight (a phenomenon known as confabulation). To remember this condition, make **ANTON** stand for **A**dmit **N**ot **T**o **O**ccipital **N**on-function.

Bilateral damage to the occipital cortex can result in a state of **cortical blindness** with accompanying **denial of blindness** known as **Anton's syndrome**.

*ANTON: **A**dmit **N**ot **T**o **O**ccipital **N**on-function.*

THE TEMPORAL CORTEX

Finally, the **temporal lobe** is the lowest part of the cerebrum, located to the sides just above the **ears**. This placement makes sense, as the temporal lobe is the site of the **auditory cortex**. Like the visual cortex in the occipital lobe, the auditory cortex receives special sensory information from the ears and processes it into the sound that we actually "hear." You can remember the association of the temporal cortex with hearing by thinking that the **tempo**-ral cortex helps you to hear the **tempo** of music. (The temporal cortex has a variety of other functions in addition to processing sound, including generating emotions and storing memories. We will talk about these later on in this chapter when we discuss the limbic system.)

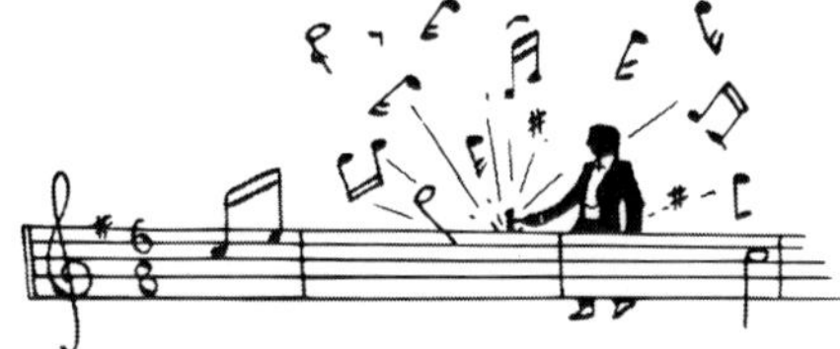

The **temporal lobe** is the site of the **auditory cortex**.

*The **tempo**-ral cortex helps you hear the **tempo** of music.*

LANGUAGE CENTERS

Using language is an incredibly complex task, so it should come as no surprise that it involves multiple regions of the brain. While these **language centers** are spread throughout the various lobes of the cerebrum, they ultimately work together as a coherent unit. (It's important to note that language centers are not only involved in speech but also play a role in any form of language-based communication, including reading, writing, and using sign language!)

The first language center we will discuss is **Broca's area** which is located in the frontal lobe of the dominant hemisphere and is responsible for **language production**. Someone who sustains damage to Broca's area will have trouble producing language, a condition known as an **expressive aphasia**. While some people with an expressive aphasia are completely mute, others are able to speak but only with great effort to produce even a few words. (For example, when asked to repeat the sentence, "The orange cat walked through the open door," someone with an expressive aphasia may only be able to say, "Cat........... door..........") To remember the association of Broca's area with an expressive aphasia, think of a **pull string doll** that is supposed to talk when you pull the string. If the doll is **Broca** (broken), then it won't talk.

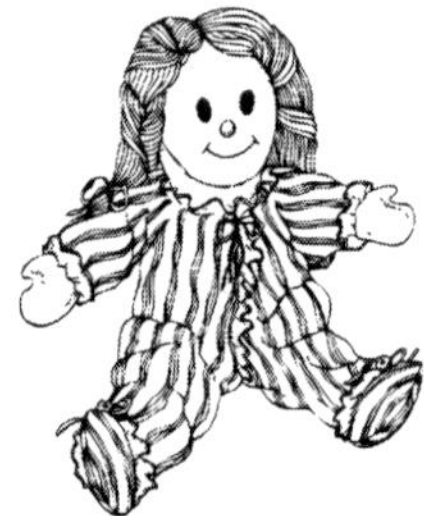

Broca's area is responsible for **language production**.
Damage to this region results in an **expressive aphasia**.

*Think of a **pull string doll**. If the doll becomes **Broca** (broken), then it **won't talk**.*

The second language center is **Wernicke's area** which is located where the temporal and parietal lobes meet. Wernicke's area is responsible for language **comprehension**, so damage to this area will result in difficulty understanding other people's words, a condition known as a **receptive aphasia**. Someone with a receptive aphasia may still be able to speak with the normal rhythm, tone, and musical flow that most speech has, although the content of what is being said is often nonsensical and may even incorporate made-up words known as **neologisms** (as in the sentence "Shemucker froos be sunt."). You can remember the association of receptive aphasia with Wernicke's area by thinking that someone with receptive aphasia can still be quite **Wer**-dy (even if the words don't actually make sense most of the time).

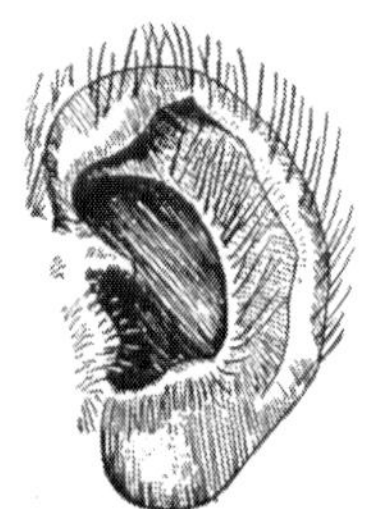

Wernicke's area is responsible for **language comprehension**.
Damage to this region results in a **receptive aphasia**.

*Someone with **Wer**nicke's aphasia can still be quite **Wer**-dy.*

A bundle of axons known as the **arcuate fasciculus** connects Broca's area to Wernicke's area and allows someone to use what is being said to them to inform what they say back. Someone with a damaged arcuate fasciculus will be able to both speak and understand language, but they will not be able to accurately repeat something that is spoken to them (known as a **conduction aphasia**).

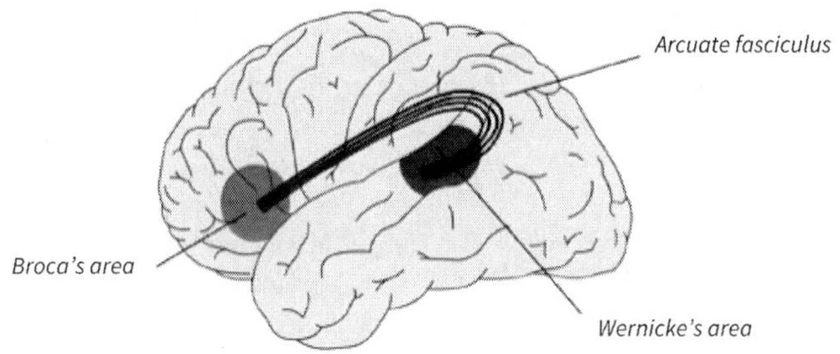

The **arcuate fasciculus** connects Wernicke's area to Broca's area.
Damage to this area results in a **conduction aphasia**.

*Without an **accurate** fasciculus, you cannot **accurately** repeat what someone just said.*

Finally, someone who sustains damage to multiple language centers at the same time can develop a **global aphasia** where language production and comprehension are both impaired. Keep the various forms of aphasia in mind, as they can be key to localizing a lesion (for example, someone who comes into the hospital for a stroke and is unable to speak has likely sustained damage in a different part of the brain compared to someone who is unable to understand what you're saying to them).

THE LIMBIC SYSTEM

Our final stop in this chapter is the **limbic system**. The word "limbic" is Latin for "border," and this region is so-named because it lies at the border between the upper brain (the cerebrum) and lower structures like the brainstem. The limbic system is not an *anatomically* distinct region but rather one whose various parts are united by a shared *function*: specifically, regulation of **emotion**, **memory**, **motivation**, and **behavior**. Because the boundaries of this system are functional rather than anatomic, not everyone agrees on which parts of the brain that are classified as being in the limbic system, with many regions having been considered. However, for the sake of simplicity we will limit our discussion to just a core few that are universally considered to be a part of the limbic system: the amygdala, the hippocampus, the mammillary bodies, the nucleus accumbens, and the anterior cingulate cortex. While some of these structures lie in "lower" areas that we haven't talked about yet (such as the subcortex and the brainstem), overall they all contribute to the "higher order" cognitive processes of emotion, memory, and behavior, so we will cover them here.

THE AMYGDALA

The **amygdala** is a paired group of neuronal cell bodies lying on the inner part of the temporal lobe that determines our **emotional response to stimuli**. For example, if a mountain lion suddenly jumps out at you from behind the bushes while you are out camping in the woods, you will likely feel an immediate rush of fear. This is because your amygdala has judged this situation to be potentially dangerous and has activated parts of your body (such as the sympathetic nervous system and its "fight or flight" response) to take action. More than just being involved with our *immediate* response to stimuli, the amygdala is directly involved in the formation of **long-term memory and decision-making**. Indeed, any situation in which we are emotionally activated is likely to be remembered strongly so that we can make different decisions in the future! The amygdala exerts a powerful effect on our lives through its effect on our emotions. You can remember the function of the amygdala by thinking of it as the **emo**-gdala to associate it with our **emo**-tional response to certain stimuli.

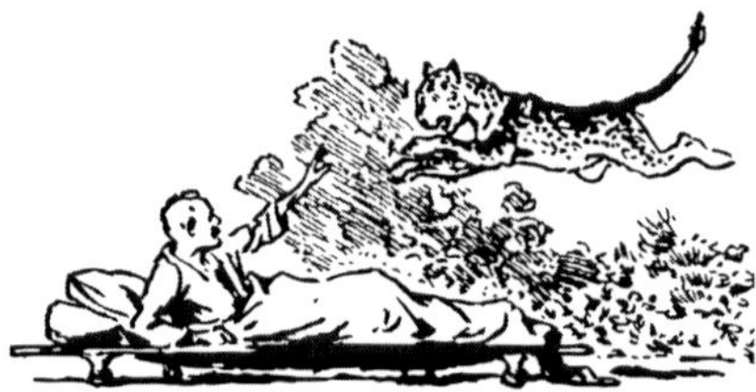

The **amygdala** is involved in determining our **emotional response to stimuli** as well as forming **long-term emotional memories**.

*The **emo**-gdala is strongly involved in our **emo**-tions.*

Damage to the amygdala can result in **Klüver-Bucy syndrome**. One of the most common findings in Klüver-Bucy syndrome is a **diminished or absent fear response** to frightening stimuli (often described as a "docility" or "tameness"). There is also an **inability to form new memories or recall old ones** which further underscores the amygdala's role in memory formation. Klüver-Bucy syndrome can also present with **hyperorality** (a tendency to put non-food objects in the mouth) and **hypersexuality**, two features that are also shared with disorders involving the frontal lobe.

THE HIPPOCAMPUS

The **hippocampus** is a pair of seahorse-shaped structures that, like the amygdala, lies on the inner side of the temporal lobe and is involved in the formation of memories. In particular, the hippocampus helps to **consolidate short-term memories into long-term ones**. All of us have the ability to keep track of information for a short amount of time (such as needing to keep a phone number in mind only long enough to dial it). Without the need to remember this for more than a few seconds, this information is quickly forgotten. In contrast, if the information is deemed important (for example, if it is the phone number of someone that we are very attracted to) then we will be much more likely to commit that information to long-term memory.

Someone who sustains bilateral damage to their hippocampi will often be unable to form new memories. The hippocampus is also one of the first structures to show evidence of damage in disorders like Alzheimer's disease in which loss of memory plays a key role. You can remember the function of the hippocampus by thinking of going to a school dance and seeing that someone has brought a hippopotamus as their date. If you saw a "**hippo** on **campus**," you would almost certainly **remember** it!

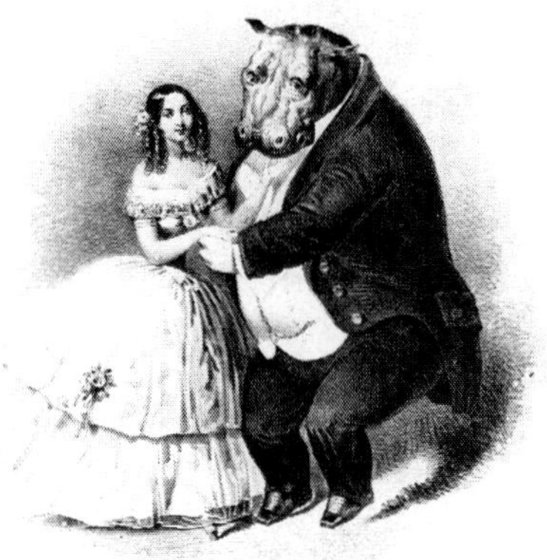

The **hippocampus** is involved in **forming new memories** and **recalling old ones**.

*If you saw a "**hippo** on **campus**," you would almost certainly **remember** it.*

THE MAMMILLARY BODIES

The **mammillary bodies** are a pair of round structures that lie on the underside of the brain (not the cortex!) and are connected to both the amygdala and the hippocampus. Given the involvement of both of these structures, it shouldn't be too surprising that the **mam**millary bodies are closely involved with the processes of recall and **mam**ory.

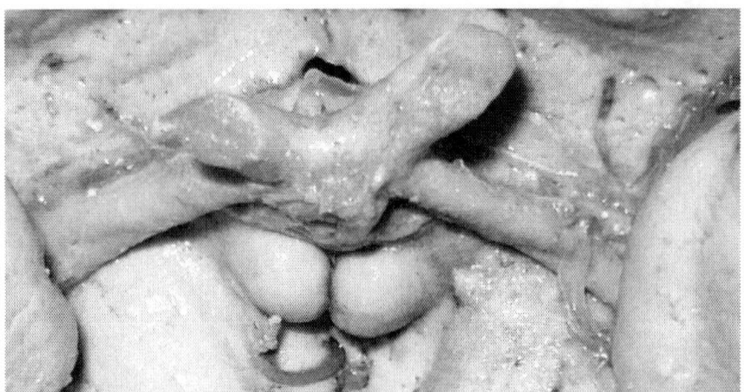

*A pair of round **mammillary bodies** as seen during an autopsy.*

The **mammillary bodies** are connected to both the **amygdala** and the **hippocampus** and play a key role in **memory formation**.

*The **mam**millary bodies are important for **mam**ory formation.*

On a clinical level, the mammillary bodies are perhaps most notable for their role in **Wernicke-Korsakoff syndrome**, a disorder that prominently features impaired memory formation, including both **anterograde amnesia** (an inability to form new memories) and **retrograde amnesia** (a loss of previously formed memories). Wernicke-Korsakoff syndrome is often associated with a long history of excessive alcohol intake, as chronic exposure to alcohol can result in a deficiency of vitamin B_1 (also known as thiamine). Atrophy of the mammillary bodies is often seen in these patients on autopsy.

THE CINGULATE CORTEX

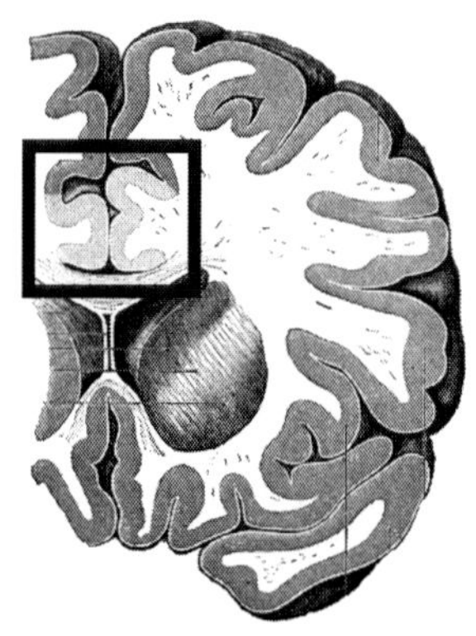

Sitting on the inside of the canyon formed by the longitudinal fissure, just above the corpus callosum, lies the **cingulate cortex**. The cingulate cortex does not belong to any one lobe but rather spans various lobes, like a belt. (In fact, the word "cingulum" is Latin for belt!) The front-most part of the cingulate cortex, or the **anterior cingulate cortex**, is often considered to be a part of the limbic system and in particular seems to play a role in **error recognition**. This can involve many different kinds of errors, whether it is a simple mistake (like seeing a word that has been misspelled) or a moral wrong (such as seeing a rich person steal money from a beggar on the street). Recognizing something as an error prompts the anterior cingulate cortex to generate a strong emotional response which then motivates us to act on the situation (such as correcting the spelling of the word or confronting the thief). Because of its key role in error recognition, the anterior cingulate cortex frequently comes up when discussing various psychiatric conditions such as obsessive-compulsive disorder in which error recognition plays a large role. You can remember the function of the **A**nterior **c**ingulate **c**ortex by thinking of someone being disgusted and exclaiming, "**Acc**!" when coming upon an error.

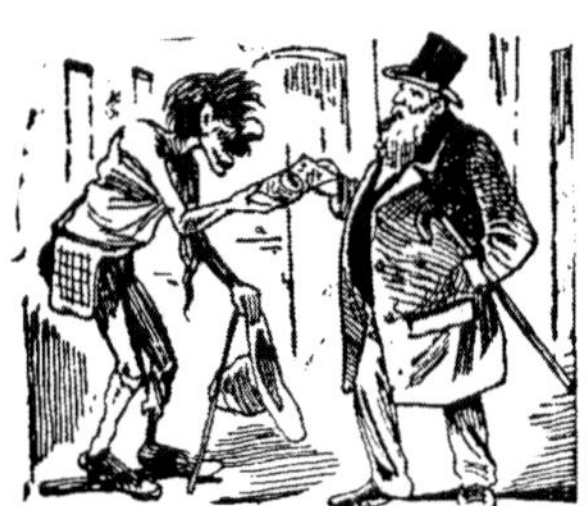

The **anterior cingulate cortex** is involved not only in **recognizing errors** but also in **motivating** us to act to fix them.

*Think of someone coming across an **error** and exclaiming, "**Acc**!"*

THE NUCLEUS ACCUMBENS

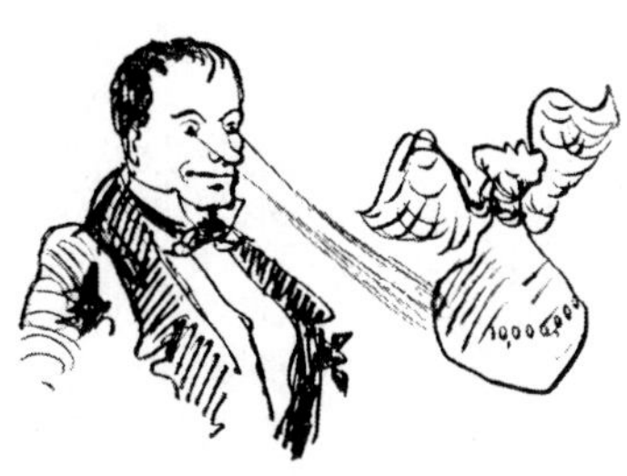

The last part of the limbic system we will talk about is the **nucleus accumbens**. Like the mammillary bodies, the nucleus accumbens is *not* located in the cortex, but because it contributes to higher cognitive functions, it is still considered to be a part of the limbic system. In particular, the nucleus accumbens appears to play a key role in **motivation and reward**. Activities such as eating food, having sex, earning money, and using addictive drugs like cocaine or heroin have direct effects on the nucleus accumbens, leading to pleasurable feelings that increase the chance that someone will engage in more of that same behavior in the future (a process known as **reinforcement**). While reward-oriented behavior is not in and of itself pathological, the nucleus accumbens has been found to play a role in addiction and other behavioral disorders. You can remember the function of this region by remembering that the nucleus **accum**bens helps you to **accum**ulate money and other rewards.

The **nucleus accumbens** governs **motivation** and **pleasure** and appears to play a key role in processes like **addiction.**

*The nucleus **accum**bens helps you to **accum**ulate money and other rewards.*

PUTTING IT ALL TOGETHER

And thus concludes our whirlwind tour of the cerebral cortex! We've covered four lobes (the **frontal**, **parietal**, **occipital**, and **temporal** lobes) as well as two systems (the **language centers** and the **limbic system**) that span those lobes.

When talking about the four lobes of the brain, it's important to point out that in this chapter we have focused exclusively on the functions of each lobe that are found in the *cortex*! However, each lobe has additional *sub*cortical structures that have their own functions, so don't go around thinking that the entirety of the temporal lobe is there *only* to allow you to hear the tempo of music. There are many more functions that are associated with the cerebrum than just the ones in the cortex, which we will learn about more in the next couple of chapters as we dive deeper into the brain by going to the subcortex!

REVIEW QUESTIONS

1. A 68 y/o left-handed F is recovering from a recent stroke. During an appointment, a physical therapist notices that she consistently does not use assistive devices that are placed on her left side and will even ignore the therapist's motioned instructions when he is standing to her left. She responds appropriately to objects placed to her right. The patient denies any difficulties understanding instructions when she is asked. Later, when the physical therapist is reviewing some forms that the patient filled out, he notices that the left half of the page is often blank, with only the right half filled out. Which of the following areas of the brain did this patient most likely sustain damage from her stroke?
    A. Left frontal cortex
    B. Right frontal cortex
    C. Left parietal cortex
    D. Right parietal cortex
    E. Left occipital cortex
    F. Right occipital cortex
    G. Left temporal cortex
    H. Right temporal cortex
    I. More than one of the above
    J. None of the above

2. A 55 y/o M is brought to his primary care doctor's office by his wife. The patient denies that there is anything wrong. However, his wife insists that over the past 3 months there has been a noticeable change in his behavior. He retired 2 years ago and initially spent his time attending to his garden. However, recently he has begun eating large amounts of candy and other sweet food, including two large tubs of ice cream that his wife had bought for a party. He has taken to stockpiling candy bars in his closet where he thinks his wife cannot find them. His wife says that he has been "throwing tantrums like a 5-year-old" when he does not get his way. He narrowly avoided having the police called on him after he was found in the mall putting his hand down his pants in the middle of a walkway. This patient's changes in behavior are most consistent with abnormalities in which of the following regions?
    A. Frontal cortex
    B. Parietal cortex
    C. Occipital cortex
    D. Temporal cortex
    E. None of the above

3. A 70 y/o right-handed M experienced a stroke one year ago. Initially he presented with loss of motor control of his right arm and leg, but this recovered with time and physical therapy. However, since his stroke he has been unable to engage in conversation and often looks puzzled and confused when others speak to him. Following an evaluation with a speech and language pathologist, he is diagnosed with Wernicke's aphasia. Given the nature of his deficits, which of the following tasks is he *most* likely to be able to perform?
    A. Pointing at the correct picture when someone says "Show me a lion"
    B. Being able to order a pizza when he gets hungry
    C. Answering the question "Why did they go up the hill?" after being told the story of Jack and Jill
    D. Being able to sing the melody of a song that he knows from childhood
    E. Repeating the sentence "She blazed around the dusty field"

4. A 12 y/o M has had recurrent seizures over the past year. Electroencephalography reveals bursts of neuronal activity originating in the occipital lobe without subsequent spread to other areas of the brain. Which of the following is the most likely sign or symptom that would appear during a seizure for this patient?
    A. Repetitive behaviors such as twisting, turning, or grimacing
    B. Hearing loud sounds despite being in a quiet area
    C. Sudden episodes of blurred vision
    D. Feeling electrical sensations running down one's arms and legs
    E. Inability to speak

5. A 44 y/o M with a long history of alcohol use is brought to the hospital by an ambulance after he was found wandering into traffic on a busy city street. He is admitted to the hospital and given intravenous fluids as well as oral thiamine. Several days later, he is discharged to a local substance abuse rehabilitation program. However, the staff there begin reporting that he has trouble engaging in treatment due to high distractibility, poor attention, and disorganized behavior. He is referred for neuropsychological testing which reveals significant deficits in both short-term and long-term memory. Which of the following limbic structures has most likely been damaged in this patient?
    A. Amygdala
    B. Hippocampus
    C. Mammillary bodies
    D. Nucleus accumbens
    E. Anterior cingulate cortex

1. **The best answer is D.** This vignette describes a case of hemineglect as evidenced by the patient's lack of awareness of information in one half of her sensory field. Given the parietal lobe's role in processing sensory information, damage to the parietal lobe is responsible for most cases of hemineglect, typically on the side opposite of the neglect. While the patient is left-handed, that does not mean that she is right dominant, as around 70% of left-handed individuals are still left dominant, making this still the most likely situation (answer C).

2. **The best answer is A.** This patient's behavior shows a startling lack of self-inhibition that is consistent with deficits in the part of the brain that says "no": the frontal lobe. This case describes a disease known as frontotemporal dementia in which damage to the frontal and temporal lobes accumulates over time. While both the frontal and temporal lobes are implicated, the patient's behavior as described in this case are clearly due to insufficient inhibition from the frontal lobe rather than damage to the temporal lobe (answer D). The parietal cortex is involved in attention, awareness, and receiving somatosensory signals (answer B) while the occipital cortex is the site of visual processing (answer C); neither would account for the behavioral changes described in this vignette.

3. **The best answer is D.** Receptive aphasia results in deficits in language comprehension. For this reason, any tasks that involve understanding the content of what someone else is saying will be impaired, including language comprehension (answers A and C) and repetition (answer E). However, receptive aphasia tends to produce deficits in speech production as well. While patients with this condition are still able to speak, the words they produce are often nonsensical, making it difficult to complete tasks like ordering a pizza (answer B). In contrast, the flow, rhythm, and musical tone of language is often preserved, so someone with this condition will often still be able to sing a melody.

4. **The best answer is C.** This vignette describes a case of occipital lobe seizures characterized by recurrent episodes of visual abnormalities, which can include blurriness, blindness, and hallucinations. Repetitive movements would be most likely in a seizure involving the motor cortex in the frontal lobe (answer A), while sudden sensory abnormalities would be more likely observed in a parietal lobe seizure (answer D). Auditory hallucinations are more often related to a seizure in the temporal cortex (answer B), while speech impairment would likely involve the language centers, none of which are located in the occipital lobe (answer E).

5. **The best answer is C.** A deficiency of thiamine, often related to chronic alcohol abuse, is known to damage the mammillary bodies, a pair of structures involved in memory. While the hippocampus is also involved in memory, its role more specifically involves consolidating short-term memories to long-term ones, in contrast to this patient who had pronounced deficits in both short-term and long-term memories (answer B). The amygdala is involved in generating fear and other emotions (answer A), while the nucleus accumbens is involved in reward-driven behavior (answer D). Finally, the anterior cingulate cortex appears to be involved in error recognition (answer E).

4 THE THALAMUS, EPITHALAMUS, AND HYPOTHALAMUS

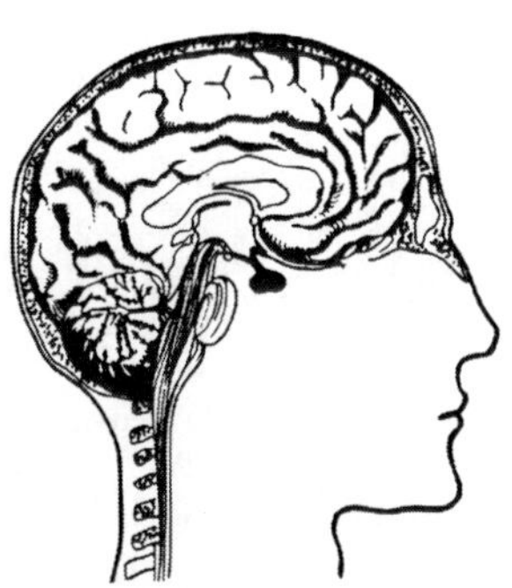

Let's go deeper into the brain to reach the structures that lie underneath the cortex, fittingly called the **subcortex**. While much of the subcortex is made up of white matter, there are pockets of grey matter in this area as well that carry out some vitally important functions. The jobs that these subcortical structures perform are perhaps less sophisticated than the complex decision-making and executive-functioning done by the cortex, but what they lack in sophistication they more than make up for in necessity. Indeed, many of the subcortex's functions are ultimately more important for survival, including the **epithalamus** and **hypothalamus** which regulate such basic functions as hunger, thirst, and sleep. The subcortex also plays a key role in fine-tuning signals coming to and from the cortex, with the **thalamus** sorting sensory information on its way to the parietal cortex and the **basal ganglia** smoothing out motor signals coming down from the frontal cortex. We'll go over the thalamus, epithalamus, and hypothalamus in this chapter, then cover the basal ganglia as well as a related structure called the internal capsule in the next chapter.

As we discuss these regions, you may see the word **nucleus** pop up from time to time (for example, the caudate nucleus or the subthalamic nucleus). It's important not to confuse this with the DNA-filled *cell* nucleus! In neurology, the term "nucleus" is used to describe a cluster of neuronal cell bodies that are grouped together and share a similar function. The term nucleus is specifically used for clusters that are located in the *central* nervous system, while the term **ganglion** is used to describe similar neuron clusters when they are found in the *peripheral* nervous system.

THE THALAMUS

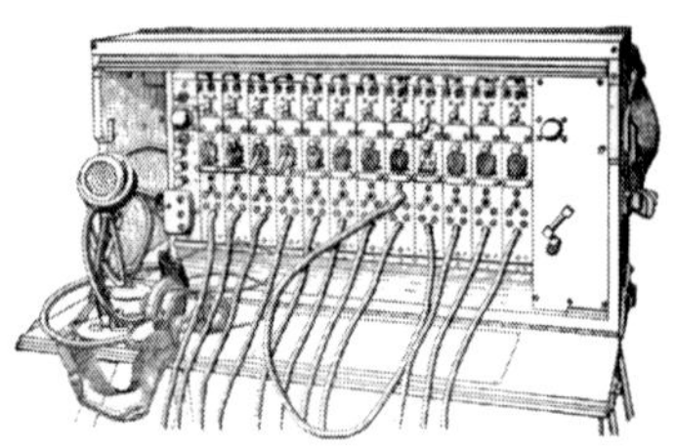

Okay, onto the specific areas of the subcortex! We're first going to talk about the **thalamus**. The thalamus acts as a **relay station for sensory information** by routing afferent neurons traveling from various areas of the body to the appropriate part of the cerebral cortex, such as sending information from the body to the parietal cortex, visual information from the eyes to the occipital cortex, and auditory information from the ears to the temporal cortex. In this way, the thalamus acts like a **switchboard** to make sure that relevant sensory information gets where it needs to go. When damage to the **th**alamus occurs, this often produces **th**evere **th**en**th**ory defici**th** such as numbness. The thalamus also appears to play a key role in determining a person's overall level of consciousness, awareness, and wakefulness. Indeed, in cases of severe damage to the thalamus, a permanent state of unresponsiveness known as a **coma** can result.

The **thalamus** acts as a **relay station** for **sensory information** traveling to the cerebral cortex.

*The **th**alamus is all about **th**en**th**ation.*

The manner in which afferent neurons pass through the thalamus is neither messy nor disorganized—quite the contrary, in fact! Like other parts of the brain, the thalamus is not a single uniform area but instead consists of specific nuclei where the cell bodies of neurons serving similar purposes have gathered together. We'll go over a few of the most clinically relevant nuclei here.

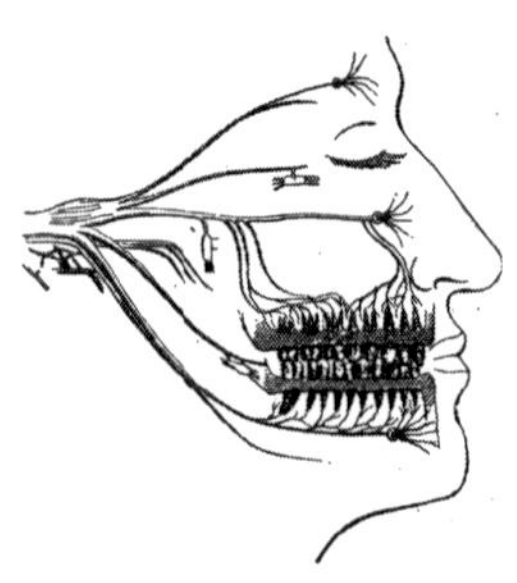

The **ventral posterolateral nucleus** and **ventral posteromedial nucleus** are both involved in relaying sensory information to the primary somatosensory cortex in the parietal lobe. In particular, **V**entral **P**ostero**L**ateral nucleus receives sensory information from the arms and legs, which means that neurons coming up from **V**ery **P**ainful **L**imbs will go through the **VPL**. In contrast, the **V**entral **P**ostero**M**edial nucleus receives input from the **face and mouth**, so neurons coming from a **V**ery **P**ainful **M**outh will pass through the **VPM**.

The **ventral posterolateral nucleus** receives sensory information from the **arms and legs**, while the **ventral posteromedial nucleus** receives sensory information from the **face and mouth**.

__V__entral __P__ostero__L__ateral nucleus = __V__ery __P__ainful __L__imbs.
__V__entral __P__ostero__M__edial nucleus = __V__ery __P__ainful __M__outh.

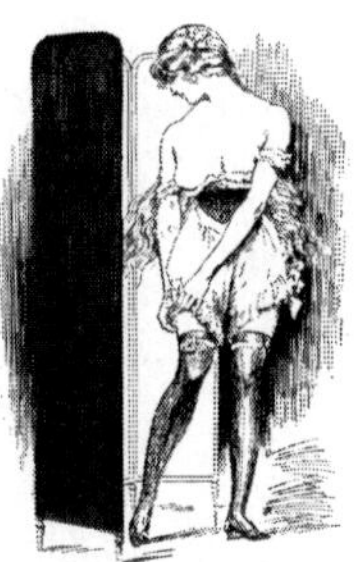

While the ventral posterolateral and ventral posteromedial nuclei process sensory information from the body, two other nuclei in the thalamus process special sensory information from the **eyes and ears**. The **L**ateral **G**eniculate **N**ucleus is the primary relay center for **visual information** and is therefore important for checking yourself in the mirror to make sure you are **L**ooking **G**ood **N**aked. In contrast, the **M**edial **G**eniculate **N**ucleus serves the same purpose for **auditory information** and is therefore important for hearing someone **M**aking **G**reat **N**oise.

The **lateral geniculate nucleus** receives **visual information** from the **eyes**, while the **medial geniculate nucleus** receives **auditory information** from the **ears**.

__L__ateral __G__eniculate __N__ucleus = __L__ooking __G__ood __N__aked (__visual__ pathway).
__M__edial __G__eniculate __N__ucleus = __M__aking __G__reat __N__oise (__auditory__ pathway).

THE EPITHALAMUS

The **epithalamus** (Greek for "above the thalamus") is mostly made up of white matter, although it also contains a tiny structure known as the **pineal gland**. The pineal gland secretes the hormone **melatonin** in response to low light levels at night which helps to regulate the **sleep-wake cycle** by inducing a tired feeling. Due to its location above a structure known as the vertical gaze center, a tumor of the pineal gland (known as a **pinealoma**) can cause an inability to move the eyes upward, leading to a state of down-looking eyes (or "sunset eyes") known as **Parinaud's syndrome**. You can remember the meaning of Parinaud's syndrome by thinking of it whenever you are examining someone and find their "**peerin' odd**."

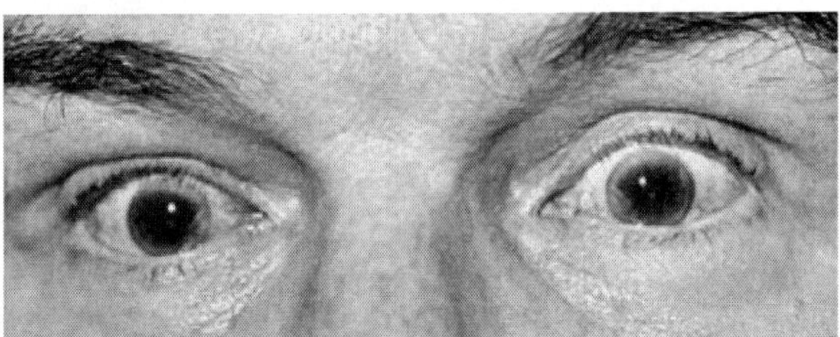

This patient with a __pineal gland tumor__ is being asked to look up but cannot.

The **epithalamus** contains the **pineal gland**. A **pinealoma** can cause **Parinaud's syndrome** which is an **inability to look up**.

Ep__i__thalamus = __pi__neal gland.
Consider __Parinaud's__ syndrome when you find someone's __peerin' odd__.

THE HYPOTHALAMUS

The **hypothalamus** (Greek for "below the thalamus") is found—wait for it—*below the thalamus*. It is made up of a collection of nuclei that each perform various activities important to survival. In addition, the hypothalamus has direct control over the release of hormones from the pituitary gland (which we will discuss in the next section). To remember the most clinically relevant functions of the **H**ypothalamus, think of the **6 H's**: **H**ot (temperature regulation), **H**ungry (food intake), **H**ourly (circadian rhythm), **H**ydrated (water balance), **H**orny (reproduction), and **H**ormonal (hormone release).

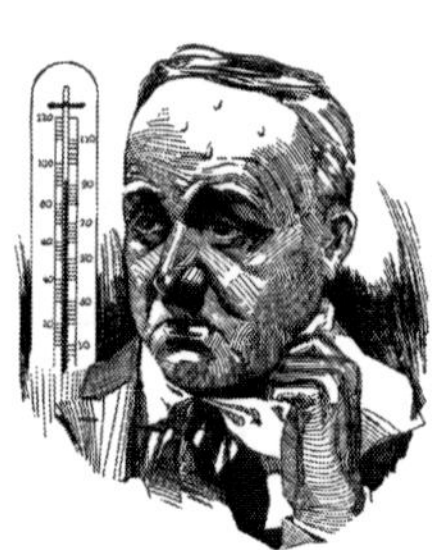

H is for Hot. The first two pairs of nuclei we will talk about each have opposing functions, with the **anterior and posterior hypothalamic nuclei** both being involved in **temperature regulation**. The **A**nterior hypothalamic nucleus helps to initiate **C**ooling mechanisms such as sweating and panting (think of an **A/C** unit cooling down a house on a hot day). In contrast, the **posterior hypothalamic nucleus** works to **heat up** the body through shivering and other mechanisms (think of the phrase "You've got a **hot posterior**!"). These two nuclei work together to regulate body temperature by cooling down and heating up the body, respectively.

The **anterior and posterior hypothalamic nuclei** work to **regulate temperature**.

*The **A**nterior hypothalamic nucleus is for **C**ooling (**A/C** = **A**ir **C**onditioning).*
*The **P**osterior hypothalamic nucleus is for **H**eating ("You've got a **hot posterior**!").*

H is for Hungry. The second pair of nuclei we will discuss regulates food intake. In particular, the **lateral hypothalamic nucleus** is responsible for the sensation of **hunger** (the lateral nucleus will make you **fatter**-al), while the **ventromedial nucleus** is associated with a feeling of satiety (eating a ventro-**meal** will make you full).

The **lateral and ventromedial hypothalamic nuclei** regulate **food intake**.

*The **later**al nucleus will make you **fatter**-al,*
*while the ventro-**meal** nucleus will make you feel **full**.*

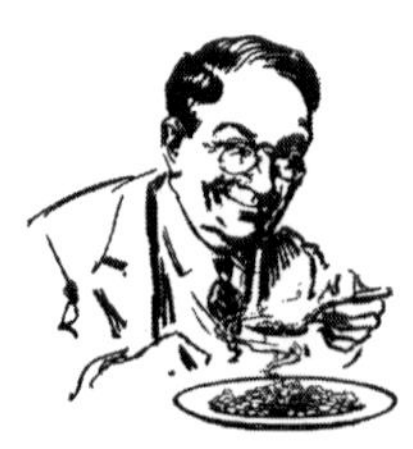

Several hormones act on these two nuclei to influence the feeling of hunger. **Ghrelin** (released by the stomach when it anticipates a meal) acts on the lateral nucleus to induce hunger, while **leptin** (released by fat cells) acts on the ventromedial nucleus to induce satiety. You can remember the function of each of these hormones by thinking that **ghrelin** is released when the stomach is **growlin'** while lep-**thin** will make you **thinner**.

Ghrelin and **leptin** are hormones that **increase and decrease hunger**, respectively.

__Ghrelin__ is released by a __growlin'__ stomach,
while lep-__thin__ will make you __thin__ner.

H is for Hourly. We've already talked about the role of the epithalamus and its pineal gland in regulating the sleep-wake cycle, but the hypothalamus plays a role here as well. In particular, the **suprachiasmatic nucleus** acts as an internal clock that regulates various processes in a consistent 24-hour cycle known as the **circadian rhythm**. The suprachiasmatic nucleus communicates with other regions of the brain (including the aforementioned pineal gland) to regulate body temperature and the production of certain hormones according to this daily cycle. To remember the function of the suprachiasmatic nucleus, remember that someone who doesn't get enough sleep is likely to be grumpy. If you get enough sleep, however, you can be charming and **chiasmatic** (charismatic).

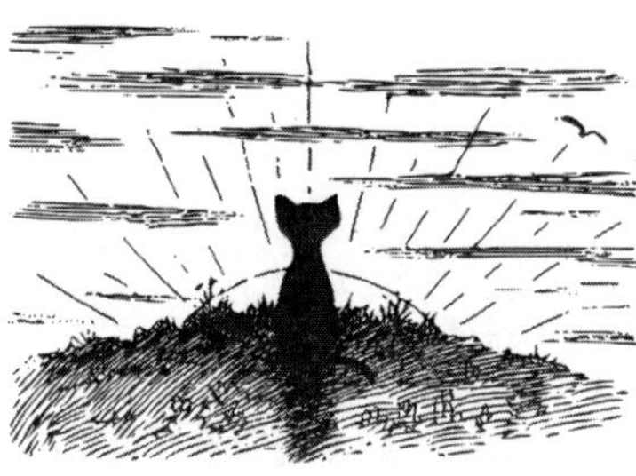

The **suprachiasmatic nucleus** maintains a daily sleep-wake cycle known as the **circadian rhythm**.

If you get enough __sleep__, you can be charming and __chiasmatic__ (charismatic).

H is for Hydrated. Control over **thirst** and **urine production** is also located in the hypothalamus. A region known as the **supraoptic nucleus** produces a hormone called **vasopressin** that works to maintain fluid balance by decreasing urine volume in the kidneys when the hypothalamus detects that the osmolality of the plasma is too high (this effect gives vasopressin its older name: **antidiuretic hormone**). In this way, vasopressin has the effect of diluting the blood by retaining more water and thereby lowering serum concentrations of sodium and other electrolytes. Vasopressin is one of two hormones that is produced in the hypothalamus and released in the **posterior pituitary** (the other being oxytocin, discussed next). To remember the function of the supraoptic nucleus, think about looking ("-optic") at the clouds above you ("supra-") to see if it's going to rain (water).

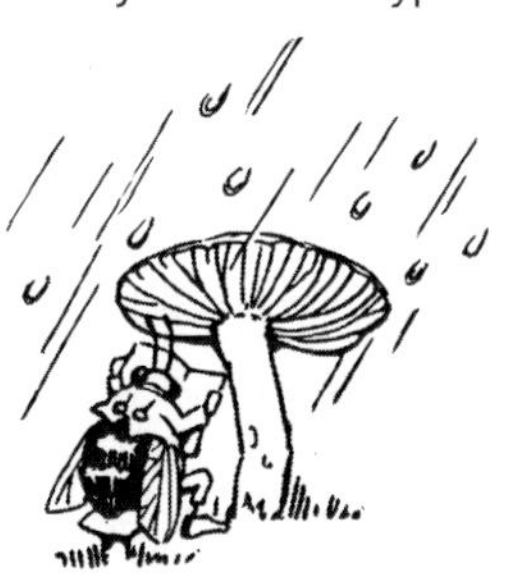

The **supraoptic nucleus** produces **vasopressin** to regulate **thirst** and **fluid balance**.

***Look** ("__-optic__") at the clouds __above__ you ("__supra-__") to see if it's going to __rain__ (water).*

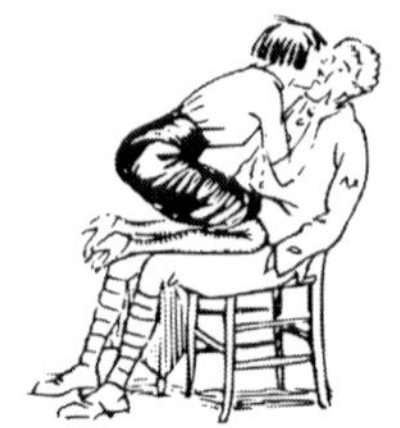

H is for Horny. Besides vasopressin, the other hormone that is produced by the hypothalamus is **oxytocin**. Oxytocin is produced in the **paraventricular nucleus** and is released in response to a variety of situations involving **interpersonal bonding and reproduction** such as hugging, skin-to-skin contact, sexual activity, and orgasm. In general, release of oxytocin during these events helps to promote trust, generosity, attachment, and other **prosocial behaviors**. It has specific functions in child rearing as well, as it helps the uterus to contract during birth and stimulates the release of breast milk after birth. You can remember the function of this nucleus but thinking that **Par**ental **V**iewing is **N**eeded for the "mature themes" that the **Para****V**entricular **N**ucleus is involved in.

The **paraventricular nucleus** produces **oxytocin**, a hormone involved in **bonding** and **reproduction**.

Par**ental **V**iewing is **N**eeded for the "mature themes" of the **Para*V**entricular **N**ucleus.*

H is for Hormonal. Finally, the hypothalamus interacts with the **pituitary gland** to release hormones that govern a variety of processes throughout the body. The pituitary gland is made up of two parts: the **anterior pituitary** and the **posterior pituitary**. We have already talked about the two hormones (vasopressin and oxytocin) that are produced in the hypothalamus, travel down the pituitary stalk, and are released in the posterior pituitary. In contrast, the hormones released by the *anterior* pituitary are not made in the hypothalamus. Rather, the hypothalamus releases its own hormones that then diffuse downstream to the pituitary gland to cause the release of *additional* hormones from the anterior pituitary. Look at the following image to gain a better understanding of the relationship between these structures, then jump to the next section to learn more about what these hormones actually do!

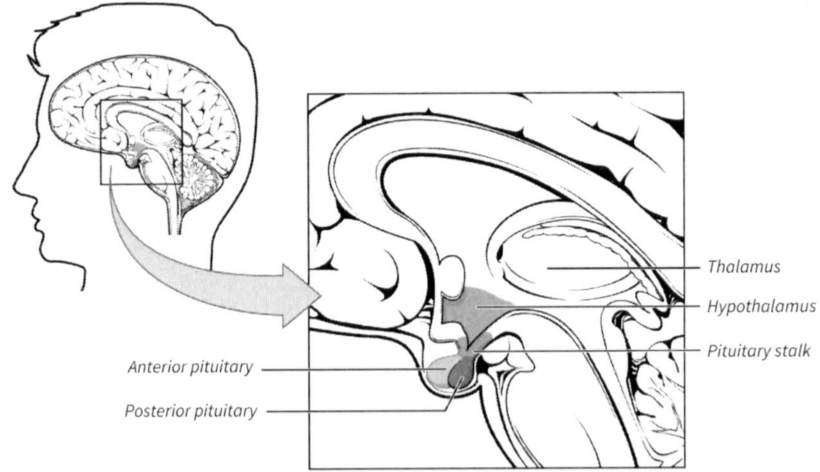

*Anatomic relationship between the **hypothalamus** and the **pituitary gland**.*

The **hypothalamus** performs a wide variety of **essential functions** in the body.

*The **6 H's** of the **H**ypothalamus:*
***H**ot (temperature regulation)*
***H**ungry (food intake)*
***H**ourly (circadian rhythm)*
***H**ydrated (water balance)*
***H**orny (reproduction)*
***H**ormonal (hormone release)*

THE PITUITARY GLAND

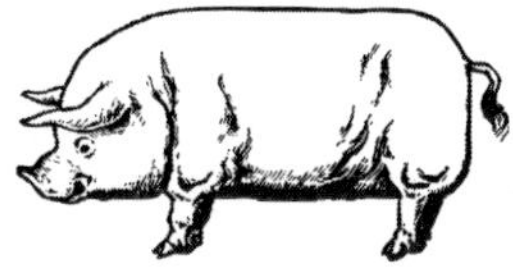

The nervous system is great at rapidly effecting change through lightning-fast transmission of action potentials. However, sometimes it needs to slow things down and create longer-lasting changes by releasing hormones throughout the body. This is where the **anterior pituitary gland** comes in. The anterior pituitary gland releases 6 hormones which you can remember using the mnemonic **FLAT PiG**:

F is for Follicle-stimulating hormone. Follicle-stimulating hormone (FSH) is involved in regulating the **reproductive processes** of both men and women. In men, follicle-stimulating hormone is involved in stimulating sperm production, while in women it stimulates the growth of ovarian follicles.

L is for Luteinizing hormone. Like follicle-stimulating hormone, luteinizing hormone (LH) is concerned primarily with reproduction. In men, LH stimulates the production of testosterone, while in women a surge in the level of this hormone triggers ovulation.

A is for Adrenocorticotropic hormone. Adrenocorticotropic hormone (ACTH) acts on the adrenal cortex to stimulate the release of **cortisol**, a hormone that allows the body to respond to stress by releasing sugar into the blood and altering electrolyte balance (such as increasing serum levels of sodium). Cortisol is also very effective at reducing inflammation, making it a great treatment for a wide variety of neurologic conditions involving an overactive immune system (as we will see in later chapters).

T is for Thyroid-stimulating hormone. Thyroid-stimulating hormone (TSH) acts on the **thyroid gland** to stimulate the production of thyroid hormones which then work throughout the body to increase the basal metabolic rate, stimulate blood flow, raise the core body temperature, and increase the speed of metabolism.

P is for Prolactin. Prolactin is primarily involved in stimulating **breast development** and the production of **breast milk**.

i is for ignore. You can ignore this one (it's just there for the mnemonic!).

G is for Growth hormone. As its name implies, growth hormone (GH) stimulates the growth of various cells and organs throughout the body, leading to muscle growth and bone lengthening. The effects of growth hormone are illustrated dramatically in the following picture:

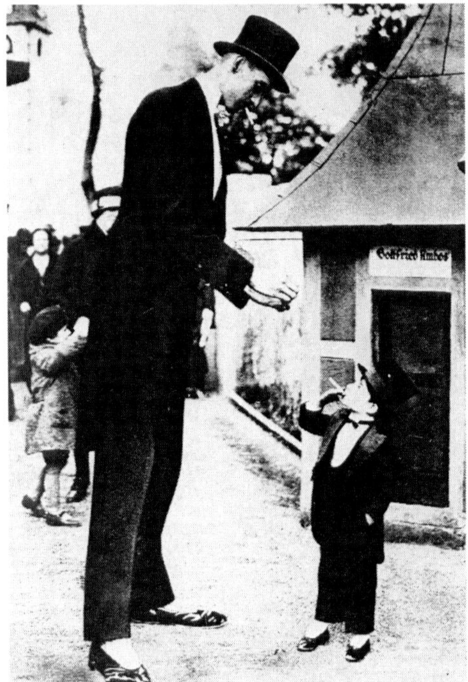

***Too much growth hormone** on the left, **too little** on the right.*

Each of these six hormones is either stimulated or inhibited by an upstream hormone released from the hypothalamus. In this way, there is a **three-part axis** formed between the hypothalamus, the pituitary, and the target organ. A summary of each hormone axis is found in the following table. One exception worth noting here is the hypothalamic–pituitary–mammary axis, as the hormone released by the hypothalamus (dopamine) actually *inhibits* rather than stimulates the release of the downstream hormone! Other than that, however, the pattern is pretty consist across all six of the hormones released by the anterior pituitary.

First, the hypothalamus releases:	**...to make the anterior pituitary secrete:**	**... which acts on the:**	**... and causes it to release:**
Thyrotropin-releasing hormone (TRH)	Thyroid-stimulating hormone (TSH)	Thyroid gland	Thyroid hormone
Corticotropin-releasing hormone (CRH)	Adrenocorticotropic hormone (ACTH)	Adrenal gland	Cortisol
Gonadotropin-releasing hormone (GnRH)	Follicle-stimulating hormone (FSH) and luteinizing hormone (LH)	Gonads	Testosterone and estradiol
Growth hormone-releasing hormone (GHRH)	Growth hormone (GH)	Liver and other organs	Insulin-like growth factor 1 (IGF-1)
Dopamine	Prolactin (inhibited, not secreted!)	Mammary glands	Breast milk

The **anterior pituitary gland** releases **six hormones** that each play an essential role in the **endocrine system**.

FLAT PiG:
__F__ollicle-stimulating hormone (FSH)
__L__uteinizing hormone (LH)
__A__drenocorticotropic hormone (ACTH)
__T__hyroid-stimulating hormone (TSH)
__P__rolactin
__i__gnore
__G__rowth hormone (GH)

PUTTING IT ALL TOGETHER

At first glance, the cerebral cortex appears to be the most complex and intricate part of the brain. However, the more you learn about the subcortex, the more it becomes clear that the cortex would be hopelessly lost without the guidance and support of the structures beneath it. The parietal, occipital, and temporal cortices wouldn't be able to receive sensory information without the **thalamus** there to route information to them. Even the prefrontal cortex (the "smartest" part of the brain) would be inept at its primary task of making decisions without the **hypothalamus** maintaining the basic processes that are central to survival such as eating, drinking, and sleeping. For this reason, don't underestimate the sophistication of the regions in the subcortex, many of which will come into play when we transition into learning about clinical neurology!

REVIEW QUESTIONS

1. A 56 y/o F with a history of hypertension experiences a sudden sense of dizziness and loss of vision while bending down to pick up a magazine. She calls an ambulance and is taken to the hospital. On admission, her blood pressure is 186/102 with otherwise normal vital signs. A neurological exam including a full motor and sensory evaluation is normal except for loss of visual acuity in the right visual fields. Which of the following structures is most likely to have been damaged during this episode?
    - A. Nucleus accumbens
    - B. Lateral geniculate nucleus
    - C. Medial geniculate nucleus
    - D. Ventral posterolateral nucleus
    - E. Ventral posteromedial nucleus

2. A 21 y/o F college student goes to see her primary care doctor after noticing an increase in how often she needs to urinate. Over the past month, she has been waking up several times per night to use the bathroom which has caused some tension between her and her roommate. At present, she notes that she urinates about once per hour during the day and once every other hour at night. She notes that the urine is usually clear with no trace of yellow coloration. She has been drinking copious amounts of water to offset an increase in her thirst that she has noticed over the same time period. Her doctor orders blood work which reveals elevated sodium levels and a normal glucose level. Imaging reveals a small tumor in the region of the hypothalamus. Which of the following hypothalamic nuclei appears to be most affected in this case?
    - A. Anterior hypothalamic nucleus
    - B. Posterior hypothalamic nucleus
    - C. Lateral hypothalamic nucleus
    - D. Ventromedial nucleus
    - E. Suprachiasmatic nucleus
    - F. Supraoptic nucleus
    - G. Paraventricular nucleus

3. A 45 y/o F sees her primary care doctor reporting that over the past several months she had felt “extremely bothered” by a variety of symptoms including frequent headaches, a “racing heart,” and constant diarrhea. She also reported a 15 lbs weight loss in the past several months but denies making active attempts to lose weight. Her exam is notable for a diffuse tremor. The doctor orders blood work as well as an MRI of the brain which reveals a pituitary adenoma as seen in the following image:

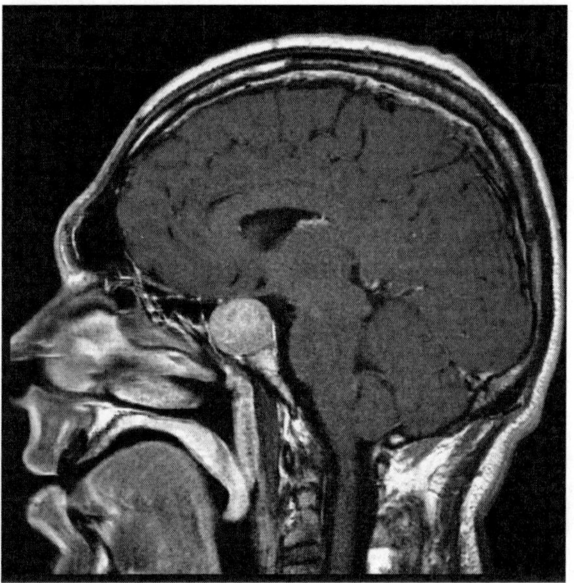

Levels of which of the following hormones are most likely to be elevated in this patient?

A. Follicle-stimulating hormone
B. Luteinizing hormone
C. Adrenocorticotropic hormone
D. Thyroid-stimulating hormone
E. Prolactin
F. Growth hormone
G. None of the above

1. **The best answer is B.** The lateral geniculate nucleus, medial geniculate nucleus, ventral posterolateral nucleus, and ventral posteromedial nucleus are all located in the thalamus. Each processes a different kind of sensory information. Given that this patient presented with visual disturbances, a lesion in the lateral geniculate nucleus, which is responsible for vision, is most likely. The medial geniculate nucleus processes auditory information, so a lesion here would most likely present with deficits in sound processing (answer C). The ventral posterolateral nucleus and ventral posteromedial nucleus process sensory information from the limbs and face, respectively, so a lesion here would result in numbness of these areas (answers D and E). The nucleus accumbens is a part of the limbic system and is not directly involved in visual processing (answer A).

2. **The best answer is F.** This vignette describes a case of diabetes insipidus related to dysfunction of the supraoptic nucleus of the hypothalamus. Under normal conditions, vasopressin helps to reduce urination and retain water in the bloodstream. When vasopressin is not produced, however, a state of excessive urination (polyuria) with resultant excessive drinking (polydipsia) can result. Around a quarter of all cases of central diabetes insipidus (those related to dysfunction of the brain rather than the kidneys) involve a brain tumor. The anterior and posterior hypothalamic nuclei are involved in temperature regulation and autonomic nervous system activation (answers A and B). The lateral and ventromedial hypothalamic nuclei are involved in regulation of hunger and satiety (answers C and D). The suprachiasmatic nucleus is involved in the circadian rhythm (answer E), while the paraventricular nucleus is involved in social bonding through the production of oxytocin (answer G).

3. **The best answer is D.** This vignette describes a case of hyperthyroidism related to a pituitary adenoma. Signs of symptoms of hyperthyroidism include diarrhea, weight loss, palpitations, and tremor, all of which are described in this case. Excess release of follicle-stimulating hormone or luteinizing hormone (answers A and B) would lead to hypergonadism and high levels of testosterone or estrogen. Excess release of adrenocorticotropic hormone (answer C) would lead to elevated cortisol levels resulting in hypertension, poor immune function, fatigue, and irritability; notably, weight *gain* rather than weight loss would be seen. Excess release prolactin (answer E) would cause breast development and/or milk release from the breasts. Finally, excess release of growth hormone (answer F) would result in enlargement of body parts such as the hands and feet.

5 THE BASAL GANGLIA AND INTERNAL CAPSULE

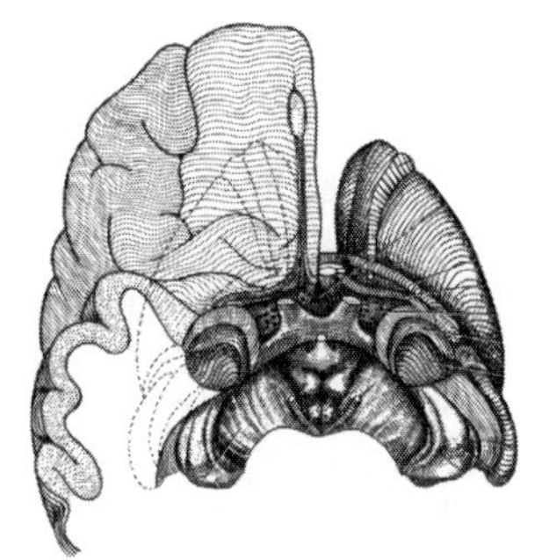

In the last chapter we talked about the thalamus, epithalamus, and hypothalamus, all of which are located in the cerebral subcortex. For this chapter, we're sticking in the subcortex but shifting our attention to a couple of other structures that are primarily involved in **movement**: the basal ganglia and the internal capsule.

Let's start with the **basal ganglia** which are a collection of nuclei that live in the subcortex and are involved in regulating **voluntary motor movements**. The primary role of the basal ganglia is to take an initial signal from the motor cortex in the frontal lobe and then modify it as it passes through them on its way down to muscles in various parts of the body. This helps to smooth out the somewhat coarse initial motor signals that are generated in the frontal cortex. For this reason, lesions in the basal ganglia often lead to movement disorders which are defined by rough, uncoordinated, and gangly motions.

Basal ganglia dysfunction leads to **uneven and uncoordinated movements**.

*A broken basal **gangli**a leads to **gangly** movements.*

Once the initial motor signal has been refined by the basal ganglia, it needs a way to get down to the muscles that will carry it out. This is where the **internal capsule** comes in! The internal capsule contains the two pathways (the corticospinal tract and the corticobulbar tract) that carry the signal to its destination.

Now that we have an overall sense of what each of these structures does, let's dive into each of them in more detail.

THE BASAL GANGLIA

The basal ganglia are not a single unit but are instead made up of several structures that all have their own unique role to play. These structures include the **striatum** (which is itself composed of two parts known as the **caudate** and the **putamen**), the **globus pallidus** (which is divided into an internal and external part), the **subthalamic nucleus**, and the **substantia nigra** which are all seen in the following image:

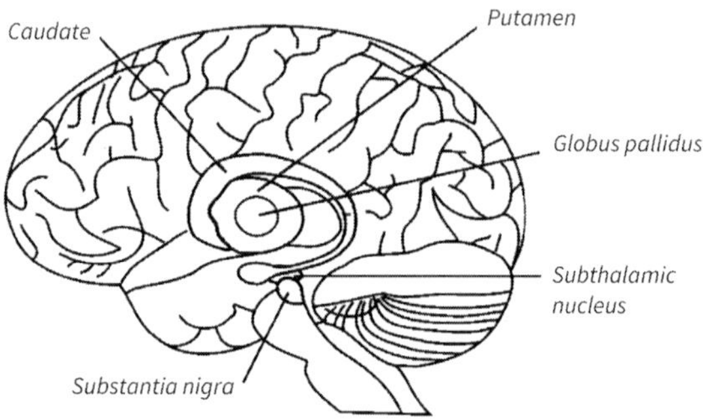

*Components of the **basal ganglia**.*

These structures do not operate independently but rather work as part of two interconnected pathways known as the **direct pathway** and the **indirect pathway** as seen in the image below. (Don't worry about understanding it just yet! We'll break it down in the next few paragraphs.)

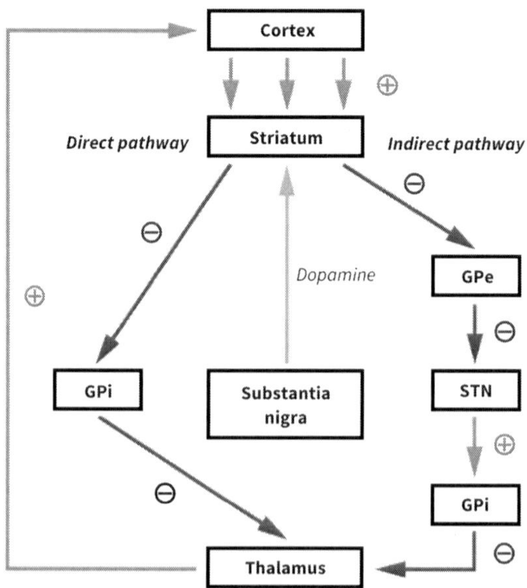

*The **direct** and **indirect pathways** found in the **basal ganglia**.*

First, let's look at the overall pattern. Each part of the basal ganglia either boosts the motor signal (indicated by a ⊕) or inhibits it (a ⊖). However, each pathway as a whole also has an *overall* effect, with the direct pathway amplifying the signal and the indirect pathway diminishing it. The logic here follows the rules of math when multiplying positives and negatives. For example, in the direct pathway the striatum and the internal globus pallidus both have an inhibitory effect, but these cancel each other out (like multiplying two negatives), making for an overall excitatory effect.

Second, you will notice that both the direct and indirect pathways end up at the thalamus before looping back to modify motor signals in the cortex. From this, we can infer that the effects of the basal ganglia are **reliant upon sensory information**. Let's illustrate this with an example: petting a dog. If we are petting the dog too hard, we can pick up that the dog doesn't like this on this via sensory information traveling through the thalamus from our eyes and hands. By getting input from the thalamus, our basal ganglia can modify the strength of our movement to be softer and more in line with what we are trying to do in the first place: pet the dog and make it happy.

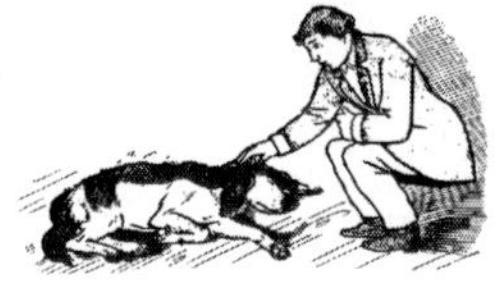

Now that we have some organizing principles in mind, let's look at the direct and indirect pathways in more detail. The **direct pathway** generally has an amplifying or **excitatory effect** on the initial motor signal (for example, if we are not petting the dog hard enough and need to pet it harder). The direct pathway travels from the **C**ortex to the **S**triatum into the **I**nternal globus pallidus and finally to the **T**halamus which sends the signal back to the cortex for further refining. You can remember this sequence by thinking that the direct pathway **C**omes **S**traight **I**nto the **T**halamus.

The **direct pathway** works to **amplify the initial signal** from the motor cortex.

*The direct pathway **C**omes **S**traight **I**nto the **T**halamus:*
*Cortex → **S**triatum → **I**nternal GP → **T**halamus.*

In contrast, the **indirect pathway** generally exerts a diminishing or **inhibitory effect** on the initial motor signal (for example, if we are petting the dog too hard and should back off a little). The indirect pathway starts out similarly to the direct pathway in that the signal is generated in the **C**ortex and travels to the **S**triatum. However, it then exits the direct pathway into the ***E**xternal* globus pallidus before traveling to the **S**ubthalamic nucleus, the **I**nternal globus pallidus, and finally the **T**halamus. You can remember this route by thinking that the indirect pathway **C**omes **S**traight, **E**xits, then **S**idesteps **I**nto the **T**halamus.

The **indirect pathway** works to **inhibit the initial signal** from the motor cortex.

*The indirect pathway **C**omes **S**traight, **E**xits, then **S**idesteps **I**nto the **T**halamus:*
*Cortex → **S**triatum → **E**xternal GP → **STN** → **I**nternal GP → **T**halamus.*

*The **in**direct pathway is **in**hibitory!*

We now have a general sense of what all of the structures in the basal ganglia are doing (whether they are inhibitory or excitatory) and the overall role they play in both the direct and indirect pathways. However, there's more nuance to these structures than that, so we'll now look at each component one by one.

THE STRIATUM

In both the direct and indirect pathways, the initial signal from the motor cortex first travels to the dorsal **striatum**. The striatum is itself composed of two things (the caudate nucleus and the putamen) which then work to amplify or inhibit the signal.

The **caudate nucleus** is highly involved in any form of **goal-directed activity** and plays an important role in other cognitive functions such as memory and sleep. You can think of the **cau**date as the most **cau**gnitive part of the basal ganglia!

The **caudate** is involved in both **motor** activity as well as more **cognitive functions.**

*The **cau**date nucleus is the most **cau**gnitive part of the basal ganglia.*

In contrast, the **putamen** is more exclusively dedicated to **motor functions** and plays a role in both preparing and executing voluntary movements. This is illustrated clinically in patients who develop bleeding in the area of the putamen (known as a **putaminal hemorrhage**) who will often present with weakness or even complete paralysis of muscles throughout their body. So whenever you see the word "putamen" on an exam, look for the answer involving **M**otor functions and "**put-an-M**" for **M**otor.

The **putamen** is primarily involved in **motor** activity.

*When you see **put-am-en** on an exam, "**put-an-M**" for **M**otor.*

THE GLOBUS PALLIDUS

The direct and indirect pathways both continue with the **globus pallidus**. The globus pallidus has both an internal part (GPi) and an external part (GPe). The internal part is found in the both the direct and indirect pathways, while the external part is found in the indirect pathway only. Regardless, both parts have **inhibitory effects** on the motor signals passing through it. You can remember the inhibitory effect of the globus pallidus by thinking of it as the **"slow bus"** pallidus.

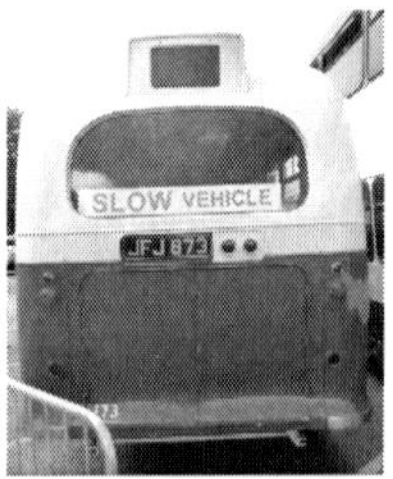

The **globus pallidus** acts to **inhibit the motor signal** passing through it.

*The "**slow bus**" pallidus **slows** down the motor signal.*

THE SUBTHALAMIC NUCLEUS

The **subthalamic nucleus** (or STN) is found only in the indirect pathway. While it releases an excitatory neurotransmitter, it acts on the inhibitory internal globus pallidus to ultimately produce inhibition of movement.

The subthalamic nucleus's inhibitory effects are illustrated in a movement disorder known as **hemiballismus** which involves dramatic movements of the limbs, almost like the patient is throwing a football or swinging a golf club. This occurs after the subthalamic nucleus becomes damaged, as the inhibitory effect of the indirect pathway has been removed, resulting in excessive movements. While rare, hemiballismus often shows up on tests, so it's helpful to think of someone swinging their arm while throwing a **ball** during **Su**nday **N**ight Football to remember hemi**ball**ismus and the **Su**bthalamic **N**ucleus.

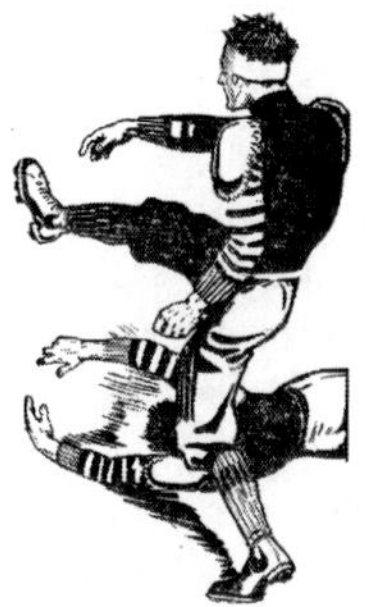

Hemiballismus is a disorder involving **involuntary flailing movements** of the limbs. It is related to damage of the **subthalamic nucleus**.

*The flailing arm movements look like **throwing a football**, so you can think of **Su**nday **N**ight **football** to associate hemi**ball**ismus and the **Su**bthalamic **N**ucleus.*

THE SUBSTANTIA NIGRA

The final part of the basal ganglia, known as the **substantia nigra** (Latin for "black substance"), is located not in the subcortex but in the midbrain of the brainstem. As you can see in the diagram on page 48, the substantia nigra is not immediately involved in either the direct or indirect pathway, but it still plays a role in modifying movement by acting on the striatum directly through the **nigrostriatal pathway**. The substantia nigra uses the neurotransmitter **dopamine** to influence the basal ganglia. Dopamine is best thought of as being like grease: it does not *cause* movements but rather *facilitates* them. Just like you would use grease to turn a rusted hinge into a smooth gliding one, dopamine makes someone's movements fast, fluid, and smooth.

On the flipside, someone with reduced production of dopamine in the substantia nigra (such as a person who has Parkinson's disease) will be much less able to initiate movements, leading to muscle stiffness, rigidity, and slowness.

The **substantia nigra** produces **dopamine** to help make movements **smoother**.

*Dysfunction in the **N**igro**S**triatal **P**athway leads to i**N**voluntary movements like **S**tuttering and **P**arkinsonism.*

THE INTERNAL CAPSULE

To finish this chapter, we will briefly talk about the **internal capsule** which is another subcortical structure that is involved in movement. The internal capsule is named "internal" because it runs inside of some important surrounding structures, including parts of the basal ganglia such as the caudate, putamen, and globus pallidus.

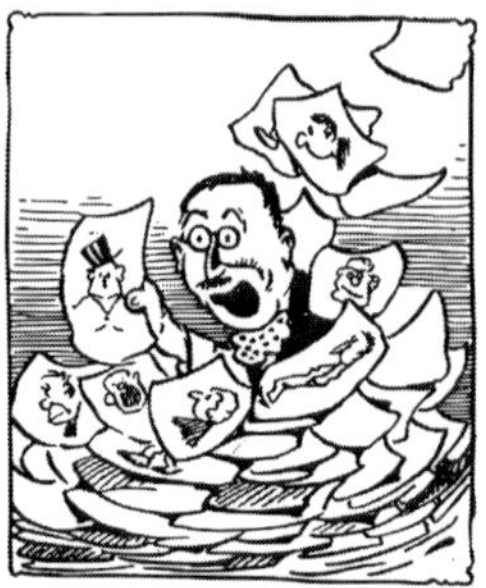

If you think about it, the structures of the basal ganglia are basically a bunch of bureaucrats: if left to their own devices, they would take the initial signal generated by the motor cortex and talk about it, debate it, and modify it until the cows come home, and the signal would never actually get where it needs to go! However, what happens when the motor cortex gets fed up with all the basal ganglia's red tape and *just wants to send a signal to the muscle it wants to already*? For this, the motor cortex has to send the signal through the **internal capsule**, a V-shaped collection of white matter that brazenly travels right through the middle of the basal ganglia on its way to the spinal cord (probably flashing a middle finger to onlookers while doing so) in order to link up with the muscles directly.

The V-shape makes the internal capsule easy to split up into three sections consisting of the **anterior limb**, the **posterior limb**, and the **genu** making up the bend between them:

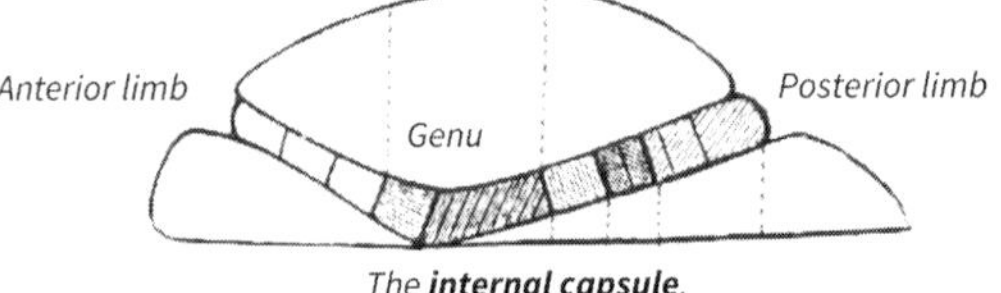

*The **internal capsule**.*

We'll start with the posterior limb. The posterior limb contains a pathway known as the **corticospinal tract**, so-named because it carries motor impulses from the cortex to muscles throughout the body via the spinal cord. For this reason, an injury to the posterior limb of the internal capsule often results in contralateral **hemiparesis** (or weakness of muscles on the opposite side of the body) or even **hemiplegia** (or a complete loss of movement). You can remember the core function of the posterior limb of the internal capsule (to bypass the bureaucracy of the basal ganglia) by thinking of a **PoLICe** (**Po**sterior **L**imb of the **I**nternal **C**apsul**e**) man who has gone rogue and is flipping the bird to the basal ganglia as it drives by on its way to the spinal cord.

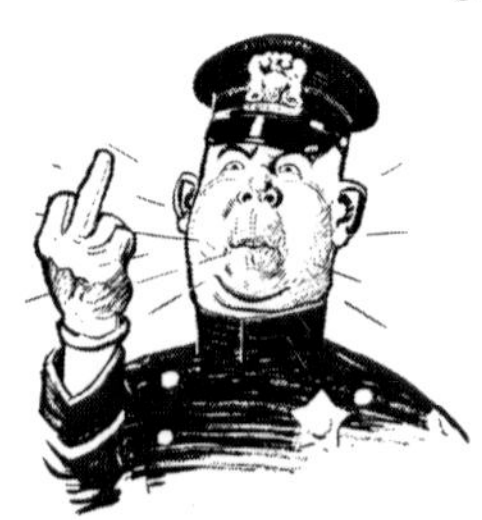

The **posterior limb of the internal capsule** contains the **corticospinal tract** which sends motor signals directly to the muscles of the body.

*The **PoLICe** (**Po**sterior **L**imb of the **I**nternal **C**apsul**e**) man bypasses the basal ganglia.*

The bend in the middle of the internal capsule is known as the **genu** (Latin for "knee"). Unlike the corticospinal tract which travels to muscles in the *body*, the genu contains the **corticobulbar tract** which travels to muscles in the *face* via the cranial nerves branching off of the brainstem. You can remember the function of the corticobulbar tract by thinking of a **genu**-ius who gets an idea in their **cranium**. What happens? A light **bulb** goes on! This will help you associate the cortico**bulb**ar tract with the **genu** of the internal capsule and the **cranial** nerves.

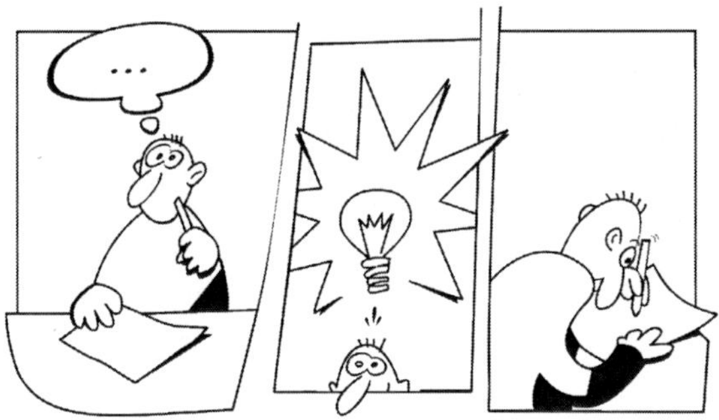

The **genu** of the **internal capsule** contains the **corticobulbar tract** which sends motor signals to facial muscles via the **cranial nerves**.

*Think of a **genius** who gets an idea in their **cranium**, making a light **bulb** go on!*

Finally, the **anterior limb** of the internal capsule contains a variety of nerve fibers connecting different parts of the brain, but honestly it doesn't really come up that much clinically so we won't spend much time on it.

PUTTING IT ALL TOGETHER

As with the other subcortical structures we talked about in the last chapter, the basal ganglia and the internal capsule are essential to the proper functioning of the human brain, even if they don't get as much credit for it as their cortical co-stars! The frontal lobe could technically make movements on its own, but without the basal ganglia these motions would be clumsy and ineffective. Without the internal capsule, motor signals from the cortex would be endlessly lost in a sea of bureaucracy and red tape that would prevent them from ever getting to the muscles to carry out the plan. The fact that they do this all without our conscious effort or input is even more amazing!

Before we move on, it's worth pointing out that you wouldn't expect to find full-on weakness or paralysis resulting from a lesion in the basal ganglia, as they are not involved in *producing* motor signals directly (this comes from the cortex) or *carrying* the signals to their destination (that would be the internal capsule). Instead, think of the basal ganglia whenever you see **uneven, uncoordinated, or rough movements** (more to come on this in Chapter 19!).

REVIEW QUESTIONS

1. A 63 y/o M with a history of atrial fibrillation is admitted to the hospital following a stroke in a branch of the left middle cerebral artery that primarily affected the posterior limb of the internal capsule. Which of the following deficits is he most likely to have from this point forward?
    A. Weakness of his right facial muscles
    B. Weakness of his left facial muscles
    C. Weakness of his right arm and leg
    D. Weakness of his left arm and leg
    E. Numbness of his right facial muscles
    F. Numbness of his left facial muscles
    G. Numbness of his right arm and leg
    H. Numbness of his left arm and leg

2. A 44 y/o M is involved in a motor vehicle accident and loses consciousness after he is hit in the right side of the head. Upon awakening in the hospital, he is confused and disoriented, with profound memory difficulties. Over the next several weeks, he begins to regain his mental abilities. However, he then begins to experience odd movements. A neurologist orders a magnetic resonance imaging scan of his brain which shows a focal lesion in the external globus pallidus. Which of the following is *least* likely to describe his movements?
    A. Recurrent spasms of his hand
    B. Tremor in his arm
    C. Involuntary tensing of his fingers
    D. Inability to flex the wrist
    E. Painful contraction of the neck and shoulders

3. A 64 y/o F is seen by her primary care doctor after being discharged from the hospital following a fall. During her hospitalization, she was noted to have poor balance and an unsteady gait. Her neurologic exam is notable for rigidity in her major joints including her elbows. Her husband notes that she has become "less emotional" over the past few months, and he has needed to take over more of her usual daily activities such as cooking meals and managing finances. After a full work-up, she is diagnosed with Parkinson's disease. Her disease progresses over the next several years, and she becomes increasingly immobile despite adequate treatment. She is enrolled in an investigational research study to assess the effect that implanting a deep brain stimulator could have on the severity of her disease. She undergoes surgery to implant the stimulator as seen in the following image:

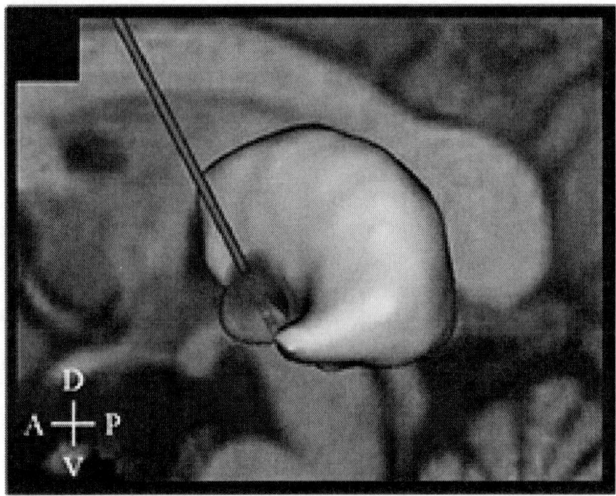

Following implantation of the stimulator, the patient begins experiencing sudden involuntary swinging motions of her left arm and leg. This goes away after the stimulator is adjusted. Which of the following structures was the deep brain stimulator most likely implanted into?

A. Caudate
B. Putamen
C. Internal globus pallidus
D. External globus pallidus
E. Subthalamic nucleus
F. Substantia nigra
G. Anterior limb of the internal capsule
H. Posterior limb of the internal capsule
I. Genu of the internal capsule

1. **The best answer is C.** The posterior limb of the internal capsule contains the corticospinal tract, a group of neurons traveling to skeletal muscles of the body. For this reason, ischemic damage to this area can result in contralateral weakness due to the crossing of these fibers in the medulla. Therefore, a stroke in the left posterior limb of the internal capsule would lead to weakness of the right extremities, not the left (answer D). Facial muscles are controlled by the corticobulbar tract which passes through the genu of the internal capsule, not the posterior limb (answers A and B). A stroke in the thalamus, rather than the internal capsule, would result in numbness (answers E—H).

2. **The best answer is D.** An injury in the external globus pallidus would lead to dysfunction of the indirect pathway. As the indirect pathway typically plays an inhibitory role in the motor pathway, this would likely result in excessive or unrestrained movements such as spasms (answer A), tremor (answer B), tension (answer C), and dystonia (answer E). Of the options listed, only wrist drop involves too little muscle contraction rather than too much.

3. **The best answer is E.** Treatment for Parkinson's disease can sometimes include implantation of a deep brain stimulator into the subthalamic nucleus when conventional treatments have not worked. The emergence of hemiballismus is the largest clue that the subthalamic nucleus is involved, as this is known to be an effect of changes to the function of this nucleus. The substantia nigra (answer F) is also implicated in Parkinson's disease and could be a potential treatment target, although this would not be expected to produce hemiballismus. None of the other options listed are implicated in the development of hemiballismus.

6 THE CEREBELLUM

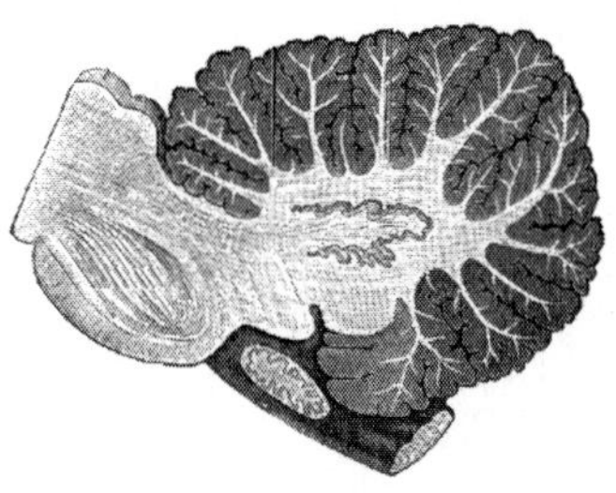

We've covered the cerebrum, including both the outer cortex as well as the subcortical structures in the middle. Now let's move onto an adjacent part of the brain that sits behind and below the cerebrum known as the **cerebellum**. On first glance, the cerebellum appears to be a miniature version of the cerebrum! It has a familiar folded appearance, the pattern of grey matter on the outside and white matter on the inside, and several divisions into multiple lobes. Despite its appearance, however, the cerebellum isn't just a smaller copy of the cerebrum. Instead, it has its own unique functions, primarily in the realm of **balance** and **motor coordination**.

The cerebellum itself does not *generate* motor impulses (recall that those come from the motor cortex in the frontal lobe). Instead, the cerebellum *coordinates* motor actions by taking into account proprioceptive information about the position of various parts of the body in space. For example, when climbing a set of stairs, your legs can't simply repeat the same action over and over. Instead, you need to know when to lift one leg up while putting the other down as well as the timing of alternating between the two legs. Your body does this automatically and instinctually by sending proprioceptive and other sensory information to the cerebellum. The cerebellum then compares the position of each body part with its intended movement and adjusts the motor signal in a way that irons out the kinks, resulting in a **smooth and coordinated** set of movements. In this chapter, we'll learn about the anatomy that enables the cerebellum to do this as well as look at what happens when the cerebellum stops working.

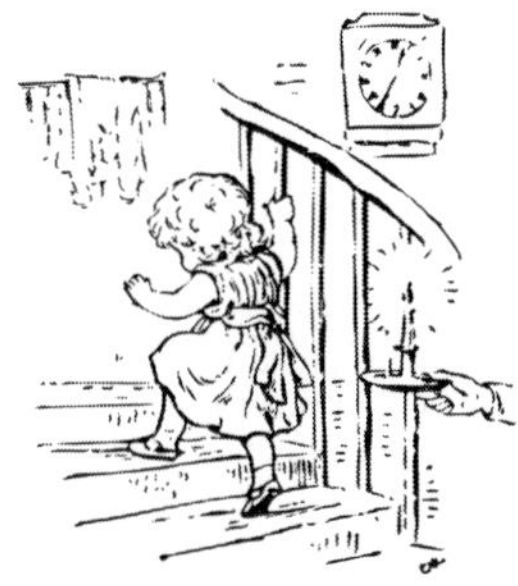

CEREBELLAR ANATOMY

The cerebellum is divided into three lobes: the **anterior lobe**, the **posterior lobe,** and the **flocculonodular lobe**. The anterior and posterior lobes are responsible for maintaining balance and coordination for the body by both sending signals *to* and receiving signals *from* the cerebral cortex and spinal cord. Notably, the medial aspect of the cerebellum, known as the **vermis**, coordinates the middle of the body (such as the trunk and proximal limbs), while the more lateral aspects of the cerebellum coordinate the lateral parts of the body (such as the hands).

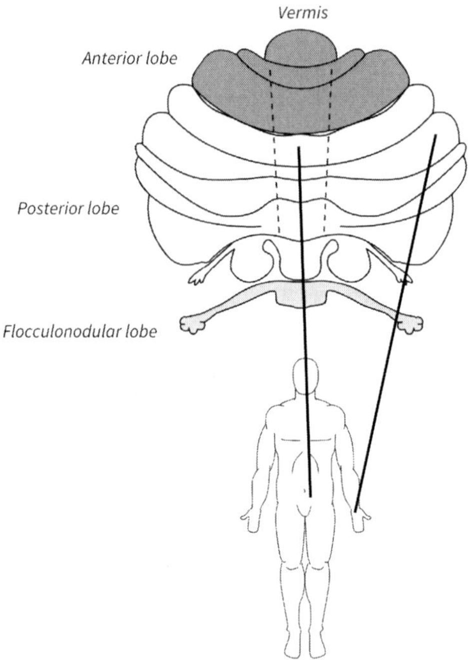

*The **medial cerebellum** controls the **trunk**, while the **lateral cerebellum** controls the **limbs**.*

Compared to anterior and posterior lobes, the flocculonodular lobe is the odd one out. Rather than involving itself with coordinating the movements of the *body*, it instead works to coordinate **eye movements** using sensory information about spatial orientation from the **vestibular system** in the inner ear (which we'll cover in more detail in Chapter 11!). You can remember the association between the **flocc**ulonodular lobe and movement of the eyes by thinking of a **flock** of **see**-gulls.

The **flocculonodular lobe of the cerebellum** is involved in coordinating **eye movements** based on sensory information from the **vestibular system**.

*Think of a **flock** of **see**-gulls to link the **flocc**ulonodular lobe and the **eyes**!*

CEREBELLAR PEDUNCLES

The lobes of the cerebellum connect to the rest of the body by way of three **cerebellar peduncles** (peduncles meaning "stalks" or "stem"), as seen in the following image:

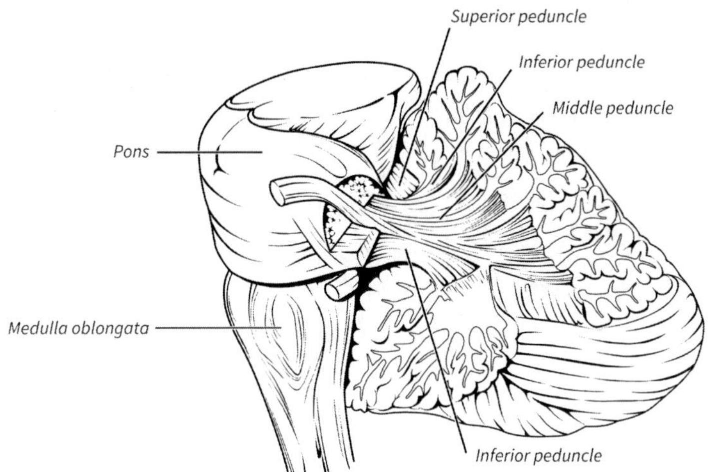

*The **cerebellum** is connected to the rest of the body by way of **3 cerebellar peduncles**.*

Each peduncle has its own function: the **superior cerebellar peduncle** *sends* information from the cerebellum to the cortex via the thalamus, while the **middle cerebellar peduncle** and **inferior cerebellar peduncle** both *receive* input (from the pons and spinal cord, respectively). Importantly, nerve tracts coming from the superior cerebellar peduncle cross from left-to-right and right-to-left so that, by the time they get to the brainstem, nerve fibers from the *left* side of the cerebellum are travelling in the *right* midbrain and vice versa. You can remember this by thinking that the **S**uperior **C**erebellar **P**eduncle **S**ends **C**rossed **P**athways.

The **superior cerebellar peduncle sends signals** to the cortex, while the **middle and inferior cerebellar peduncles receive information** from the pons and spinal cord.

***S**uperior **C**erebellar **P**eduncle = **S**ends **C**rossed **P**athways.*

However, the neurologic deficits seen in cases of unilateral cerebellar damage still end up being **ipsilateral** to (on the same side as) the lesion. This is because motor signals from the cerebellum are **dirty double crossers**: they not only cross when they leave the cerebellum in the superior cerebellar peduncle but then cross *again* in the medulla, a part of the brainstem that we will talk about in the next chapter.

Cerebellar damage produces deficits that are **ipsilateral** to the side of the lesion.

*Write it as **cerebe⤫um** to remind yourself that it's a **dirty double crosser**!*

CEREBELLAR SIGNS

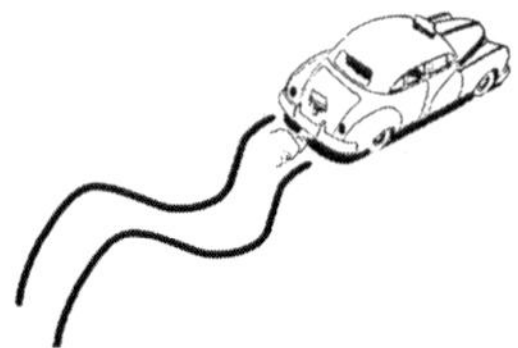

One of the best ways of understanding the function of the cerebellum is to see what happens when it stops working. In contrast to injuries of the motor cortex or internal capsule, injuries of the cerebellum do *not* generally lead to motor weakness or paralysis! Instead, cerebellar damage is associated with specific deficits in the areas of balance, posture, and coordination that are collectively known as **cerebellar signs**. The hallmark cerebellar sign is known as **ataxia** which means a lack of motor coordination and control. To remember the meaning of a**taxi**a, think of a **taxi** swerving wildly all over the road!

> **Cerebellar dysfunction** leads to a **lack of motor coordination** known as **ataxia**.
>
> *To connect a**taxi**a with poor coordination, think of a **taxi** swerving all over the road!*

Ataxia can affect many different parts of the body, including the arms, legs, eyes, and even the muscles in the throat that produce speech. Depending on the areas involved, ataxia can appear as various findings on a neurologic exam. To remember these findings, let's build on that swerving taxi mnemonic! Imagine that your aunt is heading to meet you at a family reunion. She has been tasked with bringing a few plates of food for the potluck. However, she ends up getting on the taxi with the crazy driver! By the time she arrives at the reunion, she is completely dizzy and ends up tripping and spilling all three dishes. Use this image of a **dizzy AUNT with 3 dishes** to remember the signs and symptoms of ataxia:

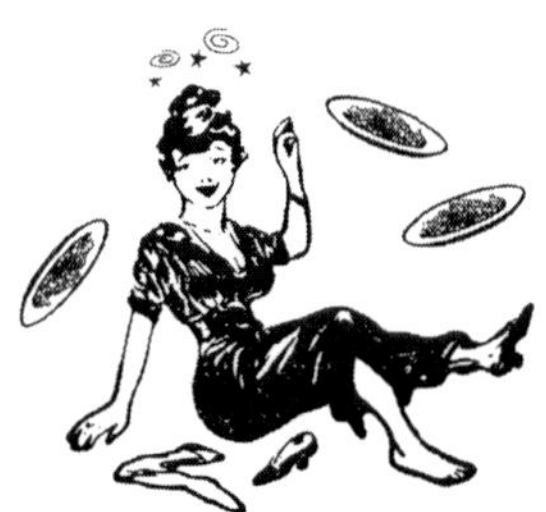

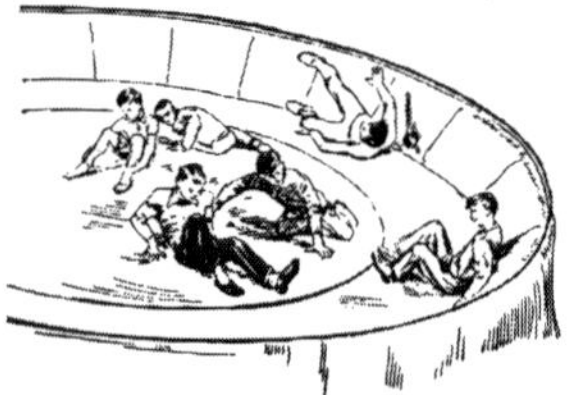

Dizzy is for Dizziness and vertigo. In addition to the objectively observable signs that we will discuss shortly, someone with cerebellar dysfunction will often experience the *subjective* symptom of **vertigo** as well. Vertigo is a form of dizziness in which someone experiences a distinct sense that things are moving even when they are not (often described as a sensation of "room spinning"). It can sometimes be accompanied by nausea or even vomiting when severe. While there are many possible causes of vertigo, those that involve the cerebellum are often called **central vertigo** (in contrast to cases of *peripheral* vertigo which are instead related to dysfunction of the inner ear, as we will talk about in Chapter 11).

A is for Ambulation. Difficulties with walking are often seen in people with ataxia. Often this takes the form of a slow and cautious gait, though staggering, lurching from side to side, and even outright falling can sometimes be seen as well. To compensate, people with cerebellar damage will often attempt to widen their stance or use their arms to balance themselves while walking, as seen below:

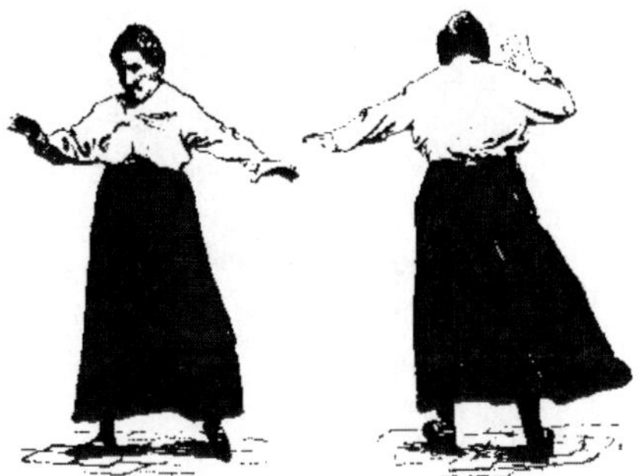

*An **ataxic gait**.*

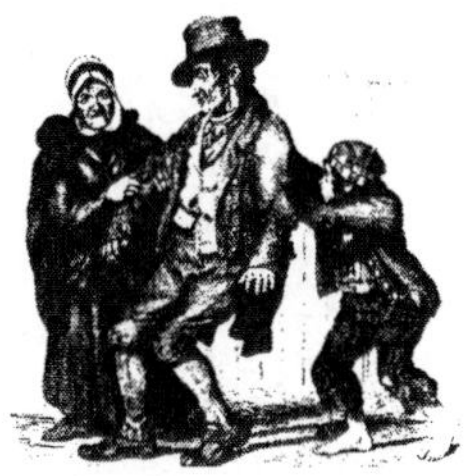

U is for Unsteadiness. Even when they are not walking (such as when standing or sitting in a chair), people with ataxia can have trouble keeping themselves upright. A common example of this phenomenon is the swaying posture of a person who is intoxicated with alcohol. This unsteadiness makes for a high risk of falling, and many patients who experience chronic ataxia have injured themselves due to falls.

N is for Nystagmus. Nystagmus is a hard concept to explain using just words, so the first order of business is to pull out your phone and look up some videos of nystagmus online! Take a few minutes to search for "nystagmus videos," then come back.

As you saw in the videos, nystagmus is an involuntary twitch-like movement of the eyes (sometimes called "dancing eyes"). To understand why nystagmus happens, we first need to understand a few key points about eye movement. Under normal circumstances, the vestibular system in the ear helps to detect when the head is moving. The vestibular system then sends signals to the flocculonodular lobe of the cerebellum to move the eyes in such a way that they can maintain their gaze rather than being moved by the motion of the head. To see if this process is working, focus on the center of the following image, then shake your head back and forth a few times:

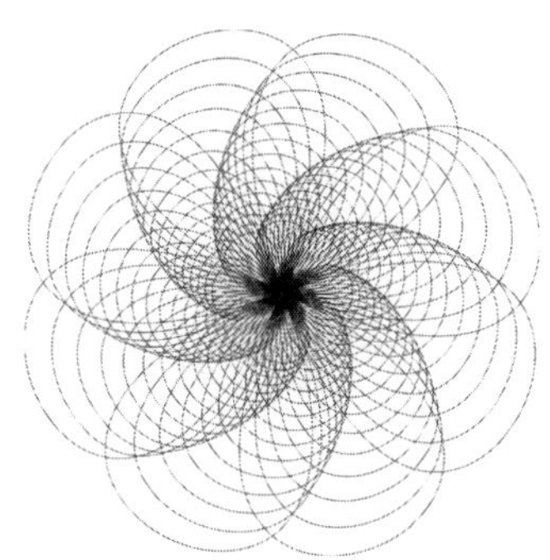

If your eyes were able to keep focused on the center despite the movement of your head, then congratulations! Your cerebellum is intact (as are a few other systems). Relative to their position in your head, your eyes were moving, but because they moved in a direction exactly *opposite* to the movement of your head, the overall effect was that your eyes were able to stay still relative to what they were looking at.

In cases of nystagmus, however, this process has broken down to the extent that the eyes try to move *even in the absence of head movement*. The eyes will usually catch themselves doing this and try to correct, but then just fractions of a second later they will begin doing it again, leading to the characteristic back-and-forth twitching motion of nystagmus. Nystagmus can at times be severe enough that it causes shaky vision for the patient!

T is for Tremor. Because the cerebellum acts to smooth out movements, dysfunction of the cerebellum can cause an involuntary, rhythmic, repetitive movement known as **tremor**. (To be clear, tremor can be caused by other things as well, which we will discuss further in Chapter 19.) Consider the image below, in which a person with cerebellar damage produced the bottom figure when asked to draw the top figure:

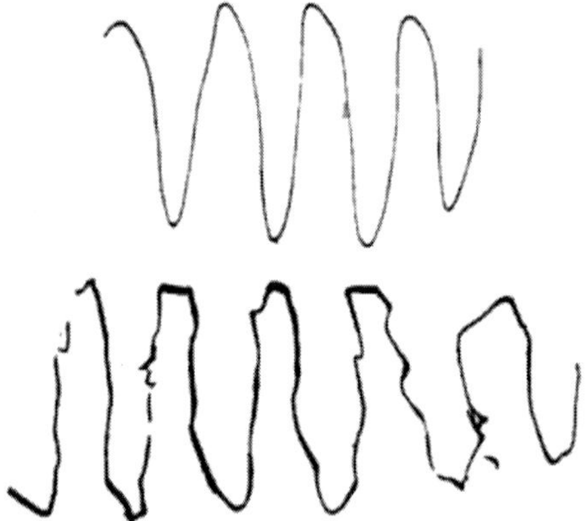

Drawing sample from a patient with ***tremor****.*

3 Dishes is for Dysdiadochokinesia, Dysarthria, and Dysmetria. Finally, we will talk about the three dishes (**dys**'es) of cerebellar dysfunction. **Dysdiadochokinesia** refers to an inability to engage in **rapid alternating movements** (for example, using your hand to screw in a light bulb). These sorts of motions require a high degree of motor coordination which will be lacking in someone with cerebellar damage. **Dysarthria** refers to an unsteadiness in the pitch or rhythm of speech. Because the cerebellum coordinates movements of the vocal cords, someone with cerebellar dysfunction will have unsteadiness that can be *heard* rather than just seen. Finally, **dysmetria** refers to an inability to accurately judge distances when moving, leading to either overshooting or undershooting the amount of movement required (such as when you embarrass yourself by trying to give someone a high-five and missing!). Dysmetria can be tested clinically using the **finger-to-nose test** which involves asking the patient to use their fingers to alternate between touching your finger and their nose several times while you move your finger around.

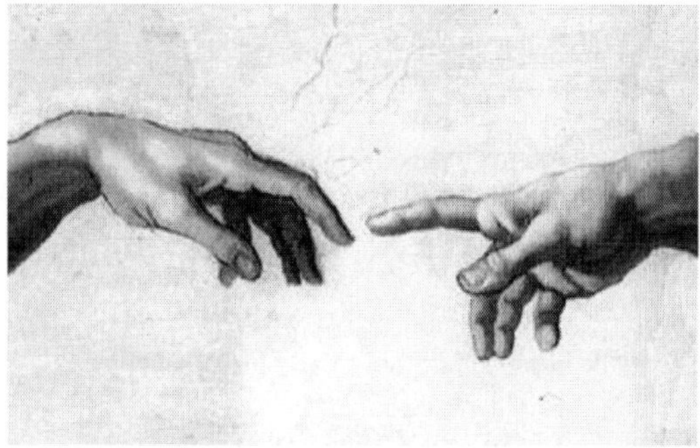

*The world's first **finger-to-nose test**.*

Ataxia can manifest through a **variety of neurologic signs and symptoms** depending on the specific parts of the body that are involved.

*Think of a **dizzy AUNT** with **3 dishes** who just got off the crazy a**taxi**a:*
Dizziness
***A**mbulation*
***U**nsteadiness*
***N**ystagmus*
***T**remor*
***D**ysdiadochokinesia*
***D**ysarthria*
***D**ysmetria*

PUTTING IT ALL TOGETHER

To gain a better understanding of the cerebellum, let's compare it to the basal ganglia, another part of the brain that also modifies movements (rather than creating them). While the basal ganglia help movements to be **smooth** and **fluid**, the cerebellum instead tries to promote **coordination** and **balance**. You can see this difference most clearly by looking at the disorders involving each of these areas, as a person with a dysfunctional cerebellum (such as someone who is intoxicated with alcohol) will likely be stumbling around and falling over, even if the individual muscle movements they're making are still smooth and fluid. In contrast, someone with a dysfunctional basal ganglia (such as a patient with Parkinson's disease) will often have slow, jerky, and stiff movements even if the movements are technically well coordinated. This is a bit of an oversimplification, but it helps to illustrate the complementary roles that each of these systems plays in the motor system!

As we continue on throughout our study of the nervous system, we will see the cerebellum popping up from time to time. Whenever someone presents with ataxia (as captured in the **dizzy AUNT with 3 dishes** mnemonic) and/or vertigo, you should think of the cerebellum!

REVIEW QUESTIONS

1. A 24 y/o M is pulled over by a police officer after he was swerving erratically across the road while driving. A breathalyzer device estimates a blood alcohol content of 0.18, over two times the legal limit for driving. Which of the following tasks will this man likely have the *least* difficulty completing?
   A. Sticking his tongue straight out from his mouth
   B. Alternating his index finger between touching his nose and the police officer's moving finger
   C. Speaking in a smooth and unbroken manner
   D. Standing upright with his eyes closed for one minute without falling
   E. Walking in a straight line by touching the heel of the stepping foot to the toes of the other foot
   F. Repeatedly flipping his hands from palms-up to palms-down

2. A 69 y/o F is brought to the hospital by ambulance after she calls 911 reporting the sudden onset of "world spinning" dizziness, blurry vision, and vomiting. She has a history of hypertension and diabetes mellitus. Neuroimaging revealed a stroke in the right posterior inferior cerebellar artery with ischemic damage to the right lateral cerebellum as seen in the following image:

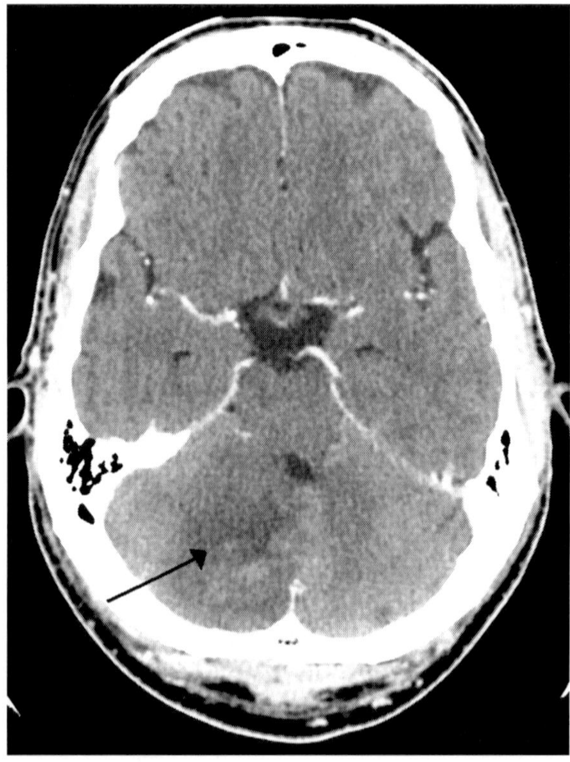

Which of the following is most likely to be observed on clinical examination?

A. Weakness of right-sided movement
B. Slow, jerky movements on the right
C. Inability to mime screwing in a light bulb with her right hand
D. Weakness of left-sided movement
E. Slow, jerky movements on the left
F. Inability to mime screwing in a light bulb with her left hand
G. Swaying of the body when standing upright with her eyes closed

1. **The best answer is A.** Alcohol has deleterious effects on the cerebellum, so any movements that require the balance and coordination that the cerebellum provides will likely be impaired in someone who is intoxicated. Point-to-point movement requires coordination between the eyes and the fingers and would likely be impaired during alcohol intoxication, known as dysmetria (answer B). Heel-to-toe walking is also likely to be impaired (answer E). Standing upright without falling requires coordination between multiple senses, including vision and proprioception, and is likely to be impaired as well (answer D). Unsteadiness of speech, known as dysarthria, is a sign of cerebellar dysfunction (answer C). Inability to perform rapid alternating motions, known as dysdiadochokinesia, is a characteristic cerebellar sign (answer F). In contrast to the other motions, sticking one's tongue out is a simple movement that does not require the coordination abilities of the cerebellum and is likely to be preserved during alcohol intoxication.

2. **The best answer is C.** A cerebellar stroke will produce cerebellar signs on the side ipsilateral to the lesion due to the double crossing of cerebellar pathways (once in the superior cerebellar peduncle and again in the medulla oblongata). For a right cerebellar stroke, dysdiadochokinesia is likely to be observed in the right hand, not the left (answer F). Weakness of movement is not typically seen in cases of cerebellar damage (answers A and D). Slow, jerky movements are more suggestive of damage to the basal ganglia (answers B and E). Truncal ataxia is less likely to be seen in cases of lateral cerebellar damage, as the trunk is controlled medially in the cerebellum (answer G).

7 THE BRAINSTEM

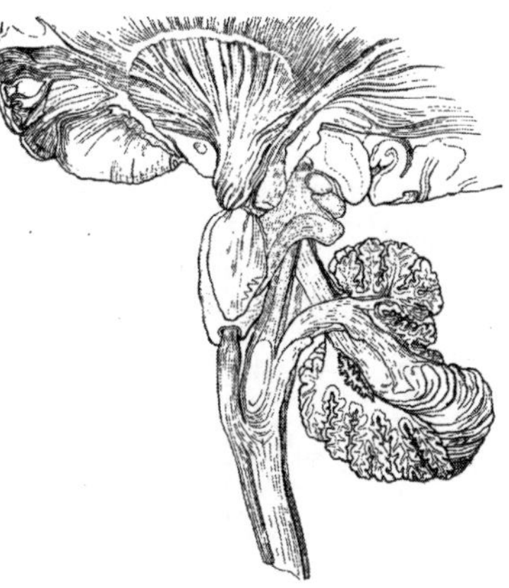

Moving down from the cerebrum and the cerebellum, we at last arrive at the final frontier of the brain: the **brainstem**! The brainstem is appropriately named, as visually it really *does* look like the stem of a plant on which the brain has grown. The brainstem can be further subdivided into three unique parts: the **midbrain**, the **pons**, and the **medulla oblongata** (or just "medulla"). The midbrain is the uppermost part and connects directly to the cerebrum before continuing down as the pons and then as the medulla before finally turning into the spinal cord at the point where it exits the skull.

On a functional level, we learned in Chapter 2 that the brainstem acts as a "bridge" connecting the brain to the spinal cord and the rest of the body. However, it's so much more than just that! Use the mnemonic "**B**rainstem **C**an **D**o **I**t **A**ll" to remember the various functions of this part of the brain:

B is for Bridge. All three parts of the brainstem contain both **motor and sensory pathways** traveling between the brain and the spinal cord. Importantly, these nerves are grouped in such a way that specific types of nerves are traveling together in predetermined "lanes." For example, nerve tracts carrying motor signals travel in the middle of the brainstem while those carrying epicritic sensory information travel more to the side. Pay attention to how these structures are organized, as this will come into play in later chapters when we talk about how damage in different parts of the brainstem will present clinically!

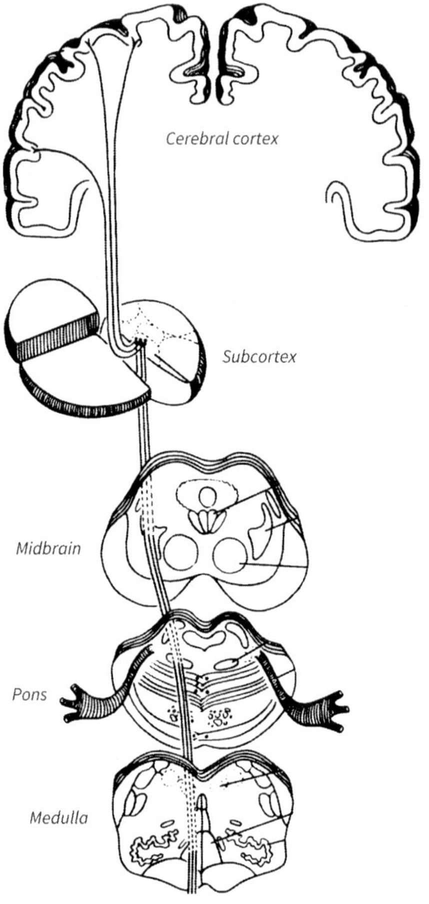

*Anatomic relationship between the **cerebrum** and the **brainstem** showing its "bridge" function.*

C is for Cranial Nerves. The brainstem is the origin of ten of the twelve cranial nerves. We will talk about each of the cranial nerves more in Chapter 9, but for now just remember them in the context of the "Rule of 4": the first 4 come out of the brain and midbrain, the middle 4 exit from the pons, and the last 4 originate in the medulla. (We'll go over the clinical implications of this more in Chapter 14 when we talk about brainstem strokes.)

Ten of the twelve cranial nerves arise from the **brainstem**.

*The cranial nerves follow the "**Rule of 4**":*
*The **first 4** (1-4) exit from the **brain and midbrain***
*The **middle 4** (5-8) exit from the **pons***
*The **last 4** (9-12) exit from the **medulla***

D is for Distinct functions. The midbrain, pons, and medulla all contain unique nuclei that carry out specific activities, each of which we will talk about more in their respective sections later on in this chapter.

I is for Integral functions. Many of the duties carried out by the brainstem are absolutely vital for survival, including control over **breathing** and **blood flow**. For this reason, injuries to the brainstem can be deadly, more than earning the designation of "integral functions."

A is for Arousal. While each of the three parts of the brainstem have their own unique roles, they can also work together to perform shared functions as well! In particular, all three parts help to regulate states of **arousal and consciousness** (including alertness and awareness) through a shared group of nuclei known as the **reticular formation**. The reticular formation plays a vital role in sorting sensory signals and deciding which are sent up to the brain for conscious processing and which are ignored. For example, someone living on a busy city street can often sleep through the night despite the sound of cars honking or the brightness of the street lights outside, as the reticular formation is filtering out irrelevant stimuli. However, if something *unexpected* happens (such as someone **tickling** them while sleeping), the reticular formation determines that this isn't just the usual background noise and sends the signal into conscious awareness, waking the person up. In this way, the re-**tickler** formation helps govern which information is consciously processed and which is ignored.

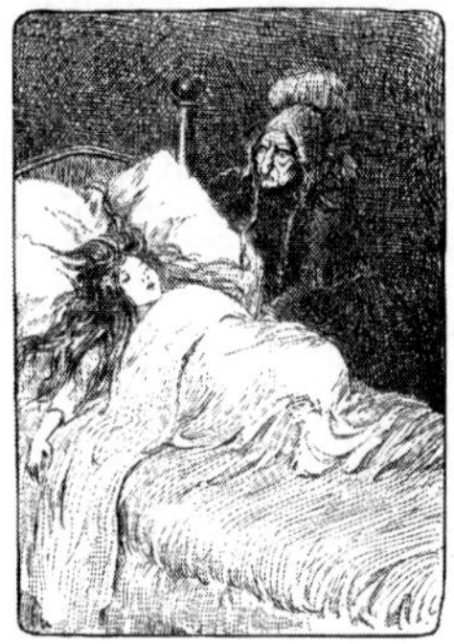

The **reticular formation** is involved in **conscious awareness** and **sensory filtering**.

*Like someone **tickling** you, activation of the re-**tickler** formation will wake you up.*

Now that we know about the functions of the brainstem as a *whole*, let's now learn about each *part* of the brainstem in more detail, starting with the **midbrain**.

The **brainstem** acts not only as a **bridge** carrying motor and sensory neurons between the brain and the spinal cord but also carries out many **vital functions**.

***B**rainstem **C**an **D**o **I**t **A**ll:*
***B**ridge between cerebrum/cerebellum and spinal cord*
***C**ranial nerves*
***D**istinct functions*
***I**ntegral functions*
***A**rousal*

THE MIDBRAIN

The **midbrain** is often divided into a few main regions: the **tectum** on the dorsal side, the **cerebral aqueduct** in the middle, the **tegmentum** on the ventral side, and two **cerebral peduncles** jutting out from the tegmentum. When slicing horizontally across the midbrain to make a cross-section, an image like a teddy bear's face appears (flip the book upside-down to see it!). We can use this basic shape to describe the relevant neuroanatomy here.

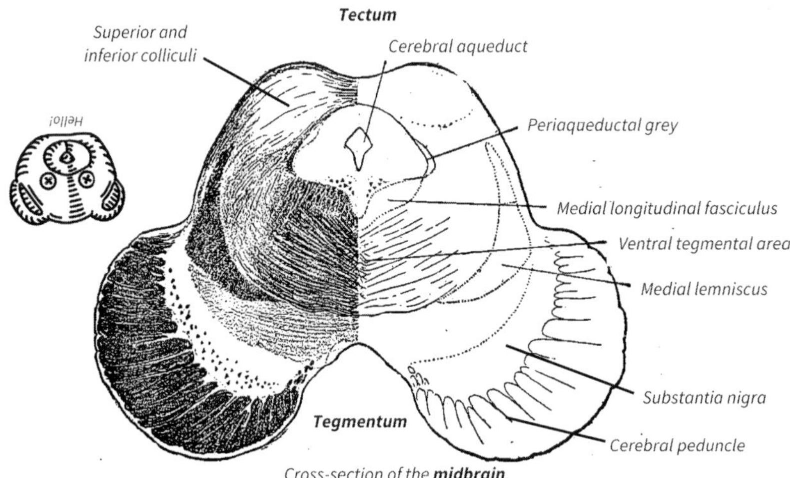

Cross-section of the **midbrain**.

The "chin" of the bear is the **tectum** which contains two paired structures that are involved in processing vision and sound. The higher pair (the **superior colliculi**) are involved in controlling eye movement in response to **visual information**, while the lower pair (the **inferior colliculi**) are involved in relaying **auditory signals** to the thalamus (and in particular the medial geniculate nucleus). We'll talk about both the superior and inferior colliculi further in Chapters 10 and 11.

The "nose" of the bear is the central **cerebral aqueduct**. This is a cavity that contains cerebrospinal fluid and forms part of the ventricular system which we will discuss further in Chapter 12. The area immediately surrounding the cerebral aqueduct (the "snout") is the **periaqueductal grey** which contains a collection of cell bodies that plays an important part in the perception and regulation of **pain**.

The "bridge" of the nose is the **medial longitudinal fasciculus**, a structure that is heavily involved in **eye movement**. Specifically, the medial longitudinal fasciculus serves as the connection point between the three cranial nerves that innervate the various muscles surrounding the eyes. We will talk about the medial longitudinal fasciculus more in Chapter 10.

The bulk of the bear's "upper face" (roughly where the eyes and forehead would be) is made up of the **tegmentum**. The tegmentum contains much of the aforementioned **reticular formation** as well as sensory fibers traveling from the spinal cord to the thalamus. In addition, there are a couple of "colorful" structures to note! The first are the paired **red nuclei** (roughly located at the "eyes") which play a role in **motor functioning** (although to a much lesser extent than the neurons traveling in the "ears" which we will discuss in a bit). The second is the **substantia nigra** (Latin for "black substance") which is found at the *base* of the "ears." As you'll recall from Chapter 5, the substantia nigra is part of basal ganglia (and in fact is the only part of the basal ganglia that lies *outside* of the cerebrum) and supplies the basal ganglia with dopamine to act as "grease" for facilitating movement. Finally, this area also contains the **medial lemniscus** which carries information about vibration and proprioception on epicritic sensory neurons to the thalamus, as we'll talk about more in the next chapter.

The "face" of the tegmentum contains the **ventral tegmental area**, a collection of cell bodies that, like the substantia nigra, produces dopamine. The dopamine produced in the ventral tegmental area goes to the cerebral cortex and limbic system where it helps to govern **reward-driven behaviors**.

Finally, the tips of the "ears" are known as the **cerebral peduncles** and consist largely of motor neurons traveling from the motor cortex to skeletal muscles (the **corticospinal tract**) as well as to the muscles of the face via the cranial nerves (the **corticobulbar tract**). Two cranial nerves branch off of the midbrain as well: III (the oculomotor nerve) and IV (the trochlear nerve), both of which are involved in **eye movement**. For this reason, damage to the anterior part of the midbrain can lead to an inability to move the eyes in particular directions.

To put this all together, you can use the mnemonic **IMPRESSV** to remember the structures that are *unique* to the midbrain (as opposed to things like the corticospinal tract, medial lemniscus, or cerebral aqueduct that run through all three parts). This stands for the **I**nferior colliculi, the **M**edial longitudinal fasciculus (which, it should be noted, is also found in the pons and medulla), the **P**eriaqueductal grey, the **R**ed nuclei, the cranial nerves involved in **E**ye movement, the **S**ubstantia nigra, the **S**uperior colliculi, and finally the **V**entral tegmental area. You can connect this to the midbrain by thinking that the midbrain is at the **top** of brainstem, having climbed up over the pons and the medulla—an **IMPRESSiVe** feat!

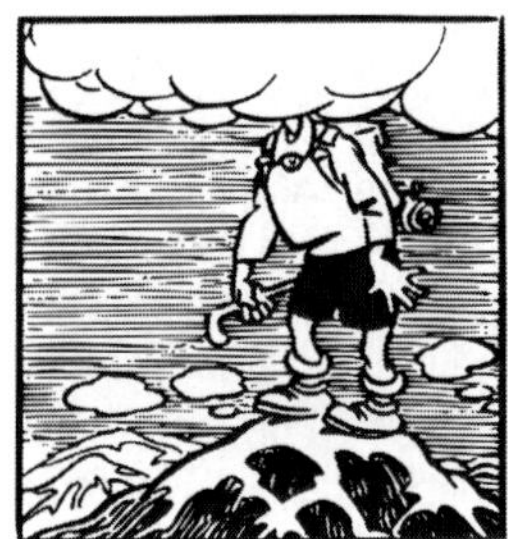

The **midbrain** has several **unique areas** in addition to the **motor, sensory, and awareness functions** it shares with the other parts of the brainstem.

***IMPRESSV*:**
***I**nferior colliculi*
***M**edial longitudinal fasciculus*
***P**eriaqueductal grey*
***R**ed nuclei*
***E**ye movement cranial nerves*
***S**ubstantia nigra*
***S**uperior colliculi*
***V**entral tegmental area*

THE PONS

Moving down from the midbrain, we next hit the **pons**. Unlike the cute-'n-cuddly bear face of the midbrain, a cross-section of the pons looks like… well, not much of anything at all. However, we've already talked about many of the structures here, so it hopefully shouldn't be too intimidating to explore!

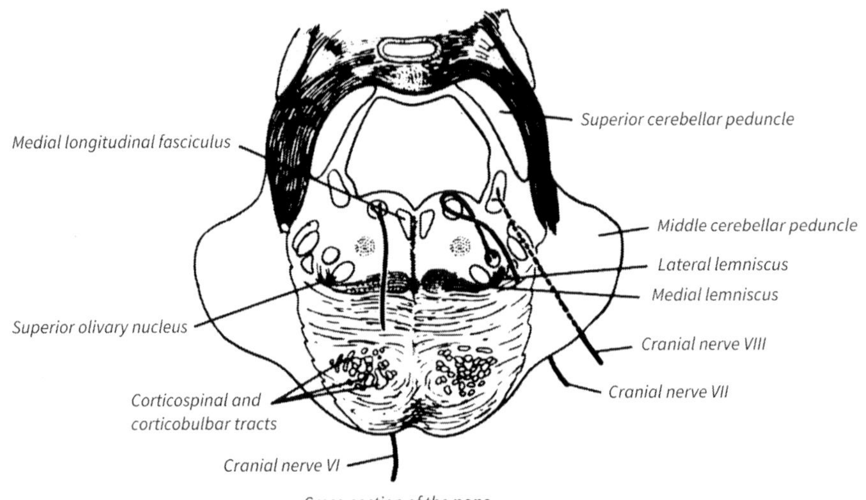

*Cross-section of the **pons**.*

Let's start with the things we already know, as they were found in the midbrain as well. Both the **corticospinal and corticobulbar tracts** (which carry motor neurons to the body and cranial nerves, respectively) and the **medial lemniscus** (which carries epicritic sensory neurons to the thalamus) continue their journey here in the pons.

Following the "Rule of 4," the **middle four cranial nerves** branch off here: V (the trigeminal nerve, not pictured), VI (the abducens nerve), VII (the facial nerve), and VIII (the vestibulocochlear nerve). We'll cover these in more detail in Chapter 9.

The pons also makes connections with the cerebellum by way of the **superior cerebellar peduncle** (which **S**ends **C**rossed **P**athways *from* the cerebellum) and the **middle cerebellar peduncle** (which passes sensory information *to* the cerebellum).

Finally, the pons contains a few unique structures that perform several vital functions (not all of which are pictured on the diagram above). Let's use the word **PONS** itself to illustrate them:

P is for Pneumotaxic and apneustic centers. The pons contains the **pontine respiratory center** which is one of three areas in the brainstem (the other two being in the medulla) that help to regulate the rate and depth of breathing. The pontine respiratory center is itself made up of two subareas. The first is the **pneumotaxic center** which stops inspiration when the lungs have stretched too far. The second is the **apneustic center** which helps to promote inspiration when the lungs are empty. Cycling between the pneumotaxic center and the apneustic center creates the usual rhythm of breathing.

O is for Ocular movement. Within the pons is the **paramedian pontine reticular formation** which is an important center for coordinating **eye movements**.

N is for Neurotransmitters. The pons contains two major sites of neurotransmitter production. The first is the **locus ceruleus** which produces **norepinephrine**, a neurotransmitter that you should be familiar with already through its role in the sympathetic nervous system. The second is the **raphe nucleus** which produces **serotonin**, a neurotransmitter involved in mood and emotion.

S is for Sound. Finally, the pons contains two structures that are important for the sense of sound: the **superior olivary nuclei**, which receive sensory neurons from the ears, and the **lateral lemniscus**, which is a tract of nerves connecting the superior olivary nuclei to the inferior colliculi of the midbrain. Take a moment to locate these on the diagram. We'll learn more about all three of these structures when we talk about the auditory pathway in Chapter 11!

The **pons** contains the continuation of **motor and sensory pathways** from the midbrain as well as areas involving **vital functions** such as breathing.

PONS:
***P**neumotaxic and apneustic centers*
***O**cular movements*
***N**eurotransmitter production*
***S**ound (superior olivary nuclei and lateral lemniscus)*

CENTRAL PONTINE MYELINOLYSIS

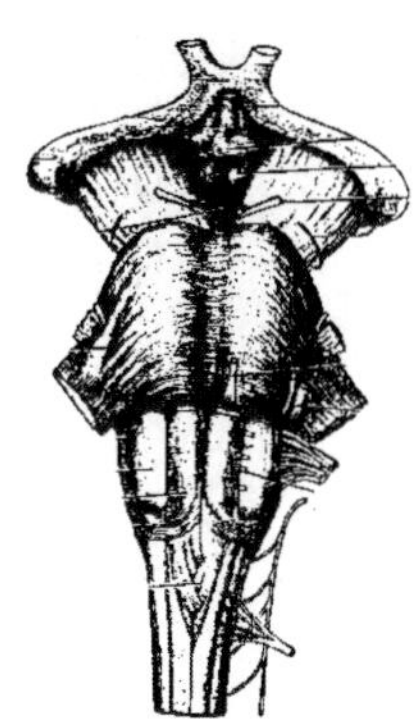

The functions of the pons are illustrated in a disease known as **central pontine myelinolysis**. In this condition, the myelin sheaths of nerves in the pons becomes damaged due to **rapid correction of hyponatremia** with intravenous fluids. This results in respiratory distress (the pneumotaxic and apneustic centers), paralysis (the corticospinal and corticobulbar tracts), ataxia (the superior and middle cerebellar peduncles), and altered consciousness (the reticular formation). Central pontine myelinolysis is a deadly disease with a poor prognosis. While some survivors make a full recovery, others are left with lasting neurologic deficits. It can be avoided by making sure to correct hyponatremia slowly. You can remember the cause of this condition by thinking of the rhyme, "From low to high, the pons will die."

Central pontine myelinolysis is a syndrome of **pontine dysfunction** resulting from **overly rapid correction of hyponatremia**.

*From **low to high** (sodium), the **pons will die**.*

THE MEDULLA OBLONGATA

The **medulla oblongata** is the lowest part of the brainstem. Let's take a closer look!

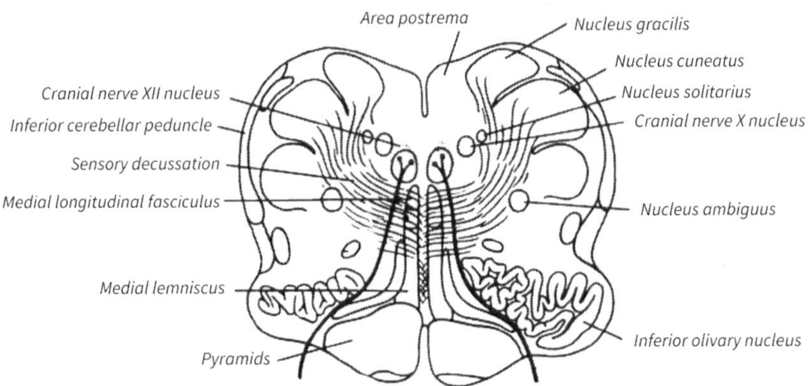

*Cross-section of the **medulla oblongata**.*

If you know the "Rule of 4," it should come as no surprise that the medulla shoots off a few cranial nerves of its own: IX (the glossopharyngeal nerve), X (the vagus nerve), XI (the spinal accessory nerve), and XII (the hypoglossal nerve).

The medulla contains several **reflex centers**, most of which involve either keeping good things *in* (the **swallowing reflex**) or pushing bad stuff *out* (the **vomiting**, **coughing**, and **sneezing** reflexes). The vomiting reflex lies in an area known as the **area postrema** which initiates this process when it detects a potential toxin in the mouth. You can remember the function of the area **postrema** by thinking of it as **p.o. streamer** (with p.o., or *per os*, being medical jargon for "by mouth").

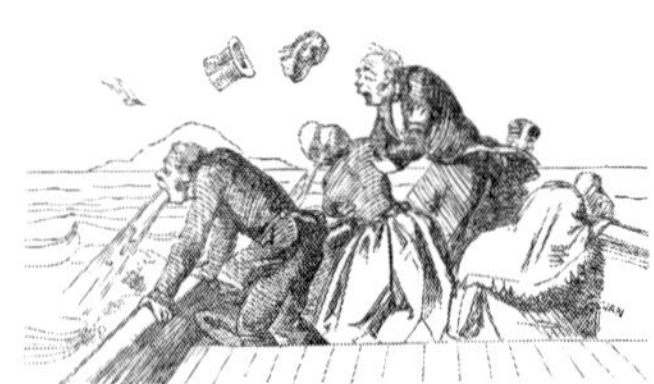

The **area postrema** regulates **vomiting** and other responses to **potential toxins**.

*A **p.o. streamer** (postrema) will have a **stream of vomit** exiting **by mouth**.*

In addition, the medulla oblongata contains the **nucleus ambiguus** which connects to the muscles involved with **speech** and **swallowing**. Damage to the nucleus ambiguus can lead to **dysphagia** (difficulty chewing), **dysarthria** (trouble speaking), and **dysphonia** (a hoarse voice). You can remember the function of the nucleus ambig-**uh-uh's** by pronouncing it with two uh's at the end, which should help to remind you of someone giving a **speech** who keeps saying lots of uh's.

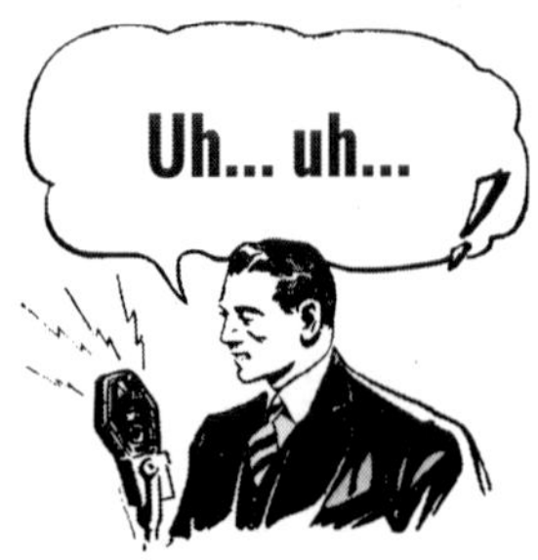

The **nucleus ambiguus** controls the muscles involved in **speech** and **swallowing**.

*Think of the nucleus ambig-**uh-uh**'s when someone is having trouble giving a **speech**.*

The medulla also contains the **nucleus solitarius** which receives input from the tongue about **taste** and is involved in the **gag reflex**. In addition, the nucleus solitarius is involved in the **baroreceptor reflex** that regulates **blood pressure**. While most people think that you need a fancy sphygmomanometer to measure blood pressure, your body is actually quite adept at measuring it naturally using pressure sensors in various arteries throughout the body. This information is sent to the nucleus solitarius which then regulates both heart rate and vascular tone using the sympathetic and parasympathetic nervous systems. Because of its dual function, a lesion at the nucleus solitarius can result in a characteristic combination of **loss of taste** as well as instability of **blood pressure** and other vital signs. You can remember this by thinking of it as the nucleus **sole-lick**-tarius. Imagine being asked to **lick** the **sole** of someone's foot. This would likely make you want to **gag** and would cause your **heart rate and blood pressure to go up**.

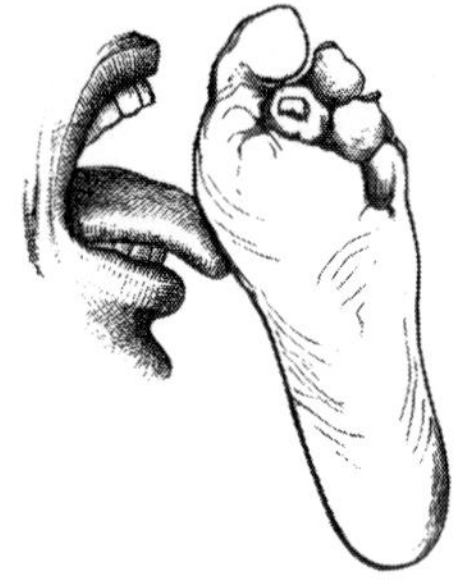

The **nucleus solitarius** is involved in **taste sensation**, the **gag reflex**, and regulation of **blood pressure**.

*The nucleus **sole-lick**-tarius is like licking the sole of someone's foot. The **taste** would make you **gag**, and your **heart rate** and **blood pressure** would increase.*

Vitally, the **cardiovascular center** lies within the medulla, with the sympathetic and parasympathetic nervous systems working here to increase and decrease the heart rate, respectively. The rest of the **respiratory center** is also found in the medulla, with the **dorsal respiratory group** starting the process of inspiration and the **ventral respiratory group** controlling expiration. (Neither the cardiovascular center nor the respiratory groups are pictured on the diagram.) You can remember these core functions of the medulla oblongata by thinking of someone getting a gold **medul** pinned onto them as a reward—the **medul**(la) goes right over their **heart** and **lungs**.

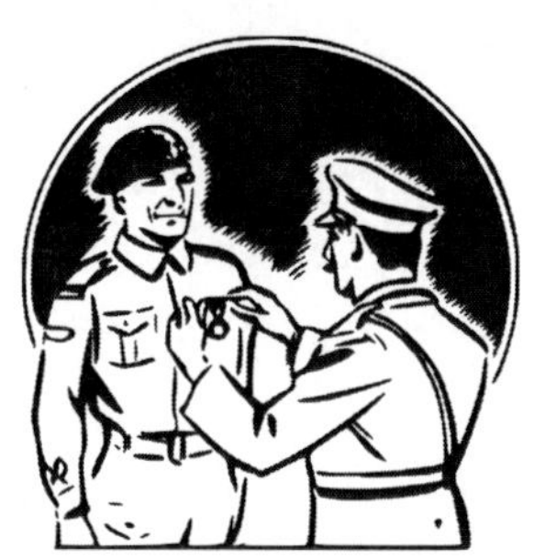

"Cross my heart."

The **medulla oblongata** contains the **cardiovascular and respiratory centers**.

*Think of someone getting a gold **medul**(la) placed over their **heart and lungs**.*

Like the midbrain and pons, the tracts carrying **motor and sensory information** continue here. *Unlike* the midbrain and pons, however, these tracts do some weird things in the medulla.

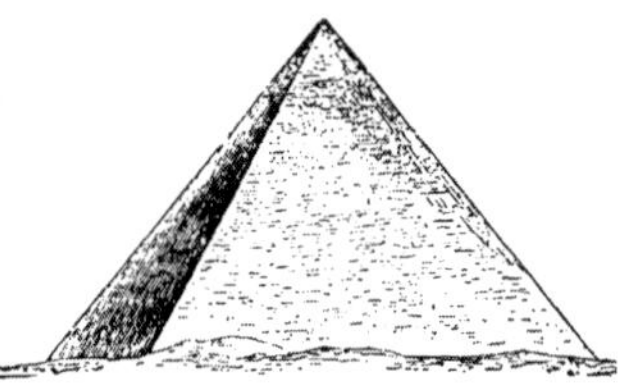

Let's start with the corticospinal tract carrying motor neurons down to the body as well as what's left of the corticobulbar tract (as many cranial nerves have already exited at this point). These motor neurons run along the anterior side of the medulla and jut out from the landscape like pyramids, so they were called "**pyramidal tracts**." At the bottom of the medulla, the **pyramidal decussation** occurs. (This is a key part of understanding the motor pathway, so pay close attention!) At the pyramidal decussation, the nerve fibers in the motor pathway cross over from left-to-right and right-to-left. This is the reason why damage to the *left* side of the brain produces weakness on the *right* side of the body and vice versa!

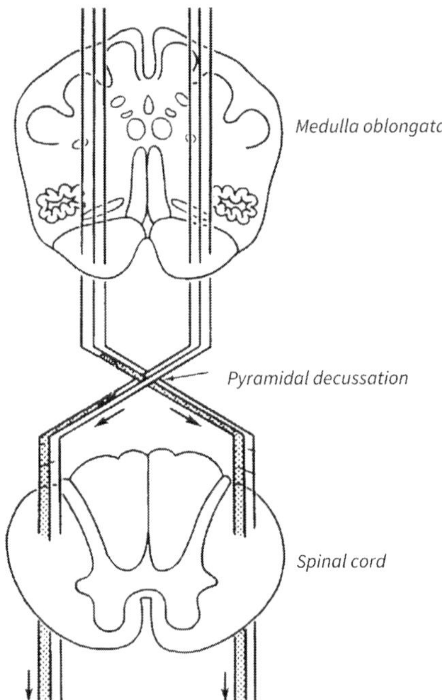

The ***crossing*** *of the* ***corticospinal tract*** *in the* ***medulla oblongata****.*

Efferent motor pathways are not the only ones that decussate in the medulla! Epicritic sensory neurons carrying vibration and proprioceptive information also cross over here in an area known as the **sensory decussation**. Of note, protopathic neurons carrying crude touch, pain, and temperature do *not* cross over here! We will talk more about the implications of this in the next chapter.

After these decussations occur, the brainstem ends and the spinal cord officially begins! Let's take a moment to remember some of the core functions of the medulla. Use the mnemonic **SCARPH** to remember the nucleus **S**olitarius, the **C**rossing of motor and epicritic pathways, the nucleus **A**mbiguus, the **R**espiratory center, the area **P**ostrema, and the cardiovascular center controlling the **H**eart. You can remember this by thinking that the medulla is the **lowest** part of the brainstem, so it is closest to the neck where you would wear a scarf.

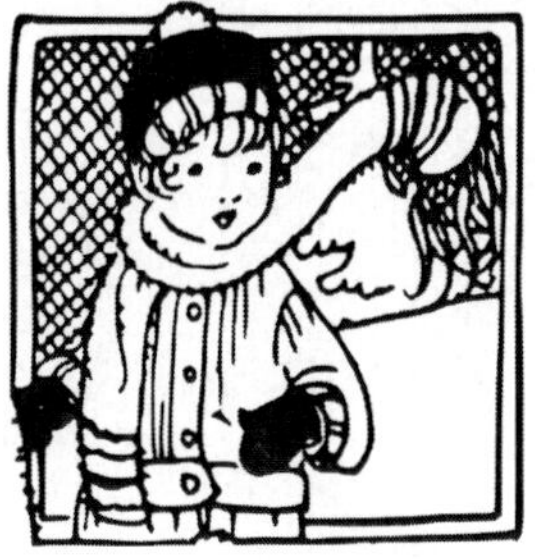

The **medulla oblongata** contains several areas that perform **unique functions** including **speech and swallowing reflexes** as well as **cardiorespiratory centers.**

SCARPH:
*Nucleus **S**olitarius*
***C**rossing of motor and epicritic pathways*
*Nucleus **A**mbiguus*
***R**espiratory center*
*Area **P**ostrema*
***H**eart (cardiovascular) center*

PUTTING IT ALL TOGETHER

And with that, we have officially crossed the "bridge" from the brain to the spinal cord! As with so much in neurology, the best way to put all of this information together is to use it clinically. We will do this in earnest in Chapter 14 when we talk about strokes, as ischemic damage in different parts of the brainstem leads to clinically distinct presentations. For now, take a moment to review the key structures that are found in each part of the brainstem using our **IMPRESSV**, **PONS**, and **SCARPH** mnemonics. It's not so important right now that you memorize the exact location of each structure in the cross-sectional diagrams! As we learn more about brainstem dysfunction in upcoming chapters, we will revisit the parts that we'll need to know.

REVIEW QUESTIONS

1. A 43 y/o M with a history of excessive alcohol intake and malnutrition presents after a fall in which he lost consciousness for approximately one minute. By the time he arrived at the hospital, he had regained consciousness. Initial neurological exam is unremarkable. Laboratory analysis reveals hyponatremia, hypokalemia, and abnormal liver function tests. Intravenous fluids are started which result in improvement in his electrolyte abnormalities within 24 hours. Several days later, he suddenly develops diffuse muscle weakness, including poor respiratory effort. This weakness progresses to complete paralysis of all muscles except for eye blinking and movement. An MRI scan of his head reveals the following:

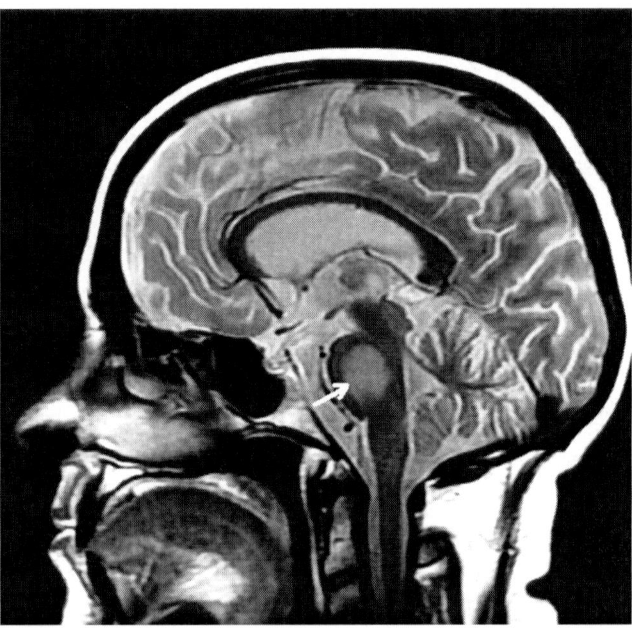

Which of the following mechanisms likely accounts for the neuronal damage observed in this case?

A. Ischemic damage in the midbrain
B. Ischemic damage in the pons
C. Ischemic damage in the medulla oblongata
D. Osmotic demyelination in the midbrain
E. Osmotic demyelination in the pons
F. Osmotic demyelination in the medulla oblongata
G. Autoimmune destruction in the midbrain
H. Autoimmune destruction in the pons
I. Autoimmune destruction in the medulla oblongata

2. A 52 y/o F is undergoing chemotherapy for breast cancer. During her initial treatment, she develops severe nausea and vomiting. Before her next treatment, she is prescribed ondansetron, an anti-nausea medication. The anti-nausea effect of ondansetron can most likely be explained by its interaction with chemical receptors in which part of the brainstem?
    A. Nucleus ambiguus
    B. Area postrema
    C. Pyramidal decussation
    D. Ventral tegmental area
    E. Paramedian pontine reticular formation
    F. Nucleus solitarius

3. A 37 y/o M military veteran is seen in a pain management clinic. He suffers from chronic pain due to multiple points of embedded shrapnel from exposure to an improvised explosive device while serving overseas. Despite several years of treatment involving medications, physical therapy, and alternative practices, he remains disabled by his pain. His pain management specialist offers to enroll him in a clinical trial of a new treatment for chronic pain involving implantation of a neurostimulator, or a device that is surgically inserted into the brain that activates neurons in nearby areas. Implantation of the neurostimulator into which of the following areas is most likely to result in pain relief for this patient?
    A. Periaqueductal grey
    B. Substantia nigra
    C. Medial longitudinal fasciculus
    D. Apneustic center
    E. Red nuclei

1. **The best answer is E.** This vignette describes a case of central pontine myelinolysis, a potentially deadly condition in which overly rapid correction of hyponatremia results in demyelination of neurons in the pons due to osmotic fluid shifts. Ischemic damage (answers A—C) and autoimmune mechanisms (answers G—I) are not believed to be involved. Damage to the midbrain (answer D) or medulla (answer F) would produce different signs and symptoms.

2. **The best answer is B.** Many chemotherapy drugs are notorious for causing severe nausea by activating chemoreceptors in the area postrema of the medulla oblongata. Ondansetron is believed to block this effect by antagonizing serotonin receptors in this area. None of the other areas listed are thought to be involved in the vomiting reflex, with the nucleus ambiguus involved in speaking and swallowing (answer A), the pyramidal decussation involved in the crossing over of the motor pathway (answer C), the ventral tegmental area involved in reward-driven behaviors (answer D), and the paramedian pontine reticular formation involved in eye movements (answer E). The nucleus solitarius is involved in the gag reflex which shares a similar purpose as the vomiting reflex (to keep potentially toxic substances out of the body); however, the mechanisms and neuroanatomical centers by which they do so are different (answer F).

3. **The best answer is A.** The midbrain contains the periaqueductal gray, a nucleus that plays a critical role in modulating pain perception. Indeed, several studies have shown that the periaqueductal gray appears to be the most promising site for deep brain stimulators in patients with chronic pain. The substantia nigra and red nuclei are involved in movement (answers B and E), the medial longitudinal fasciculus helps to control eye movements (answer C), and the apneustic center helps to regulate the respiratory cycle (answer D).

8 THE SPINAL CORD

If the brain is the capital city and the brainstem is the bridge, then the **spinal cord** is the highway on which nerves travel to and from their destination. Just as cars exit from the highway to take side streets, nerves traveling in the central nervous system branch off of the spinal cord and exit the vertebral column when they get close enough to their destination, at which point they continue their journey as **peripheral nerves**. In this chapter, we will learn about the spinal cord in more detail, with the next chapter devoted to the peripheral nervous system in all of its glory.

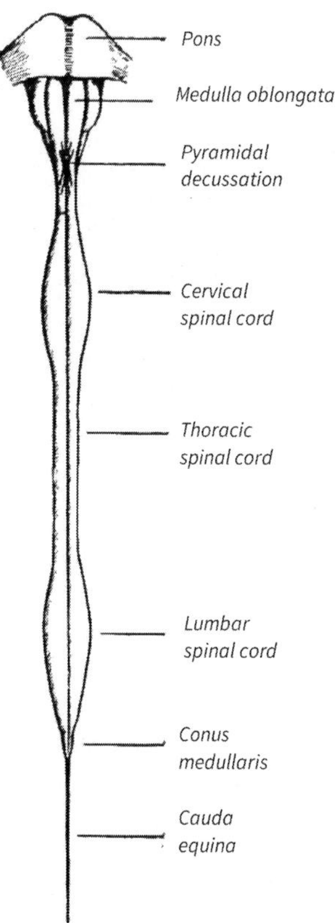

The spinal cord is traditionally divided into three regions, with the **cervical** spinal cord in the neck, the **thoracic** spinal cord in the chest, and the **lumbar** spinal cord in the abdomen. As you can see in the diagram on the right, there are enlargements in both the cervical and lumbar regions that correspond to the increased number of nerves shooting off here to go to the arms and legs, respectively. After the lumbar enlargement, the spinal cord begins to thin into a tapered region known as the **conus medullaris**. The spinal cord officially ends around the first or second lumbar vertebrae. However, even after the spinal cord ends, many of the nerves that have branched off from it continue to run downwards in a cluster of nerves known as the **cauda equina** (Latin for "horse's tail," which makes sense given its appearance).

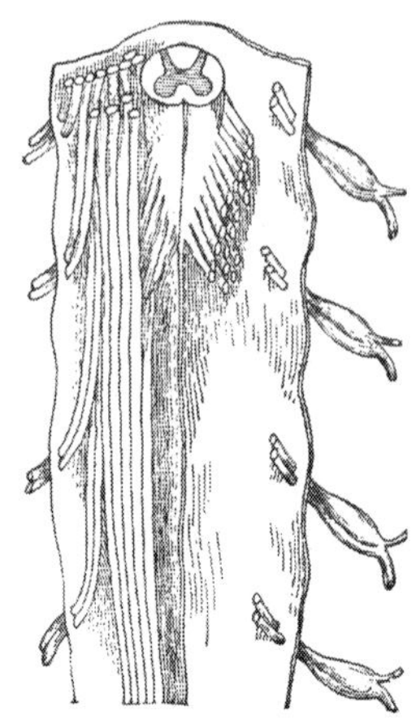

When talking about the spinal nerves that exit from the spinal cord, it's important to note that the place where a nerve branches off of the spinal cord is *not* the same place where it exits from the vertebral column! Instead, these nerves generally travel in the vertebral column for a while before exiting (as seen in the image to the right). For example, the T1 spinal nerve exits the vertebral column below the first thoracic vertebra, but it likely split off from the spinal cord somewhere in the cervical region. This is something that is easy to get confused about, but it's important to grasp as it explains why there are spinal nerves from the sacral and coccygeal regions (in the pelvis) even though the spinal cord ends up in the lower back (as these nerves exit the *spinal cord* before its termination at L1/L2 but do not exit the *vertebral column* until the sacral region).

Spinal nerves are **mixed nerves** containing both sensory and motor neurons. While the two kinds of neurons intermingle for most of the length of the nerve, close to the spinal cord the two types separate, with efferent motor neurons exiting on the *anterior* side of the spinal cord and afferent sensory nerves entering on the *posterior* side (somewhat like the on-ramps and off-ramps of a highway like we talked about back in Chapter 2).

Another difference between sensory and motor nerves involves the position of their cell bodies. The cell bodies of *sensory* nerves lie *outside* the spinal cord in clusters known as **dorsal root ganglia**, while the cell bodies of *motor* nerves lie *inside* the spinal cord in a region known as the **anterior horn**. You can use the word "**SO-MA**" (another name for neuronal cell bodies) to keep this pattern straight. The soma of **S**ensory nerves are **O**utside the spinal cord in the dorsal root ganglia, while for **M**otor nerves they are inside in the **A**nterior horn!

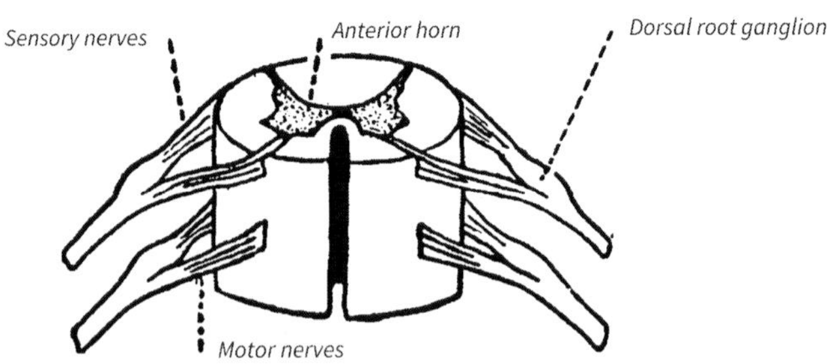

Spinal nerves *connecting to the* ***spinal cord****.*

Sensory nerves enter in the **posterior spinal cord**,
while **motor nerve** exit from the **anterior spinal cord**.

SO-MA*:*
Sensory cell bodies on the ***O****utside (in dorsal root ganglia),*
M*otor cell bodies on the inside in the* ***A****nterior horn.*

SPINAL CORD ANATOMY

The spinal cord is not a disorganized tangle of nerves thrown together in a haphazard fashion. Instead, the spinal cord features a surprising degree of organization owing to the fact that, as in the other parts of the nervous system we have discussed so far, **nerves that do similar things tend to travel together**. This allows us to understand and name the various parts of the spinal cord that we see.

When you cut horizontally across the spinal cord to make a cross-section, the first difference you'll notice is the separation between grey and white matter. Unlike the cerebrum (where the grey matter is on the outside and the white matter is on the inside), the spinal cord features the opposite arrangement, with the white matter on the *outside* and the grey matter on the *inside* in a butterfly-like shape as seen below:

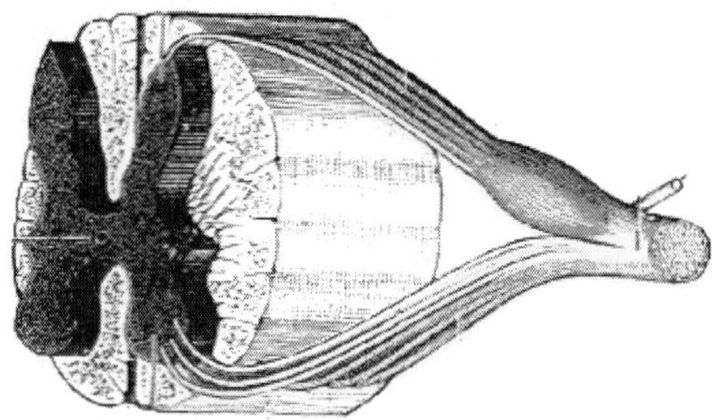

*The **spinal cord**, with **grey matter** on the inside and **white matter** on the outside.*

While the composition of the grey and white matter changes depending on which region of the spinal cord you are in, overall this butterfly-like appearance remains remarkably consistent down the entire length of the cord:

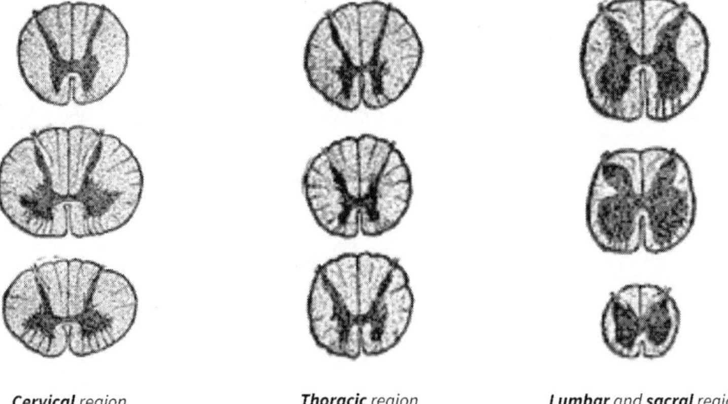

***Cervical** region* | ***Thoracic** region* | ***Lumbar** and **sacral** regions*

Within the grey and white matter are further subdivisions based on function. To understand these, we'll need to look at the various pathways traveling through the spinal cord in more detail, starting with the two sensory pathways and then moving onto the motor tract.

THE DORSAL COLUMN—MEDIAL LEMNISCUS PATHWAY

Recall from Chapter 2 that there are two kinds of sensory neurons: **protopathic neurons** (which carry crude touch, pain, and temperature) and **epicritic neurons** (which carry fine touch, vibration, and proprioception). We'll focus first on epicritic neurons which travel in the **dorsal column—medial lemniscus pathway**.

Epicritic neurons travel in the spinal cord within the **dorsal column** (located between the two upper wings of the butterfly). The dorsal column is further split into two parts known as the **gracile fasciculus** and the **cuneate fasciculus**. There are two important things to note here! First, information from the *lower* body is carried in the **gracile fasciculus**, while information from the *upper* body is carried in the **cuneate fasciculus**. Use the phrase, "**Walk grac**efully and **eat** with your **hands**" to associate legs with the **grac**ile fasciculus and hands with the cune**ate** fasciculus. Second, the gracile fasciculus is *medial* to the cuneate fasciculus, so injuries to the middle of the cord will result in sensory loss in the legs, while injuries to the side will instead cause sensory loss in the arms. (This is different from the other two pathways we will talk about in this chapter where the pattern is reversed!) To associate this pattern with this particular pathway, think of it as the dorsal column—**medial leg**-niscus pathway.

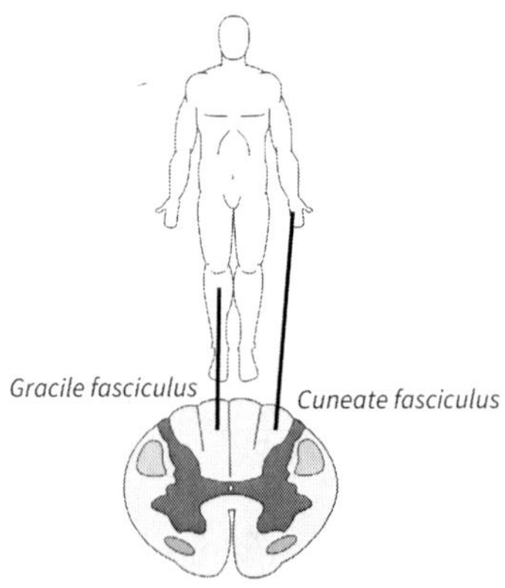

Epicritic neurons from the **legs** travel **medially** in the **gracile fasciculus**, while those from the **arms** travel **laterally** in the **cuneate fasciculus**.

***Walk grac**efully and **eat** with your **hands**.*
*In the dorsal column—**medial leg**-niscus pathway, the **legs** are **medial**!*

These neurons travel in the dorsal column of the spinal cord until they hit the medulla where they join with a cluster of cell bodies known as the **nucleus gracilis** and **nucleus cuneatus**. After synapsing here, these neurons **cross over** from left-to-right and right-to-left in the **sensory decussation** (just like we talked about in the last chapter). From there, these neurons continue their journey through the brainstem on a bundle of axons known as the **medial lemniscus** before hitting the **thalamus** (which you'll recall is the brain's "switchboard" for *th*en*th*ory information) and in particular the ventral posterolateral nucleus (since the VPL is where a Very Painful Leg is sensed). From the thalamus, the signal is passed on to its final target: the **somatosensory cortex** in the parietal lobe. You can remember the order of these steps using the phrase "**D**iscover **N**ew **D**irections for **M**oving **V**ibration & **P**roprioception."

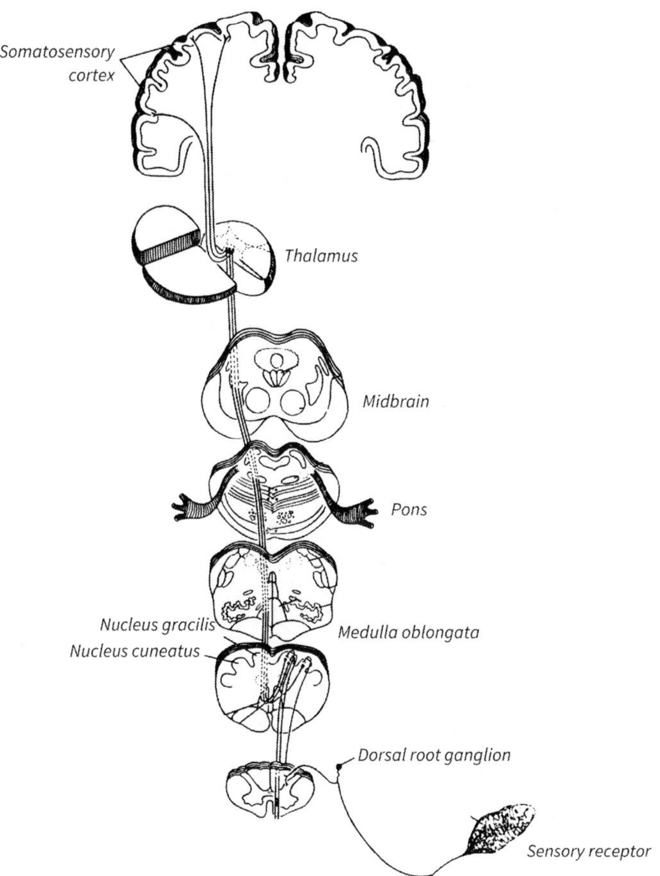

*The **dorsal column—medial lemniscus pathway**.*

The **dorsal column—medial lemniscus pathway** carries **epicritic neurons**.

***D**iscover **N**ew **D**irections for **M**oving **V**ibration & **P**roprioception:*
***D**orsal columns (gracile fasciculus and cuneate fasciculus)*
***N**ucleus gracilis and nucleus cuneatus*
***D**ecussation*
***M**edial lemniscus*
***V**entral posterolateral nucleus of the thalamus*
***P**arietal lobe*

THE SPINOTHALAMIC TRACT

The dorsal column—medial lemniscus pathway is just one of the two possible routes that sensory information can take through the central nervous system. The other route, known as the **spinothalamic tract**, carries information about **crude touch**, **pain**, and **temperature** and has its own way of doing things!

Peripheral nerves carrying protopathic neurons first enter the spinal cord on the posterior side. They initially enter an area known as the **posterolateral tract** or **Lissauer's tract**. Lissauer's tract features an interesting quirk: nerves here often move up or down a spinal level or two (seemingly for no good reason other than to confuse students!). Because of this, protopathic sensory loss related to a spinal cord injury is often "off" a level or two from what you would expect (either too high or too low).

After passing through Lissauer's tract, these neurons then enter into one of two areas that are both contained in the upper wings of the butterfly: the **substantia gelatinosa** (which is named for the "goopy" gelatin-like texture of this tissue caused by the lack of myelin in these nerves) and the **nucleus proprius**.

Unlike the nerves traveling in the dorsal column (which wait until the medulla to cross over), the nerves in the spinothalamic tract cross over soon after entering the spinal cord in a bundle called the **anterior white commissure**. You can remember this by thinking that **F**ine touch, **V**ibration, and **P**roprioception are **F**eeling **V**ery **P**atient (they can wait until the medulla to cross over), while **N**on-discriminative touch, **T**emperature, and **P**ain are **N**ot **T**hat **P**atient and want to cross over *immediately*.

Protopathic neurons cross over immediately in the **anterior white commissure** of the spinal cord, while **epicritic neurons wait** to cross over in the **medulla oblongata**.

__F__ine touch, __V__ibration, and __P__roprioception are __F__eeling __V__ery __P__atient,
while __N__on-discriminative touch, __T__emperature, and __P__ain are __N__ot __T__hat __P__atient.

Because the dorsal column—medial lemniscus pathway and the spinothalamic tract cross over at different places, a patient with damage to their spinal cord can have **crossed findings** with numbness of crude touch, pain, and temperature on the right half of their body and numbness of fine touch, vibration, and proprioception on the left (or vice versa). This occurs if the injury is located *after* the spinothalamic tract has crossed over but *before* the dorsal column-medial lemniscus pathway has crossed.

After crossing over in the anterior white commissure, the spinothalamic tract travels upwards in the white matter surrounding the anterior horn of the spinal cord, with information from *lower* in the body being carried on the most *lateral* aspect while information from the *upper* body is carried more *medially*. (Note that this is the *opposite* pattern of what we saw with the dorsal column—medial leg-niscus pathway!) They then travel to the brainstem where they *don't* cross over in the medulla (as they have done this already in the spinal cord since they're **N**ot **T**hat **P**atient!). They then synapse in the ventral posterolateral nucleus of the **thalamus** before completing their journey in the somatosensory cortex of the **parietal lobe**.

Like with the dorsal column—medial lemniscus pathway and its "**D**iscover **N**ew **D**irections for **M**oving **V**ibration & **P**roprioception" mnemonic, we can use another phrase here to remember the steps of the spinothalamic tract: "**L**ist **S**ome **P**roper **A**venues for **S**ending **T**emperature & **P**ain."

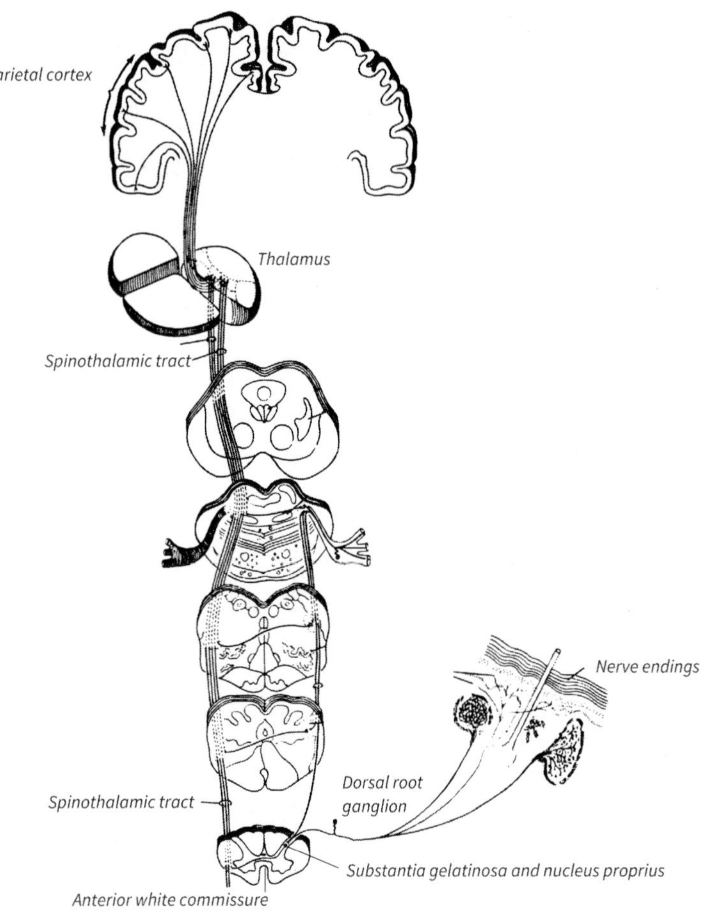

The ***spinothalamic tract****.*

The **spinothalamic tract** carries **protopathic neurons** from the body to the brain.

L*ist* ***S****ome* ***P****roper* ***A****venues for* ***S****ending* ***T****emperature &* ***P****ain:*
L*issauer's (posterolateral) tract*
S*ubstantia gelatinosa and nucleus* ***P****roprius*
A*nterior white commissure*
S*pinothalamic tract*
T*halamus*
P*arietal lobe*

THE CORTICOSPINAL TRACT

Now that we have covered both sensory pathways, we will shift our attention to the motor neurons that make up the other half of nerves flowing through the spinal cord. The vast majority of motor neurons travel through the spinal cord in the **corticospinal tract**. The corticospinal tract is itself divided into two parts: the *lateral* corticospinal tract and the *anterior* corticospinal tract. The lateral corticospinal tract is the larger of the two, accounting for around 90% of all motor neurons in the spinal cord. In general, motor neurons going towards the upper extremities travel more *medially* while those going to the lower extremities are found more *laterally*. (This is the *same* pattern as the spinothalamic tract but the *opposite* pattern of the dorsal column—medial lemniscus pathway!)

When it comes time to exit the highway and take the side streets to their final destination, nerves in the lateral corticospinal tract synapse onto motor neurons in the **anterior horn** of the spinal cord (the bottom half of the butterfly's wings). This marks the position of a clinically important divide between **upper motor neurons** and **lower motor neurons**. The neurons that carry the motor signal at any point from the motor cortex in the cerebrum up until the anterior horn cell are considered *upper* motor neurons, while those that carry the signal down from the anterior horn cell to the muscle itself are considered *lower* motor neurons (as seen in the diagram on the opposite page). On a clinical level, damage to upper motor neurons produces different signs and symptoms compared to damage to lower motor neurons (a concept that we will revisit in more detail in Chapter 18).

After picking up the signal from the upper motor neurons in the anterior horn, lower motor neurons then exit the spinal cord as the anterior nerve root (remember "SO-MA"!) before joining afferent nerves from the dorsal root to form a spinal nerve.

And with that, the motor pathway is done! (If you've made it this far, use your corticospinal tract to give yourself a high-five.) A visual summary of the corticospinal tract is found on the next page. You can use the phrase, "**F**lexing **I**nvolves **P**yramids, **C**ords, and **H**orns" to remember each step on this path!

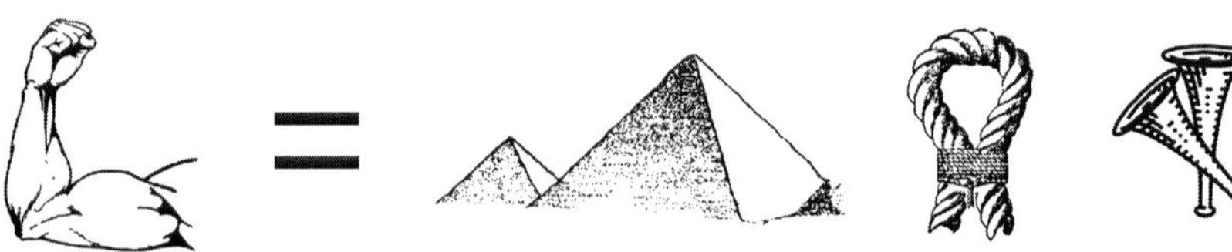

The **corticospinal tract** carries **motor signals** from the brain to the body.

***F**lexing **I**nvolves **P**yramids, **C**ords, and **H**orns:*
***F**rontal lobe*
***I**nternal capsule*
***P**yramidal decussation*
***C**orticospinal tract*
*Anterior **H**orn*

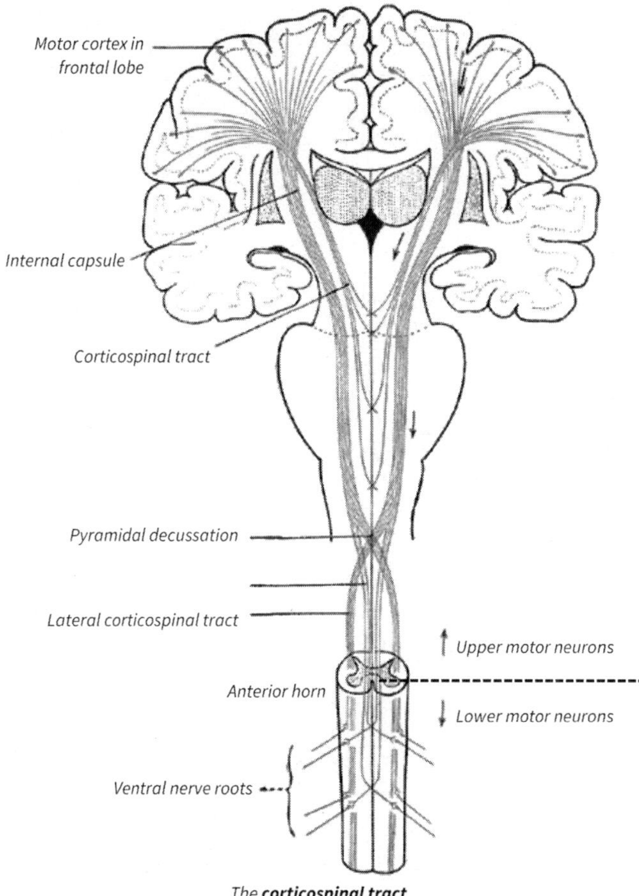

The **corticospinal tract**.

SPINAL REFLEXES

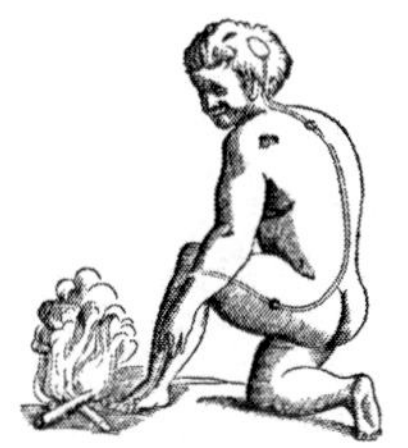

Thus far, we have primarily talked about neurons traveling between the brain and the rest of the body by way of the spinal cord, including both motor and sensory neurons. However, the spinal cord also contains connections between neurons that *don't* involve the brain at all and are instead contained entirely within the spinal cord itself! These connections are responsible for several **spinal reflexes** that occur without conscious effort. Someone who receives a sensory stimulus (say, by accidentally stepping into a fire) will activate sensory neurons in the skin. Signals from these neurons will first travel along their axons to their main cell bodies in the dorsal root ganglion before entering the spinal cord. While some neurons will continue up to the brain via the spinothalamic tract, others will instead synapse with **interneurons** (or neurons that connect neurons to each other) that then synapse directly onto motor neurons in the anterior horn. These neurons will send motor signals to leg flexors that will then act to quickly withdraw the foot from the fire. Because this reflex arc only involves a few neurons and takes place entirely at the level of the spinal cord, it can occur with lightning-fast speed. In fact, the person may find that they have already moved their foot by the time their brain registers any conscious sensation of pain!

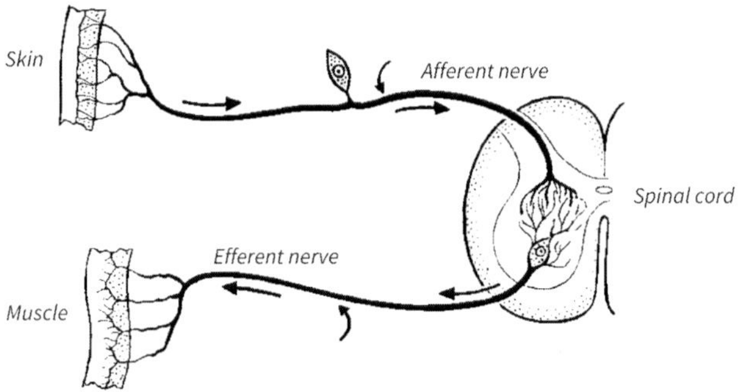

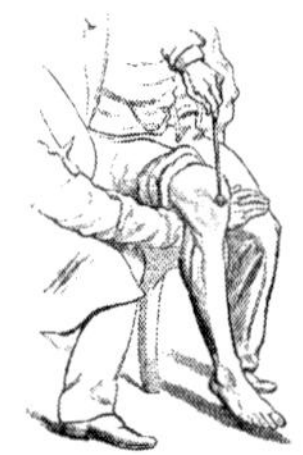

A number of **stretch reflexes** activate certain muscles in response to that muscle being stretched. This phenomenon should be familiar to anyone who has been to a doctor, as testing reflexes by tapping on them is very common! As we will cover in Chapter 13, testing these reflexes can be helpful for localizing where damage to the spinal cord has occurred, as each specific reflex maps to a particular level of the spinal cord. The absence of a particular reflex suggests damage to some aspect of the reflex arc (either the sensory nerves, the motor nerves, or the spinal cord connecting them) at or around this level.

Before we move on, let's recap what we've learned about the anatomy of the spinal cord using this diagram. Feel free to refer back to this image as often as needed!

Dorsal columns

Gracile fasciculus

Cuneate fasciculus

Substantia gelatinosa and nucleus proprius

Lateral corticospinal tract

Anterior horn

Spinothalamic tract

Central canal

Anterior white commissure

SPINAL CORD PATHOLOGY

The best way to reinforce everything we've learned about the anatomy of the spinal cord so far is to look at what happens when something goes wrong. Injuries to the spinal cord can come from various sources, from mechanical injuries like a car crash to infectious diseases like polio. When looking at the effects of spinal cord injuries, the column-like nature of the spinal cord introduces a new complication. It's no longer enough to simply say *what part* of the spinal cord we are talking about. Instead, we also need to specify at *what level* of the spinal cord the damage has occurred. While the *nature* of the deficits (such as whether there are motor deficits, sensory deficits, or both) can help us to figure out the structures involved, the *location* of the deficits in the body (such as whether they are in the arms or legs) will help us figure out the level. For example, someone who sustains an injury at the level of their chest will likely lose all sensory and motor ability in their legs (but will retain these abilities in their arms). This is because the spinal nerves for the upper extremities have already exited the spinal cord in the neck, while those traveling to the legs have yet to depart.

The simplest kind of spinal cord injury to understand is a **complete spinal injury** in which all function below the level of the lesion is lost. In cases of **incomplete spinal injury**, however, only a part of the spinal cord has been damaged, so some functions will be lost while others will be retained. As we talk about the different forms of incomplete spinal injury, refer back to the cross-section of the spinal cord on the previous page to link the findings to everything that we've learned so far!

ANTERIOR CORD SYNDROME

An injury to the anterior half of the spinal cord causes a **motor paralysis** as well as **numbness of crude touch, temperature, and pain** sensation below the level of the lesion. The paralysis is due to the fact that motor neurons are found in the *anterior* horn of the spinal cord, while the numbness is due to the placement of protopathic neurons within both the (anteriorly located) spinothalamic tract as well as their crossing in the anterior white commissure. Notably, fine touch, vibration, and proprioception remain intact, as epicritic neurons travel in the (posteriorly located) *dorsal* columns!

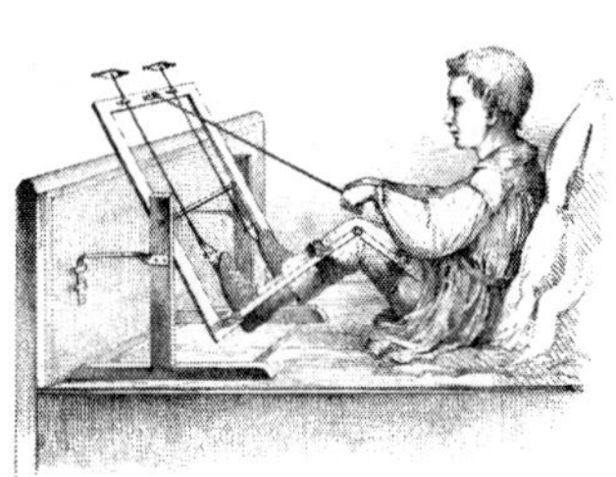

POSTERIOR CORD SYNDROME

Logically, posterior cord syndrome involves the *opposite* findings as anterior cord syndrome! Because the dorsal columns are located in the posterior spinal cord, an injury here results in deficits of **fine touch, vibration, and proprioception** below the level of the injury. Importantly, crude touch, temperature, and pain sensation as well as motor function all remain intact! Due to the loss of proprioception, people with posterior cord syndrome often develop a "stomping" gait as a way to compensate for their inability to sense posture and position. Posterior cord syndrome is most often caused by metabolic or inflammatory insults. As one example, infection with syphilis can lead to demyelination of the dorsal columns, resulting in a permanent posterior cord syndrome known as **tabes dorsalis**.

BROWN-SÉQUARD SYNDROME

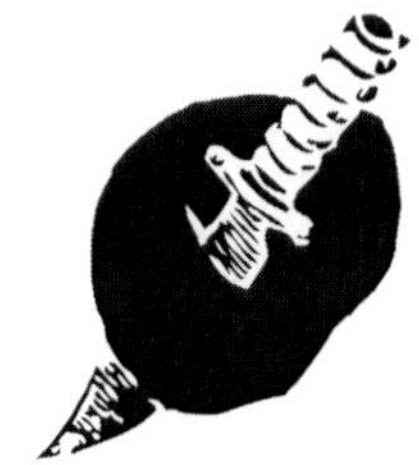

Brown-Séquard syndrome (also known as **spinal hemiplegia**) occurs when one half of the spinal cord (either the right or the left) is injured more than the other half. In these cases, motor function and fine touch, vibration, and proprioception are compromised on the *same* side as the injury, while crude touch, temperature, and pain are affected on the *opposite* side from the lesion. (Remember that, of all the motor and sensory nerves in the spinal cord, only those carrying **N**on-discriminative touch, **T**emperature, and **P**ain are **N**ot **T**hat **P**atient and want to cross over immediately, which is why these are the specific deficits that are found *contra*lateral to the lesion.)

While Brown-Séquard syndrome can occur due to any process that injures the spinal cord, the most common cause is direct penetrating trauma as in a gunshot or stab wound. You can remember this by thinking that **B**rown-**S**équard is what happens when someone tries to **B**ack**S**tab you but only does it **halfway**.

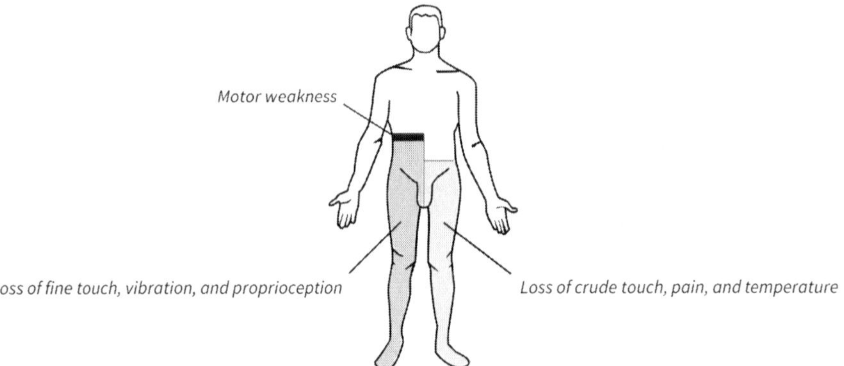

Crossed findings as seen in ***Brown-Séquard syndrome****.*

> **Brown-Séquard syndrome** is a **unilateral spinal cord injury** resulting in **ipsilateral motor weakness** and loss of **epicritic sensation** as well as loss of **contralateral protopathic sensation**.
>
> ***B**rown-**S**équard is when someone tries to **B**ack**S**tab you but only does it **halfway**.*

CENTRAL CORD SYNDROME

An injury to the center of the spinal cord causes greater weakness of the **arms** compared to the legs (remember that the motor neurons traveling to the arms are *medial* to those traveling to the legs!). Loss of crude touch, pain, and temperature sensation below the level of the injury is often seen as well due to the proximity of the spinothalamic tract to the center of spinal cord, although some degree of **sacral sparing** is often seen (as these fibers are going lower in the body and are therefore located *laterally* away from the center). Common causes of a central cord syndrome include tumors (such as an ependymoma or astrocytoma) which can arise from *within* the spinal cord.

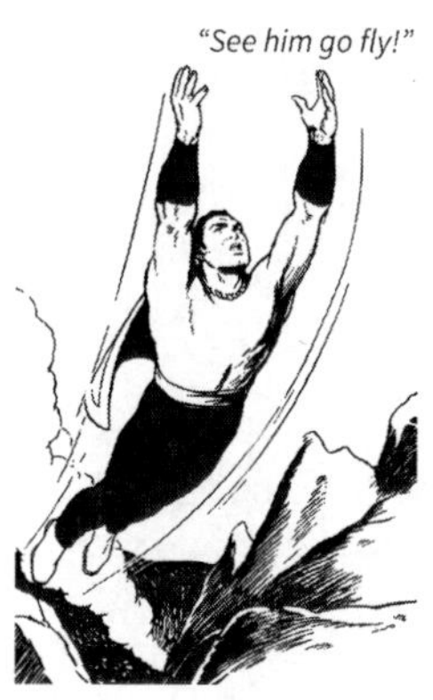
"See him go fly!"

Another potential cause of central cord syndrome that is frequently tested is **syringomyelia**, a condition in which a fluid-filled cavity (known as a syrinx) forms within the spinal cord. The classic presentation of syringomyelia involves **bilateral weakness** as well as **crude touch, pain, and temperature numbness** in the chest, back, and upper arms (often referred to as a "**cape-like distribution**"). This is due to the cyst forming from the cerebrospinal fluid-filled central canal and impinging upon the anterior white commissure and spinothalamic tract. (This also explains why fine touch, vibration, and proprioception are spared, as these travel in the dorsal columns.) Protopathic sensation in the lower extremities is not affected, as these neurons travel more laterally in the spinothalamic tract than those coming from the upper extremities. You can remember to associate syringomyelia and a cape-like distribution by renaming it to **"see-him-go-fly"-lia**. This should put the image of a **flying superhero** with a **cape** into your mind when you hear the word!

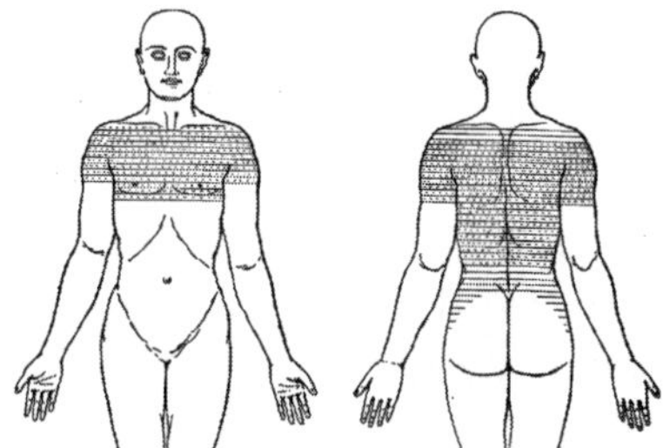

***Syringomyelia** causes weakness and numbness in a "**cape-like distribution.**"*

Syringomyelia typically presents as a **bilateral weakness** and **crude touch, pain, and temperature numbness** in a **cape-like distribution**.

"See-him-go-fly"-lia:
*Visualize a **flying superhero** wearing a **cape**!*

SUBACUTE COMBINED DEGENERATION OF THE SPINAL CORD

Subacute combined degeneration is a condition in which the myelinated tracts of the spinal cord (the dorsal columns and the corticospinal tract) slowly lose their myelin, leading to **poor balance and falling** (due to demyelination of the dorsal columns) and **muscle weakness** in the arms and legs (due to demyelination of the corticospinal tract). Because the nerves in the spinothalamic tract are already unmyelinated by default, crude touch, pain, and temperature sensation remains intact. The most common cause of subacute combined degeneration is a **deficiency of vitamin B_{12}** which you can remember by thinking that a lack of B**12** leads to damage in not ***1*** but ***2*** areas of the spinal cord!

Subacute combined degeneration of the spinal cord results in **demyelination** of both the **dorsal columns** and **corticospinal tract**, with sparing of the spinothalamic tract. **Vitamin B_{12} deficiency** is a common cause.

*Lack of vitamin B**12** leads to not **1** but **2** forms of spinal cord injury!*

CAUDA EQUINA SYNDROME

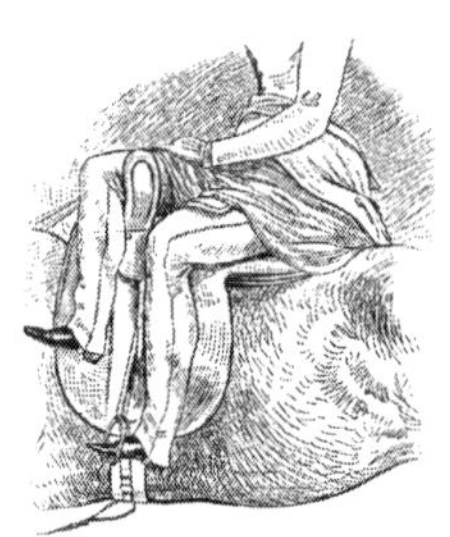

While intuitively it would make sense that the nerves coming out of the cauda equina (the "horse's tail" at the lowest end of the spinal cord) would go to the lowest part of the body (the feet), in reality these nerves instead travel to the pubic and anal areas. (We'll go over the reasons for this in the next chapter!) For this reason, **cauda equina syndrome** leads to deficits in both motor and sensory function in the **pelvic region**, including loss of bowel and bladder control, muscle paralysis and hyporeflexia in the lower body, and numbness around the perineum (sometimes called **"saddle anesthesia"** because the numbness is in the same area that would be in contact with a horse's saddle). It's not hard to use a little bit of mental imagery to connect an injury in the **horse**'s tail with a **saddle** distribution.

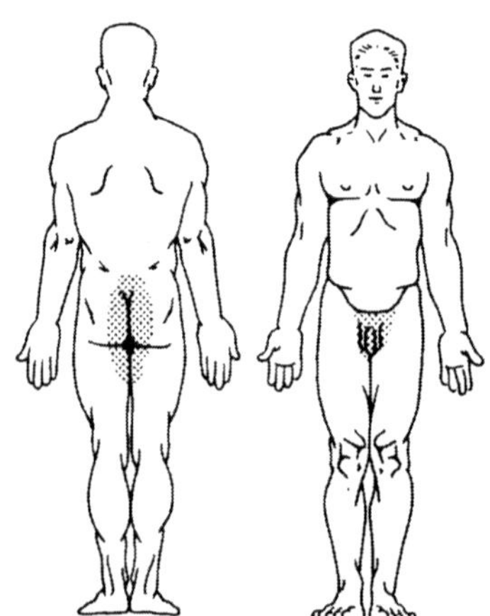

*"**Saddle anesthesia**" as seen in cases of **cauda equina syndrome**.*

An injury to the **cauda equina** leads to **bowel and bladder incontinence**, **muscle paralysis** in the lower body, and **saddle anesthesia**.

*Connect the **horse**'s tail (cauda equina) with numbness in a **saddle** distribution.*

PUTTING IT ALL TOGETHER

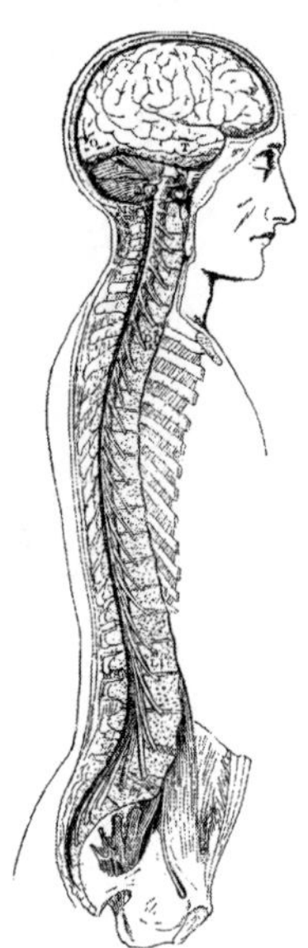

And with that, it's time to exit the central nervous system and head for the peripheral nervous system! Before we go, let's review each of the three pathways we have covered in this chapter: the **dorsal column—medial lemniscus pathway** (large myelinated epicritic neurons carrying fine touch, vibration, and proprioception), the **spinothalamic tract** (small unmyelinated protopathic neurons carrying crude touch, temperature, and pain), and finally the **corticospinal tract** (large myelinated motor neurons carrying motor signals from the brain).

For the dorsal column—medial lemniscus pathway, the phrase "**D**iscover **N**ew **D**irections for **M**oving **V**ibration & **P**roprioception" will help you remember that these nerves first travel in the **D**orsal columns (with information from the legs in the gracile fasciculus and information from the arms in the cuneate fasciculus). Next, they synapse in the **N**ucleus gracilis and nucleus cuneatus within the medulla before **D**ecussating (crossing over). They then travel in the **M**edial lemniscus before synapsing in the **V**entral posterolateral nucleus of the thalamus before finally reaching their destination in the **P**arietal cortex.

For the spinothalamic tract, the phrase "**L**ist **S**ome **P**roper **A**venues for **S**ending **T**emperature and **P**ain" can remind you that protopathic neurons first enter via **L**issauer's tract, often going up or down a level or two before synapsing in the **S**ubstantia gelatinosa or nucleus **P**roprius. These neurons then cross over in the **A**nterior white commissure before traveling in the **S**pinothalamic tract in the lateral spinal cord. They then synapse again in the ventral posterolateral nucleus of the **T**halamus before traveling on to the **P**arietal cortex.

Finally, for the corticospinal tract, the phrase "**F**lexing **I**nvolves **P**yramids, **C**ords, and **H**orns" will allow you to recall that motor neurons originating in the **F**rontal cortex first pass through the posterior lib of the **I**nternal capsule and then into the brainstem before crossing over in the **P**yramidal decussation within the medulla. They then continue on in the spinal cord as the **C**orticospinal tract before synapsing on an interneuron entirely within the spinal cord which itself synapses onto the third and final neuron in the Anterior **H**orn. This lower motor neuron then exits the spinal cord on its anterior aspect and completes its journey to the muscle as a spinal nerve.

Make sure you know each of these pathways down cold before moving on!

REVIEW QUESTIONS

1. A 78 y/o M makes an appointment to see a doctor. He reports no significant medical history. On exam, the doctor notices that his ability to sense the position of his toes with his eyes closed is impaired. He does not detect a vibrating tuning fork when it is applied to his feet. Which of the following pathways is most likely damaged?
    A. Gracile fasciculus
    B. Cuneate fasciculus
    C. Spinothalamic tract
    D. Posterolateral (Lissauer's) tract
    E. Lateral corticospinal tract
    F. Anterior corticospinal tract

2. A 52 y/o F comes to the hospital after sustaining second-degree burns on her right hand. While cooking dinner, she did not notice that her hand was touching a pot of boiling water. On exam, she is noted to have absent pain and temperature sensation in both arms as well as the back and shoulders, with motor weakness in a similar distribution. Pain and temperature sensation is normal throughout the lower extremities. Vibration and proprioception are intact throughout as well. Magnetic resonance imaging reveals the following image:

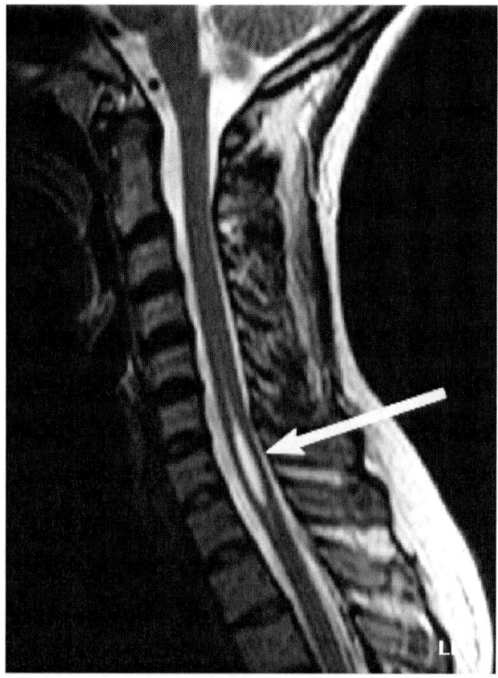

Which region of the spinal cord has most likely been affected?

A. Anterior
B. Posterior
C. Center
D. Periphery
E. Left
F. Right

3. A 27 y/o F is brought to the hospital for a neurological evaluation. She is noted to have significant motor weakness in both her right arm and right leg, with an inability to make a fist with her right hand or raise her right foot off of the ground. Sensory exam is notable for loss of fine touch and vibration on the right side, with loss of pain and temperature on the left. Which of the following is the most likely event that precipitated this presentation?
   A. Sudden onset following a focal bacterial infection
   B. Slow onset due to a nutritional deficit
   C. Rapid onset following significant blood loss during childbirth
   D. Onset at birth due to a genetic mutation
   E. Immediate onset following complete transection of the spinal cord during a motor vehicle accident

1. **The best answer is A.** The gracile fasciculus is the part of the dorsal columns that carries sensory information about fine touch, vibration, and proprioception from the lower extremities to the brain. While the cuneate fasciculus also carries this information, it connects to the upper extremities, not the lower (answer B). The spinothalamic tract and posterolateral tract both carry crude touch, pain, and temperature sensation (answers C and D), while the lateral and anterior corticospinal tract carry motor signals to voluntary skeletal muscles (answers E and F).

2. **The best answer is C.** This patient's loss of motor strength and protopathic sensation occurs in a cape-like distribution which combined with the intact epicritic sensation should make you think of syringomyelia. Syringomyelia is often caused by a cyst forming in the central canal of the spinal cord, which is why the dorsal columns on the periphery are generally spared (answer D). While anterior spinal cord syndrome involves the same combination of deficits as syringomyelia (motor weakness with intact epicritic sensation), the cape-like distribution helps to differentiate this, as an anterior cord syndrome would instead show these deficits below the level of the lesion in the lower extremities but not the upper (answer A). The intact epicritic sensation effectively rules out posterior cord syndrome (answer B). A spinal injury on either the right or left side would present as Brown-Séquard syndrome (answers E and F).

3. **The best answer is A.** This vignette describes a case of Brown-Séquard syndrome in which one-half of the spinal cord (either the right or left side) is injured. This results in a characteristic combination of ipsilateral motor weakness, ipsilateral loss of epicritic sensation, and contralateral loss of protopathic sensation. While Brown-Séquard syndrome is most classically associated with stab injuries to the back, it can occur as a result of any lesion that affects one side of the spinal cord over the other (in the case of this vignette, a focal bacterial abscess that is located in only one side of the spinal cord). Systemic causes of spinal cord damage such as nutritional deficits (answer B), shock (answer C), and genetic diseases (answer D) would be expected to affect both sides of the spinal cord equally. Complete transection of the spinal cord would result in bilateral loss of all movement and sensation in areas below the lesion (answer E).

9 THE PERIPHERAL NERVOUS SYSTEM

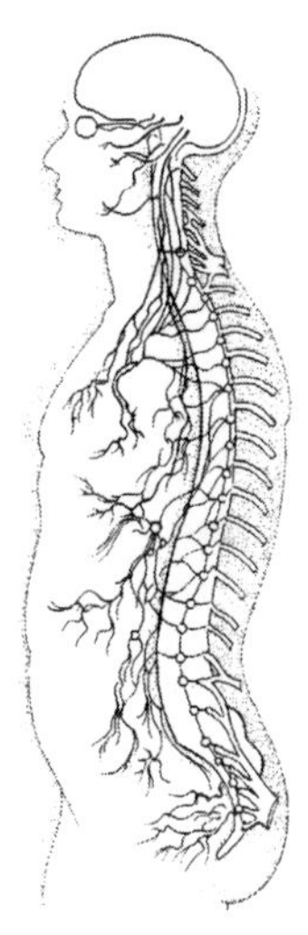

If the brain is the capital city and the spinal cord is the highway coming out of it, then the **peripheral nervous system** consists of the many side streets connecting the highway to the cities and towns scattered across the countryside. Peripheral nerves attach to the organs of the body directly and help to both receive sensory information (via afferent neurons) and transmit motor impulses (via efferent neurons). As a reminder from Chapter 2, the efferent division of the peripheral nervous system is further divided into the **somatic nervous system**, which innervates skeletal muscles to exert voluntary control over movement, and the **autonomic nervous system**, which exerts unconscious control over various muscles and glands via two opposing systems: the **sympathetic nervous system** (which kicks in the "fight or flight" response) and the **parasympathetic** nervous system (which activates when it is time to "feed and breed, then rest and digest"). If any of this feels unfamiliar to you, take a few moments to review Chapter 2!

In this chapter, we will take our understanding of the peripheral nervous system to the next level by looking not only at the organization of the system as a whole but also at some of the individual nerves within it, including the twelve **cranial nerves** that branch off of the brain to supply the structures of the face, neck, and shoulders as well as the **spinal nerves** that emerge from the spinal cord to supply the rest of the body. We will not necessarily talk about *every single peripheral nerve in the entire body*, as there are so many of them that this would require a whole book on its own! Instead, we will go into enough detail so that you are able to understand what happens on a clinical level when diseases of the peripheral nervous system arise.

CRANIAL NERVES

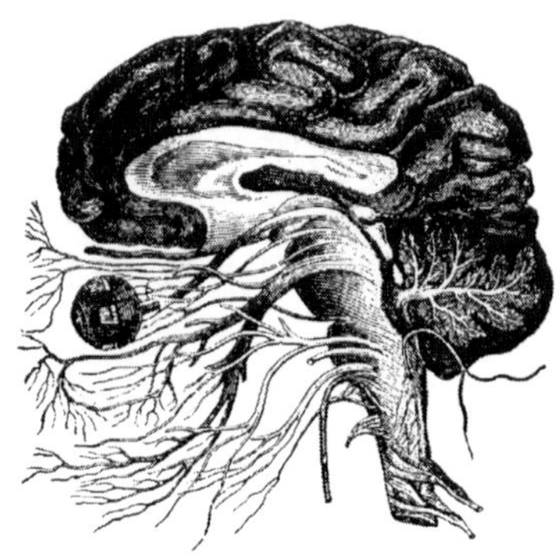

The **cranial nerves** are a collection of 12 peripheral nerves which branch directly off of the brain rather than from the spinal cord like the rest of the peripheral nervous system. (Technically speaking there are *24* cranial nerves as each one comes in a pair! However, for the sake of simplicity we will refer to each of them in the singular.) Recall from Chapter 7 that the cranial nerves follow a "Rule of 4," with the first 4 coming out of the brain and midbrain, the middle 4 exiting from the pons, and the last 4 branching off of the medulla.

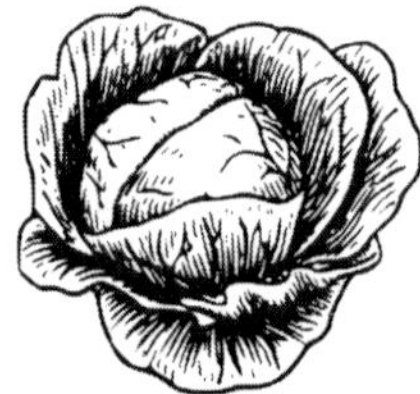

The cranial nerves are frequently tested in clinical settings, as various forms of dysfunction in these nerves can indicate specific types of diseases. In addition, they are frequently tested on board exams, so make sure to learn them well! A variety of mnemonics exist to help you memorize them. We'll go with, "**O**oh, **O**oh, **O**oh, **T**o **T**ouch **A**nd **F**eel **V**ery **G**reen **V**egetables, **AH**!" to remember the cranial nerves in order:

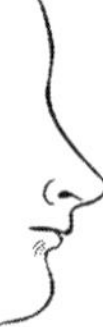

O is for Olfactory. The **olfactory nerve** is a **sensory** nerve that carries information about **smell**. Unlike most other sensory nerves, the olfactory nerve does *not* pass through the thalamus before going to the cortex but rather goes to parts of the cerebral cortex and subcortex directly (which may explain why our response to smells tends to be much more immediate and emotional compared to other sensory modalities).

O is for Optic. The **optic nerve** is a **sensory** nerve that is responsible for **eyesight**. Like the olfactory nerve, it branches off of the brain directly (rather than the brainstem). We will cover the process by which light entering the eyes is converted into a conscious visual image in more detail in Chapter 10.

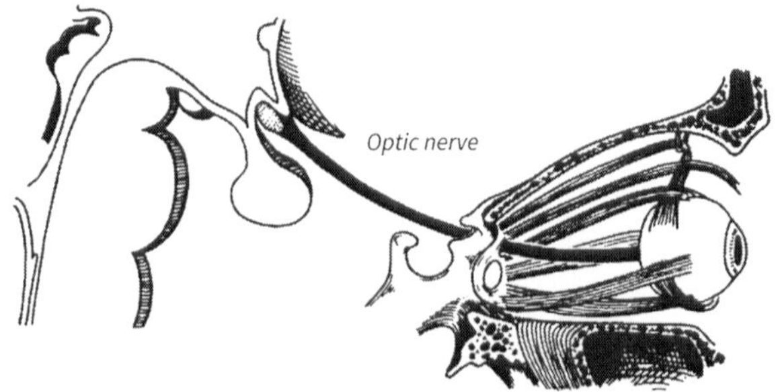

*The **optic nerve** connecting the eye to the brain.*

O is for Oculomotor. The **oculomotor nerve** is a **motor** nerve that branches off of the midbrain. It is one of three cranial nerves that are responsible for **eye movement** (the other two being the trochlear nerve and the abducens nerve). Together, these nerves control the six **extraocular muscles** as seen below:

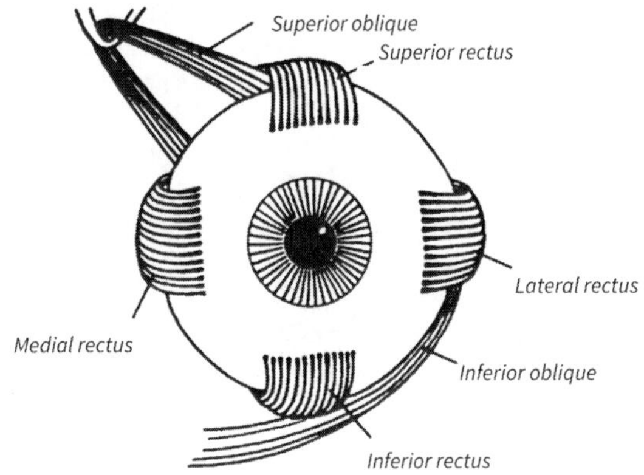

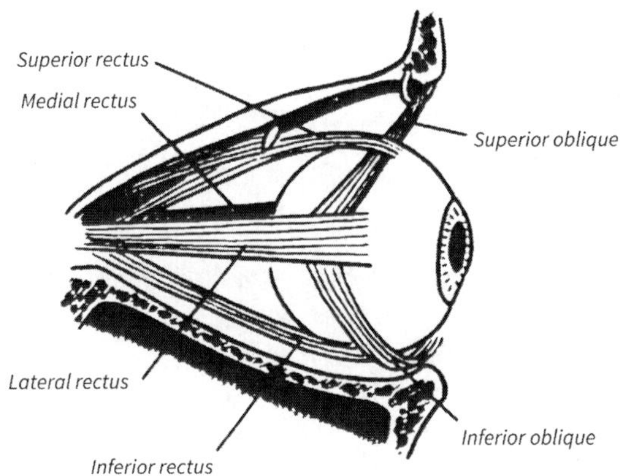

The oculomotor nerve innervates four out of these six muscles, making it by far the biggest contributor to extraocular movement. This nerve also contains the nerve fibers going to the **pupillary sphincter** (which constricts the pupils to change the amount of light entering the eye) as well as those going to the **ciliary muscle** (which changes the shape of the lens to allow the eye to focus on nearby objects), making it a powerful contributor to multiple functions in the eyes.

T is for Trochlear. The **trochlear nerve** is a **motor** nerve that controls the **superior oblique** muscle which is responsible for moving the eyes at a downward medial angle. Interestingly, the superior oblique exists as a "pulley" system of sorts (as seen on the image above) which is why it pulls the eye at an angle rather than in a simple left-right or up-down direction.

T is for Trigeminal. The **trigeminal nerve** is a **mixed** nerve that contains both motor and sensory neurons. It carries sensory information from the **face** as well as controls the muscles responsible for **chewing**. The trigeminal nerve splits into three branches: the **ophthalmic nerve** (which carries sensation from the upper third of the face), the **maxillary nerve** (which carries sensation from the middle third of the face), and the **mandibular nerve** (which not only carries sensation from the lower third of the face but also exerts motor control over chewing).

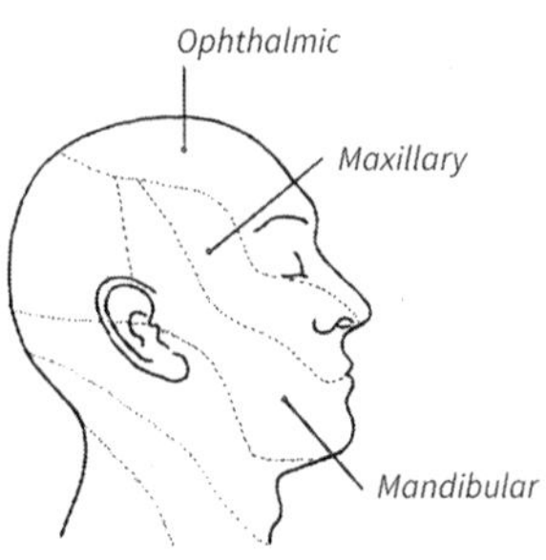

A is for Abducens. The **abducens nerve** is a **motor** nerve that is the third and final nerve responsible for extraocular movements. It controls the **lateral rectus** muscle that makes the eye look outward towards the ears (rather than inward towards the nose). You can remember which cranial nerves move which extraocular muscles by thinking of the phrase **LR_6SO_4** which, despite being nonsense, has a strange way of sticking in the brain.

The **trochlear nerve** supplies the **superior oblique**, the **abducens nerve** supplies the **lateral rectus**, and the **oculomotor nerve** supplies the rest.

***LR_6SO_4**: **L**ateral **R**ectus is the **6**th cranial nerve, **S**uperior **O**blique is the **4**th cranial nerve.*

F is for Facial. The **facial nerve** is a **mixed** nerve that splits into several branches as it progresses, with the temporal, zygomatic, buccal, mandibular, and cervical branches each traveling to various regions controlling the muscles of **facial expression** from the forehead down to the chin. The facial nerve also carries sensory information about **taste** from the anterior **two-thirds** of the tongue. Finally, a branch of the facial nerve travels to the **stapedius**, a small muscle (in fact, the *smallest* one in the body!) that helps to stabilize and reduce the noise traveling on the stapes bone in the inner ear.

Dysfunction of the facial nerve is known as **Bell's palsy**. Bell's palsy presents with a loss of motor ability on one side of the face resulting in facial asymmetry. A change in the ability to taste and an increased volume of auditory sensations (known as **hyperacusis**) may both occur as well given the facial nerve's role in taste sensation and noise reduction. You can remember the definition of **Bell**'s palsy by linking it to the clinical finding of lost **Bell**-lateral (bilateral) face symmetry!

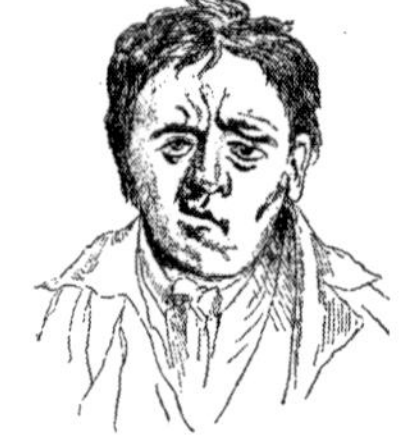

Bell's palsy is a form of **facial nerve dysfunction** that results in **unilateral loss of facial movement**, changes in **taste sensation**, and **hyperacusis**.

***Bell**'s palsy shows up as a loss of **Bell**-lateral (bilateral) face symmetry!*

V is for Vestibulocochlear. The **vestibulocochlear nerve** is a **sensory** nerve that carries two different types of sensory information from the inner ear. It splits into two main divisions: the **cochlear nerve** (which carries information about **sound** from the cochlea) and the **vestibular nerve** (which carries information about **balance and spatial orientation** from the vestibular system).

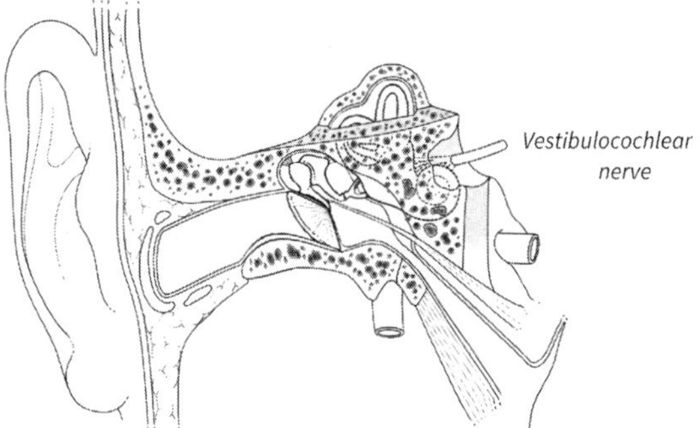

G is for Glossopharyngeal. The **glossopharyngeal nerve** is a **mixed** nerve, although its sensory functions far outweigh its motor roles, as it innervates only a single muscle (the stylopharyngeus, which assists in **swallowing**). Its primary responsibility is to convey sensory information from the **inside of the mouth** as well as **taste** from the **posterior third of the tongue** (remember that the facial nerve covers taste from the anterior two-thirds!). One of its keys roles is to detect the presence of objects in the mouth that shouldn't be there and to initiate the **gag reflex** (the motor component of which is carried out by the vagus nerve, discussed next).

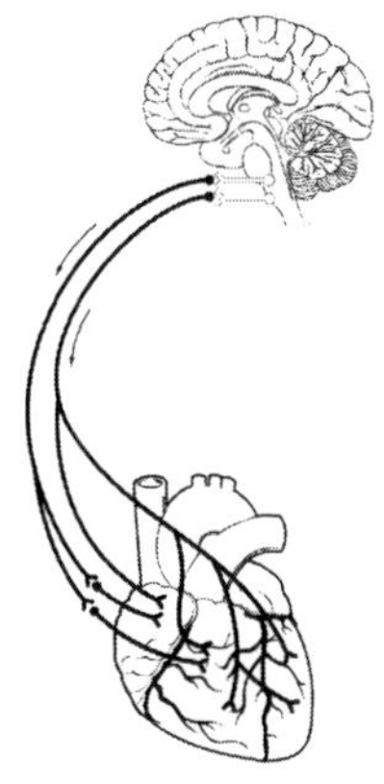

V is for Vagus. The **vagus nerve** is a **mixed** nerve that innervates various muscles of the head and neck, including those used for **speaking** and **swallowing** as well as the motor component of the **gag reflex**. Unlike most cranial nerves, however, the **vagus nerve** doesn't involve itself *only* with the head and neck but instead travels across the **entire body** to innervate various organs including the heart, lungs, and gastrointestinal tract. (In fact, the only major organ that *doesn't* receive signals from branches of the vagus nerve in some way is the adrenal gland!) The vagus nerve is responsible for delivering **parasympathetic output** to these organs, putting them in a state where they support "feeding and breeding, then resting and digesting." The vagus nerve also regulates **vital signs** such as heart rate and blood pressure through its parasympathetic effects. Finally, the vagus nerve relays **sensory signals** from these organs back to the brain. Overall, the vagus nerve is a hugely important nerve given its widespread effects throughout the body! You can remember its core functions using the word **VEGAS** (as in "Las Vegas") to remind you of this nerve's involvement in **V**ital signs, the **E**ntire body (not just the head and neck), the **G**ag reflex, **A**utonomic (parasympathetic) output, and motor control of both **S**peaking and swallowing.

The **vagus nerve** innervates not only the areas of the head and neck but also the **entire body**! It is involved in delivering **parasympathetic output**.

VEGAS:
***V**ital signs*
***E**ntire body*
***G**ag reflex*
***A**utonomic (parasympathetic)*
***S**peaking and swallowing*

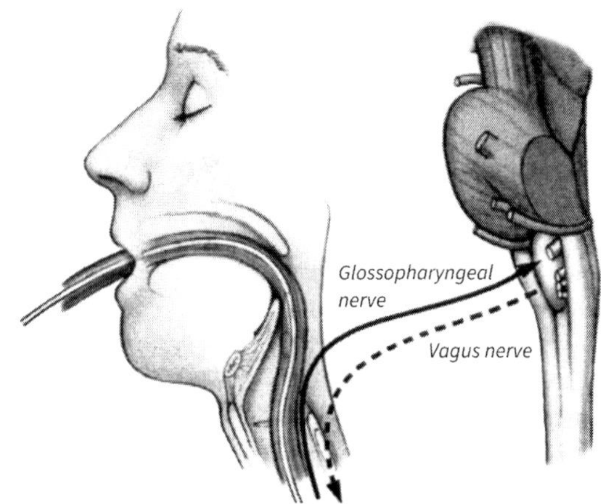

*The **glossopharyngeal nerve** (top, solid) and **vagus nerve** (bottom, dashed) enacting the **gag reflex**.*

A is for Accessory. The **accessory nerve** (also called the spinal accessory nerve) is a **motor** nerve that supplies two muscles in the neck: the **sternocleidomastoid** (which turns the head from side to side) and the **trapezius** (which shrugs the shoulders).

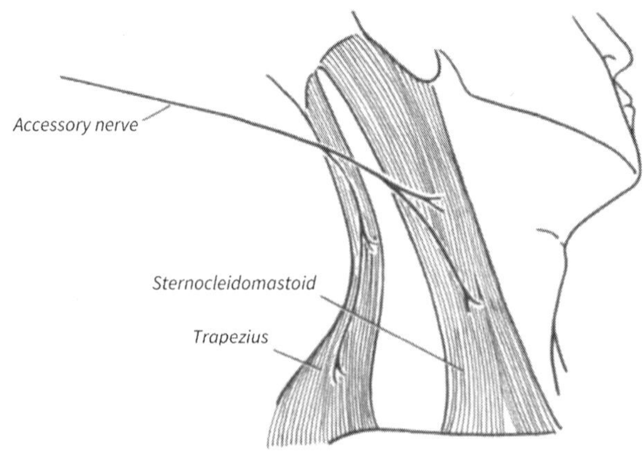

*The muscles innervated by the **accessory nerve**.*

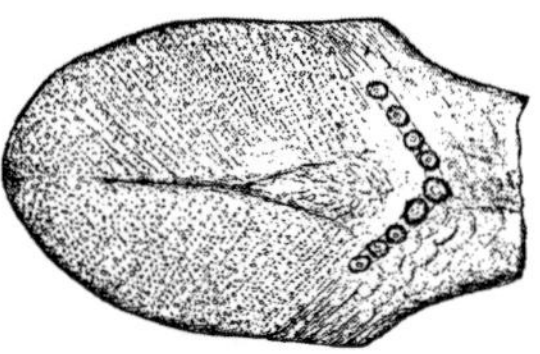

H is for Hypoglossal. Finally, the **hypoglossal nerve** is a **motor** nerve that innervates nearly all muscles involved with movement of the **tongue** (which makes sense as "glossal" comes from the Greek word for tongue). It is *not* involved in taste sensation (recall that this function is covered by the facial and glossopharyngeal nerves).

Putting it all together, it can be helpful to remind yourself of the general function of each of the cranial nerves (specifically, whether it is a sensory nerve, a motor nerve, or both). You can use the phrase "**S**ome **S**ay **M**arry **M**oney **B**ut **M**y **B**rother **S**ays **B**ig **B**rains **M**atter **M**ore" to remember the function of each nerve in order, with words beginning with **S** being **S**ensory nerves, those beginning with **M** being **M**otor nerves, and those beginning with **B** having **B**oth motor and sensory functions.

The **twelve pairs** of **cranial nerves** generally innervate the **head and neck**.

__O__oh, __O__oh, __O__oh, __T__o __T__ouch __A__nd __F__eel __V__ery __G__reen __V__egetables, __AH__!
__O__lfactory
__O__ptic
__O__culomotor
__T__rochlear
__T__rigeminal
__A__bducens
__F__acial
__V__estibulocochlear
__G__lossopharyngeal
__V__agus
__A__ccessory
__H__ypoglossal

Each **cranial nerve** is either a pure **motor**, pure **sensory**, or **mixed** nerve.

__S__ome __S__ay __M__arry __M__oney __B__ut __M__y __B__rother __S__ays __B__ig __B__rains __M__atter __M__ore:
__S__ensory (olfactory)
__S__ensory (optic)
__M__otor (oculomotor)
__M__otor (trochlear)
__B__oth (trigeminal)
__M__otor (abducens)
__B__oth (facial)
__S__ensory (vestibulocochlear)
__B__oth (glossopharyngeal)
__B__oth (vagus)
__M__otor (accessory)
__M__otor (hypoglossal)

SPINAL NERVES

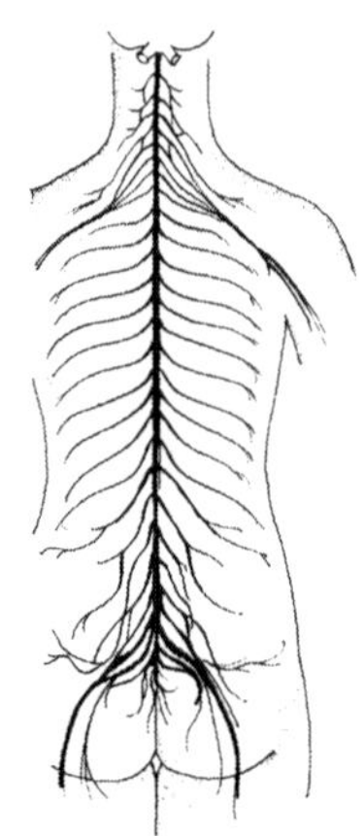

As the central nervous system exits from the skull and becomes the spinal cord, it continues to shoot off nerves supplying the rest of the body. These paired nerves are known as **spinal nerves** and are **mixed** nerves containing both sensory and motor neurons. Spinal nerves are named according to the region of the spine they come from, with 8 pairs of **cervical nerves**, 12 pairs of **thoracic nerves**, 5 pairs of **lumbar nerves**, 5 pairs of **sacral nerves**, and 1 pair of **coccygeal nerves**. These spinal nerves emerge from the vertebral column in between two vertebrae. Just to make things confusing, all spinal nerves are named for the vertebra *above* where they exit *except* for cervical nerves 1 through 7 (this is because there is no vertebra above C1, as it exits between the first vertebra and the skull). Each region of the spine sends out nerves to specific parts of the body, with the cervical nerves innervating the **neck**, upper **chest**, and **upper limbs**; the thoracic nerves innervating the **trunk** and **back**; the lumbar nerves innervating the **upper legs** and **buttocks**; the sacral nerves innervating the **hips**, **thighs**, **legs**, and **feet**; and the single pair of coccygeal nerves innervating the skin on the back of the **coccyx**.

When learning about each set of spinal nerves, we'll be paying particular attention to its sensory and motor functions. Recall from Chapter 2 that the specific area of the skin innervated by a particular spinal nerve is known as its **dermatome**. The specific dermatome of each spinal nerve is shown in the drawing below:

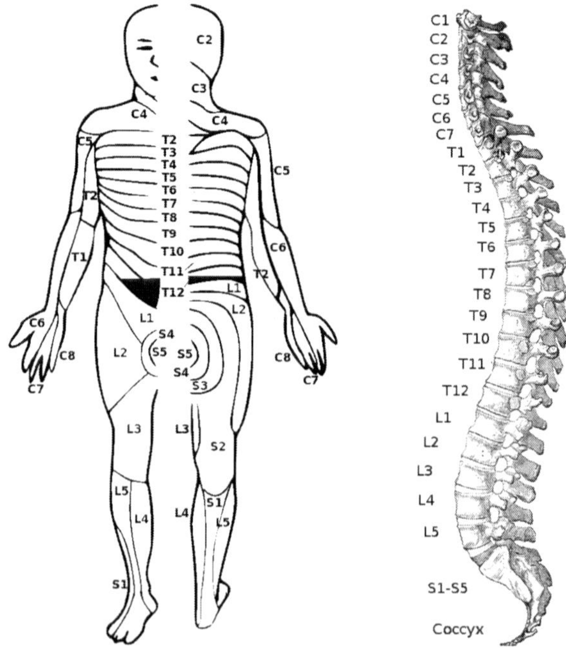

Dermatomes *associated with each spinal nerve.*

When looking at the dermatomes, they initially seem to make sense, with the first few cervical dermatomes proceeding in an orderly fashion down the neck. However, things quickly begin to break down. Why do C5 and C6 innervate the *lateral* portions of the arm while C8 and T1 innervate the *medial* parts? Why does L1 cover the skin over the buttocks, but the genitals and anus aren't covered until the sacral nerves? Why is the area covered by S2 (the back of the legs) *higher up* than what is covered by S1 (the foot)? If you try to apply the order of the dermatomes to a human in a standing position, it won't make sense. However, if you instead put them in a *bent over* position (as if they were a dog or a cat), things start to come together a little more! Suddenly it's clear why the lateral arm is innervated by higher spinal nerves (it's closer to the head) or why the anus is innervated by lower spinal nerves compared to the legs (it's farther back). When trying to memorize dermatomes, always bend the patient forward!

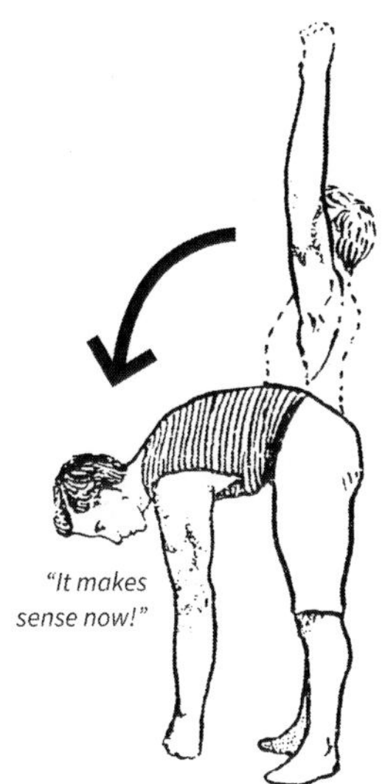

Dermatomes are the specific **area of skin** innervated by each spinal nerve. They are organized based on a **quadrupedal position**.

Visualize someone ***bending over*** *to pick up a heavy (derma)****tome*** *off the floor!*

Each spinal nerve is also responsible for innervating specific groups of muscles which are known as its **myotome**. Knowing the myotome for each spinal nerve can help to localize injuries to the spinal cord or to specific nerves branching off of it (as we will discover throughout the rest of this chapter).

When learning about spinal nerves, it's important to know that the dermatome and myotome for a particular spinal nerve do not necessarily overlap, as a muscle may be innervated by a completely different spinal nerve than the skin overlying it! For example, the spinal nerve C6 innervates the biceps muscle in the upper arm as part of its *myo*tome but its *derma*tome covers the hand. Don't get confused on this point!

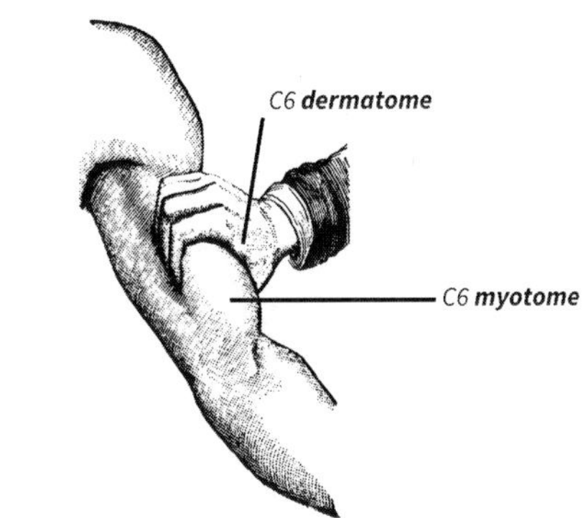

The ***dermatome*** *and* ***myotome*** *of spinal nerve C6.*

CERVICAL NERVES

Now that we've introduced some broad themes about spinal nerves, let's look at each region in more detail, starting with the cervical nerves. The 8 pairs of cervical nerves emerge from the spinal cord in the neck and form **two networks** of nerves.

The first is known as the **cervical plexus** and is made up of the first four nerves (C1-C4). Nerves from the cervical plexus innervate the skin over the **back of the head** as well as the **muscles of the neck**. For this reason, injuries to the neck can result in sensory deficits in the back of the head as well as motor weakness in the neck.

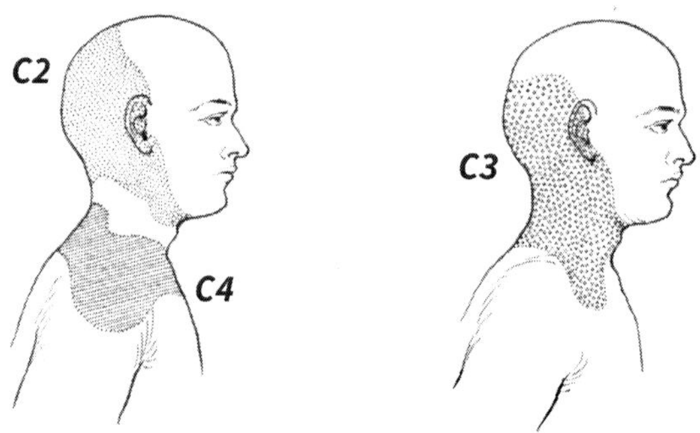

***Dermatomes** of the **cervical plexus**.*

The second network arising from cervical nerves (specifically C5-C8) is known as the **brachial plexus** and lies in the deep tissue between the neck and the armpit. Nerves from the brachial plexus innervate the **shoulders, arms, and hands**. For this reason, damage to these cervical nerves can produce numbness in the hands and arms as well as muscle weakness in the elbow, forearm, wrist, and fingers.

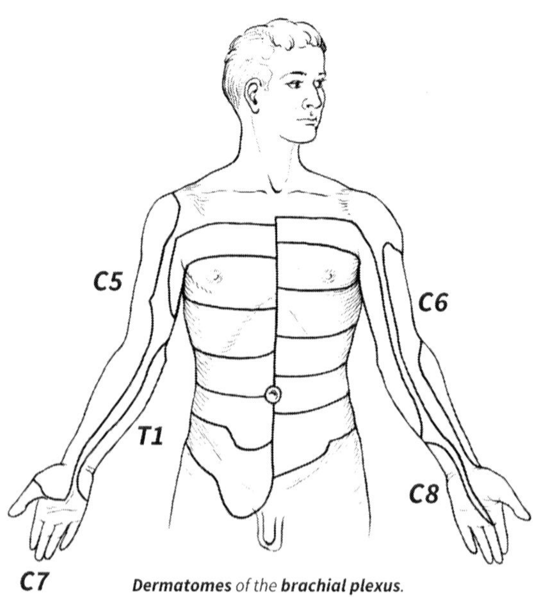

***Dermatomes** of the **brachial plexus**.*

Damage to the brachial plexus can produce several characteristic motor deficits on exam. One common finding is **wrist drop** or an inability to extend the hand at the wrist. This is commonly (though not always) due to dysfunction in C7 or its branches, including the **radial nerve**. Another finding known as a **winged scapula** can occur due to damage of the **long thoracic nerve** which branches off of C5, 6, and 7 and travels to the **serratus anterior muscle**. Damage to the nerve can lead to an unnatural protrusion of the shoulder blade, especially when raising the arms.

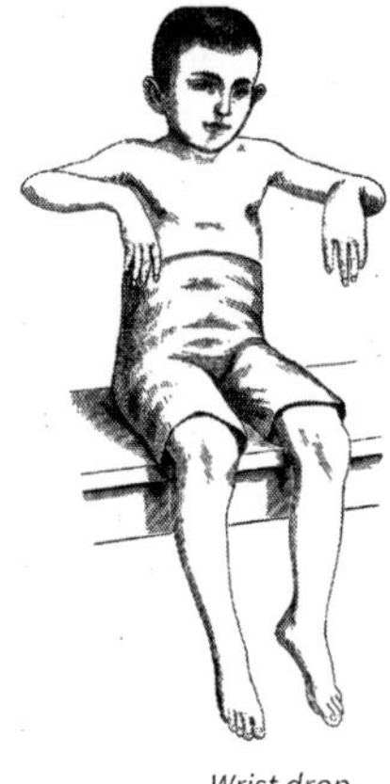

Wrist drop

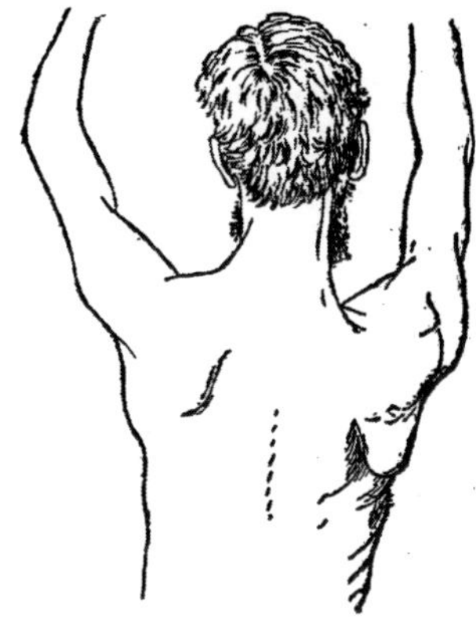

Winged scapula

Finally, nerves from both the cervical and brachial plexuses (specifically C3-C5) innervate the **diaphragm** or the large flat muscle that helps to bring air into the lungs. Damage to these nerves can compromise respiratory function. You can remember this using the rhyme, "C3, 4, and 5 keep the diaphragm alive."

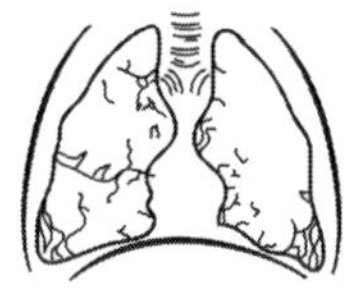

The **third through fifth cervical nerves** innervate the **diaphragm**.

C3, 4, and 5 *keep the* ***diaphragm*** *alive.*

THORACIC NERVES

The 12 pairs of thoracic nerves run between the ribs and are known as **intercostal nerves** (except for the last thoracic nerve which runs *under* the last rib, earning it the name **subcostal nerve**). The thoracic nerves supply the regions of the **chest** and **upper back**. You can remember the general distribution of dermatomes by keeping in mind a few landmarks. For example, if you know that **T4** innervates the skin near the nipples ("T4 does the **teat pore**") and **T10** innervates the skin around the umbilicus ("T10 does the belly but-**TEN**"), you can estimate approximately which thoracic nerve is involved in an injury resulting in pain or numbness in any region between them.

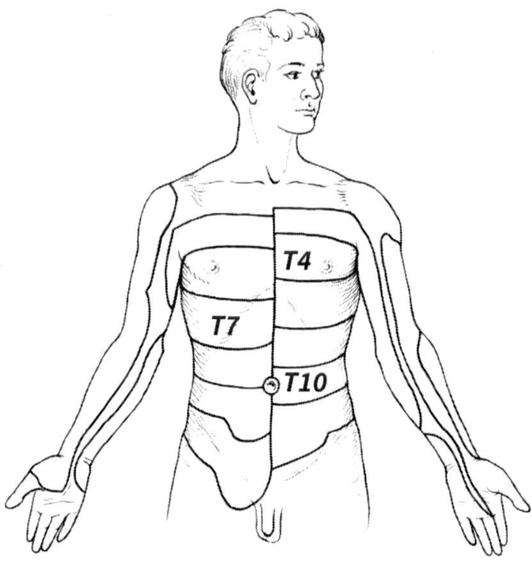

***Dermatomes** of some **thoracic nerves**.*

Dermatomal landmarks include the **nipple (T4)** and the **umbilicus (T10)**.

***T4** does the **teat pore**, while **T10** does the belly but-**TEN**.*

LUMBAR NERVES

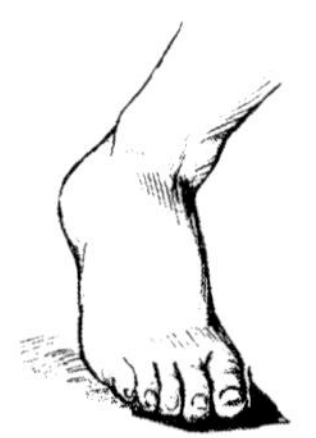

The 5 pairs of lumbar nerves generally cover the **lower back**, **outer buttocks**, and **front of the legs**. Like the cervical nerves, the lumbar nerves have a tendency to form mesh-like networks. The first few pairs form the **lumbar plexus** which innervates the muscles of the **thigh**, while the latter pairs combine with sacral nerves from the next vertebral region to form the **lumbosacral trunk** which innervates the skin and muscles of the **buttocks and pelvis**. Lumbar nerves also innervate the muscles of the lower **leg and foot**, which is why damage to this region (and in particular the L5 nerve root) can result in **foot drop**.

There are a few helpful dermatomal landmarks to remember here. One is that **L1** helps to innervate the skin over the **Inguinal Ligament** or the band that helps form the "V" leading from the abdomen to the pubic region. The other is that **L4** helps to innervate the thigh leading down to the **knee**, which you can remember by thinking that L4 is activated when you get down on **all fours** (L4s).

Dermatomal landmarks in the **lumbar region** include the **inguinal ligament (L1)** and the **knee (L4)**.

***L1** does the **1**nguinal **L**igament, while **L4** is for when you get down on **all fours** (L4s).*

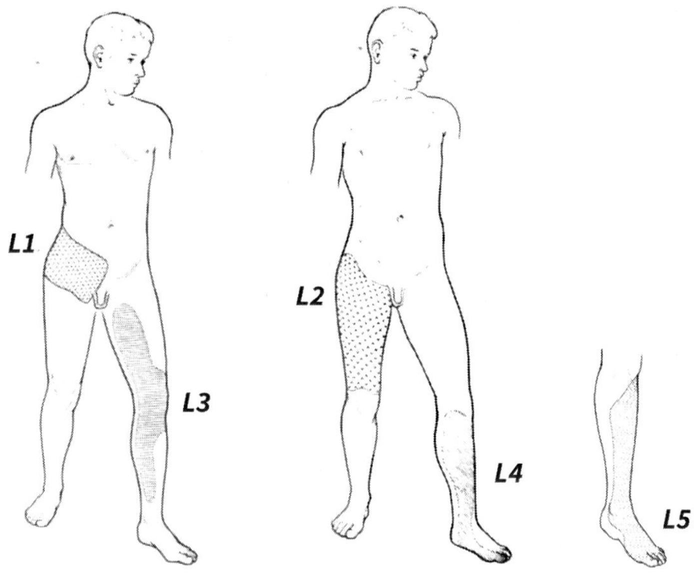

***Dermatomes** of the **lumbar nerves**.*

SACRAL NERVES

The 5 pairs of sacral nerves form a **sacral plexus** which goes on to supply the muscles of the **hip**, **thigh**, **leg**, and **foot** as well as innervate the skin on the **back of the leg** and the **anogenital** region. The **pudendal nerve** arises from S2, S3, and S4 and gives parasympathetic input to the gastrointestinal, urinary, and reproductive systems. You can remember the significance of S2 through S4 by using the rhyme, "S2, 3, and 4 let the urine hit the floor" (or the alternative, "S2, 3, and 4 keep the penis off the floor").

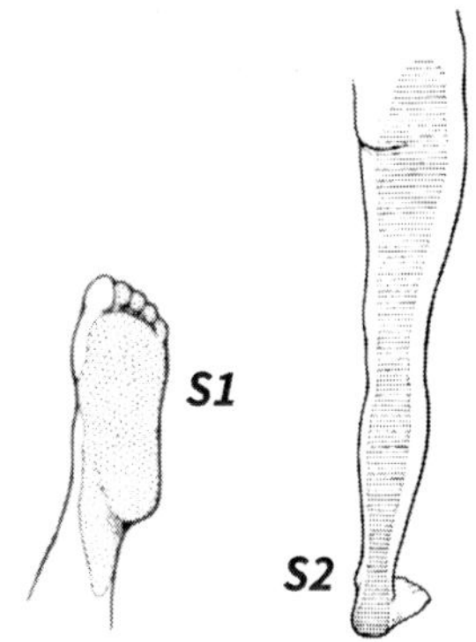

***Dermatomes** of some **sacral nerves**.*

COCCYGEAL NERVE

Finally, the single pair of coccygeal nerves arises from the conus medullaris and helps to provide sensation to the skin over the **coccyx**.

THE SYMPATHETIC TRUNK

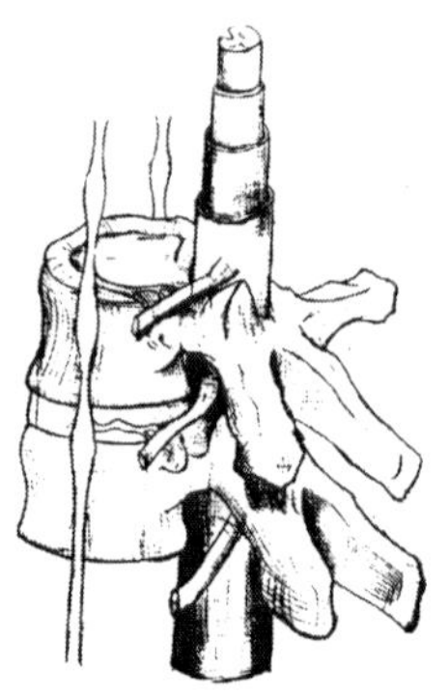

Before we finish off this chapter, let's talk about one last part of the peripheral nervous system known as the **sympathetic trunk**. Unlike the *para*sympathetic nervous system which largely works through just a few nerves in the cranial and sacral regions (like the vagus and pudendal nerves), the sympathetic nervous system is instead spread out across a bundle of nerve fibers that runs alongside the vertebral column for most of its length (although it is most pronounced in the **thoracic** and **lumbar** regions). Because the sympathetic trunk provides sympathetic activation to the entire body, some nerve fibers will actually shoot *upwards* from the thorax to return to the muscles of the *face*!

This becomes clinically important when trying to determine the source of dysfunction in the sympathetic nervous system. One high-yield condition you must be able to recognize promptly is **Horner's syndrome**. When the upper part of the sympathetic trunk becomes damaged, it causes a set of findings in the face including constricted pupils (**miosis**), a lack of sweating (**anhydrosis**), and a drooping eyelid (**ptosis**). (Why is the eyelid involved? The superior tarsal muscle responsible for raising the upper eyelid receives its innervation not only from the facial nerve but from the sympathetic nervous system as well.)

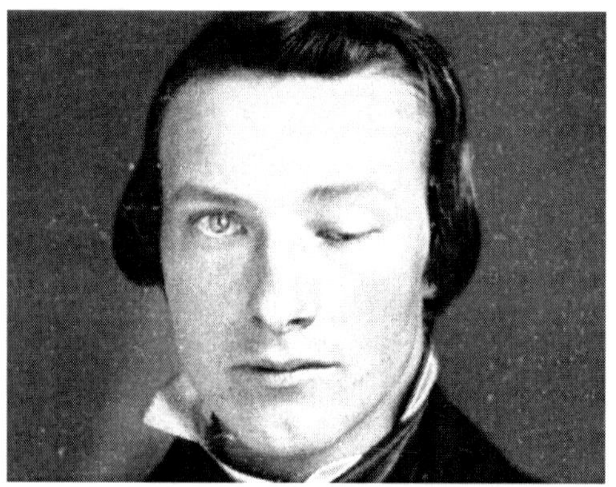

A case of ***ptosis*** *related to* ***Horner's syndrome****.*

Horner's syndrome can be caused by any lesion that interferes with normal functioning in the sympathetic nervous system, and we will return to it a few times throughout this book. For now, just remember h**O**rner's syndrome by thinking of **Sympa** Claus saying, "H**O** h**O** h**O**!" This should remind you of pt**O**sis, mi**O**sis, and anhydr**O**sis as well as the **sympa**thetic nervous system.

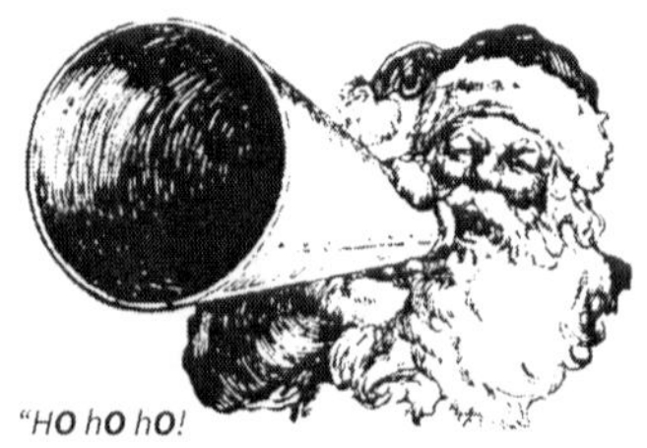

*"H**O** h**O** h**O**!*
*Pt**O**sis, mi**O**sis, anhydr**O**sis!"*

Horner's syndrome is a combination of **ptosis**, **miosis**, and **anhydrosis** caused by damage to the **sympathetic trunk**.

***Sympa** Claus says, "H**O** h**O** h**O**!" (pt**O**sis, mi**O**sis, and anhydr**O**sis).*

The location of the sympathetic trunk in the thoracic region explains why lesions in the chest can lead to sympathetic dysfunction. Another high-yield condition to learn is a **Pancoast tumor** which is an abnormal growth in the uppermost part of the lung that leads to Horner's syndrome. Initially it can seem strange to learn this ("Why does a *lung* tumor lead to issues in the *face*?"), but now that we know that the sympathetic trunk arises from the thoracic and lumbar regions (with some fibers turning around to head back up to the face), it makes much more sense. You can remember this diagnosis by making an acronym out of **PANCOAST**: a **P**ulmonary **A**pex **N**eoplasm **C**ausing **O**'s (ptOsis, miOsis, and anhydrOsis) **A**ttributable to the **S**ympathetic **T**runk.

A **Pancoast tumor** is a **tumor in the lungs** that compresses the **sympathetic trunk**, leading to **Horner's syndrome**.

***PANCOAST**:*
*A **P**ulmonary **A**pex **N**eoplasm **C**ausing **O**'s **A**ttributable to the **S**ympathetic **T**runk.*

PUTTING IT ALL TOGETHER

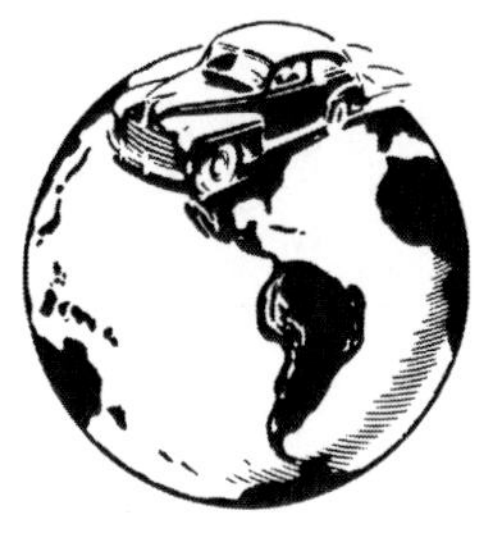

Peripheral nerves are tricky to learn, but perhaps this should come as no surprise! If they are truly the "side streets" of the nervous system, then trying to memorize them would be like trying to learn the roadmap of an entire country. Like side streets, peripheral nerves don't just proceed in an orderly fashion to their final destination but instead form networks, take detours, join up with (and then depart from) nerves in other regions, and generally do everything they can to resist an easy understanding.

Given this complexity, let's do what we can to keep things simple. Rather than trying to memorize each and every individual nerve (which would be as pointless as memorizing each street on a map), instead try to learn as much about the peripheral nervous system as is **reasonable**. There are 12 cranial nerves, each of which serve an important function, so this is a realistic amount to memorize! For the 31 spinal nerves, however, there are too many to possibly keep track of, so it's enough to remember them in terms of general **regions** (perhaps memorizing a few landmarks like T4 and T10 that will help to orient you when working with patients). Do your best not to get bogged down by the overwhelming amount of information! For now, just know the specific functions of each cranial nerve and the general mapping of dermatomes and myotomes covered by each spinal region, and we will fill in additional details as we go.

REVIEW QUESTIONS

1. A 54 y/o M with no prior medical history is referred to a neurologist after he notices increasing weakness in his legs, with pain and cramping if he walks for more than a few minutes. He recently has had several episodes where he has the sensation of "choking" while trying to swallow food. After a thorough evaluation he is diagnosed with amyotrophic lateral sclerosis, a disease that selectively causes degeneration of motor neurons. Which of the following nerves is *least* likely to be affected by this disease?
    A. Trigeminal nerve
    B. Facial nerve
    C. Vestibulocochlear nerve
    D. Glossopharyngeal nerve
    E. Hypoglossal nerve

2. A 27 y/o M sees a sports medicine specialist after he notices increasing weakness of his right wrist over the past week. He is a professional body builder and is distraught about the prospect of missing his normal workout routine as a result of this deficit. On exam, he is unable to extend his wrist as seen below:

    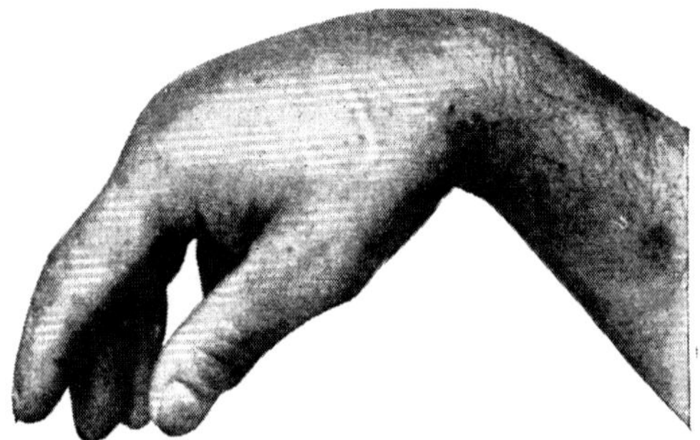

    Physical examination shows atrophy of muscles in the forearm and hand, with preservation of the triceps. Which of the following regions is most likely to show signs of numbness on further examination?
    A. Neck
    B. Arm
    C. Forearm
    D. Hand
    E. Chest

3. A 51 y/o M sees his primary care doctor complaining of pain in his left shoulder and arm. He first noticed it one month ago, but it has slowly gotten worse since that time. He reports numbness and tingling in his left forearm and fingers. His only other symptom is a persistent cough which he attributes to smoking one pack of cigarettes every day for the past 30 years. He is diagnosed with musculoskeletal pain and sent home with instructions to rest his shoulder. One

week later, he presents to the emergency department of the hospital believing he is having a stroke. Vital signs are HR 118, BP 146/90, RR 28, and T 100.1°F. His oxygen saturation is decreased to 84%. A chest x-ray is obtained:

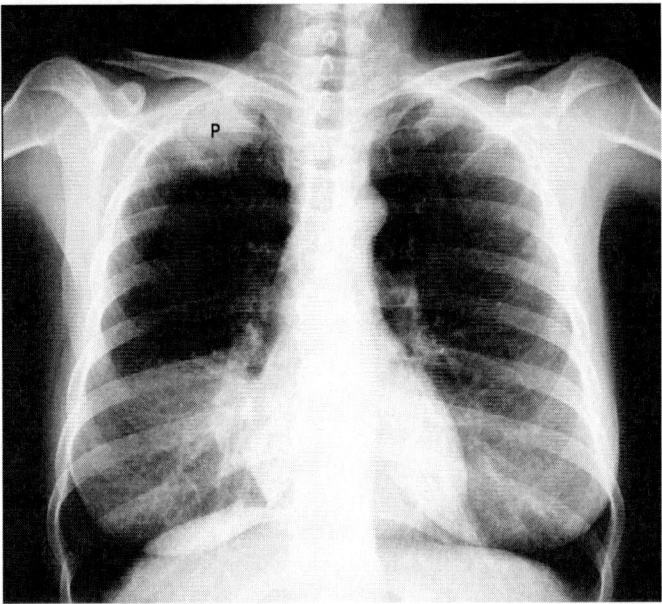

Upon further work-up, he is diagnosed with an apical lung tumor that has spread to the preganglionic neurons ascending to the cervical sympathetic chain. Which of the following signs and symptoms is *least* likely to be seen in this patient?

A. Weakness of the muscles of chewing
B. Unequal diameter of the left and right pupils
C. Asymmetry of muscles innervated by the facial nerve
D. Changes in facial sweat production
E. All of the following are equally likely to be seen

4. A 58 y/o F comes to see her neurologist for a follow-up appointment. She has had difficulty speaking and vocal hoarseness which is related to dysfunction of her vagus nerve. Which of the following regions of the brain connects to the vagus nerve and is most likely implicated in her symptoms?

A. Broca's area
B. Wernicke's area
C. The cerebellum
D. The inferior colliculi
E. The nucleus ambiguus

1. **The best answer is C.** Given that amyotrophic lateral sclerosis only affects motor neurons, any nerves that do not have a motor component will not be affected. Out of the listed cranial nerves, all but one have a motor component and are therefore candidates for being affected by amyotrophic lateral sclerosis, with the trigeminal nerve (answer A) controlling the muscles of chewing, the facial nerve (answer B) controlling the muscles of facial expression, the glossopharyngeal nerve (answer D) controlling swallowing muscles, and the hypoglossal nerve (answer E) controlling the tongue muscles. In contrast, the vestibulocochlear nerve has only a sensory component.

2. **The best answer is D.** Damage to C7, either at its root or in one of the nerves that it contributes to, is a potential cause of wrist drop as most of the muscles of wrist extension originate at this level. The sensory dermatome of C7 includes the hands. The neck is generally C3 and C4 (answer A), the arm and forearm is C5 and C6 (answers B and C), and the chest gets into thoracic territory (answer E).

3. **The best answer is A.** This vignette describes a case of Horner's syndrome related to a Pancoast tumor. A Pancoast tumor is a form of lung cancer that develops in the apex of the lung. Some of the neurons traveling through the lung apices ascend in the cervical sympathetic chain to return to the face. For this reason, a tumor in this location can lead to the specific facial abnormalities seen in Horner's syndrome, including ptosis (answer C), miosis (answer B), and anhydrosis (answer D). The muscles involved in chewing are not directly innervated by the sympathetic nervous system.

4. **The best answer is E.** The vagus nerve branches off from the medulla which also houses the nucleus ambiguus, a region of the brain involved in speech. Broca's area is also involved in speech, but it is not in the medulla (answer A). Wernicke's area is involved in speech comprehension, not production (answer B). The cerebellum is involved in the steadiness and pitch of speech, but the vagus nerve does not branch off of it directly (answer C). Finally, the inferior colliculi are involved in sound processing, not speech production (answer D).

10 VISION

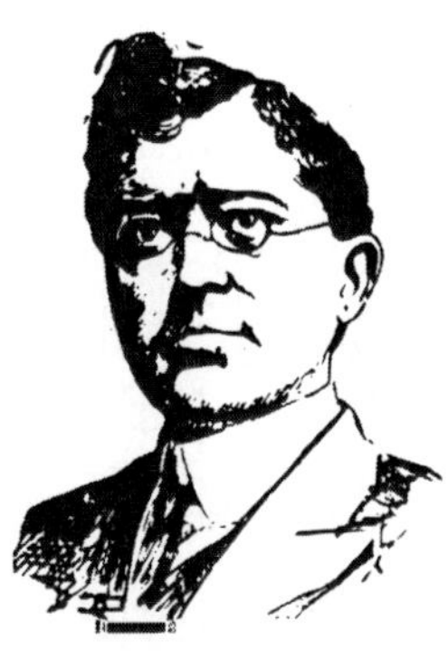

Now that we have covered both the central and peripheral nervous systems, we have the tools necessary to learn about the pathways involved in each of the **special senses**, including **vision**, **hearing**, **balance**, **taste**, and **smell**. These senses each require a specialized organ to process, which results in the ability to take in more detailed information from the outside world and convert them into rich, complex sensations such as sight or sound. Each of these senses relies upon an intricate pathway that carries the signal from the time the sense organ first picks it up to the point at which it is processed into conscious awareness in the cerebral cortex. Despite the complexity of these pathways, our task at hand is to make this process understandable, so onward we go! We will start by devoting an entire chapter to vision (as it is easily the most complex of the special senses) before moving on to talk about hearing, balance, taste, and smell in the next chapter.

Vision is the process of interpreting the patterns of light reflecting off of objects surrounding us in order to make sense of our environment. Our eyes are unique for a sense organ in that they do not just passively absorb information from the environment. Instead, they play an active role in controlling what information is available by moving in different directions, focusing on some objects rather than others, and controlling how much light enters. (While one could argue that this applies to other special senses as well, such as moving the head to better hear a sound, this process is nowhere near as complex as it is in vision.) For this reason, we will need to examine *multiple* processes (not just one) in order to understand vision. First we will talk about the **visual pathway** which carries sensory information from the eyes back to the brain, then we'll talk about the centers that control **eye movements**, and finally we will go over the nerves involved in regulating **pupillary size**.

THE EYES

Vision begins in the **eyes**. The eyes are a pair of specialized sensory organs whose primary function is to convert light from our environment into neural signals that can travel to the cortex and enter our conscious awareness. Light initially hits the **cornea** and then travels through the **lens** which focuses it onto the **retina** at the back of the eye. The retina is filled with **photoreceptor cells** that are responsible for translating light into a neural signal. These photoreceptor cells contain proteins known as **opsins** that absorb light and transmit them into neuronal signals.

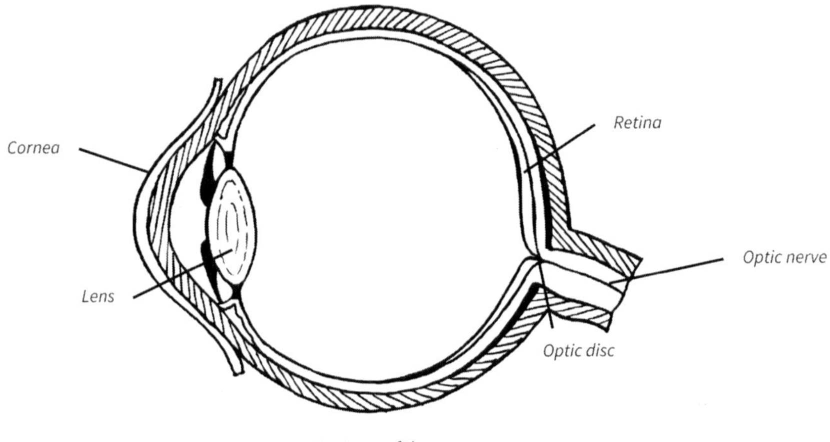

*Anatomy of the **eye**.*

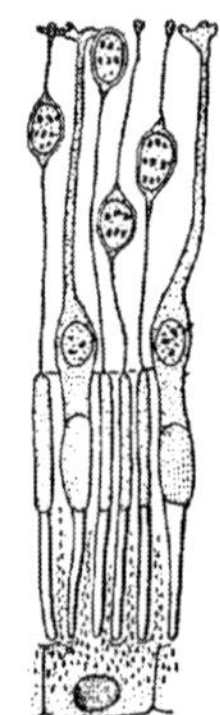

There are two main types of opsins that are involved in creating a visual image: **cones** (which can discriminate between different wavelengths to generate color) and **rods** (which cannot distinguish between different colors but are better adapted to see at low levels of light). Rods and cones are spread all across the retina, although they are highly concentrated in an area known as the **macula**. (The macula covers the center of one's vision, with damage to the macula producing a loss of central vision.) After a lot of processing, this visual information begins its journey to the brain on the second cranial nerve, also known as the **optic nerve**. (Interestingly, the point at which the optic nerve leaves the retina, known as the **optic disc**, does *not* contain photoreceptor cells and is considered a visual blind spot.)

The **retina** contains both **cones**, which are responsible for **color vision**, and **rods**, which can pick up on **lower intensity light**.

***Co**nes add **co**lor to an image.*

THE VISUAL PATHWAY

Once the optic nerve departs from the eye, the visual pathway has officially begun. (It's worth noting that the visual pathway is best understood through images, not text! Follow along with the diagram on the next page as you read.) The optic nerve first travels to the **optic chiasm** which sits just under the hypothalamus and pituitary gland. Visual information from the *medial* part of the retina **crosses over** here, while information from the *lateral* part of the retina stays on the same side. However, because the light has already crossed over once when entering the eye via the lens, the medial part of the retina actually receives light from the *lateral* visual fields.

Following the optic chiasm, visual information continues its journey via the **optic tract** which now contains visual information from *both* eyes corresponding to the *opposite* field of view (so the left optic tract contains visual information from the patient's right field of view and vice versa). The optic tract then travels to the **L**ateral **G**eniculate **N**ucleus of the thalamus (remember that this is involved in ***L**ooking* **G**ood **N**aked) before traveling further via **optic radiations** to finally reach its destination in the visual cortex of the **occipital lobe**. Of note, the optic radiations on each side are divided into halves, with the **superior division** carrying visual information from the *upper* retina (or the *lower* part of the visual field, since the image is reversed when it enters the eye) while the **inferior division** carries information from the *lower* retina (or the *upper* part of the visual field).

To remember this entire pathway, use the phrase "**2 Ch**arismatic **Tra**velers **L**ooking **G**ood **N**aked at the **Radia**nt **Oc**ean." This will remind you of the optic nerve (cranial nerve **2**), the optic **Ch**iasm, the optic **Tra**ct, the **L**ateral **G**eniculate **N**ucleus of the thalamus, the optic **Radia**tions, and finally the visual cortex in the **Oc**cipital lobe.

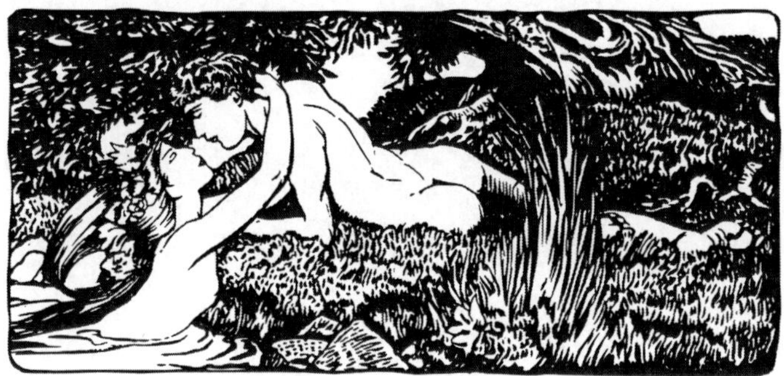

The **visual pathway** carries signals from the **retina** to the **occipital cortex**.

***2 Ch**arismatic **Tra**velers **L**ooking **G**ood **N**aked at the **Radia**nt **Oc**ean:*
*Optic nerve (cranial nerve **2**)*
*Optic **Ch**iasm*
*Optic **Tra**ct*
***L**ateral **G**eniculate **N**ucleus of the thalamus*
*Optic **Radia**tions*
***Oc**cipital cortex*

A summary of the visual pathway is found below. When learning about this pathway, refer back to this page as often as needed to make sure you have a good understanding of what is happening at each step along the way!

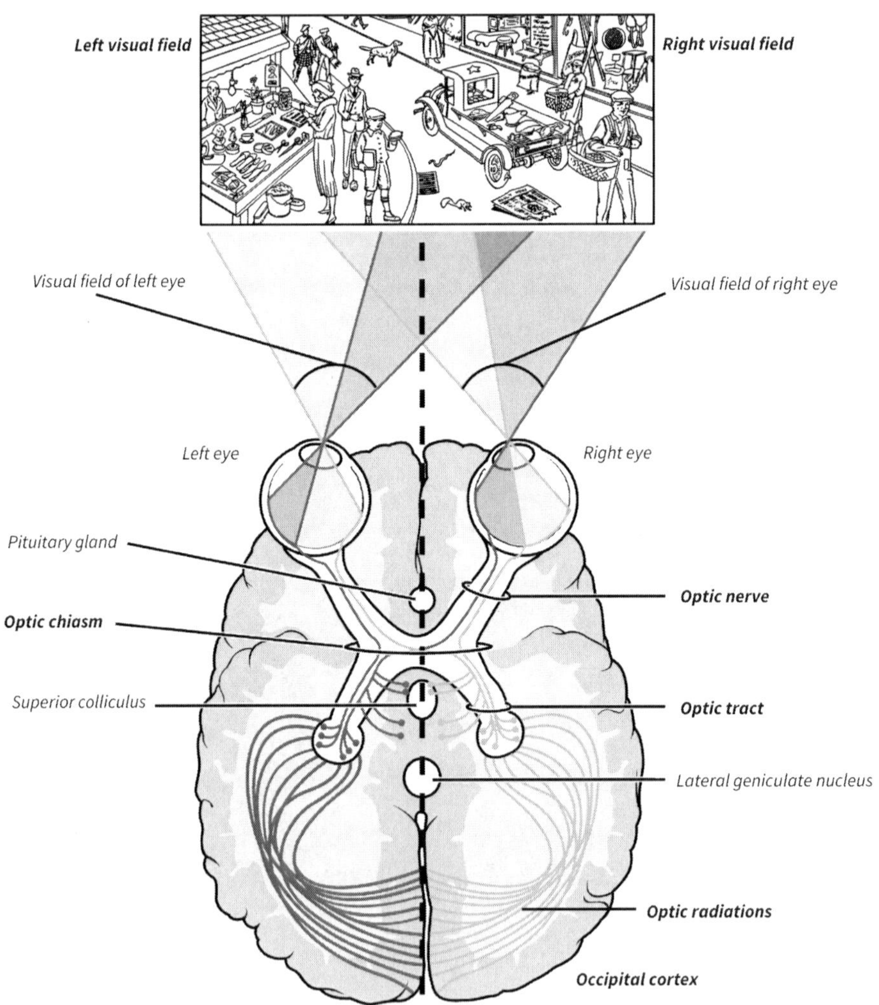

The **visual pathway**.

VISUAL FIELD DEFICITS

Because visual information travels from the retina to the occipital lobe in an organized way, we can predict how any given lesion will affect eyesight based on its precise location in the pathway. The table on the opposite page summarizes each of these changes for easy reference! Don't worry about understanding it all at first glance, as we will break it down step by step on the next few pages.

Damage to the:	... will produce:	... which looks like:
Optic nerve	Unilateral blindness	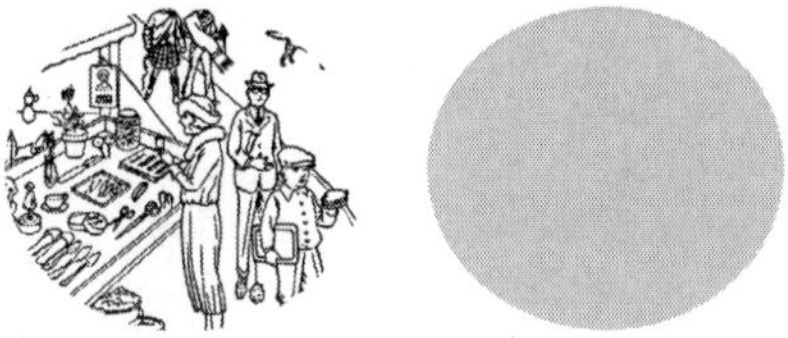
Optic chiasm	Bitemporal hemianopsia	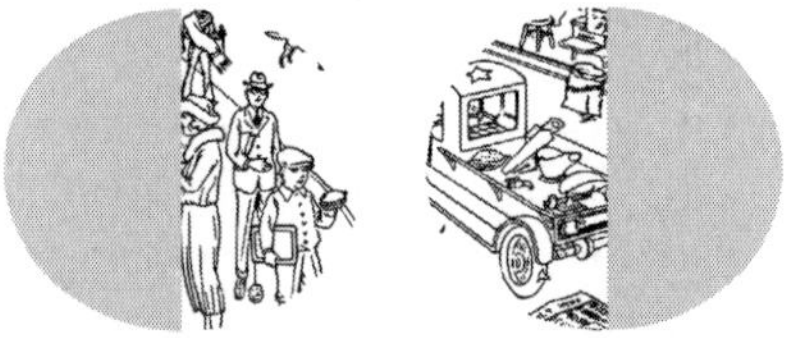
Optic tract	Homonymous hemianopsia	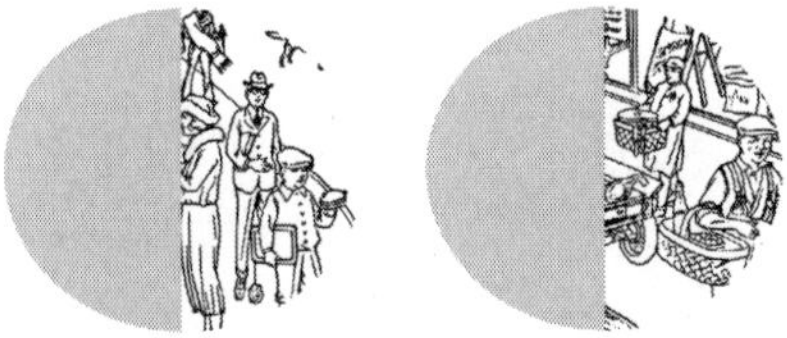
Optic radiations (superior division)	Quadrantanopsia	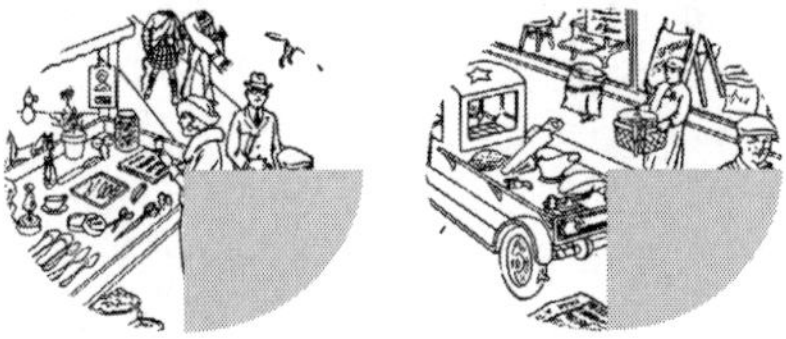
Optic radiations (inferior division)	Quadrantanopsia	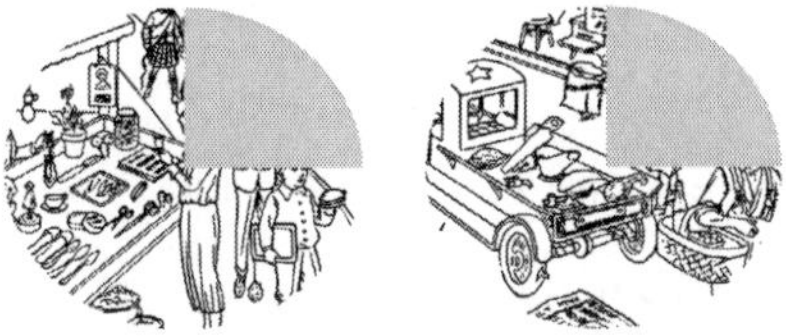
Occipital cortex	Homonymous hemianopsia with macular sparing	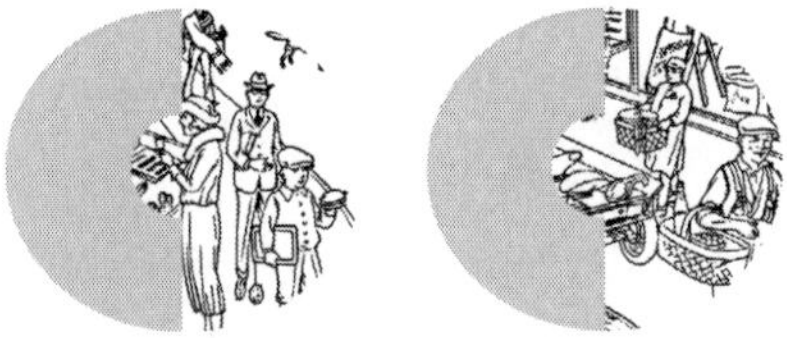

If someone has normal eyesight, they will see this:

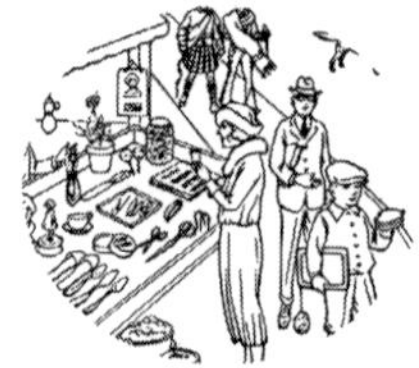
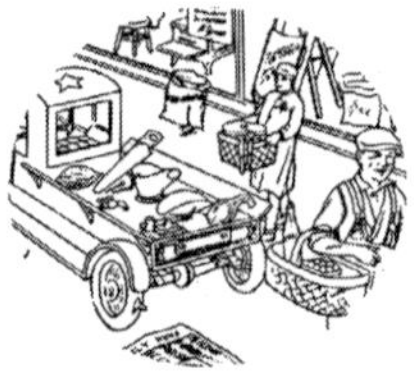

If a lesion occurs in the **optic nerve**, they will have unilateral blindness as below (note that all of these images reflect damage to the *right* side of the visual pathway):

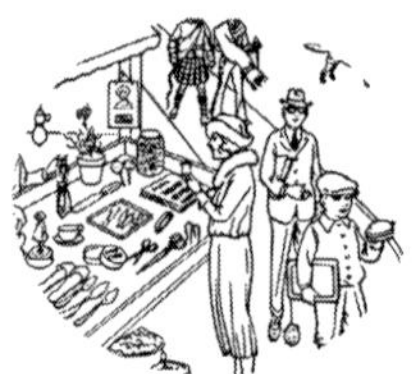

If damage occurs in the **optic chiasm**, it would instead result in **bitemporal hemianopsia** in which visual information is missing from the *lateral* fields of view (those closer to the temples of the head, which gives this condition its name):

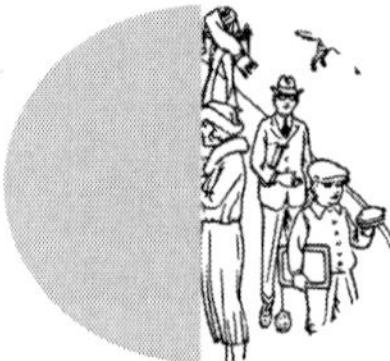
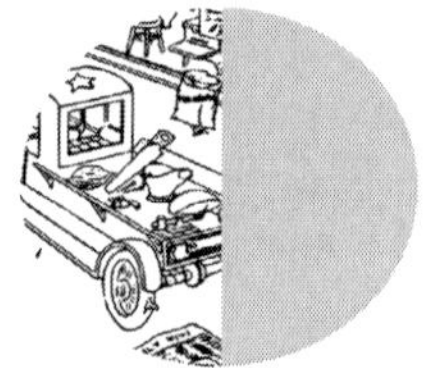

If instead the **optic tract** instead were to become damaged, a **homonymous hemianopsia** would result:

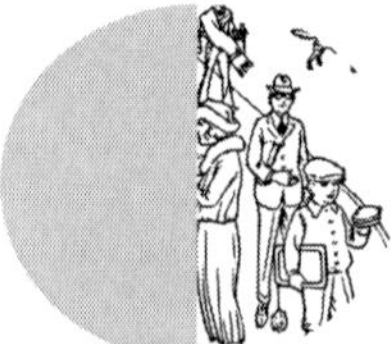
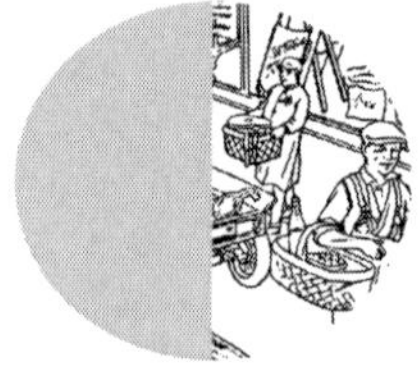

Damage to the **optic radiations** would produce **quadrantanopsia** in which a fourth of the visual field is missing. Due to various crossings, damage to the *superior* division of the right optic radiations produces a loss of *inferior* visual fields…

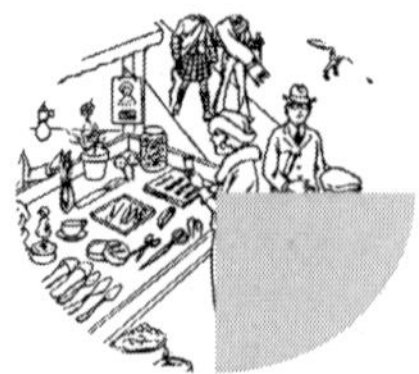
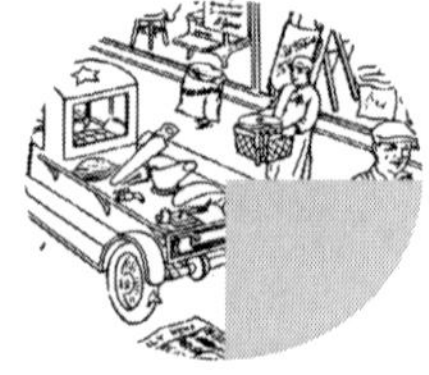

... while damage to the *inferior* division produces a loss of *superior* visual fields:

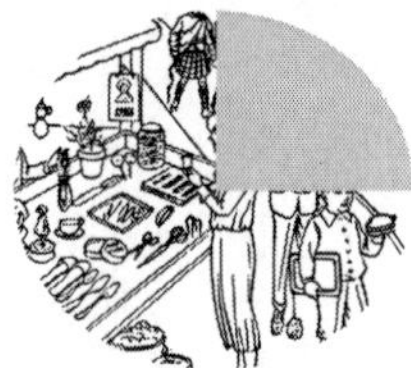
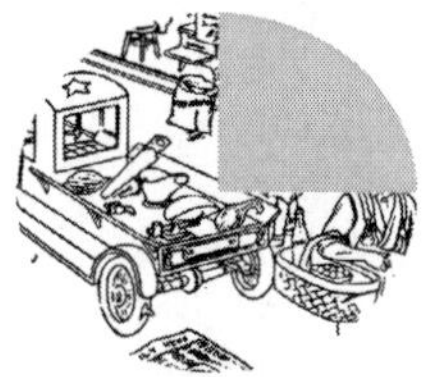

Finally, damage to the visual cortex in the occipital lobe will produce either a homonymous hemianopsia or quadrantanopsia. The key defining feature here is that the center of the visual field is preserved, a phenomenon known as **macular sparing**:

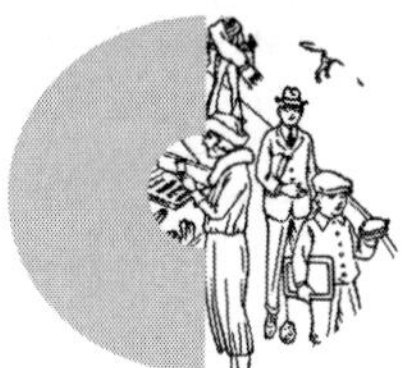
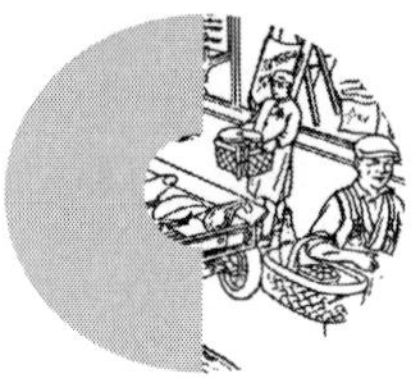

Why does macular sparing occur? The brain has lots of collateral circulation (meaning that there are many redundant arteries) which helps to prevent complete blockage of blood flow to this part of the cortex. In addition, the macula is so densely innervated that the nerve connections to this part of the brain are quite widespread, further preventing against a total black out. You can remember this by thinking that damage to the **back** (of the brain) leads to sparing of the **mac**(ula)!

Damage to the occipital cortex leads to either a homonymous hemianopsia or quadrantanopsia with **preservation of central vision** due to **macular sparing**.

*Damage to the **back** leads to sparing of the **mac**(ula)!*

BRANCHES OFF OF THE VISUAL PATHWAY

When looking at the diagram on page 120, you may notice a few branches off of the main visual pathway that that are not in the "**2 Ch**arismatic **Tra**velers **L**ooking **G**ood **N**aked at the **Radia**nt **Oc**ean" mnemonic.

The first branch goes to the **superior colliculi** (which you should recognize from Chapter 7 as a structure in the midbrain). The superior colliculi takes signals from the visual pathway and uses them to move the eyes in response to various stimuli. For example, if you see a shadowy figure out of the corner of your eye, your superior colliculi will send signals to your eyes telling them to move in that direction.

The second branch involves **melanopsin** which is a third type of photoreceptor in the retina (in addition to rods and cones). Melanopsin is activated by light which causes it to send signals first to the **pretectal olivary nucleus** and then to the **suprachiasmatic nucleus** of the hypothalamus where they set the circadian rhythm in response to environmental light. (You should remember the suprachiasmatic nucleus from Chapter 4. Remember that you need sleep to be **chiasmatic**!)

EXTRAOCULAR MOVEMENTS

As mentioned before, eyes are not passive participants in the process of vision! They actively move around to focus on whatever merits the most attention at any given moment. These extraocular movements are controlled by the three cranial nerves (the oculomotor nerve, trochlear nerve, and abducens nerve) that we talked about in the last chapter. To improve our understanding, let's see what happens when each of these nerves becomes dysfunctional.

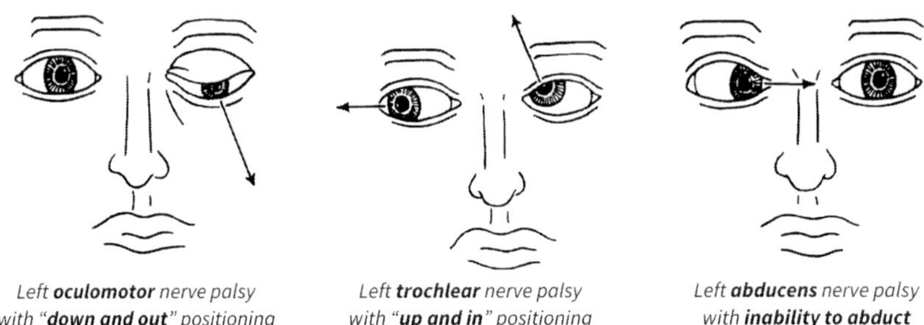

Left ***oculomotor*** *nerve palsy with "****down and out****" positioning*

Left ***trochlear*** *nerve palsy with "****up and in****" positioning*

Left ***abducens*** *nerve palsy with* ***inability to abduct***

Loss of **oculomotor nerve** function results in a "**down and out**" positioning of the eyes. This is because the two remaining extraocular muscles each are unopposed, with the lateral rectus pulling "out" and the superior oblique pulling "down."

Loss of **trochlear nerve** function leads to paralysis of the **superior oblique** muscle which normally helps to pull the eye downward at an angle, leading to an "**up and in**" positioning of the eye when asked to look inward. This may cause someone with a chronic trochlear nerve palsy to develop a compensatory head tilt as a way of using their entire head to offset the upward drift of the eye.

Finally, loss of **abducens nerve** function is probably easiest to understand, as its associated muscle (the **lateral rectus**) performs a simple function: pull the eye outwards towards the ear. For this reason, an abducens nerve palsy results in an eye that drifts inward by default and cannot be pulled outward.

THE MEDIAL LONGITUDINAL FASCICULUS

While extraocular movements can be brought under voluntary control, they also act automatically without our conscious input most of the time. This "autopilot" function for extraocular movements is largely coordinated by a structure known as the **medial longitudinal fasciculus** (MLF) that lives in the brainstem. The medial longitudinal fasciculus integrates motor signals from the frontal lobe with information about the position of the head from the inner ear in order to generate **smooth and coordinated movements** of the eyes.

Damage to the medial longitudinal fasciculus can result in a condition known as **internuclear ophthalmoplegia** (INO). To understand what this involves, let's first take a healthy patient and ask them to look left:

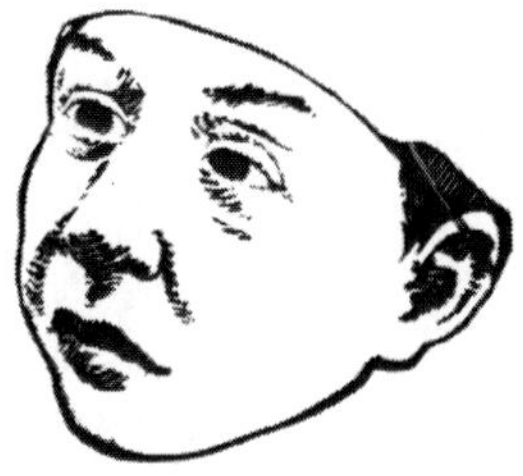

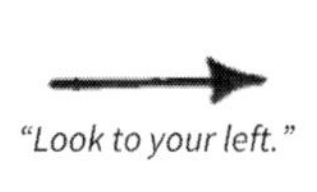

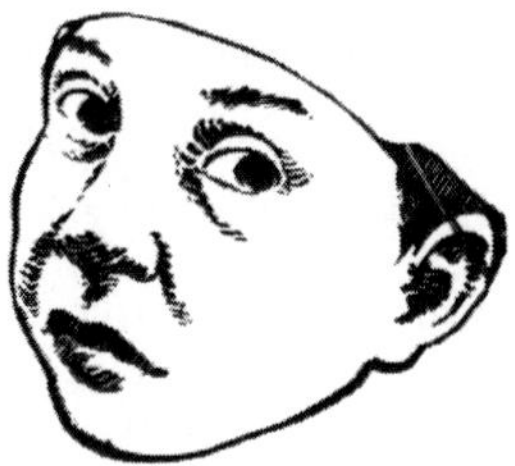

The eyes do exactly what you would expect! In contrast, if you take a patient with internuclear ophthalmoplegia and ask them to do the same thing, you'll notice a few differences. First, the eye on the same side as the lesion **cannot adduct** (look inwards towards the nose) which leads to **double vision** from the eyes looking in two different directions. Second, the eye on the *un*affected side can still look in that direction, but if you look closely you will notice a back-and-forth quivering movement known as **nystagmus** (which we covered back in Chapter 6!).

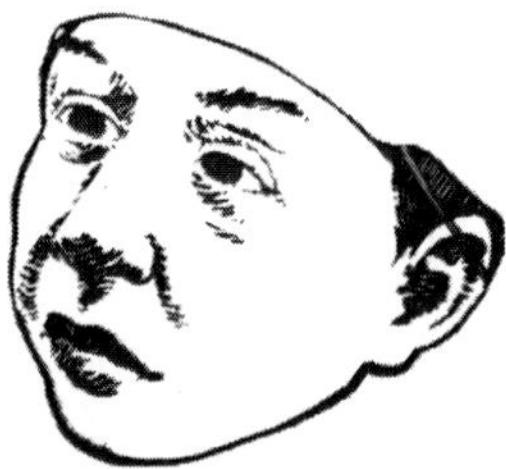

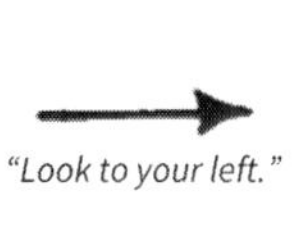

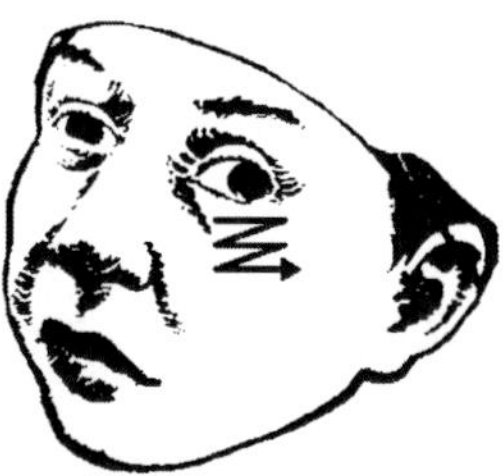

Whenever you see this particular combination of signs (an inability to adduct on one side with nystagmus on the other side), make sure you can not only connect it to dysfunction of the **M**edial **L**ongitudinal **F**asciculus but also name it as **I**nter**N**uclear **O**phthalmoplegia! Do this by repurposing the letters from **MLF** and **INO** into a new phrase the captures the clinical findings: "**M**idline **L**ook **F**ails **I**psilaterally, **N**ystagmus on **O**pposite."

Internuclear ophthalmoplegia is characterized by **ipsilateral adduction paralysis** with **contralateral nystagmus**. It is caused by damage to the **medial longitudinal fasciculus**.

*Medial **L**ongitudinal **F**asciculus + **I**nter**N**uclear **O**phthalmoplegia (**MLF** + **INO**):*
*"**M**idline **L**ook **F**ails **I**psilaterally, **N**ystagmus on **O**pposite."*

PUPILLARY REFLEXES

In addition to controlling the movement of the eyes, the body also controls how much light enters them by changing the size of the **pupil** via two pupillary reflexes.

THE PUPILLARY LIGHT REFLEX

The first of these reflexes, the **pupillary light reflex**, determines how much light enters the eye. In low light situations, the pupils will **dilate** to allow more light in (**mydriasis**). This is controlled by the **sympathetic** nervous system. In contrast, when there is *too much* light, the pupils will instead **constrict** (**miosis**) which is controlled by the ***para*sympathetic** nervous system. You can remember the difference between mydriasis and miosis because only my**D**riasis has a **D** in it to allow you to spell **D**ilate.

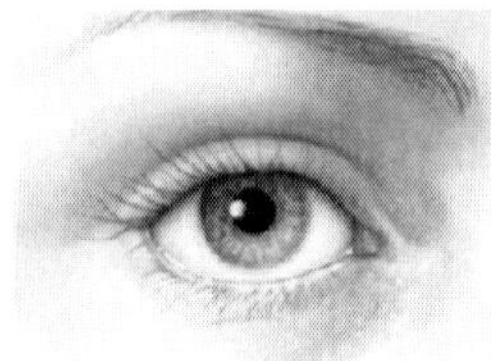

Miosis.

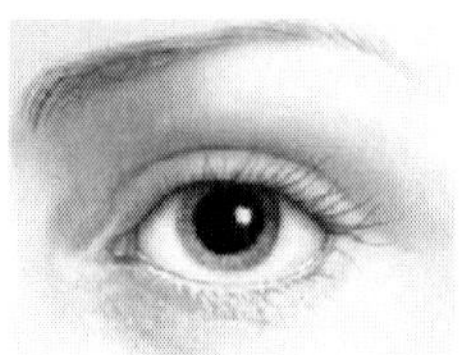

Mydriasis.

Pupil dilation (mydriasis) is controlled by the **sympathetic** nervous system, while **pupil constriction (miosis)** is controlled by the **parasympathetic** nervous system.

*Only my**D**riasis has a **D** in it to allow you to spell **D**ilation.*

You can test the pupillary light reflex by quickly shining a light into someone's eyes. This should make both pupils constrict within a few seconds. Importantly, light entering even *one* eye will cause *both* pupils to constrict!

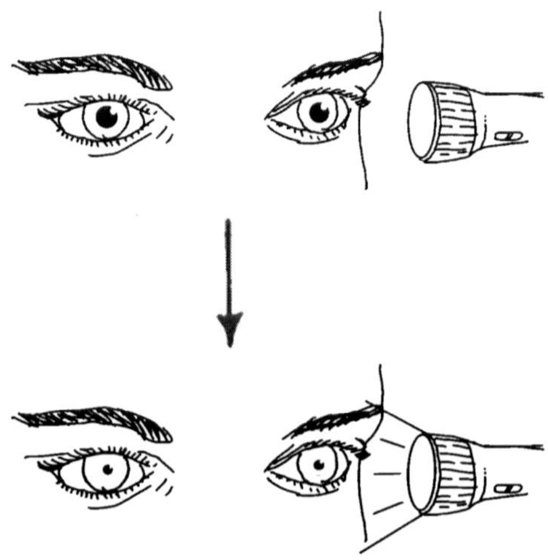

*The **pupillary light reflex**.*

An intact pupillary light reflex relies on both the afferent half (the optic nerve) and the efferent half (the oculomotor nerve) of the reflex to be intact. The reflex arc involves information from the optic nerve traveling to the **midbrain** (specifically an area known as the **pretectal nucleus**) which then sends information to the **Edinger-Westphal nuclei** (also in the midbrain) on *both* the left and the right (this is why light coming into one eye will cause both eyes to constrict). The Edinger-Westphal nuclei then sends parasympathetic signals on the oculomotor nerve which then activate the **ciliary sphincter** in the iris of the eye, causing them to contract and thereby reducing the size of the pupils. You can remember the function of the **E**dinger-**W**estphal nuclei (to constrict the pupils) by thinking of them looking at something disgusting (like a fly in your coffee) and saying, "**EW**! I don't want to look at that..."

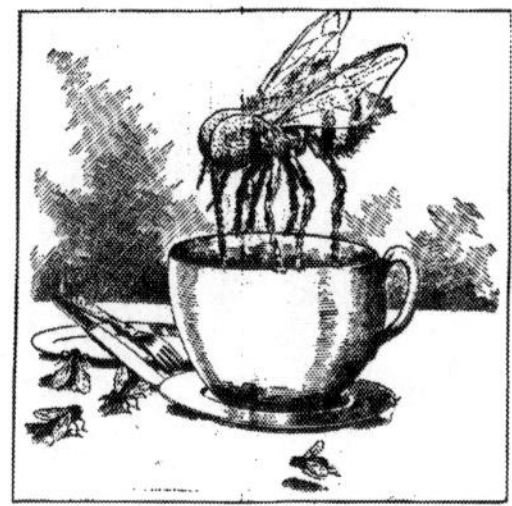

The **Edinger-Westphal nuclei** in the midbrain convert the **afferent signal** of **light entering the eye** into an **efferent signal** to **constrict the pupils**.

*The **E**dinger-**W**estphal nuclei says, "**EW**! I don't want to look at that..." and then **constricts the pupils** to block the light from coming in.*

To summarize, you can memorize the pathway for the pupillary light reflex by connecting the image of **pupils** with a **religious school** and using the phrase, "**2 pri**ests **ed**ucated **3 cili** (silly) **pupils**." This will remind you that this reflex starts with afferent signals coming in on the optic nerve (cranial nerve **2**) and connecting to the ipsilateral **pre**tectal nucleus in the midbrain. Nerves from this nucleus then synapse on the left and right **Ed**inger-Westphal nuclei which send signals on the oculomotor nerve (cranial nerve **3**) to the **cili**ary sphincter, resulting in **pupil**lary constriction.

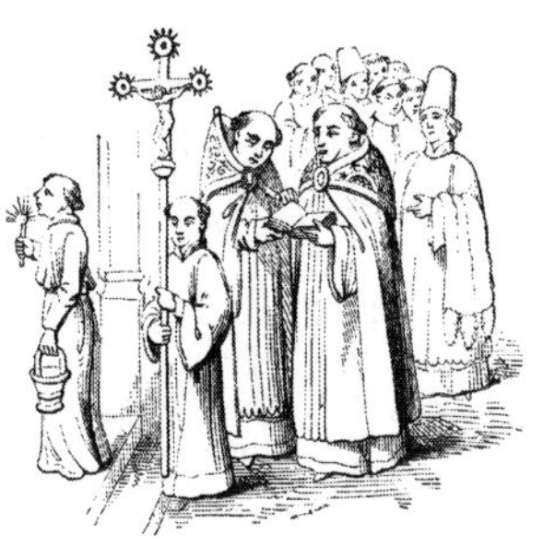

The **pupillary light reflex** involves both **afferent and efferent nerves** traveling between the **eye** and the **midbrain**.

***2 pri**ests **ed**ucated **3 cili** (silly) **pupils**:*
*Optic nerve (cranial nerve **2**)*
***Pre**tectal nucleus*
***Ed**inger-Westphal nuclei*
*Oculomotor nerve (cranial nerve **3**)*
***Cili**ary sphincter → **pupil**lary constriction*

THE ACCOMMODATION REFLEX

The second pupillary reflex, known as **accommodation reflex**, also changes the size of the pupil, but this time the goal is different. Instead of trying to alter the amount of light coming in, this time the pupils are constricting to try and change the shape of the lens so they can better **focus on nearby objects**. This process can be tested clinically by placing a finger or other object close to the space between the patient's eyes and observing for pupillary constriction.

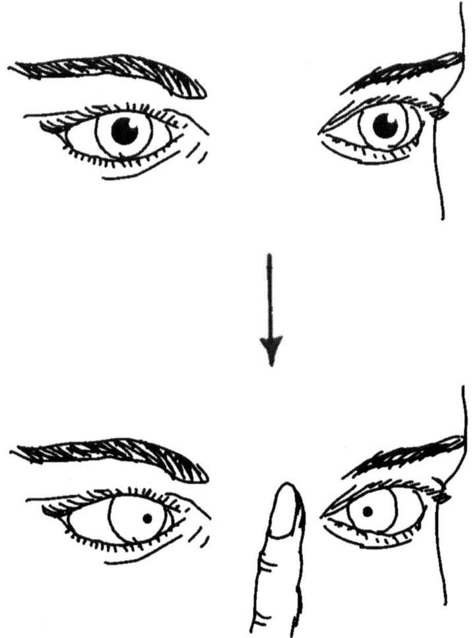

The ***accommodation reflex****.*

The accommodation reflex and the pupillary light reflex each involve different processes and pathways, so it is possible for one to be intact while the other is dysfunctional. A particular finding known as **Argyll Robertson pupils** occurs when the pupils constrict in response to a nearby object but do *not* constrict to light. Argyll Robertson pupils have historically been a sign of a **syphilis** infection within the nervous system, although in the age of easy access to antibiotics it is more often a sign of diabetic neuropathy or other types of nerve damage. (Argyll Robertson pupils are sometimes called "prostitute's pupils" both due to the association with syphilis and because they will "accommodate but not react.")

Argyll Robertson pupils is a clinical finding in which the pupils **constrict in response to a nearby object** but **not when exposed to light**.

*Argyll **R**obertson pupils will **A**ccommodate but not **R**eact.*

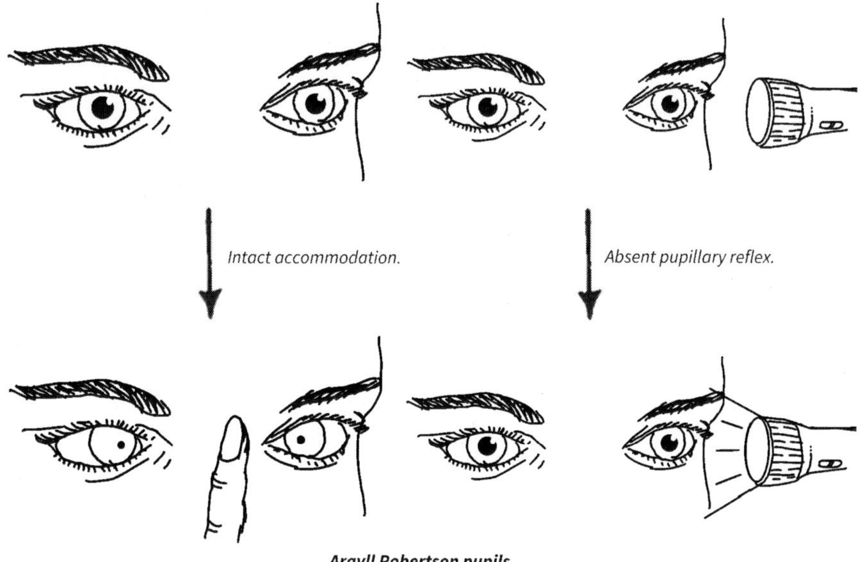

Argyll Robertson pupils.

ORGANIZATION OF THE OCULOMOTOR NERVE

Before we finish this chapter, let's go over one last note about the oculomotor nerve! Specifically, nerve fibers involved in motor output travel towards the *middle* of the nerve, while parasympathetic nerve fibers responsible for pupillary constriction travel towards the *periphery* of the nerve. You can remember this using the letters **OOMMPP**: the **O**cul**O**motor nerve has **M**otor in the **M**iddle and **P**upils on the **P**eriphery.

Nerve fibers supplying **extraocular muscles** are found in the **middle** of the **oculomotor nerve**, while nerve fibers involved in **pupillary constriction** travel towards the **outside**.

OOMMPP*: The* ***O****cul****O****motor nerve has* ***M****otor in the* ***M****iddle and* ***P****upils on the* ***P****eriphery.*

Different diseases can affect the inside or the outside of the nerve preferentially, which provides a helpful diagnostic clue! Absent extraocular movements with intact pupillary constriction suggests damage to the *middle* of the nerve, while the opposite pattern (*intact* extraocular movements with *absent* pupillary constriction) suggests damage to the *periphery* of the nerve.

The two most common things that affect the inside of the nerve more than the outside (leading to ptosis and diplopia with sparing of pupillary function) are ischemia and diabetes. In contrast, a common disease that affects the outside of the nerve more often is an aneurysm of the nearby posterior communicating artery, as the nerve is damaged through direct compression.

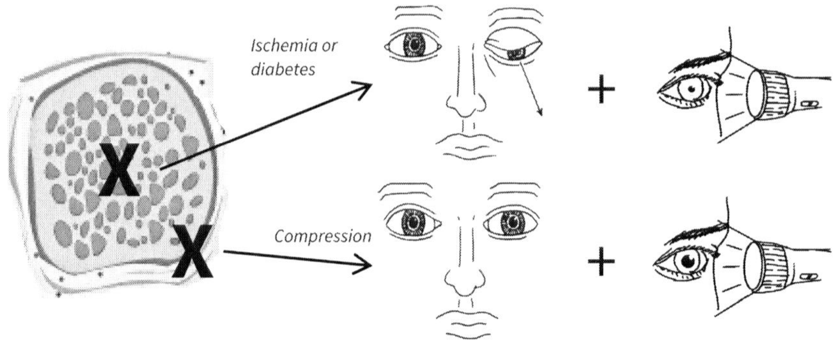

Damage to the **inner nerve fibers** of the **oculomotor nerve** can be caused by **diabetes mellitus** and **ischemia**, while damage to the **outer nerve fibers** can be caused by **compression**.

__D__iabetes __M__ellitus __D__amages the __M__iddle
__I__schemia gets the __I__nside.
Nearby __O__bjects damage the __O__utside.

PUTTING IT ALL TOGETHER

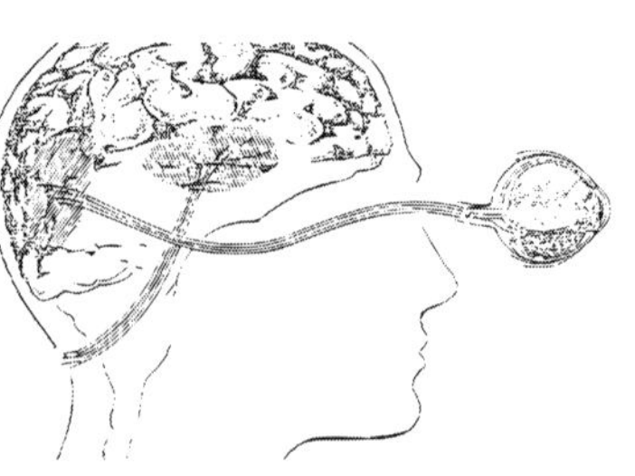

We've gone over a lot of information in this chapter, so take a moment to digest all of it! By far the most important thing in this chapter is to have a solid grasp on the visual pathway on page 120. In fact, it's so important that you should be able to draw the basics of the pathway from scratch and then label it using our "**2 Ch**arismatic **Tra**velers **L**ooking **G**ood **N**aked at the **Radia**nt **Oc**ean" mnemonic! For this reason, the next page has been intentionally left blank for you to draw it out on your own. Try to do this first *without* going back to page 120! While you will likely struggle through it, this challenge will make you more likely to remember it long term. Repeat this again every day until you have a firm grasp of it. Good luck!

REVIEW QUESTIONS

1. A 52 y/o M with no significant past medical history is brought to the emergency department following a motor vehicle accident in which he was an unrestrained passenger. He reports significant pain in his face and head as well as difficulty seeing due to double vision. Physical examination reveals bruising around both eyes but no breaks in the skin. A complete neurological exam reveals weakness of sideways gaze in the right eye as seen below:

   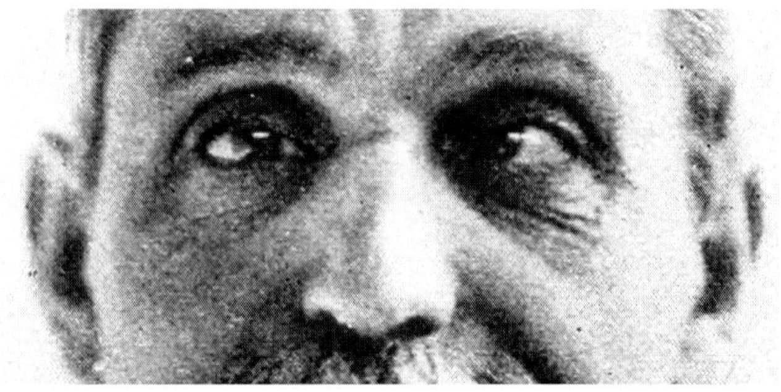

   The exam is otherwise unremarkable. Which of the following cranial nerves has most likely been affected?
   A. Optic nerve
   B. Oculomotor nerve
   C. Trochlear nerve
   D. Trigeminal nerve
   E. Abducens nerve
   F. Facial nerve

2. A 58 y/o F comes into clinic with a letter from the Department of Motor Vehicles requiring her to undergo a medical evaluation before she can get her driver's license back. She has been pulled over by police twice in the past month after hitting trash cans and mailboxes with her car. She tested negative for alcohol both times. She has no significant past medical history. Her review of systems is negative. Neurological exam is positive only for bitemporal hemianopsia on visual acuity testing. A magnetic resonance imaging scan of the brain is most likely to reveal a tumor compressing which of the following structures?
   A. Retina
   B. Optic nerve
   C. Optic chiasm
   D. Optic tract
   E. Optic radiations
   F. Occipital cortex
   G. Pretectal nucleus
   H. Edinger-Westphal nuclei

3. A 36 y/o M goes to the emergency department complaining of double vision. When asked to look to the right, both eyes move synchronously. When asked to look to the left, however, his right eye remains in the middle while his left eye moves laterally, as seen below:

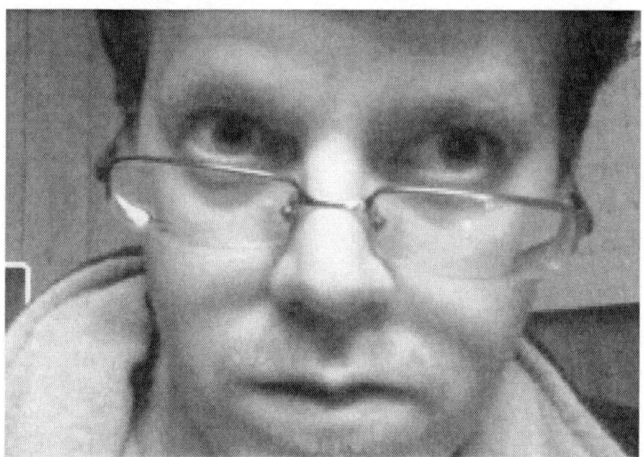

The patient exclaims, "That made everything go *really* double!" While looking to the left, his left eye is seen making quick darting movements back and forth in the horizontal axis. Visual acuity, pupillary light reflexes, convergence, and eyelid strength are all intact. Fundoscopic exam reveals normal-sized and symmetric optic discs. He demonstrates full motor strength and sensory function throughout all four limbs. A lesion is most likely to be found in which of the following structures?

   A. Optic nerve
   B. Oculomotor nerve
   C. Trochlear nerve
   D. Abducens nerve
   E. Medial longitudinal fasciculus
   F. Paramedian pontine reticular formation

1. **The best answer is E.** This patient is presenting with inability to abduct his right eye following a traumatic injury. Abduction is controlled by the lateral rectus muscle which is innervated by the abducens nerve. The other extraocular muscles are controlled by the oculomotor and trochlear nerves (answers B and C). The optic nerve is involved in processing sensory information from the eye but does not play a role in eye movements (answer A). The trigeminal nerve provides sensory information from the cornea and the skin around the eyes but does not control extraocular movements (answer D). Finally, the facial nerve controls the muscles of facial expression including blinking but does not control the movement of the eye itself (answer F).

2. **The best answer is C.** Bitemporal hemianopsia is most often related to injury of the optic chiasm through which sensory neurons from the medial retina of both eyes pass. This can occur due to a tumor of the pituitary gland which sits right above the optic chiasm at the base of the brain. Damage to the retina or optic nerve would produce monocular blindness, not bitemporal hemianopsia (answers A and B). Damage to the optic tract or optic radiations would produce a homonymous hemianopia or quadrantanopsia, respectively (answers D and E). Damage to the occipital lobe tends to produce a homonymous hemianopia or quadrantanopsia with macular sparing (answer F). Finally, the pretectal nucleus and Edinger-Westphal nuclei are involved in the pupillary reflex pathway, so damage here generally does not lead to loss of visual fields (answers G and H).

3. **The best answer is E.** This case describes a typical presentation of internuclear ophthalmoplegia as evidenced by impaired adduction of one eye with intact abduction and nystagmus of the other eye. Internuclear ophthalmoplegia is related to dysfunction of the medial longitudinal fasciculus in the brainstem. The medial longitudinal fasciculus coordinates between the oculomotor nerve, trochlear nerve, abducens nerve, and the paramedian pontine reticular formation, though an injury in any one of these individual components will generally not produce internuclear ophthalmoplegia (answers B, C, D, and F). The optic nerve is intact as evidenced by full visual acuity and pupillary light reflexes (answer A).

11 HEARING, BALANCE, TASTE, AND SMELL

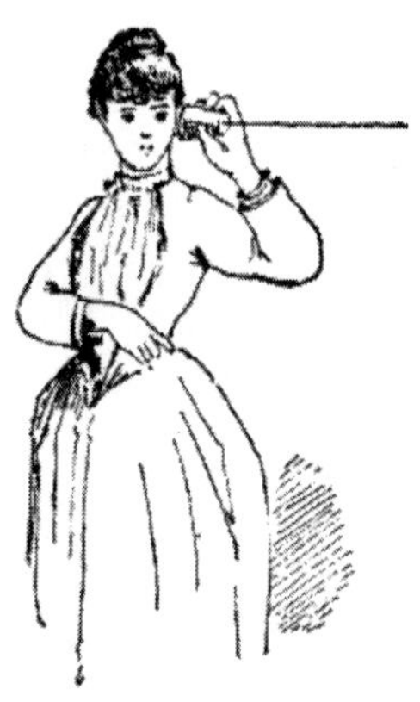

After having made our way through the complicated mess that is the visual pathway, we must now turn our attention to the other special senses: hearing, balance, taste, and smell. Luckily, all of the processes here are quite a bit simpler than those involved in vision! In addition, you will find a lot of recurring themes.

In particular, the **auditory pathway** on which information about sound travels to the brain is overall quite similar to the visual pathway, but the process is a little simpler given that the ears themselves do not move or respond to the environment as much as the eyes. Both of these pathways progress also in an orderly fashion from the sensory organ to the relevant part of the cortex in a way that must be memorized. The vestibulo-ocular reflex arc may also remind you of the pupillary reflexes we covered in the last chapter.

On the other hand, taste and smell are less about *pathways* and more about *processes*, so these sections will involve less direct memorization and more of an understanding of how a signal generated in the sensory organ travels to and is interpreted by the cerebral cortex). These latter senses are fairly "low-yield" in the sense that they don't tend to come up often in clinical settings or on tests, so we won't spend too much time on them (just a taste!).

HEARING

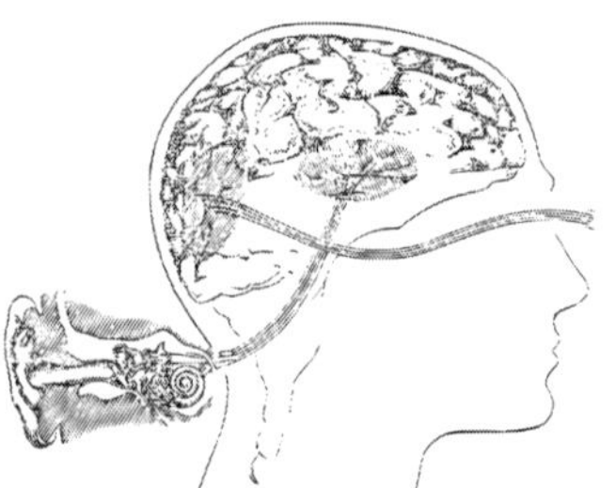

Hearing is the process by which sound waves traveling through the air are converted into signals that allow our brain to respond to the environment (such as turning our head to identify the source of a sudden loud noise). Sound waves initially travel through the **outer ear** until they hit the **eardrum** (formally known as the **tympanic membrane**). The eardrum then converts these sound waves into vibrations which travel down the three smallest bones in the body: the **malleus**, **incus**, and **stapes**. From there, these vibrations are passed onto the **cochlea** which is a highly specialized organ with a shape not unlike a snail's shell. The cochlea is filled with many sensory receptors known as **hair cells**. As the sonic vibrations travel through the cochlea, they generate action potentials in various parts depending on the pitch of the sound.

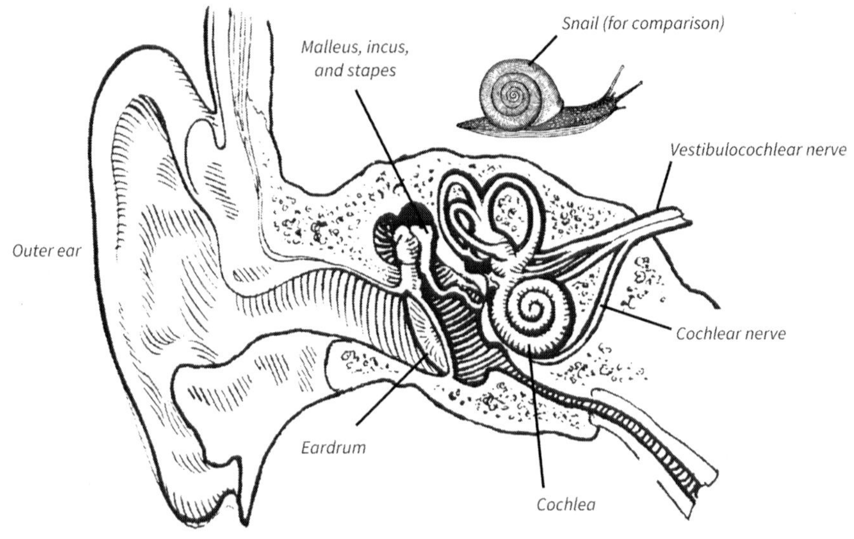

*Anatomy of the **ear**.*

These auditory signals initially travel on the **cochlear nerve** which soon meets up with the **vestibular nerve** to form the **vestibulocochlear nerve** (which you should recognize from Chapter 9 as the eighth cranial nerve!). Auditory signals then travel to the **cochlear nucleus** in the brainstem. From there, they go to the **superior olivary nuclei** (also in the brainstem) before traveling via the **lateral lemniscus** to the **inferior colliculus** in the midbrain. From there, the information travels to the **medial geniculate nucleus** of the thalamus (remember "**M**aking **G**reat **N**oise?") before finally hitting the primary auditory cortex in the **temporal lobe**.

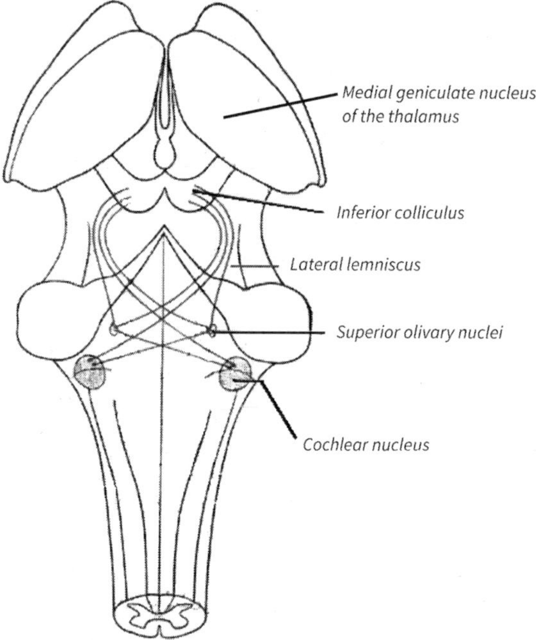

The ***auditory pathway****.*

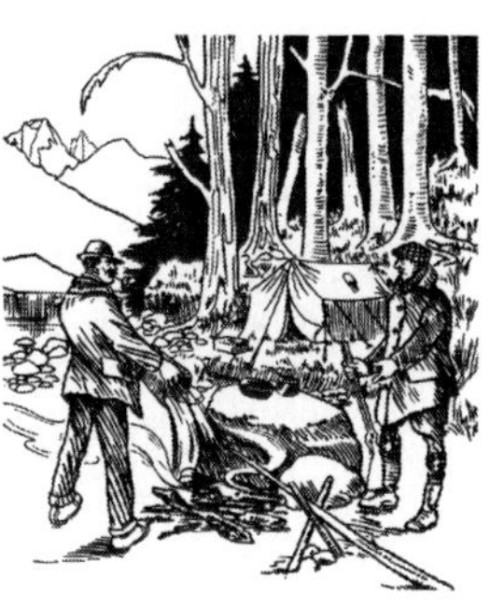

Just like we did with the visual pathway and its associated "**2 Ch**arismatic **Tra**velers **L**ooking **G**ood **N**aked at the **Radia**nt **Oc**ean" mnemonic, you can recall this long and complicated pathway by thinking about the **sound** of "**8 Coc**ky **SON**s **La**ughing '**N M**aking **G**reat **N**oise in the **Te**nt." This will help you remember that auditory signals travel on the vestibulocochlear nerve (cranial nerve **8**), the **Coc**hlear nucleus, the **S**uperior **O**livary **N**uclei, the **La**teral lemniscus, the i**N**ferior colliculus, and the **M**edial **G**eniculate **N**ucleus of the thalamus on their way to the primary auditory cortex of the **Te**mporal lobe.

The **auditory pathway** carries signals from the **cochlea** to the **temporal lobe**.

8 Coc*ky* ***SON****s* ***La****ughing '****N M****aking* ***G****reat* ***N****oise in the* ***Te****nt:*
Vestibulocochlear nerve (Cranial nerve ***8****)*
Coc*hlear nucleus*
S*uperior* ***O****livary* ***N****uclei*
La*teral lemniscus*
*i****N****ferior colliculus*
M*edial* ***G****eniculate* ***N****ucleus of the thalamus*
Primary auditory cortex of the ***Te****mporal lobe*

TESTS OF HEARING

The auditory pathway can be tested in clinical settings by using two distinctive exam maneuvers: the Weber test and the Rinne test.

The **Weber test** involves placing a vibrating tuning fork in the middle of the patient's forehead and asking if they hear the sound louder in the right ear, the left ear, or equally on both sides. A normal response is to say that the sound is equal in both ears, while saying that one side is louder than the other indicates that some degree of **hearing loss** is present on one side compared to the other.

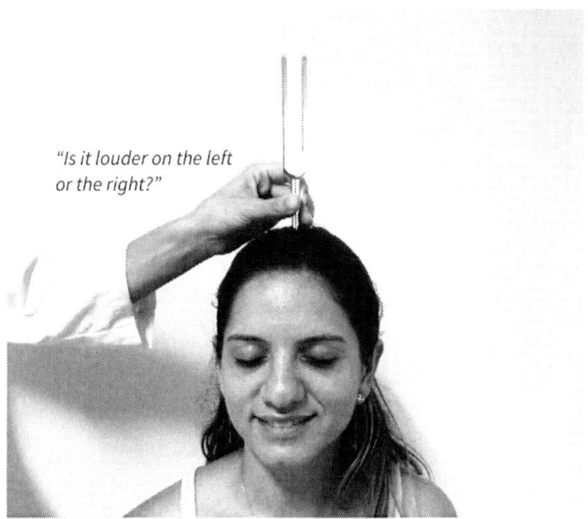

"Is it louder on the left
or the right?"

*The **Weber test**.*

However, just using the Weber test won't tell you *which* side the hearing loss is on or *what kind* of hearing loss it is. This is where the **Rinne test** comes in. The first step of the Rinne test is to place a vibrating tuning fork directly on the **mastoid bone** to test **bone conduction**. (Recall that the eardrum converts sound waves into vibrations in the three bones of the middle ear. For this reason, *any* vibrations—not just sound—can be picked up by the cochlea. This forms the basis for bone conduction.) When the patient says they can no longer hear the sound, you move the tuning fork in front of the ear to test **air conduction**.

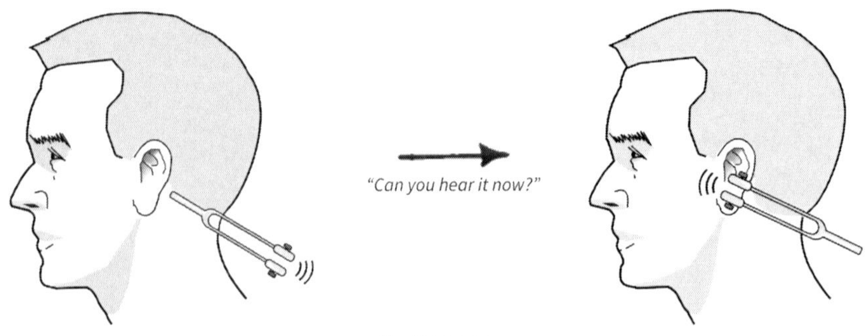

"Can you hear it now?"

*The **Rinne test**.*

Under normal circumstances, air conduction is louder than bone conduction, so someone should be able to hear the tone again once the fork is moved from the bone to the ear. If bone conduction is greater than air conduction, however, it means that something is blocking sound transmission in the ear, known as **conductive hearing loss.** (You can demonstrate conductive hearing loss on yourself by using a finger to plug your ear and then making a humming sound at a consistent volume. By doing this, you will see that sound actually becomes *louder* when you plug one ear and quieter when you remove your finger.) In cases where air conduction is greater than bone conduction but there is clear asymmetry between the right and left ears on the Weber test, the patient likely has a **sensorineural hearing loss** on the quiet side due to damage in the auditory pathway.

To remember the difference between the Weber and Rinne tests, focus on the fact that **W** is a **symmetrical** letter, so doing the **W**eber test tells you about whether hearing ability is symmetrical in both ears. In contrast, **R** is an *a*symmetric letter, so the **R**inne test can tell you whether the hearing loss is on the **R**ight or left.

The **Weber test** is used to test the **symmetry of hearing ability**, while the **Rinne test** assesses the **laterality of hearing ability**.

***W** is a **symmetric** letter, so the **W**eber test tells you about **symmetry**.*
*The **R**inne test tells you whether the damage is on the **R**ight or left.*

You can combine the results of the Weber and Rinne tests to diagnose what kind of hearing loss is present and where it is located. Under normal circumstances, the Weber test will not lateralize (both ears will hear equally well), and both ears will have stronger air conduction than bone conduction. In conductive hearing loss, the Weber test will lateralize to the *affected* or bad ear, with bone conduction greater than air conduction in that ear (this is the condition you simulated by putting your finger in your ear). In sensorineural hearing loss, the Weber test will lateralize to the *un*affected or good ear, with air conduction greater than bone conduction in *both* ears. You can use the nonsense phrase "**MAN BBC GAS**!" to remind yourself of these patterns!

If the Weber test lateralizes to:	... and Rinne test shows:	... then the likely diagnosis is:
Midline	**A**ir > Bone (both ears)	**N**ormal
Bad ear	**B**one > Air (bad ear)	**C**onductive hearing loss
Good ear	**A**ir > Bone (both ears)	**S**ensorineural hearing loss

Combining the results of the **Weber and Rinne tests** can help you to diagnose whether **hearing loss** is **conductive** or **sensorineural** in nature.

*"**MAN BBC GAS**!"*
***M**idline + **A**ir > Bone (both ears) = **N**ormal*
***B**ad ear + **B**one > Air (bad ear) = **C**onductive*
***G**ood ear + **A**ir > Bone (both ears) = **S**ensorineural*

BALANCE

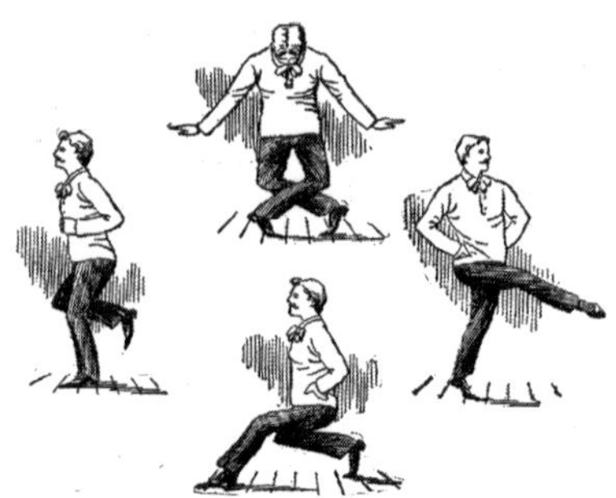

Hearing is not the only thing that the ear does! The ear also contains the **vestibular system** which is responsible for the sense of **balance**. At its most basic level, balance can be defined as the **sensory information that prevents someone from falling over**. Balance is not a single modality like vision or hearing but rather a complex integration of various senses, including **visual** information from the eyes, **proprioceptive** information from the dorsal column–medial lemniscus pathway, and signals about **movement, acceleration, and rotation** from the inner ear. We've already talked about vision and proprioception, so we will now turn to the systems found within the inner ear.

The vestibular system has two components: three **semicircular canals**, which generate information about *rotational* movements, and two **otoliths** (the utricle and the saccule) which generate information about *linear* accelerations.

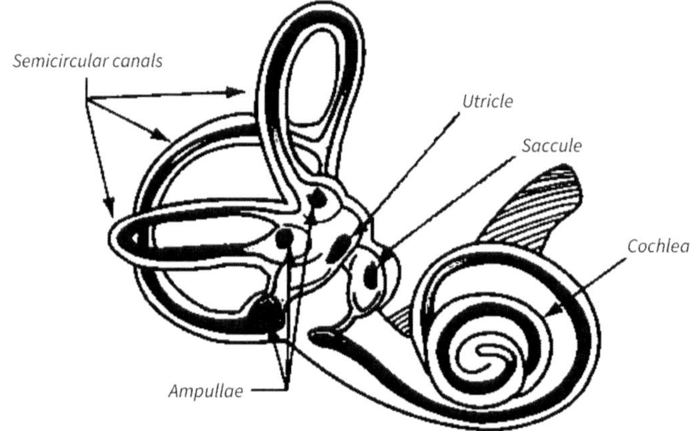

*Anatomy of the **vestibular system**.*

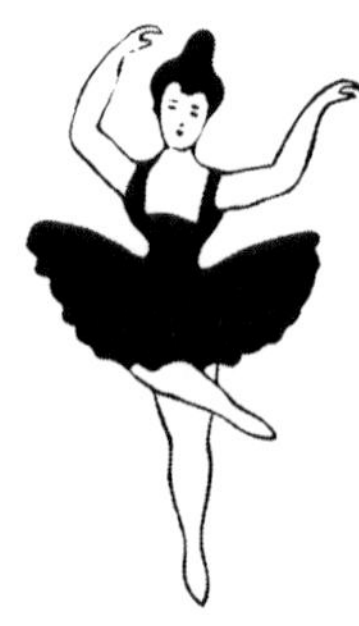

Let's talk about the semicircular canals first. Each of the three are able to detect movement in one of the three **rotational axes**, with one detecting rotation in a *vertical* plane (like when you nod your head), another detecting rotation in a *horizontal* plane (like when you shake your head back and forth to say "no"), and the third detecting rotation in a *flat* plane (like when you touch your head to your shoulder). (Go ahead and do each of these three movements now to help cement these axes in your mind!) These movements are detected by specialized **hair cells** in a sac at the base of each semicircular canal known as an **ampulla**. Together, the three semicircular canals are able to give the brain detailed information about the movement of the head in space.

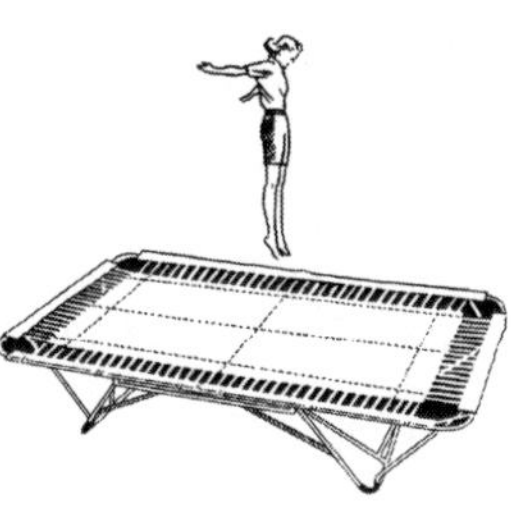

While the semicircular canals are able to sense movement in each of the three *rotational* axes, the two otolith are able to sense *linear* acceleration. The first otolith (the **utricle**) senses movement in a *horizontal* plane (such as someone going from 0 to 60 in a sports car). In contrast, the second otolith (the **saccule**) senses movement in a *vertical* plane (such as someone jumping up and down on a trampoline). You can try to remember the difference between the utricle and the saccule by thinking of the phrase "**drop** it like a **sac**k of potatoes" to associate the **sac**cule and vertical movement.

The three **semicircular canals** detect **rotational movements**, while the two **otoliths** (the **utricle** and **saccule**) detect **linear acceleration**.

*Say "**drop** it like a **sac**k of potatoes" to associate the **sac**cule and **vertical** movement.*

THE VESTIBULO-OCULAR REFLEX

Together, the three semicircular canals and the two otoliths (combined with visual information from the eyes and proprioceptive information from the body) are able to determine the body's current position in space and use this information to keep itself upright. This information is also used in the **vestibulo-ocular reflex** which helps to keep your eyes focused on a particular object even when your head is moving. When the semicircular canals detect movement, they send signals via the **vestibulocochlear nerve** to the **vestibular nuclei** in the pons and medulla. From there, motor signals are sent to the **abducens nerve** as well as the **oculomotor nerve** via the **medial longitudinal fasciculus** to correct for the movement of the head. This pathway is short and to the point, allowing for very rapid adjustments to the eyes in response to head movement. (In fact, the vestibulo-ocular reflex is among the fastest in the body!)

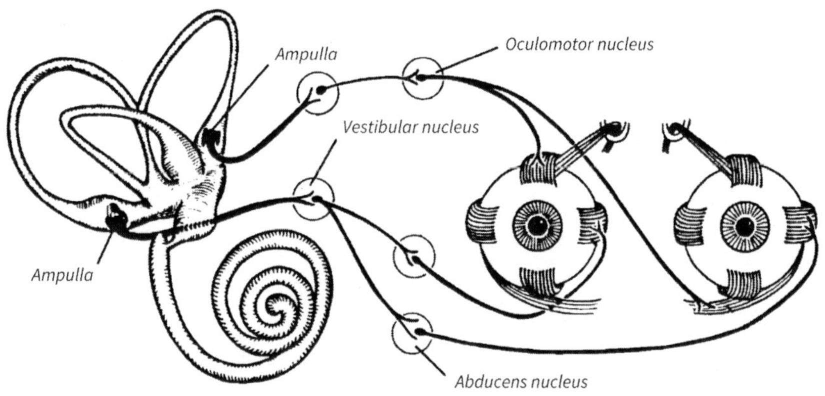

*The pathways involved in the **vestibulo-ocular reflex**, moving from left to right.*

Because the circuit for the vestibulo-ocular reflex travels through the brainstem, it is often used clinically as a test of brainstem function in patients who are comatose. If the eyes move when the head is moved, this suggests that the reflex is intact. However, if the pupils remain fixed in the middle of their eye sockets no matter what direction the head is turned (like a doll's, giving this finding the name "**doll's eyes sign**"), this is highly suggestive of brainstem damage—and a poor prognosis.

VERTIGO

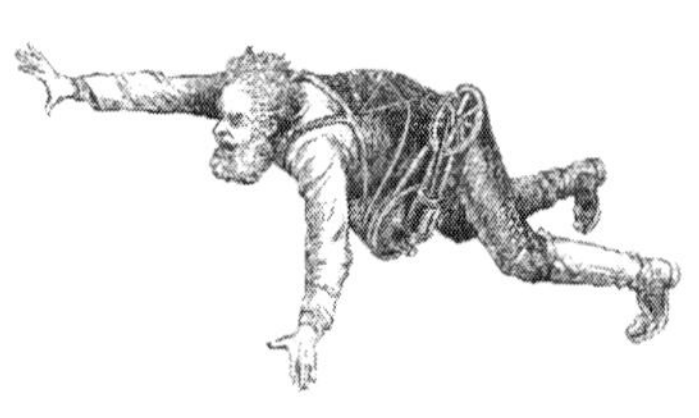

We talked about **vertigo** (the sense that things are moving when they are not) as one of the core cerebellar signs and symptoms back in Chapter 6. However, vertigo can also result from damage to the vestibular system. Cases of vertigo resulting from the brain are known as **central vertigo**, while those stemming from the inner ear are known as **peripheral vertigo**.

The most common cause of vertigo is a condition known as **benign paroxysmal positional vertigo** (BPPV) in which an otolith breaks off from its usual position and enters the semicircular canals. This "otolith on the lam" then erroneously signals that things are moving when in fact they are not, creating feelings of vertigo (especially when the patient is lying in bed or otherwise changing the position of their head, hence the word "positional" in the name). Benign paroxysmal positional vertigo is a common condition, especially in the elderly. For most people it resolves on its own within a few weeks, although for some it may become recurrent.

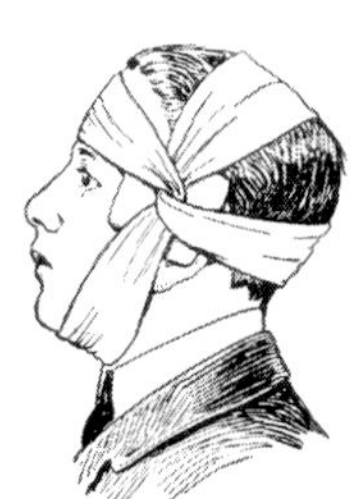

Another common cause of vertigo is **Ménière's disease** which occurs as a result of excessive fluid build-up in both the vestibular system and the cochlea. This results in a feeling of "fullness" in the ears accompanied by a classic triad of **vertigo**, **sensorineural hearing loss** (which will show up on exam as lateralization to the good ear with air conduction greater than bone conduction), and a ringing in the ears known as **tinnitus**. (Compare this to benign paroxysmal positional vertigo which only involves the vestibular system and therefore does not impact hearing at all.) You can remember the definition of **Ménière's** disease by thinking of someone yelling, "**Mine ears**!" due to their problems in both balance and hearing.

Ménière's disease causes the triad of **vertigo**, **tinnitus**, and **sensorineural hearing loss** as a result of **excessive fluid build-up** in the **inner ear**.

*Think of it as "**Mine ears!**" disease to associate it with the two senses found in the ears.*

TASTE

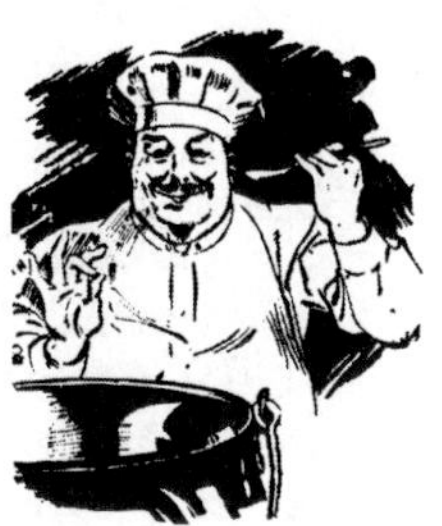

Taste is the process by which the nervous system is able to recognize what kinds of chemicals are present in the mouth before swallowing. Certain chemicals that the body needs to function (like sugar) will cause a pleasant taste, while other chemicals that could potentially harm the body (like toxins) will instead taste bad, prompting the person to spit out them out. **Taste buds** on the tongue can detect five basic tastes: **salty** (things containing alkali metals like sodium), **sweet** (things containing carbohydrates like glucose), **sour** (things containing hydrogen ions like an acid), **bitter** (a variety of compounds, some of which are toxic), and **umami** (a Japanese word roughly meaning "savory," "meaty," or "delicious" that is activated by the presence of the amino acid glutamate).

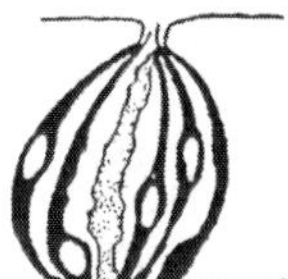
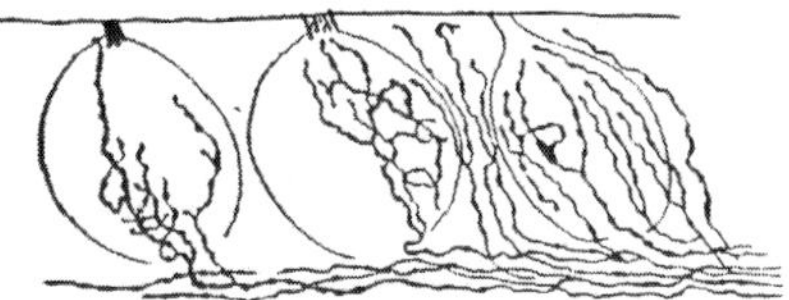

***Taste buds** on the surface of the **tongue**.*

Recall from Chapter 9 that sensory information about taste travels to the brain via two different nerves: the **facial nerve**, which covers the anterior two-thirds of the tongue, and the **glossopharyngeal nerve**, which covers the posterior one-third of the tongue. You can remember this by thinking that if a bug makes it to the *anterior* two-thirds of the tongue, you'll probably make a face (as the facial nerve is also responsible for innervating facial muscles), but if that bug makes it to the *posterior* third, you're likely to gag (as the glossopharyngeal nerve is also responsible for the gag reflex).

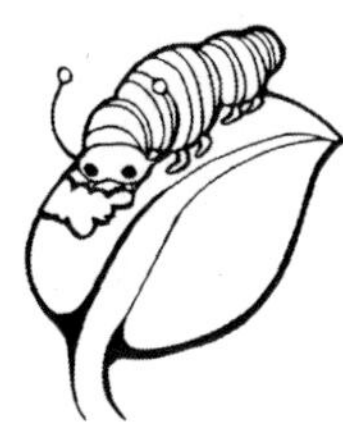

The **facial nerve** innervates the **anterior two-thirds of the tongue**, while the **glossopharyngeal nerve** supplies the **posterior third**.

*If a bug crawls on the **anterior** two-thirds of the tongue you'll probably **make a face**, but if it makes it all the way to the **posterior third** you'll likely **gag**.*

Sensory information about taste travels via these two nerves to the **solitary nucleus** in the medulla. (Remember from Chapter 7 that the **sole-lick**-tary nucleus is involved in both taste and the gag reflex!) From the solitary nucleus, information about taste then goes to various parts of the brain including neurons involved in the **parasympathetic nervous system** (which makes sense given its role in "resting and *digesting*"), the **hypothalamus** (which also makes sense since it governs hunger and satiety), and the **thalamus** (where it can then travel to the somatosensory cortex in the parietal lobe to generate the conscious sensation of taste).

SMELL

The last of the special senses we will talk about is **smell**, or the process by which the body can sense and respond to **airborne chemicals**. Smell is highly complementary to taste, as it allows us to get a sense of whether something is likely to be palatable way before we get it anywhere *near* our mouths.

Smells are sensed by the **olfactory system** which begins in the nose. In contrast to the five basic tastes that the tongue can sense, the nose is capable of picking up millions of different smells by responding to distinct combinations of chemicals. When an airborne chemical binds to sensory neurons in the nose, this sets off a process by which an action potential is generated and sent down the first cranial nerve (the **olfactory nerve**).

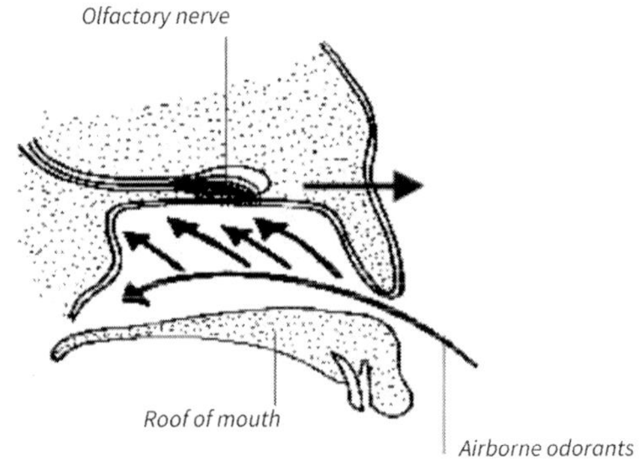

*The **olfactory system**.*

The olfactory nerve is unique in that it travels *directly* to the **olfactory cortex** rather than synapsing first in another part of the brain like the brainstem or thalamus. The olfactory cortex is strongly connected to parts of the limbic system which explains why our emotional responses to smells are often so strong and immediate (you can probably think of times in your life when a smell triggered a vivid memory or when an unpleasant smell immediately ruined your mood). Smell also appears to play a role in mate selection, with humans being able to unconsciously detect when someone's genetics are not sufficiently different from their own. All in all, olfaction is not a complex process, but it is a very important one for survival!

PUTTING IT ALL TOGETHER

On a neurological level, learning about the special senses can help to integrate much of what we have learned already, as their pathways run through many parts of both the central and peripheral nervous systems. Make sure that you have a good grasp on all of the topics we have covered so far, as we have only one more chapter to go before we move on to clinical neurology in earnest!

REVIEW QUESTIONS

1. A 15 y/o F is reading a book on a boat while vacationing overseas. While she is reading, the boat hits some rough waters, causing it to pitch and roll. Despite the movement, the girl is still able to keep her eyes fixed on the line of text that she is reading at that moment. Which of the following structures is *least* involved in the process of maintaining her line of sight while reading in this rough weather?
    A. Semicircular canals
    B. Vestibulocochlear nerve
    C. Midbrain
    D. Pons
    E. Medulla oblongata
    F. Oculomotor nerve
    G. Abducens nerve
    H. All of the above are involved in maintaining her line of sight

2. A 37 y/o F sees her primary care doctor complaining of episodes where "the world is spinning like crazy" on a daily basis for the past week. The episodes of dizziness last only a few minutes at most, but when they occur they are disabling. They are accompanied by a feeling of "fullness" in her right ear. She has also noticed some difficulty hearing out of her right ear during conversations and while watching television which has been worsening over the past few weeks. Which of these additional signs or symptoms is most likely to be reported by this patient?
    A. Transient episodes of blurry vision
    B. "Ringing" sound in her ear
    C. Abnormally low blood pressure
    D. Impaired proprioceptive ability
    E. Lack of taste from the posterior third of the tongue

3. A 80 y/o F presents to her geriatrician reporting episodes of hearing loss which are accompanied by a high-pitched "whine." On exam, she is able to hear sounds but notes that they sound "dull." She also is unable to localize where sounds are coming from with her eyes closed. Which of the following structures is *least* likely to be dysfunctional for this patient?
    A. Temporal cortex
    B. Cochlear nucleus
    C. Medial geniculate nucleus of the thalamus
    D. Superior olivary nuclei
    E. Medial lemniscus
    F. Inferior colliculus
    G. Vestibulocochlear nerve

1. **The best answer is H.** The ability to maintain a stable line of sight despite changes in the position of one's head relies upon an intact vestibulo-ocular reflex. The vestibulo-ocular reflex involves a complex pathway that nevertheless is able to act quickly. Information about head position is sent from the semicircular canals (answer A) in the vestibular system via the vestibulocochlear nerve (answer B) to the vestibular nuclei in the pons and medulla (answers D and E). Some of these pathways connect to the medial longitudinal fasciculus in the midbrain (answer C). Compensatory movements of the eyes are enacted via the cranial nerves controlling the extraocular muscles, including the oculomotor and abducens nerves (answers F and G).

2. **The best answer is B.** This vignette describes a case of Ménière's disease, a disorder characterized by a characteristic triad of vertigo, hearing loss, and tinnitus. While it is not diagnostic of this disease, a sensation of fullness in the ears is often reported as well. Ménière's disease is believed to result from distention of the fluid-filled spaces in the inner ear. While the sense of balance relies upon visual and proprioceptive information in addition to the vestibular system, these are not involved directly in Ménière's disease (answers A and D). Sensory information about taste from the posterior one-third of the tongue is carried on the glossopharyngeal nerve and is not related to the inner ear (answer E). Finally, abnormalities in blood pressure are not commonly seen in Ménière's disease (answer C).

3. **The best answer is E.** You should recognize each of these structures from the auditory pathway, as each are involved in sound processing. The only exception is the medial lemniscus which instead belongs to the dorsal column—medial lemniscus pathway that is responsible for sensing fine touch, vibration, and proprioception! Don't confuse this with the *lateral* lemniscus which *is* part of the auditory pathway.

12 THE MENINGES, VENTRICLES, AND BLOOD SUPPLY

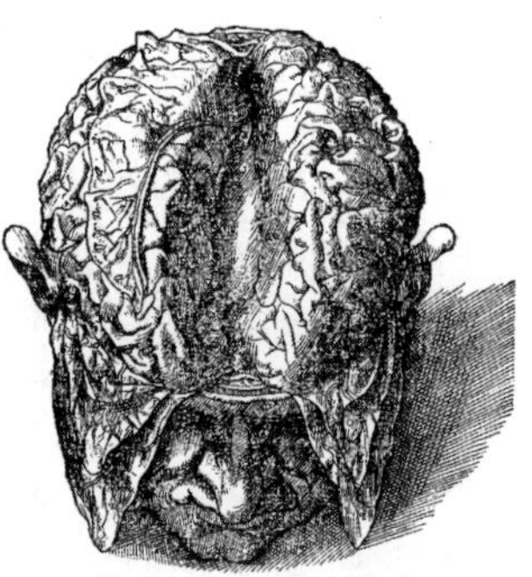

In this final chapter on neuroanatomy, we will cover a few last bits and pieces of the nervous system which didn't fit neatly into any of the other topics we've talked about so far! There is nothing that inherently unites all of these structures other than the fact that, despite being in the brain, they are *not* made up of nerves. Instead, these structures help to **support nervous tissues** in several ways, including serving as a protective cushion, filtering out toxic potentially chemicals, and delivering oxygen and other vital nutrients.

We will first talk about the **meninges** which are a series of membranes that envelope the brain. Next, we will discuss the **ventricular system** which produces and circulates cerebrospinal fluid. Finally, we will finish the chapter by talking about the **blood supply** of the central nervous system as well as its **venous drainage** (which allows all the blood and cerebrospinal fluid flowing around to go somewhere). Despite not being made of nervous tissue themselves, these structures are all incredibly important for maintaining proper functioning of the nervous system, and even small disruptions in these systems can lead to major problems, as we will see shortly!

THE MENINGES

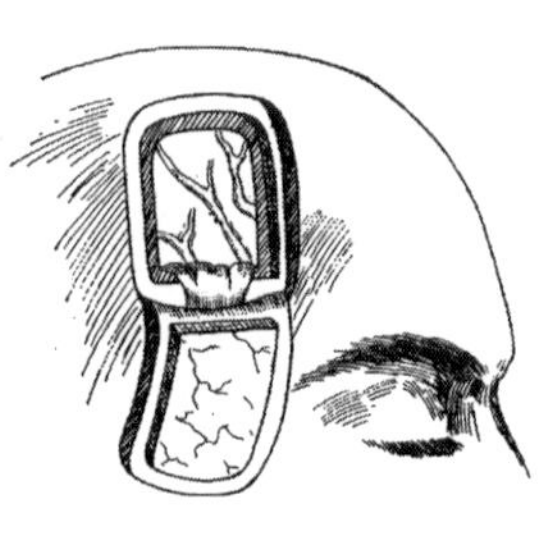

The **meninges** are the membranes that surround the brain and spinal cord, enveloping them and protecting them from injury. The meninges consist of **three distinct layers**: the **dura mater**, the **arachnoid mater**, and the **pia mater**. (Your brain is "the gift so nice they wrapped it thrice!") In between these three layers are additional spaces (like the subarachnoid space within which cerebrospinal fluid flows as part of the ventricular system, which we will discuss in the next section). Let's "unpeel" the brain to learn about each of these layers in more detail:

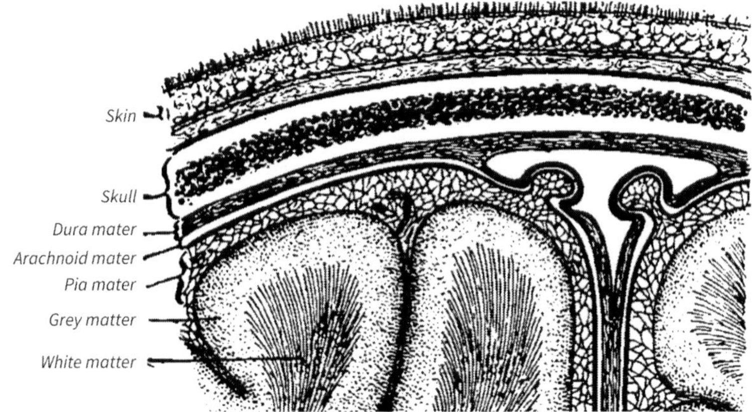

*The **meninges** lie between the skull and the brain itself.*

The first thing we hit when we attempt to lift away the layers surrounding the brain is the **skin**. Peel that away and you have the **skull** (the bony structure encasing the brain) and its associated outer covering known as the **periosteum**.

After removing those, you next hit the first layer of the meninges: the **dura mater** (Latin for "tough mother"). The dura mater is appropriately named, as it is a thick and fibrous coating that provides structural support to the brain. Under normal conditions, the dura mater is in direct contact with the structures both above it (the skull) and below it (the arachnoid mater, discussed next). However, in cases of injury the dura mater can separate from one or both of these, creating an **epidural space** above and/or a **subdural space** below.

Immediately beneath the dura mater is the next meningeal layer: the **arachnoid mater** (named for its spider web-like appearance) which is much thinner than the dura mater but still helps to cushion the central nervous system. Directly beneath the arachnoid mater is the **subarachnoid space** through which cerebrospinal fluid flows.

Finally, we reach the innermost layer of the meninges: the **pia mater** (Latin for "tender mother"). The pia mater is a delicate film that wraps the brain quite tightly. Despite being thin, the pia mater is impermeable to fluid and thereby helps to keep the cerebrospinal fluid flowing in the subarachnoid space separated from the brain itself.

Like most things in the nervous system, the meninges work great—until they don't. The meninges are vulnerable to bruising, bleeding, and tumors in each of the layers we have discussed. We'll go over these conditions in later chapters. For now, just remember the layers of the meninges in order from the inside out by thinking that the brain has a **PAD** made up of the **P**ia mater, **A**rachnoid mater, and **D**ura mater.

The **meninges** consist of three layers (the **dura mater**, **arachnoid mater**, and **pia mater**) that **envelop the central nervous system** and help to protect it.

The brain has a ***PAD****:* ***P****ia mater,* ***A****rachnoid mater, and* ***D****ura mater.*

MENINGEAL STRUCTURES

The meninges make a few unique structures of their own. In particular, the thick and fibrous dura mater is shaped into three structures that you should know: the falx cerebri, the falx cerebelli, and the tentorium cerebelli.

The **falx cerebri** is formed when the dura mater descends into the longitudinal fissure (which is the deep "canyon" dividing the left and right hemispheres of the brain). This creates a physical separation between the two hemispheres in a sickle-like shape (with the word "falx" being Latin for sickle). An equivalent structure known as the **falx cerebelli** separates the two hemispheres of the cerebellum.

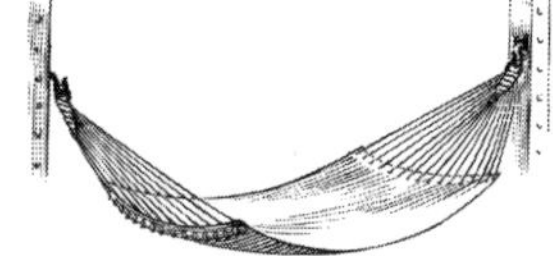

While the falx cerebri separates the left and right cerebral hemispheres, another structure known as the **tentorium cerebelli** helps to separate the cerebrum from the cerebellum. The tentorium cerebelli is an extension of the dura mater that forms a "hammock" of sorts that cradles the underside of the cerebrum (around the occipital lobes) and suspends it above the cerebellum sitting beneath it. The tentorium cerebelli thus forms a discrete physical barrier between the "upper" brain and the "lower" brain, and throughout this book you will see references to things being **supratentorial** (above the tentorium) or **infratentorial** (below the tentorium).

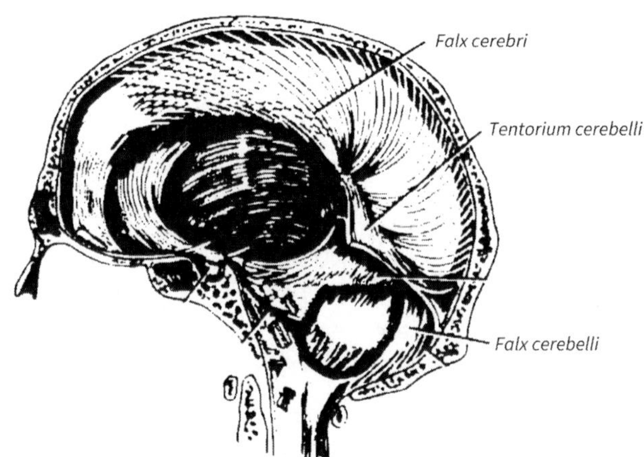

Meningeal structures *formed by the* ***dura mater****.*

THE VENTRICULAR SYSTEM

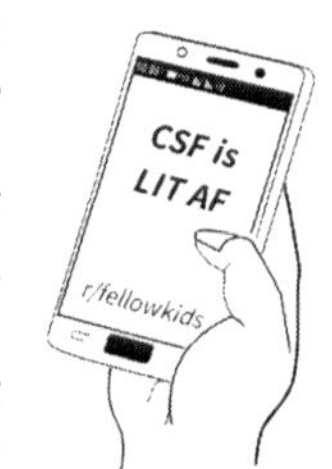

The **ventricular system** is a series of interconnected holes in the brain that are filled with **cerebrospinal fluid**. There are four ventricles in the brain, and cerebrospinal fluid flows through them in a linear fashion. To remember the order of the ventricular system, use the phrase "**C**SF is **LIT AF**." Cerebrospinal fluid is first produced in the **C**horoid plexuses found throughout all four ventricles of the brain. It then flows from the **L**ateral ventricles before flowing through the paired **I**nterventricular foramina into the **T**hird ventricle. From there, it flows down the cerebral **A**queduct into the **F**ourth ventricle. On a clinical level, a blockage in one part of the ventricular system will cause too much fluid in areas "upstream" and too little in areas "downstream" which is why it is so important to memorize the order! This is known as **hydrocephalus** (which we'll cover more in Chapter 15).

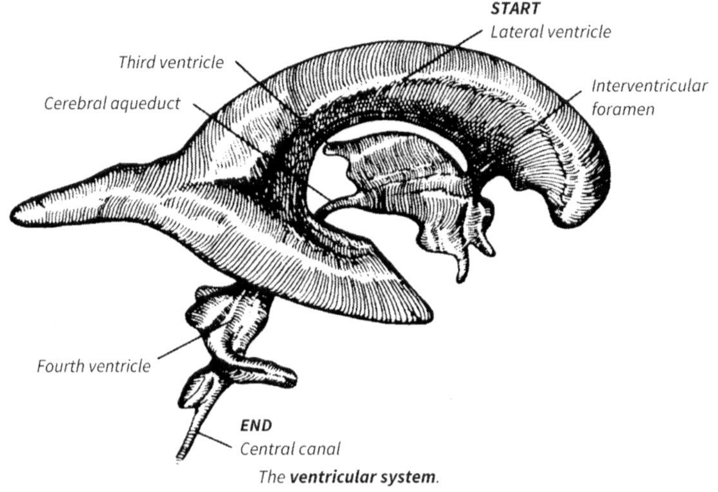

*The **ventricular system**.*

Cerebrospinal fluid travels through the **ventricular system** in a **linear fashion**.

*CSF is **LIT AF**:*
***C**horoid plexuses*
***L**ateral ventricle*
***I**nterventricular foramina*
***T**hird ventricle*
*Cerebral **A**queduct*
***F**ourth ventricle*

After arriving at the end of the ventricular system, the cerebrospinal fluid can go one of two directions: it can either continue into the spinal cord through the **central canal**, or it can pass into the **subarachnoid space** via several holes where it helps to cushion the brain as a whole.

CEREBRAL BLOOD SUPPLY

For the last part of this chapter, we will shift our focus to the blood vessels of the brain, starting first with its arterial supply and then talking about its venous drainage.

Most of the blood flow to the brain comes from the **carotid arteries** in the neck (which you can easily feel as a bounding pulse when you place a finger on either side of your neck in the soft spot just lateral to the trachea). The carotid arteries divide into the **internal carotid arteries** and the **external carotid arteries**. As the *external* carotids split off to supply blood to the face and neck, we will instead follow the *internal* carotids which go on to supply the brain.

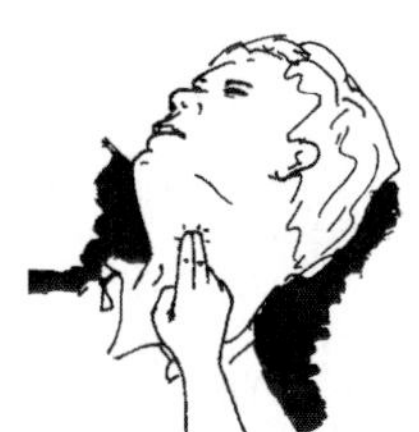

After traveling up the neck, the internal carotids reach the underside of the brain and join what is known as the **circle of Willis**. Knowing the structure of the circle of Willis is *absolutely crucial* to understanding the effects that bleeds and blockages in various arteries will have on a clinical level, so don't move on from this section until you have this down cold! First, take a look at an unlabeled circle of Willis on the left:

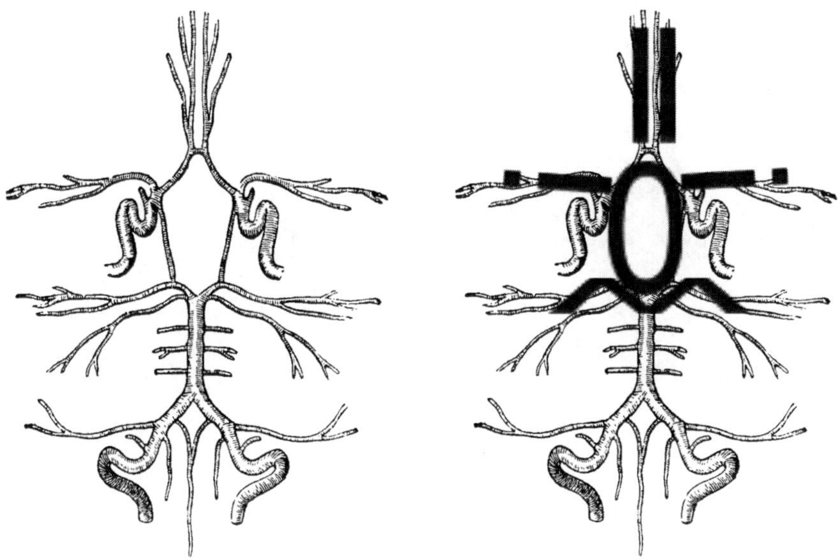

That's no joke, huh? But let's see if we can simplify it down as much as possible and maybe even be able to draw most of it from scratch entirely by memory. Start by focusing on just the *circle* part towards the top (onto which a circle has been drawn in the right image). Then, let's write the word "**Willis**" going around the circle, starting at the bottom and going clockwise. First draw an upside-down **W** at the bottom, then an **i** in the upper left, two l's together (**ll**) at the top, and another **i** in the upper right. And that's the head of the circle of Willis! Now we just need to label all the parts.

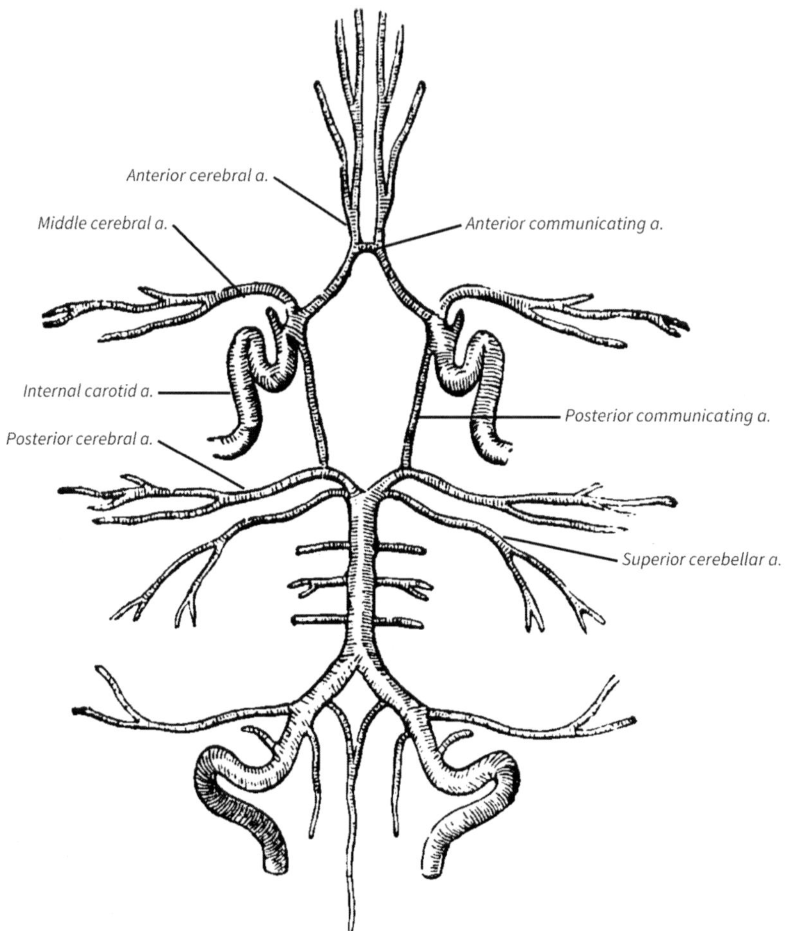

*The **circle of Willis** with major arteries labeled.*

The major components of the circle of Willis are the three pairs of **cerebral arteries**. The upside-down **W** (don't call it an M!) at the bottom represents the two **posterior cerebral arteries**, the **i**'s in the middle represent the **middle cerebral arteries** (which are direct continuations of the **i**nternal carotid artery), and the two **l**'s are the **anterior cerebral arteries**. The circle itself is made up of two communicating arteries: the short **anterior communicating artery** in between the two l's and the longer **posterior communicating arteries** making up the bottom half of the circle.

The **anterior cerebral circulation** is supplied by the **internal carotid arteries** and perfuses the **cerebrum** via a series of anastomoses known as the **circle of Willis**.

*Draw the **circle of Willis** by drawing a **circle with the word "Willi" around it**, with the letters being drawn in a **clockwise rotation** starting at the bottom.*

From here, let's transition from the *anterior* to the *posterior* circulation. For this, we're basically drawing a stick figure, with the head being the circle that we already drew. Let's name our new stick figure **Willis**.

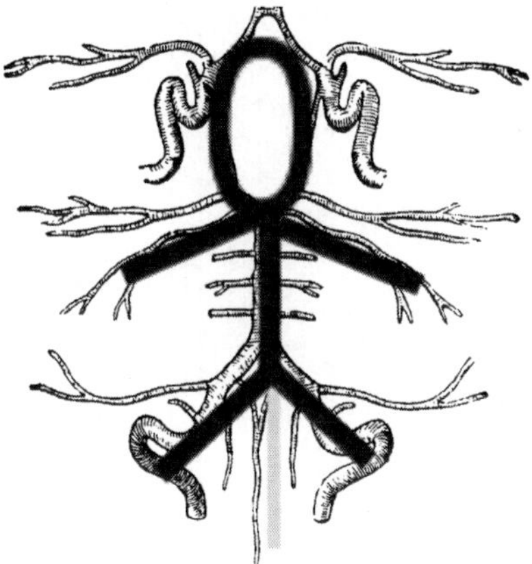

First, draw Willis's arms: these are the **superior cerebellar arteries** supplying the cerebellum. Next, draw his torso: this is the **basilar artery** from which many small **pontine arteries** branch off. Next, draw his legs: these are the **vertebral arteries** from which several smaller arteries, including the **anterior inferior cerebellar arteries** and the **posterior inferior cerebellar arteries**, branch off of. Finally, this stick figure is, um, "well-endowed" with the **anterior spinal artery** in between his legs.

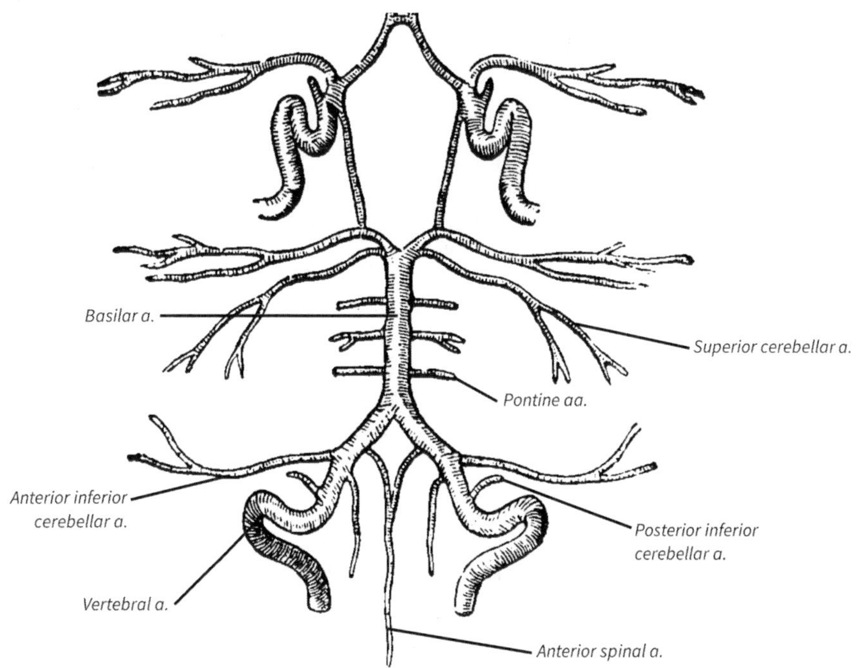

Posterior cerebral circulation.

The **posterior cerebral circulation** is supplied by the two **vertebral arteries** and helps to perfuse the **cerebellum**, **brainstem**, and **spinal cord**.

*Draw a **stick figure** with the circle of Willis as the **head**, the superior cerebellar arteries as the **arms**, the basilar artery as the **neck**, the vertebral arteries as the **legs**, and the anterior spinal artery as his **endowment**!*

And that's it! You now know how to draw the circle of Willis and the associated arteries going to the midbrain, cerebellum, and spinal cord. Before we move on, however, there is an important point to note. Despite how it may appear, the vertebral arteries are *not* a continuation of blood flowing *down* from the basilar artery. Instead, they (like the internal carotid arteries) help to bring blood *up* the neck from the heart. In this way, the circle of Willis has two primary blood supplies: the internal carotid arteries in the front and the vertebral arteries in the back. These two sets of arteries effectively form a **bridge** between the anterior circulation (the circle of Willis) and the posterior circulation.

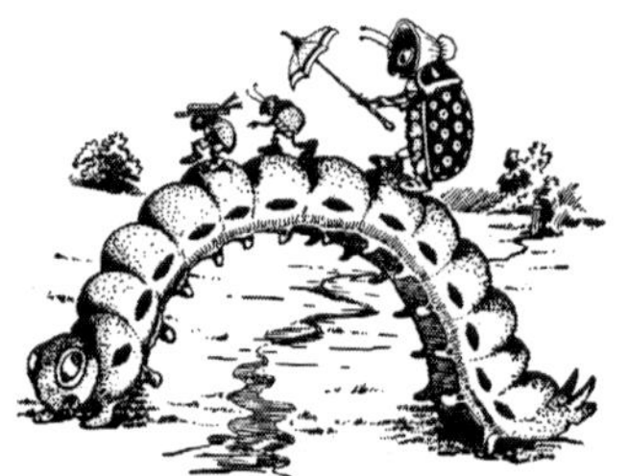

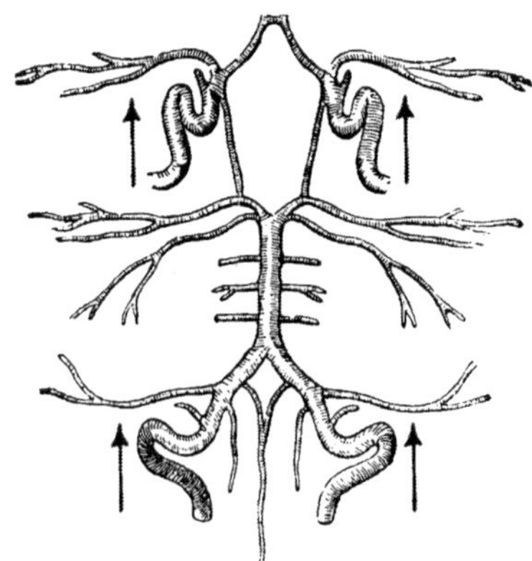

*Both the **internal carotid arteries** and the **vertebral arteries** bring blood **up from the heart**.*

This pattern of having multiple redundant connections between blood vessels (known as **anastomoses**) is common in the brain and helps to preserve such a vital organ. If blood supply were to become compromised in any one artery, the other arteries would be able to compensate for this to make sure that all parts of the brain still get the blood they need. For example, if the right internal carotid artery were to become blocked, the left internal carotid artery (as well as blood originating from the vertebral arteries and passing into the anterior circulation by way of the basilar artery) could help to make up the difference. Nevertheless, various situations can create blockages that are severe enough that not even these anastomoses can fully compensate, which can lead to injury and even death of brain tissue (known as a **stroke**, which we will learn about more in Chapter 14).

THE BLOOD-BRAIN BARRIER

While the arteries we have discussed help to bring oxygen and other vital nutrients into the central nervous system, the contents of the blood do not go to the nervous tissue directly. Instead, there exists a **blood-brain barrier** that acts as a filter to permit only *some* of what the blood is carrying to come into contact with nervous tissue directly. This helps to prevent toxic chemicals from wreaking havoc on the brain. However, the blood-brain barrier can also sometimes prevent helpful drugs from reaching where they need to go. In general, **fat soluble** chemicals are much more able to diffuse across the blood-brain barrier than water soluble ones, and this has important implications for any drug that is intended to act on the central nervous system. (Water soluble chemicals that are needed by the brain, such as glucose, are actively transported across the blood-brain barrier by transport proteins.)

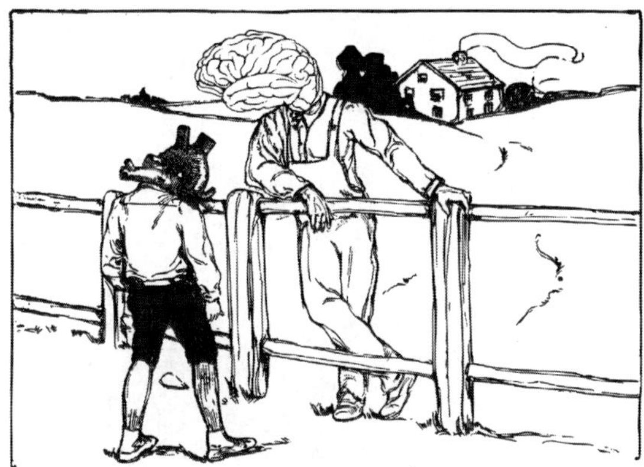

"I'm gonna need to see some ID."

VENOUS DRAINAGE

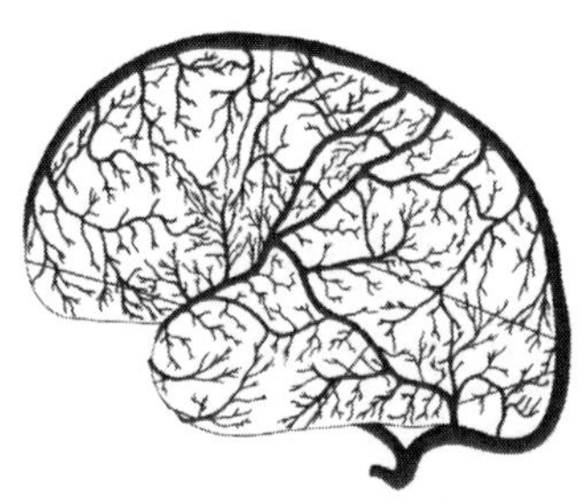

If more and more blood keeps coming into the brain via the arterial system and more and more cerebrospinal fluid keeps being produced in the ventricular system, where does all this extra fluid *go*? After all, the amount of the fluid in the skull can't keep building up in its enclosed space or else we would end up with a dangerously high pressure inside the skull! Luckily, both blood and cerebrospinal fluid are able to exit the brain through a series of **veins** scattered throughout the central nervous system, although they each exit in slightly different ways. Blood enters the venous system *immediately* after passing through the capillaries, while cerebrospinal fluid does not enter into the venous system *directly* but rather is absorbed through specialized protrusions of the arachnoid mater into the dura mater known as **arachnoid granulations**. Overall, though, the end result is the same!

There are two general systems of veins in the skull. The first, known as **cerebral veins**, carries blood from the brain itself and runs through the *subarachnoid* space. The second, known as **diploic veins**, instead carries blood from the skull and its overlying skin through the *dura* mater. There are several connecting veins running in the *subdural* space that bridge the gap between these two venous systems which are known, appropriately, as **bridging veins**. (The specific spaces that these arteries and veins run through will become clinically important when we talk about the effects of bleeding into each of these spaces in Chapter 15.)

Cerebral veins are made up of many small veins that, like rivers forming a delta, collectively merge into larger basins known as **dural venous sinuses**. Each dural venous sinus collects blood from broad areas of the brain as seen below:

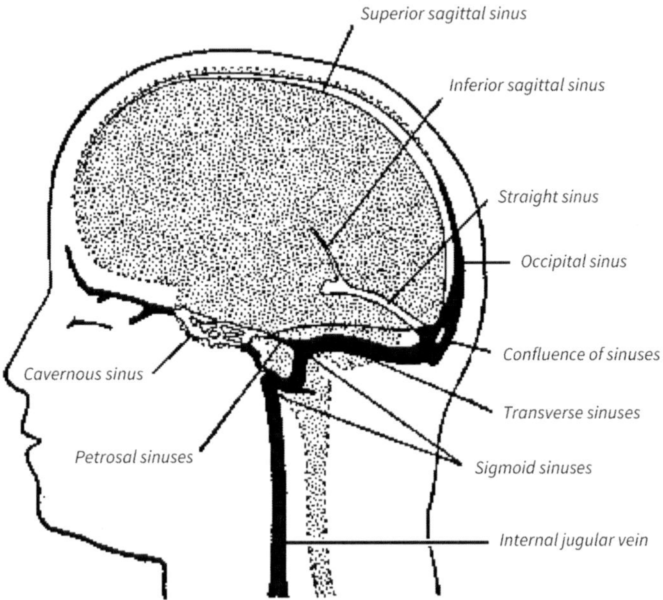

*The **venous drainage** of the brain.*

It's a lot, isn't it! It's like another circle of Willis to learn. However, let's see if we can simplify this using another mnemonic. This time, let's make a diagram using the letters from the word **VEIN** as below. First draw the V, then draw the E (with the letters overlapping), then draw the I coming down, and finally draw the N at the bottom:

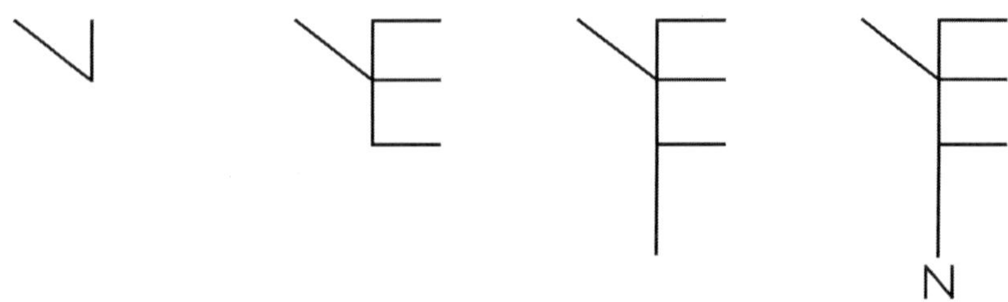

And with that, we're ready to label the parts:

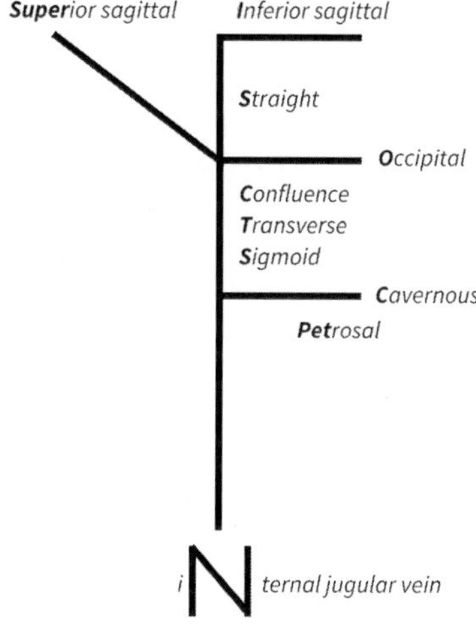

Now that we have both the anatomically correct diagram and its simplified counterpart, let's walk through the cerebral veins step by step. The *upper-middle* part of the cerebral cortex is drained by the **superior sagittal sinus** (which runs along the top of the brain right down the middle like a mohawk), while the *lower-middle* part drains to the **inferior sagittal sinus** (which runs parallel to the superior sagittal sinus but lower down) which then dumps into the **straight sinus**. The *posterior* aspect of the brain is drained by the **occipital sinus**. These three sinuses (the superior sagittal, straight, and occipital sinuses) all then merge at a point in the back of the head called the **confluence of sinuses** which lies beneath the occipital protuberance (which you can locate on yourself by placing a hand on the back of your skull and feeling for the small bump right in the middle). The confluence of sinuses then drains via the paired **transverse sinuses** (one going to the left and the other going to the right) which both run anteriorly. Along the way, the transverse sinuses become the **sigmoid sinuses** which pick up blood draining from the *lateral* parts of the brain via the **petrosal sinuses** as well as drainage from the *anterior* aspects of the brain (including the area around the eyes) via the **cavernous sinus**. All of these various drainage basins collect and then drain out of the head via the paired **internal jugular veins**. And that's it! So how can we remember all of the veins and sinuses here? Recall that the venous system is responsible for draining the brain. There's so much blood to take care of, you could almost say that it's "draining cats and dogs!" Take a moment to visualize this idiom, then connect that to a paraphrasing of it that lines up with the labeling of the VEIN diagram above: a "**S**uper **I**cy **S**hower **Of** **C**a**TS** & **C**anine **Pet**s." The **N** from VEIN will remind you that it all dumps into the i**N**ternal jugular vein!

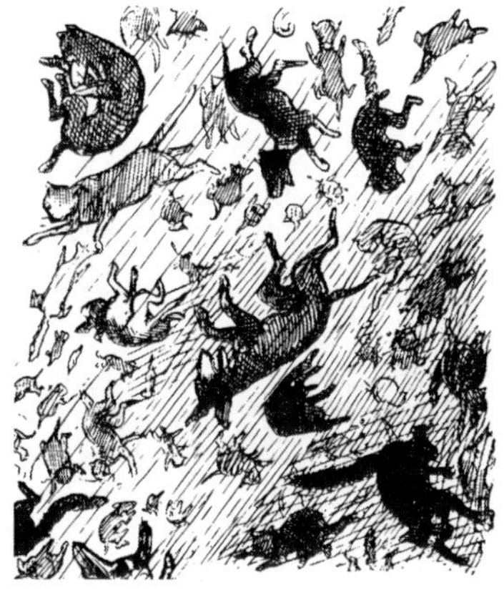

The **cerebral venous system** collects deoxygenated blood from various **sinuses** around the brain before depositing into the **internal jugular veins**.

*Draw the diagram using the word **VEIN**, then fill it in using the phrase*
*"**S**uper **I**cy **S**hower **O**f **C**a**TS** & **C**anine **Pet**s":*
***Super**ior sagittal sinus*
***I**nferior sagittal sinus → **S**traight sinus*
***O**ccipital sinus*
***C**onfluence of sinuses → **T**ransverse sinus → **S**igmoid sinus*
***C**avernous sinus → **Pet**rosal sinus*
*i**N**ternal jugular vein*

CAVERNOUS SINUS THROMBOSIS

Let's look at a clinical diagnosis involving cerebral veins that illustrates the anatomy here well. **Cavernous sinus thrombosis** occurs when a blood clot gets trapped within the cavernous sinus. Ordinarily a clot in any area of the venous drainage from the head isn't that big of a deal, as there is an extensive system of anastomoses that provide alternative routes for blood to leave the brain and return to the body. However, in the case of the cavernous sinus, a clot has the potential to cause clinically significant problems due to the sheer number of other structures that pass through the cavernous sinus. You can remember these structures using the mnemonic **Tom COAT** which stands for the **T**rigeminal nerve (specifically its **o**phthalmic and **m**axillary divisions), the internal **C**arotid artery, the **O**culomotor nerve, the **A**bducens nerve, and finally the **T**rochlear nerve. In total, four different cranial nerves and a major artery all pass through the cavernous sinus, making a clot in this region a potentially dangerous situation!

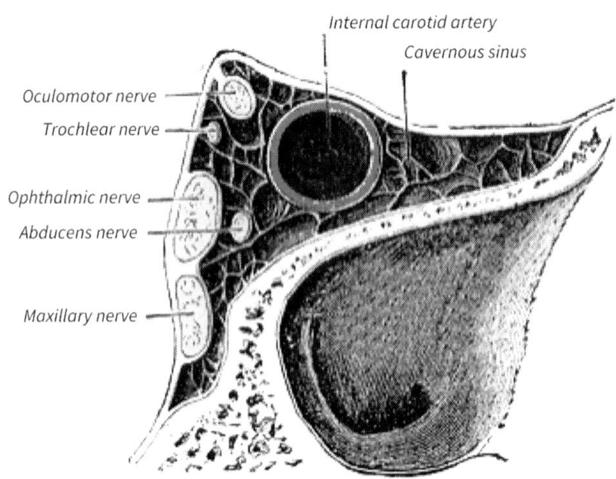

*Structures running through the **cavernous sinus**.*

Cavernous sinus thrombosis involves a **blood clot** blocking venous drainage from the **cavernous sinus** around the eyes. This has the potentially to disrupt nearby structures including **four cranial nerves** and the **internal carotid artery**.

Tom COAT:
__T__rigeminal nerve (__o__phthalmic and __m__axillary divisions)
Internal __C__arotid artery
__O__culomotor nerve
__A__bducens nerve
__T__rochlear nerve

The specific signs and symptoms you would observe in a patient with cavernous sinus thrombosis include **swelling or bulging of the eyes** (due to a blockage in fluid drainage from the eyes), changes in **vision** (due to the proximity of the cavernous sinus to the eyes), weakness of extraocular muscles (due to the involvement of the oculomotor, trochlear, and abducens nerves), and numbness of the upper two-thirds of the face (due to injury of the ophthalmic and maxillary divisions of the trigeminal nerve). By knowing the structures that course through the cavernous sinus, these signs and symptoms should not come as too much of a surprise.

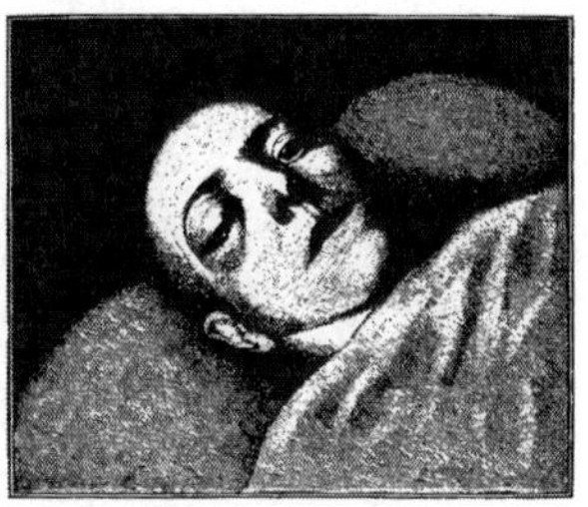

Diagnosis is based upon the presence of these signs and symptoms as well as a form of neuroimaging known as a **flow venogram** that allows for venous blood flow to be visualized and measured. Because this condition is usually associated with a local infection, treatment consists of **antibiotics**, with broad-spectrum agents used until the specific pathogen can be determined. Cavernous sinus thrombosis is a serious condition, with a very high mortality rate (up to 100% without treatment, and even as high as 20% *with* treatment)!

PUTTING IT ALL TOGETHER

Hey, we did it! At this point, we can confidently say that we've covered all the basics you'll need to know about neuroanatomy in order to understand clinical neurology. From this point forward, we are going to transition from merely *hinting* about what goes wrong in the nervous system to driving head-on into dangerous territory. All those beautiful and intricate neurologic systems we've spent time learning about are going to come crashing down in some surprising and unexpected ways. So buckle up and get ready as we transition away from the foundational anatomy of the nervous system and into a discussion of the diseases and disorders that are seen in clinical settings!

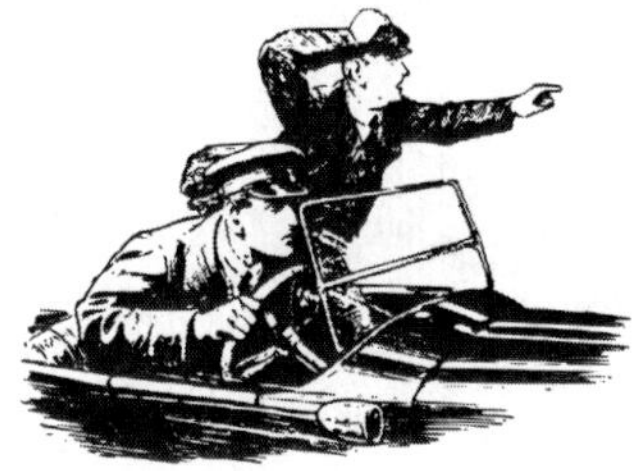

REVIEW QUESTIONS

1. A 60 y/o M comes to the emergency department after feeling dizzy for several hours. He has had two episodes of vomiting during this time. His gait is notably ataxic, and he appears increasingly lethargic as time goes on. An emergent angiogram is obtained which shows an occlusion in his basilar artery. Which of the following letters best identifies the artery involved?

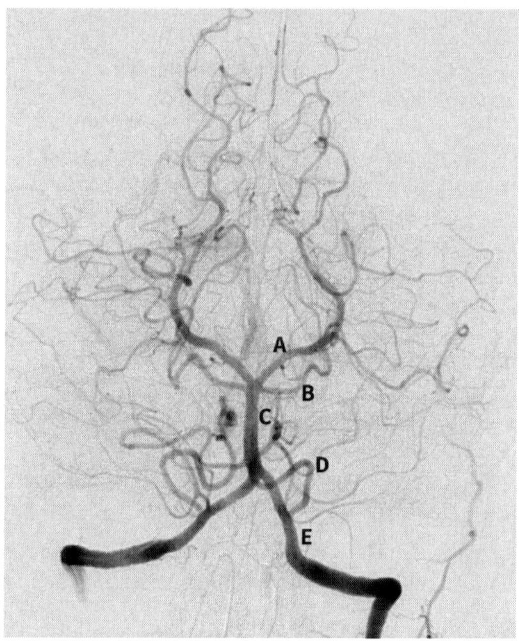

2. A 23 y/o F is prescribed propranolol, a beta-blocker, to help reduce anxiety related to public speaking. Compared to other beta-blockers, propranolol is believed to have greater effects on the central nervous system due to its ability to easily cross the blood–brain barrier. What property of propranolol likely accounts for this ability?
    A. High bioavailability
    B. Small molecular weight
    C. Tight protein-binding
    D. Low water solubility
    E. Active transport across tight junctions

3. A 33 y/o M is involved in a motor vehicle accident. He initially loses consciousness but then awakens within several minutes. In the emergency department, he complains of nausea and a severe headache. While the doctor is conducting a review of systems, the patient suddenly appears confused and stops responding to questions. Seconds later, he begins having a seizure. A CT scan is ordered

which shows bleeding in the epidural space. Which of the following is the most likely explanation for his seizure?

A. Mechanical compression of brain tissue
B. Dysfunction of grey matter due to direct exposure to blood
C. Tearing of white matter related to the injury
D. Blood mixing with cerebrospinal fluid in the ventricular system
E. Lack of mechanical protection due to loss of cerebrospinal fluid

4. A 10 y/o M is brought to his pediatrician by his parents. Over the past month he has experienced headaches, nausea, and vomiting which have all progressively worsened to the point where he is unable to attend school. His physical exam is notable for bilateral swelling of the optic discs suggestive of increased intracranial pressure. Head imaging is ordered which shows an arteriovenous malformation causing mechanical compression of the cerebral aqueduct. Which of the following areas is *least* likely to show enlargement in size?

A. Third ventricle
B. Fourth ventricle
C. Interventricular foramina
D. Lateral ventricle
E. All of the following are likely to be enlarged

5. A 68 y/o F with no significant medical history is seen in the emergency department for swelling and redness of the left eye as seen below:

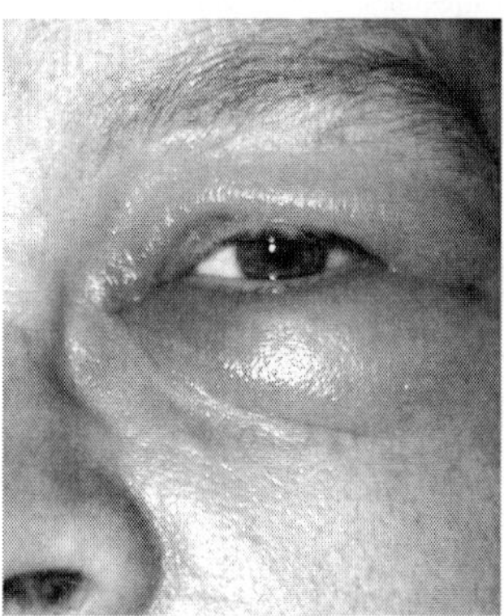

She reports that she first noticed these signs one week ago and that they have been gradually worsening since then. Review of systems is positive for fever, headache, and severe fatigue. She is diagnosed with a blood clot in the cerebral venous circulation. Given her presenting signs and symptoms, which of the following venous spaces is most likely to show filling defects on neuroimaging?

A. Superior sagittal sinus
B. Inferior sagittal sinus
C. Occipital sinus
D. Transverse sinus
E. Cavernous sinus

1. **The best answer is C.** The basilar artery is an unpaired artery in the posterior circulation of the head. Strokes here can lead to a variety of signs and symptoms, though the cerebellum and brainstem are the regions most often affected leading to signs like ataxia in this case. The posterior cerebral artery (answer A), superior cerebellar artery (answer B), anterior inferior cerebellar artery (answer D), and vertebral artery (answer E) are all paired arteries.

2. **The best answer is D.** Fat-soluble molecules are better able to cross the blood–brain barrier compared to those that are water-soluble. Out of all the beta-blockers, propranolol is unique in that it is by far the most lipophilic (making it also the most hydro*phobic*). Bioavailability refers to the amount of the ingested dose that reaches the bloodstream; however, this has no direct effect on the ability to cross the blood–brain barrier (answer A). A smaller molecular weight is only minimally helpful for allowing a drug to cross the blood–brain barrier (answer B). Protein-bound drugs cannot cross the blood–brain barrier, so a highly bound substance would be *less* able to cross it, not more (answer C). Finally, there is no evidence that propranolol is actively transported across the blood–brain barrier (answer E).

3. **The best answer is A.** Bleeding in the epidural space, known as an epidural hematoma, causes neural dysfunction due to compressive forces on the brain tissue itself. When the force is sufficiently strong, it can compress the brainstem, leading to loss of consciousness. The meninges acts to separate the brain from surrounding tissues, so bleeding in the space above the outer layer of the meninges would not lead to blood coming in direct contact with grey matter (answer B), nor would it lead to a tear injury of white matter (answer C). Cerebrospinal fluid flows in the subarachnoid space, not the epidural space (answers D and E).

4. **The best answer is B.** Compression of the cerebral aqueduct is likely to lead to enlargement of areas "upstream" due to build-up of cerebrospinal fluid. Out of the options listed, only the fourth ventricle occurs "downstream" of the cerebral aqueduct and is therefore unlikely to be enlarged. The lateral ventricles (answer D), interventricular foramina (answer C), and third ventricle (answer A) all are found "upstream" of the cerebral aqueduct.

5. **The best answer is E.** Of the listed options, only the cavernous sinus drains venous blood from areas in the front of the head, including the eyes. In contrast, the superior sagittal sinus drains the upper-middle aspect of the cerebral cortex (answer A), the inferior sagittal sinus drains the lower-middle cerebral cortex (answer B), and the occipital sinus drains the posterior aspect of the cerebral cortex (answer C). These three sinuses drain to the confluence of sinuses before continuing on as the transverse sinus (answer D).

13 THE NEUROLOGICAL EXAM

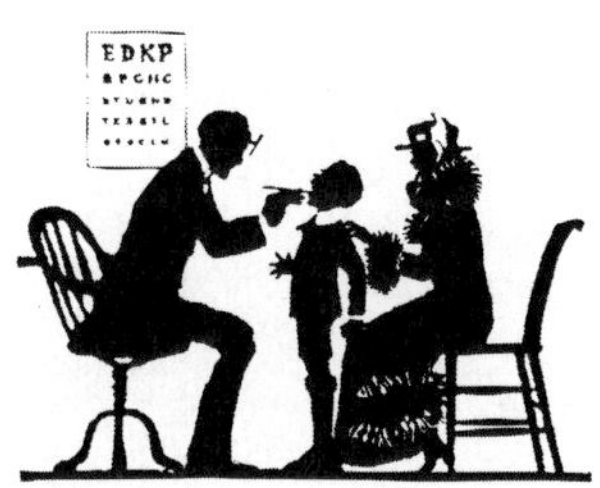

As we transition away from the foundational science of neuroanatomy into the actual practice of neurology in clinical settings, we're not leaving behind anything that we've learned so far! All of the knowledge that we've accumulated about the nervous system is still fair game to pop up for the rest of this book, so feel free to refer back to previous chapters whenever you need a refresher on a particular subject.

The goal of any clinician who is seeing a patient with a neurological complaint is two-fold: first, to find out what is going on (**diagnosis**), and second, to use this information to offer suggestions on how best to help (**treatment**). The starting point for diagnosis in neurology is to perform an **evaluation**. As in most medical fields, this typically begins with a detailed **history** and **physical** exam. In addition, neurologists will use the **neurological exam** which is a systematic series of tests to assess the function of all aspects of the nervous system across various areas of the body. This exam helps to localize dysfunction to specific parts of the nervous system, making it an invaluable tool for diagnosis.

In modern neurology, the neurological exam is just one piece of the puzzle. In many cases, it must be combined with relevant laboratory and imaging data to come up with the most accurate diagnosis. For this reason, we will briefly discuss some of the most common tools that are used in neurology to diagnose a patient's condition, including **neuroimaging** techniques such as **computed tomography** (CT) scans and **magnetic resonance imaging** (MRI) as well as **laboratory analysis** of blood and cerebrospinal fluid samples (the latter obtained using a technique known as a **lumbar puncture**).

THE NEUROLOGICAL EXAM

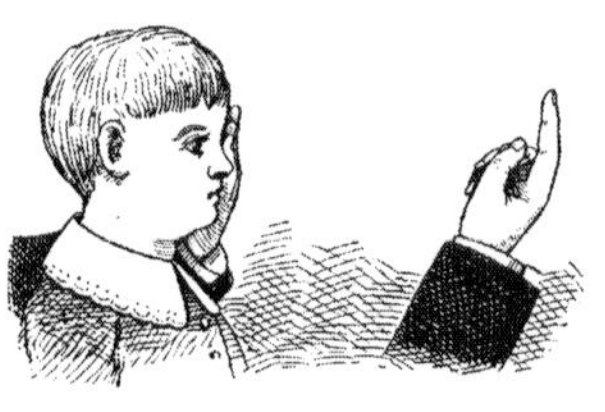

The neurological exam is a long procedure, as there is no way to systematically test every major aspect of the nervous system in multiple parts of the body without having to expend some serious time and effort! You'll need to bring a few tools with you to perform a neurological exam, including a **reflex hammer**, **tuning fork**, and **vibrating prongs**.

When performing a neurological exam, it can be helpful to have a mnemonic to remember each step to make sure you're not skipping any key components. You can use the following rhyme to keep the steps of the neurological exam in mind:

Head and **hammer**, **feet like tots**
Bulk and **tone**, **pretend we fought**
Stroking, **poking**, **shaking**, **hot**
Touch my finger, **stand** and **walk**!

Let's use this rhyme to break down these steps one by one.

MENTAL STATUS AND CRANIAL NERVES ("head")

The starting point for the neurological exam is to assess the patient's **mental status**, which includes their overall **level of consciousness** as well as **cognitive abilities** like concentration and memory. Even within the first few seconds of the exam, you can get a sense for whether the patient is fully alert or whether they are sedated, confused, or even comatose. However, if you'd like to assess this more systematically, you can ask the patient basic **orientation questions** including who they are, where they are, what time it is, and the reason for their visit (person, place, time, and purpose). Additional tests such as simple arithmetic and memory games can provide further clues. In cases where you suspect cognitive impairment, you may consider using a structured test like the Mini-Mental State Examination (MMSE) or Montreal Cognitive Assessment (MoCA) to provide a more detailed picture of the patient's cognitive abilities.

After assessing their mental status, the second part of "head" is to do a cranial nerve examination. Assessing each of the cranial nerves can help to localize specific deficits in the cerebrum or brainstem. We'll go over how to test each cranial nerve here. In clinical settings, you can use the same "Ooh Ooh Ooh To Touch And Feel Very Green Vegetables AH!" mnemonic from Chapter 9 to remember the order!

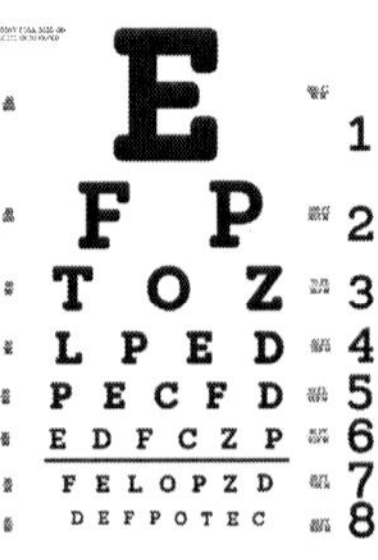

The **olfactory nerve** is difficult to assess unless if you've specifically brought something with you. Some neurologists will carry a small jar of tea leaves, coffee beans, or other objects with a distinct (but hopefully not unpleasant!) odor to test that the patient's sense of smell is intact.

The **optic nerve** can be assessed by asking the patient to cover one eye. You can then bring your finger into each of the four quadrants and ask the patient to say where your finger is. You can also test visual acuity by using a chart (such as the **Snellen chart** pictured to the right) at a fixed distance.

The cranial nerves controlling extraocular movements (the **oculomotor**, **trochlear**, and **abducens nerves**) can be tested by asking the patient to follow your finger with their eyes while keeping their head still. Move your finger in an H-shape in front of the patient's head to confirm that their eyes are able to move fully in all directions, as in the image below:

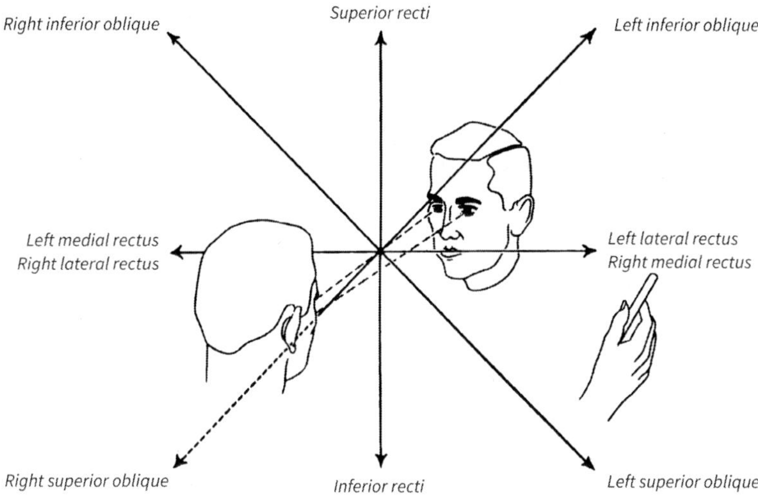

While assessing extraocular movement, look for **nystagmus** (which can indicate damage to the cerebellum, inner ear, or other systems involved in balance). Next, move your finger in towards the space between the patient's eyes to test for **accommodation**, as the patient's pupils should constrict as you move your finger inwards. Finally, test for the **pupillary light reflex** by shining a light into one eye at a time to ensure that *both* of the patient's pupils constrict in response to this.

The sensory component of the **trigeminal nerve** can be tested by lightly drawing a soft object like a cotton swab across the forehead, cheek, and jaw on both the left and the right, while the motor component can be tested by asking the patient to clench their jaw as well as open it against resistance ("Open your mouth while I try to hold it shut.").

The **facial nerve** can be tested by asking the patient to perform a variety of actions involving the muscles of the face, including raising their eyebrows, closing their eyes tightly, puffing out their cheeks, and showing their teeth. Look for weakness or asymmetry in any of these actions. You can simultaneously test both the fifth and seventh cranial nerve using the **corneal reflex** in which you try to (gently!) poke the patient's eye with a soft object. The patient should quickly shut their eye to keep out the incoming object. This reflex relies on the ophthalmic branch of the trigeminal nerve for its afferent limb and the facial nerve for its efferent limb.

A quick-and-dirty way to test the auditory component of the **vestibulocochlear nerve** is to rub your fingers together outside of each of the patient's ears and asking if they can hear the sound. If more in-depth testing is required, you can use the Weber and Rinne tests described in Chapter 11.

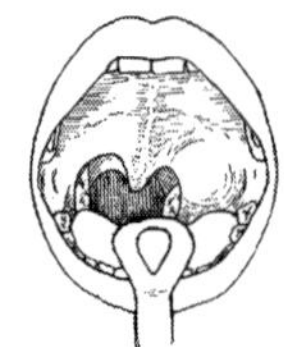

The **glossopharyngeal** and **vagus nerves** can be tested together, as they both are involved in uvula movement and the gag reflex. (This is the classic "Say ah!" moment when you visit the doctor.) If there is any unilateral weakness of these muscles, the uvula will deviate *away from* the weakness, as the non-affected side is pulling on it stronger than the affected side.

The **accessory nerve** can be quickly tested by asking the patient to shrug their shoulders as well as turn their head from side to side against your resistance.

Finally, the **hypoglossal nerve** is easily tested by asking the patient to stick out their tongue. Any weakness on one side will cause the tongue to deviate, although in contrast to the uvula, this will be *towards* the weakness. You can remember this by linking it to the phrase, "You lick your wounds."

A lesion of the **hypoglossal nerve** will cause the **tongue to deviate towards the side of lesion**.

*You **lick** your **wounds**.*

DEEP TENDON REFLEXES ("hammer")

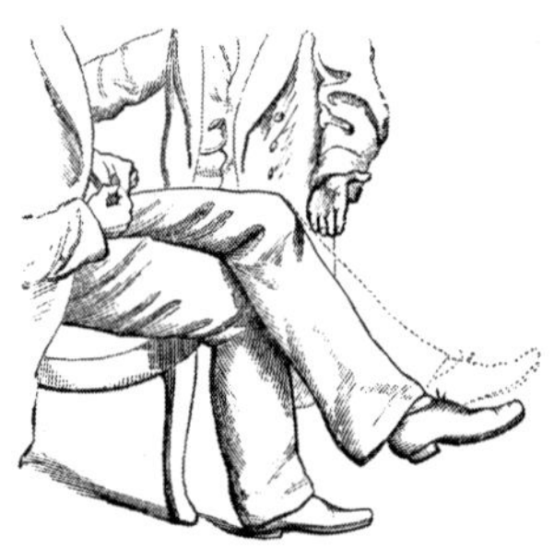

The word "hammer" should remind you of a **reflex hammer**, the tool that is commonly used to test **deep tendon reflexes**. As mentioned in Chapter 8, some sensory neurons synapse directly onto efferent motor neurons in the spinal cord to produce an automatic unconscious reaction. The prototype example of this is the **patellar or knee-jerk reflex** (pictured here on the right). When the patellar tendon is tapped, some of the sensory nerve fibers travel directly to the nerve roots of motor neurons in the spinal cord, causing an immediate "kick" of the leg. Decreased or absent reflexes (known as **hyporeflexia** and **areflexia**, respectively) tend to suggest damage in the afferent or efferent nerves involved, while brisk or hyperactive reflexes (known as **hyperreflexia**) tend to suggest involvement of either the frontal cortex or upper motor neurons. Reflexes are often graded on a scale of 0 to 4+, with 0 being absent, 1+ being below average, 2+ being average, 3+ being above average, and 4+ being very brisk and with continued rhythmic contractions known as **clonus**. If you can remember that 2+ is normal, the two grades above and two grades below will follow naturally!

Grade	Description
4+	**Hyperactive** with **clonus**
3+	**Above** average
2+	**Average**
1+	**Below** average
0	**No reflex**

There are several other reflex arcs like this in the spinal cord, and they are clinically useful for localizing at what level an injury has occurred. The primary spinal reflexes are the **biceps reflex** (C5-C6), the **triceps reflex** (C6-C7), the **patellar or knee jerk reflex** (L2-L4), and the **Achilles or ankle jerk reflex** (S1-S2). Let's learn a few memory aids to remember the spinal nerves associated with each one.

For the biceps and triceps, draw a stick figure but use the numbers 6 and 7 instead of arms, as below. The **6** looks like someone flexing their bulging **biceps** while the **7** looks like someone showing off their **triceps**:

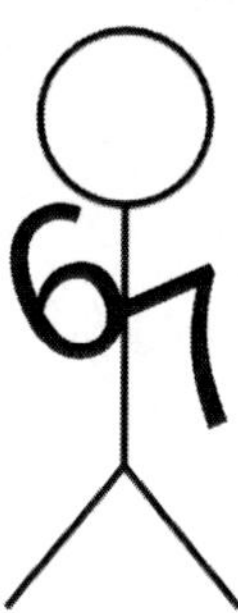

For the patellar reflex, draw a stick figure using an **L** for the lower half of the body to show that he is kneeling on two legs or even down on L4s (all fours). This should help you remember that the knee jerk reflex is between L2 and L4.

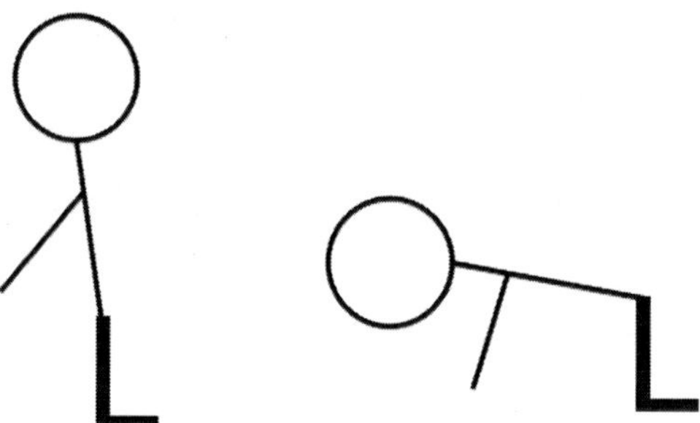

Finally, for the ankle jerk or Achilles reflex, write Achilles as Ach-**I**-**II**-e**S** (using Roman numerals **I** and **II**) to remember that it is between S**1**-S**2**.

The primary spinal reflexes are the **biceps reflex** (C5-C6), the **triceps reflex** (C6-C7), the **patellar reflex** (L2-L4), and the **Achilles reflex** (S1-S2).

*A stick figure with **6**s for arms is showing off its **biceps** (C5-C**6**).*
*A stick figure with **7**s for arms is showing off its **triceps** (C6-C**7**).*
*A stick figure with **2 Ls** for legs is either kneeling or down on **L4**s (L2-L4).*
*Ach-**I**-**II**-e**S** reflex (S**1**-S**2**).*

PRIMITIVE REFLEXES ("feet like tots")

Next, you will test a set of **primitive reflexes** which are so-named because they are typically exhibited by infants but not adults. While the underlying reflex circuits are present for people of all ages, as someone gets past one or two years of age, the frontal lobe develops to the point where it is able to automatically *inhibit* these reflexes (as it's the part of the brain that says "no"). For this reason, re-appearance of primitive reflexes in an adult is indicative of either **frontal lobe pathology** or of damage to **upper motor neurons** that carry these inhibitory signals down to the body.

By far the most commonly tested primitive reflexes is the **Babinski sign** (also known as the **plantar reflex**). To perform this test, drag an instrument (such as the sharper end of a reflex hammer) on the bottom of the foot on the lateral side from the heel to the toes. In healthy adults, the toes will naturally curve in *towards* the stimulus. In contrast, a positive Babinski sign occurs if the toes instead fan out *away* from the stimulus. This is why testing of primitive reflexes is called "feet like tots": the toes react in the same way that an infant's would. You can remember this by thinking that the **Babi**nski sign is only normal in **Babi**s.

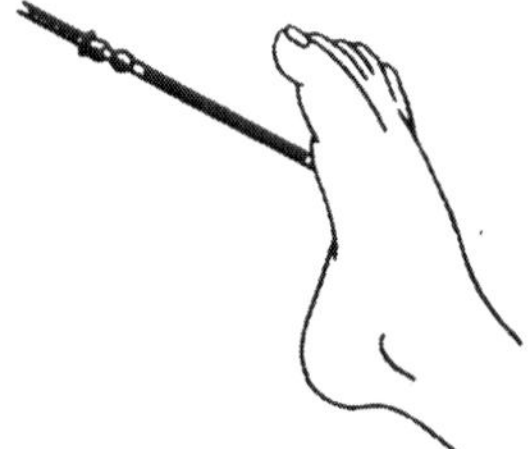

Downgoing Babinski *(normal)*

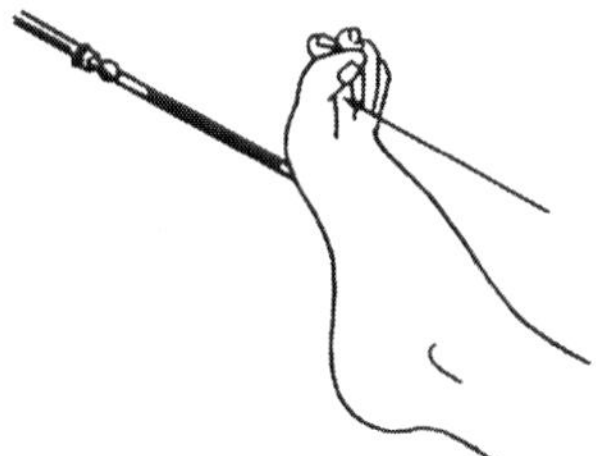

Upgoing Babinski *(abnormal)*

Presence of the **plantar reflex** in an adult is indicative of either **frontal lobe pathology** or **upper motor neuron disease**.

*The **Babi**nski sign is only normal in **Babi**s.*

While the Babinski sign is the most commonly tested primitive reflex, a few others exist as well, including the **rooting reflex** (the baby turns its head if its cheek is touched), the **Moro reflex** (the baby throws its arms out when startled), and the **palmar grasp reflex** (the baby's fingers close around an object placed in the palm). These are used clinically in a similar fashion to the Babinski sign.

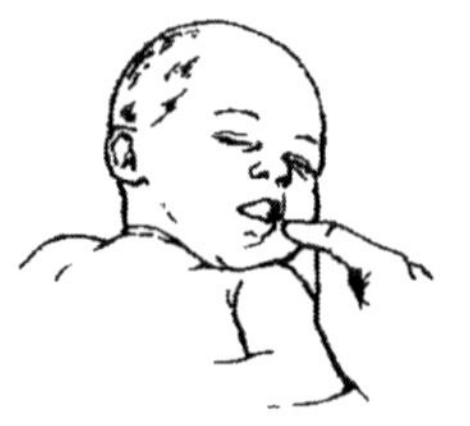

Rooting *reflex*

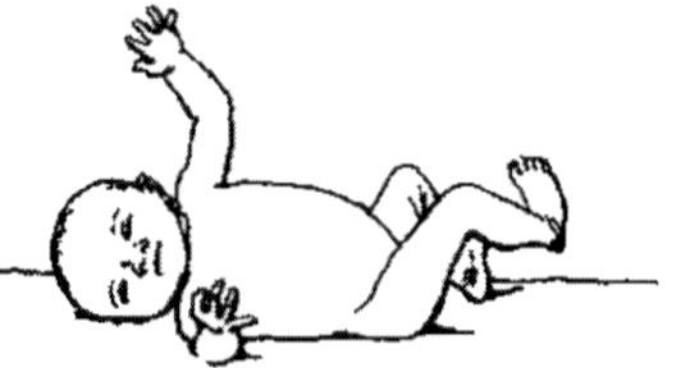

Moro *reflex*

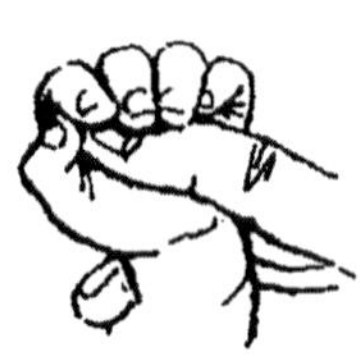

Palmar grasp *reflex*

THE MOTOR SYSTEM ("bulk and tone, pretend we fought")

Testing the **motor system** involves three components: observing the **bulk** (or overall size) of various muscles in the body, noting their **tone**, and testing their **strength**.

Determining the bulk of muscles does not require any sort of sophisticated exam maneuvers. Instead, you simply observe. Someone with focal wasting or atrophy of specific muscles may have sustained damage to the motor neurons innervating that muscle, as a lack of nerve supply tends to shrivel muscles like a flower without water. A generalized atrophy of all muscles in the body may be more suggestive of a disease in the muscle tissue itself (known as a **myopathy**, which we will cover in Chapter 16).

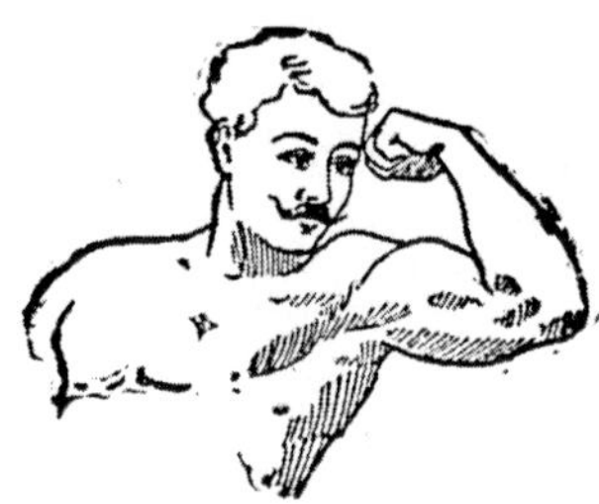

Muscle **tone** can be assessed by asking the patient to completely relax while you perform various movements on their behalf (such as holding their arm in one hand while moving their forearm with the other hand to assess muscle tone around the elbow joint). Changes in muscle tone can suggest different types of pathology. A weak or **flaccid tone** may suggest lower motor neuron damage, especially combined with wasting. In contrast, a **spastic tone** (muscles that are unusually tight, stiff, or jerky) can indicate upper motor neuron damage. A specific finding known as **cogwheel rigidity** (in which manipulating the patient's joints results in a *click-click-click*-like jerking of the joint) is suggestive of a condition known as Parkinsonism (which we will cover further in Chapter 19).

Finally, testing the **strength** of muscles can be done by asking the patient to resist you in performing various actions (hence "pretend we fought"). For example, you can test the muscles of the arm by asking the patient to bend their elbows and try to extend their arms while you push against them. Strength is traditionally graded on a scale between 0 and 5, with 5 being full strength resistance, 4 being some resistance, 3 being resistance against gravity but not the examiner, 2 being some movement but no ability to hold up against gravity, 1 being a flicker or twitching of muscles but no actual limb movement, and 0 being complete paralysis of the muscles.

Grade	Description
5	Can move against **full resistance**
4	Can move against **moderate resistance**
3	Can move **against gravity** but not against any resistance
2	Can move only if positioned so that **gravity is eliminated**
1	Contractions seen but **insufficient to produce movement**
0	**No contraction** seen

SENSATION ("stroking, poking, shaking, hot")

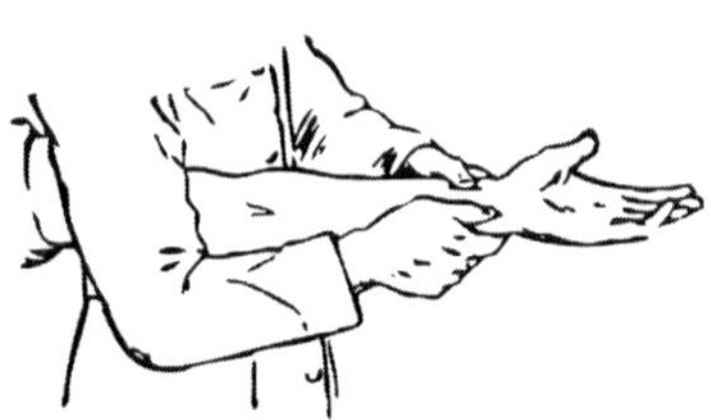

Because different kinds of sensory information travel along different pathways, we need to test each kind in order to determine where damage may have occurred. These tests will need to be repeated across various areas of the body. For example, someone may have intact sensation in their upper extremities but not their lower extremities, so if you only tested this in one location, you would miss this finding.

You can test **light touch** by gently pulling something soft against the skin ("stroking"). In contrast, **pain** sensation can be tested by applying a sharp but not dangerous object (such as a toothpick) lightly into the skin ("poking"). You can also consider testing for **discriminative touch** by placing two pins close together on the skin and asking the patient when they can discern that there are two sensations rather than just one. Under normal circumstances, two-point discrimination is stronger in areas with many sensory nerves (such as the lips or the tips of the finger) and less powerful in insensitive areas such as the back.

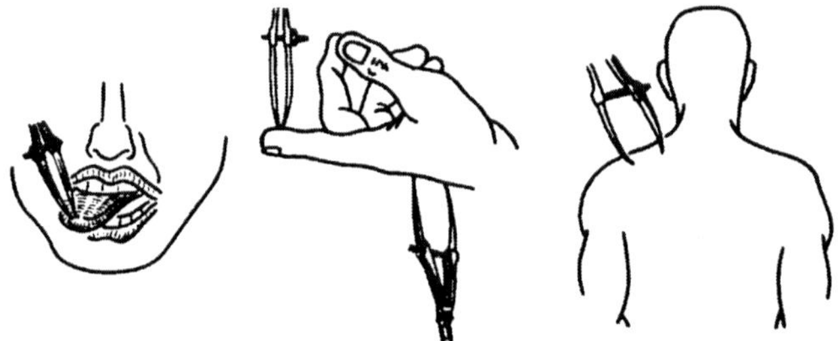

***Discriminative touch** varies in sensitivity across different parts of the body.*

Testing **vibration** ("shaking") can be done by applying a vibrating prong against the patient's skin and asking them when they feel it stop vibrating. Make sure to test **proprioception** (which also travels in the dorsal column—medial lemniscus pathway) as well by asking the patient to close their eyes and tell you if you are lifting their fingers or toes up or down (which is kind of like a slow-motion version of "shaking").

Finally, you can test **temperature** ("hot") by applying both a warm and a cold object (such as a heated blanket and a metal stethoscope) against the skin to ensure that the patient can discriminate between the two temperatures.

COORDINATION ("touch my finger")

Coordination and balance are largely reliant upon the cerebellum. Cerebellar function can be tested in a few ways. The most commonly used test is the **finger-to-nose test** in which you ask the patient to alternate between touching their nose and touching your finger while you move your finger around ("touch my finger"). This requires the cerebellum to be able to integrate visual information about the position of *your* finger with proprioceptive information about the position of *their* finger.

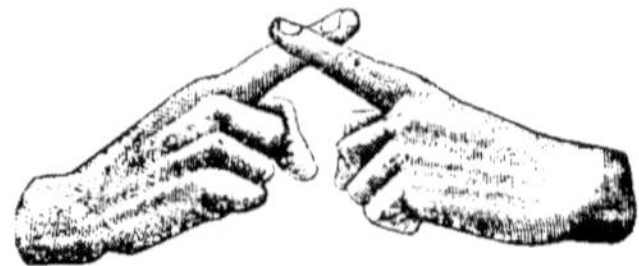

Two other ways to test cerebellar function are the **heel-to-shin test** (in which you ask the patient to place the back of their ankle against the knee of their other leg, then run their ankle down the shin to the foot and back up again) and the **rapid pronation-supination test** (in which you ask the patient to touch the palm of one hand with the front of their other hand then with the back of their other hand and repeat this movement as fast as possible). An inability to perform any of these actions can indicate cerebellar dysfunction.

THE ROMBERG TEST ("stand")

To perform the **Romberg test**, ask the patient to stand with their feet shoulder-width apart ("stand"). They should then put their arms straight out in front of them palms-up (as if they are holding an invisible platter of food). Ordinarily, someone can do this without falling over by using three senses: their sense of **sight**, their sense of **balance**, and their sense of **proprioception**. Even if one of these senses is missing, the patient can still use the other two to compensate and maintain their balance. However, to fully pass the Romberg test, the patient must close their eyes. By doing this, you are taking sight out of the equation. If they can maintain balance even after closing their eyes, then both their vestibular system and proprioception are intact. If they fall over after closing their eyes, however, you know that at least one of those functions is absent. (Make sure to stand close to the patient to steady them in case they start falling!) For this reason, a positive Romberg is indicative of problems with either **proprioception** or the **vestibular system**.

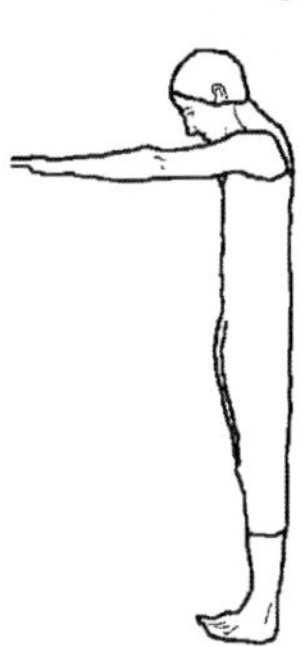

GAIT ("walk")

The final step of the neurological exam is to test the patient's **gait** ("walk"). Someone with a normal gait should be able to walk steadily without tripping or falling. They should even be able to walk when given specific conditions, such as walking only on their heels or the tips of their toes. An unsteady or **ataxic** gait can be suggestive of either upper or lower motor neuron damage, cerebellar dysfunction, or various forms of sensory pathology.

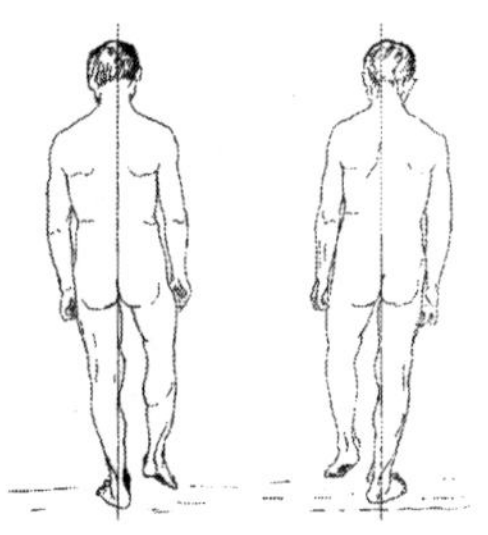

The **neurological exam** is a **systematic series of tests** of neurological function across the entire body.

Head *and* ***hammer, feet like tots***
Bulk *and* ***tone, pretend we fought***
Stroking, poking, shaking, hot
Touch my finger, stand *and* ***walk!***

Ultimately, the best way to learn the neurological exam is to just *do it*! Find someone else who is trying to learn it, then practice until it feels comfortable. You can use the rhyming mnemonic above to remind yourself of what steps come next!

NEUROIMAGING

While the neurological exam can provide you with a wealth of information about the current status of the patient's nervous system, there's something to be said about just *seeing it* with your own eyes! Using neuroimaging, it is now possible to get detailed images depicting both the structure and function of the nervous system, allowing for greater diagnostic precision and targeted treatment. There are a few different types of neuroimaging techniques, each of which can be ordered in a variety of configurations depending on the specific clinical situation.

COMPUTED TOMOGRAPHY

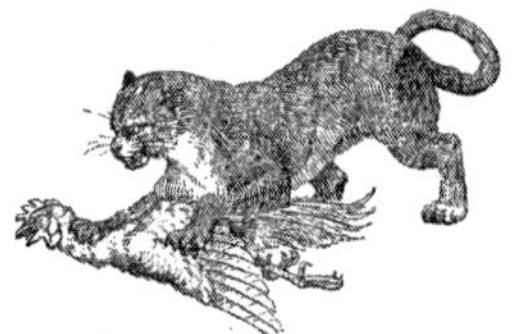

Computed tomography scans (also known as **CT** or **CAT scans**) use a series of x-rays to produce an image of the brain. CT scans have the advantage of being **quick** to produce, taking only a few minutes. This makes them ideal for **emergency situations** (like ruling out a brain bleed in a patient who hit their head in an accident). However, this speed comes at a price, as the images that are produced are often a bit muddy-looking compared to the highly detailed images you would get from an MRI. In addition, because CT scans use multiple x-rays, they expose the patient to high amounts of potentially harmful **ionizing radiation**. For this reason, it can be helpful to think of **CT** scans as being like a **C**a**T**: they are quick but can be harmful.

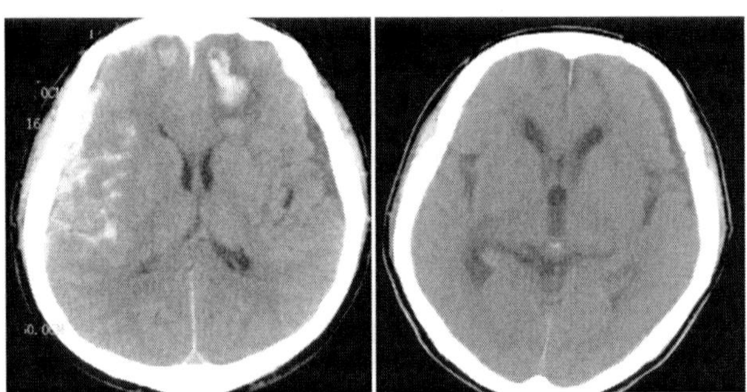

Computed tomography (CT) scan *of the head.*

CT scans are **quick to obtain**, but they **lack detail** and involve **radiation exposure**.

*CaT scans are like **cats**: they are **quick** but can be **harmful**.*

MAGNETIC RESONANCE IMAGING

Magnetic resonance imaging (or **MRI**) uses magnetic fields and radio waves to produce **high-quality images**. (Just compare the images on the next page with the CT scans on this one—there's no contest!) MRIs are particularly well-suited for visualizing structures deep in the **posterior fossa** (such as the cerebellum or brainstem) that x-rays have trouble reaching. Furthermore, because they do not use x-rays, MRIs do not expose the patient to ionizing radiation, making them much **safer** than CTs.

So if they're safer and produce better quality images than a CT, why not use them all the time? The main drawback of MRIs is that they are **slow**, with some scans taking an hour or more to produce. In addition, the patient must remain still the entire time to get a good image. Because of this, they are less useful in emergencies where a rapid diagnosis is needed.

MRI scans produce **detailed images** and do not involve ionizing radiation, but they also take **more time to make**.

***MRI**s **M**ake **R**ealistic **I**mages but you **M**ust **R**emain **I**dle.*

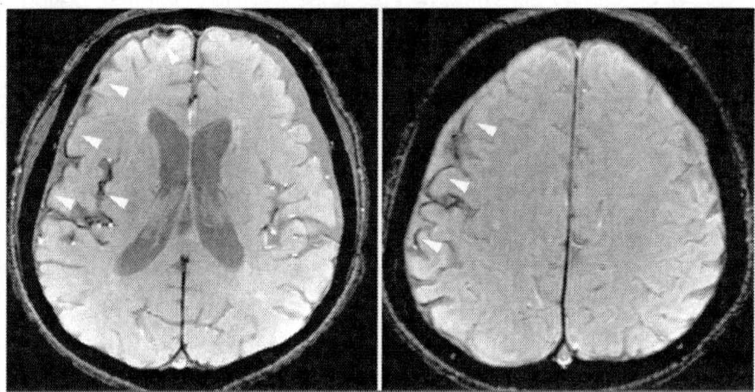

***Magnetic resonance imaging (MRI) scan** of the head.*

It's worth pointing out that both CT and MRI scans are displayed as though the patient is lying face-up on a table with their toes pointed towards the ceiling. You are standing at the patient's feet looking forward towards their head. For this reason, the patient's *left* brain is actually on the *right* side of the image and vice versa!

FUNCTIONAL NEUROIMAGING

There are various forms of **functional neuroimaging** that allow you to look at the *activity* of certain areas of the brain. One of the most common is **functional magnetic resonance imaging** (**fMRI**) which measures the difference between oxygenated and deoxygenated blood to estimate activity. Functional MRI scans are increasingly being used to diagnose strokes and other conditions involving poor blood flow.

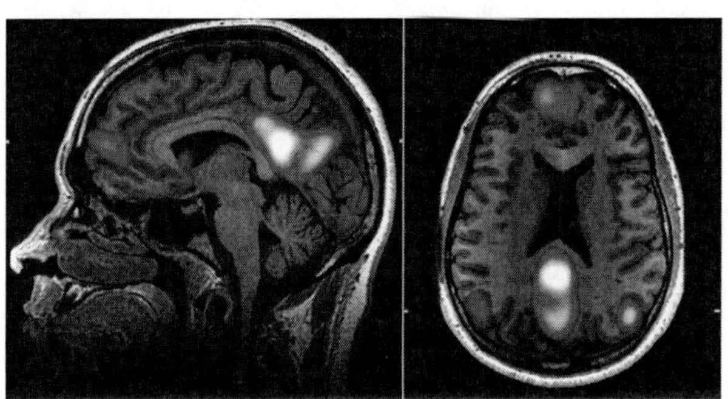

*An **fMRI** scan, with **lighter areas** showing regions of **greater activity**.*

Like fMRI, **positron emission tomography** (or **PET**) scans are able to measure the metabolic activity of specific regions rather than simply showing the structure. For this reason, they are useful for detecting diseases that involve changes in metabolic activity (either too much activity, as in a metabolically hungry brain tumor, or too little, as in certain forms of dementias). Overall, PET scans are quicker to obtain, while fMRI scans are able to produce more detailed images.

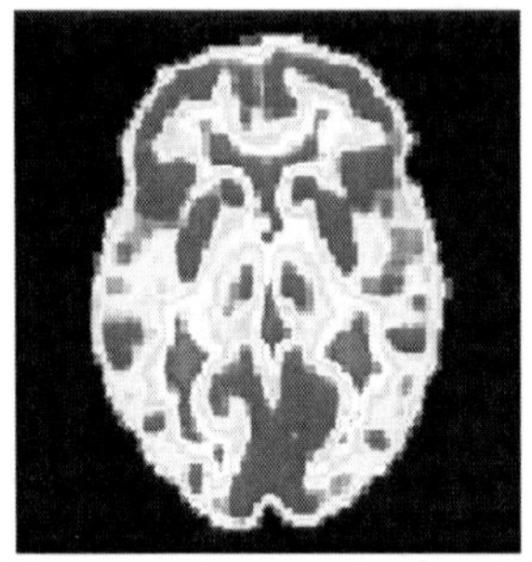
*A **PET scan** showing **normal brain activity**.*

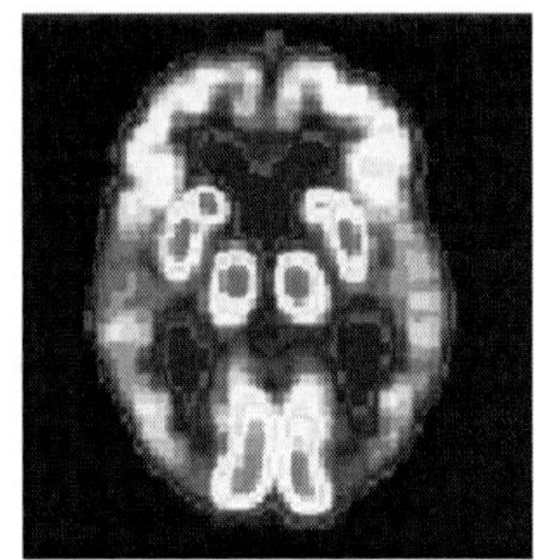
*A **PET scan** in a patient with **Alzheimer's disease**.*

LUMBAR PUNCTURE

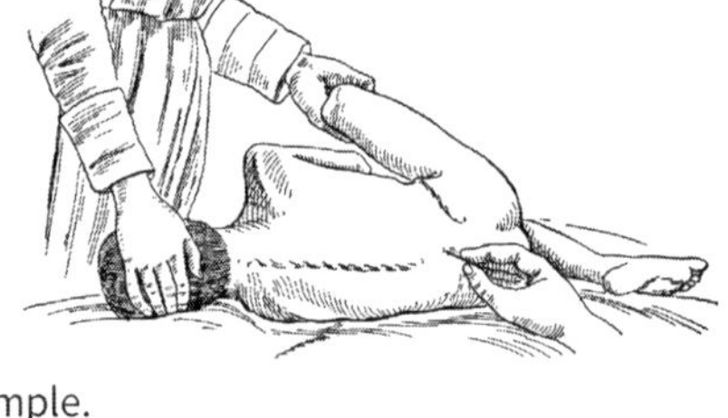

In neurology, sometimes you'll need to test a patient's **cerebrospinal fluid** to examine things that normal blood testing cannot reveal not (for example, an infection of the meninges). Because cerebrospinal fluid lies deep within the highly protected central nervous system, you will need to use a procedure known as a **lumbar puncture** (also known as a spinal tap) to obtain the sample.

You can perform a lumbar puncture by asking the patient to bend forward to help open up the intervertebral space as much as possible. Find the space between the **posterior superior iliac crests** and bring your fingers in towards the spine. This should place you at the intervertebral space between **L3-L4** which is where the needle should be inserted. (Inserting the needle at L3-L4 helps it to avoid hitting the spinal cord directly, as the spinal cord terminates into the conus medullaris around L1 or L2.) The needle can then be used to extract cerebrospinal fluid from this space.

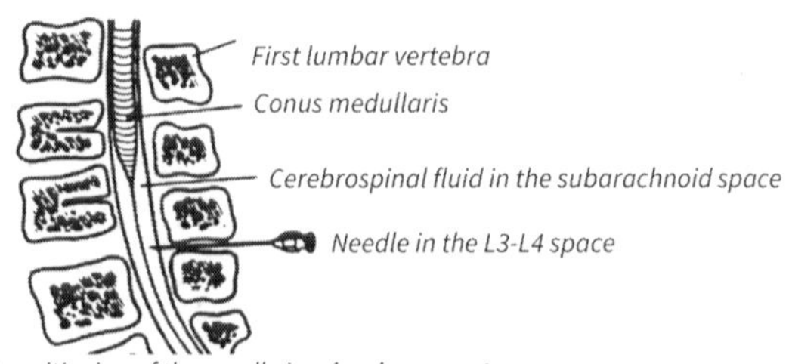

*Correct positioning of the needle in a **lumbar puncture**.*

A **lumbar puncture** can be used to obtain a sample of **cerebrospinal fluid** for **diagnosis or treatment**. The needle should be inserted between **L3-L4**.

*"**LP in L3!**" (L1, L2, L4, and L5 don't rhyme...)*

While a lumbar puncture can be an incredibly helpful procedure, it is not without risk! In addition to being uncomfortable or even painful for the patient, inserting a needle into a protected space like the central nervous system introduces the potential for infection, so **sterile technique** must be followed at all times! In addition, there is a risk that removing cerebrospinal fluid can cause the pressure in the spinal cord to drop, thereby creating a vacuum that in some cases can even suck parts of the brain down into the spine (a condition known as **cerebral herniation**). As we will discover in Chapter 15, herniation can compress parts of the brain and can even lead to permanent damage. For most people, the risk of cerebral herniation due to a lumbar puncture is incredibly low. However, in patients with high intracranial pressure, you will need to order a CT scan to assess the risk more fully before proceeding with a lumbar puncture. High-risk patients include those with a known history of **C**entral nervous system disease, any **F**ocal neurologic deficits, an **I**mmunocompromised status, evidence of **R**aised intracranial pressure (such as bulging of the optic discs on eye exam), new-onset or unexplained **S**eizures, and anyone whose **T**hinking is unclear (altered mental status). You can remember these cases by thinking that you have to **C FIRST** before doing a lumbar puncture.

In certain patients, **brain imaging** is required before performing a **lumbar puncture** to avoid **cerebral herniation**.

*In some patients, you'll want to **C** (see) **FIRST**:*
***C**entral nervous system disease*
***F**ocal neurologic deficits*
***I**mmunocompromised*
***R**aised intracranial pressure*
***S**eizures (new-onset or unexplained)*
***T**hinking unclear*

PUTTING IT ALL TOGETHER

The number of tools that neurologists and other clinicians have at their disposal for diagnosing and treating disease keeps increasing as medical technology continues to improve. At the end of the day, however, knowing how to take a good **history** and perform a thorough **neurological exam** remain vital skills that any clinician needs to have! Keep practicing the neurological exam until you feel completely comfortable doing it. When you meet a patient with a neurological complaint for the first time, you will be glad you did!

REVIEW QUESTIONS

1. A 78 y/o F is brought to the emergency department from her skilled nursing facility after a staff member noticed that she began appearing confused during a meal. In the hospital, a medical student discussing the case with his preceptor says that he believes the patient has had a stroke but wants to get an MRI to determine the exact location. What is the preceptor's most likely response?
    A. "There's no time. We should do a CT instead."
    B. "Let's do a thorough neurological exam first before subjecting the patient to such high doses of radiation."
    C. "An MRI won't produce the kind of images that we would need to localize a stroke for this patient."
    D. "We need a clearer picture of metabolic activity in this patient's brain. Let's do a functional MRI scan instead."
    E. "Before we can do that, we need to do a lumbar puncture."

2. (Continued from previous question.) During the neurological exam, the medical student drags his pen against the patient's foot. This causes the toes to fan out as seen below:

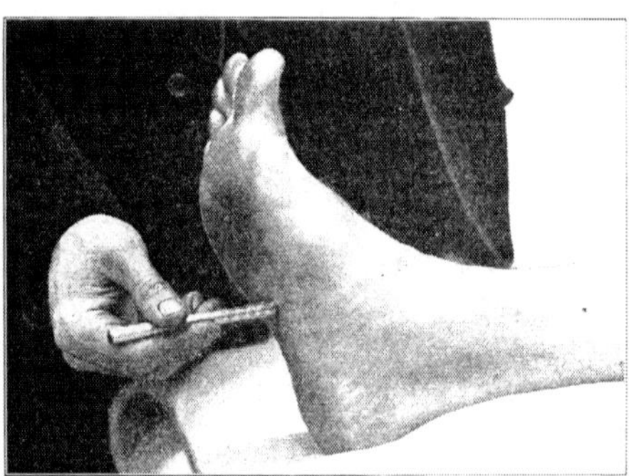

   Which of the following additional exam findings is the most likely to be seen?
    A. Brisk 4+ reflexes
    B. Flaccid muscle tone
    C. Unilateral deviation when sticking out the tongue
    D. Lack of vibration and proprioception
    E. Focal parietal lobe atrophy on neuroimaging
    F. None of the above are likely to be seen

3. A 38 y/o M is undergoing a thorough neurological exam after he has fallen several times while walking in the past week. On exam, his gait is notably ataxic. As part of the exam, the neurologist asks the patient to stand up and place his feet together. He does this without a problem. When asked to close his eyes, he sways unsteadily for the first 5 seconds. However, he is ultimately able to stay standing upright for a full minute. Based on the results of this test, where is there most likely to be a lesion in this patient?

A. Cerebellum
B. Dorsal columns of the spinal cord
C. Visual pathway
D. Vestibular apparatus in the inner ear
E. Vestibulocochlear nerve

4. A 44 y/o M presents to his primary care nurse practitioner complaining of right arm pain. He says the pain goes down his arm and "into my thumb and index finger." X-ray of the neck reveals degenerative bone changes at C5 as below:

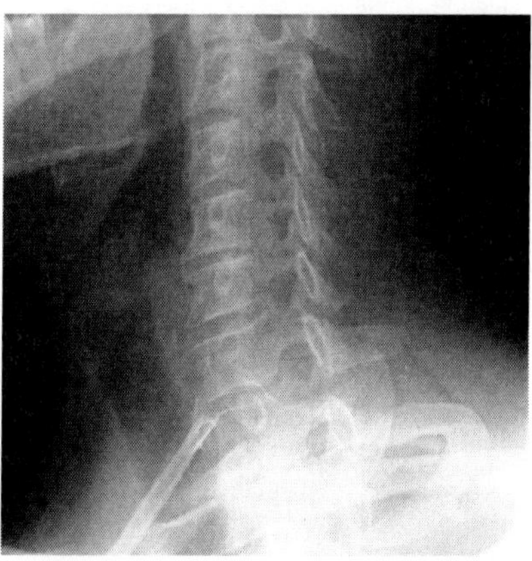

After a full history and neurological exam, he is given a presumptive diagnosis of cervical spinal stenosis at the level of C5. The patient is most likely to show an abnormality in which of the following reflexes?
A. Biceps
B. Triceps
C. Patellar
D. Ankle jerk
E. Plantar

5. An 18 y/o M is brought to the hospital after he was found lying in the hallway of his dorm appearing sleepy and confused. He is febrile with a temperature of 101.8°F. His dorm has experienced a recent outbreak of meningitis, so a lumbar puncture is ordered. A new intern is called to assist with the lumbar puncture. How should the intern demonstrate where she will place the needle?
A. Measuring the length of the back from the shoulders to the waist and inserting the needle halfway down
B. Feeling for the bottoms of the ribcage bilaterally and then marking halfway between them
C. Feeling for the tops of the pelvis bilaterally and then marking the midpoint between them
D. Ordering an x-ray of the spine to determine the location of the cauda equina
E. Asking the patient to point to where his back hurts the most

1. **The best answer is A.** Different modalities of neuroimaging each have their advantages and disadvantages. An MRI is better than a CT when it comes to producing detailed images (answer C) and does not involve ionizing radiation (answer B). A specific subtype of MRI known as functional MRI is able to show metabolic processes (answer D). The main disadvantages of an MRI are its cost and the time it takes to produce an image compared to a CT. In an emergency situation like a possible stroke, an MRI would take too long to obtain, making a CT the imaging modality of choice. In cases of suspected stroke, waiting to do a lumbar puncture before performing neuroimaging is likely to harm the patient by allowing ischemic injury to progress (answer E).

2. **The best answer is A.** A positive Babinski sign in an adult is indicative of either frontal lobe pathology or upper motor neuron damage. Both of these would also be expected to cause hyperreflexia as well. None of the other findings are clearly associated with frontal lobe pathology or upper motor neuron damage.

3. **The best answer is A.** The Romberg test assesses three things: the patient's sense of proprioception, their vestibular system, and their visual pathways. Under normal conditions, at least two of these three structures must be intact for the patient to remain upright. By asking the patient to close his eyes, the examiner is testing his proprioception and vestibular function. Some degree of swaying is normal and, provided the patient is able to remain upright, actually demonstrates intact functioning of these systems. For this reason, the patient's negative Romberg test is a sign that all three of these systems are working (answers B—E). While it is sometimes mistaken as such, the Romberg test is *not* a test of cerebellar function! Given this, a negative Romberg test suggests that the cause of this patient's ataxia is most likely to be in his cerebellum.

4. **The best answer is A.** The biceps reflex is most often associated with damage to the C5 or C6 spinal nerves or one of their branches. In contrast, the triceps reflex is associated with C6-C7 (answer B), the patellar reflex with L2-4 (answer C), and the ankle jerk or Achilles reflex with S1-S2 (answer D). The plantar reflex, or Babinski sign, is generally a sign of frontal lobe damage and would not be abnormal in a patient with cervical spinal stenosis (answer E).

5. **The best answer is C.** Proper needle placement when performing a lumbar puncture is essential to avoid injuring the spinal cord. The target of the needle is the lumbar cistern or the cerebrospinal fluid-filled space below the termination of the spinal cord known as the cauda equina. The cauda equina typically occurs around the level of L1 or L2, so needle placement is generally between L3 and L4. The posterior superior iliac crests serve as a useful anatomical landmark to identify this space. The bottom of the ribcage would be too high and would likely result in spinal cord injury (answer B), as would inserting the needle into the midpoint of the back (answer A). A spinal x-ray is not necessary for determining the location of the L3-L4 interspace (answer D), nor are patients' self-reports of back pain relevant to this (answer E).

14 STROKES

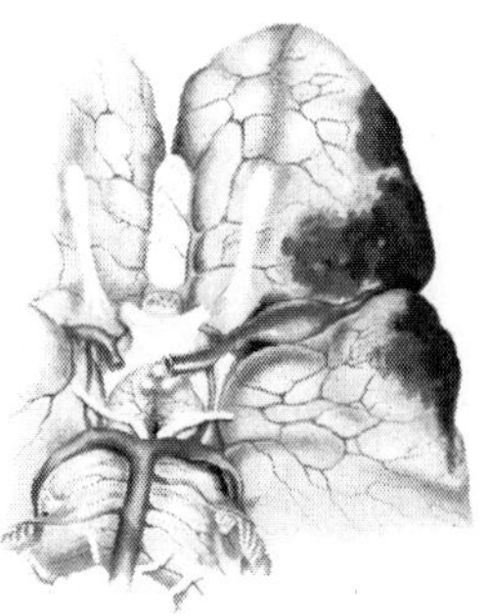

Now that we have the tools for diagnosing neurologic conditions, let's look at the diseases themselves! We'll first talk about **strokes** (also known as **cerebrovascular accidents** or CVAs). Strokes are a **neurologic emergency** related to **interruptions in oxygen supply** to the brain or other nervous tissue.

There are two primary forms of stroke. An **ischemic stroke** occurs when blood is unable to get to its destination which can occur either as a result of a **blockage** (like a tree falling across a river and creating a dam) or due to a **decrease in the amount of blood flow** (like a river drying up as the result of a drought). In contrast, a **hemorrhagic stroke** occurs when blood escapes from its intended path and goes someplace it shouldn't be going (like a pipe bursting, allowing water to flood the surrounding areas). In the case of hemorrhagic stroke, the displaced blood can also cause problems by being in areas that it shouldn't be, as blood can both irritate nervous tissue and lead to increased intracranial pressure. While the mechanism differs between the two forms of stroke, in both cases the effect is the same: the blood does not get to where it needs to go, depriving neurons of needed oxygen and leading to cell death and loss of function.

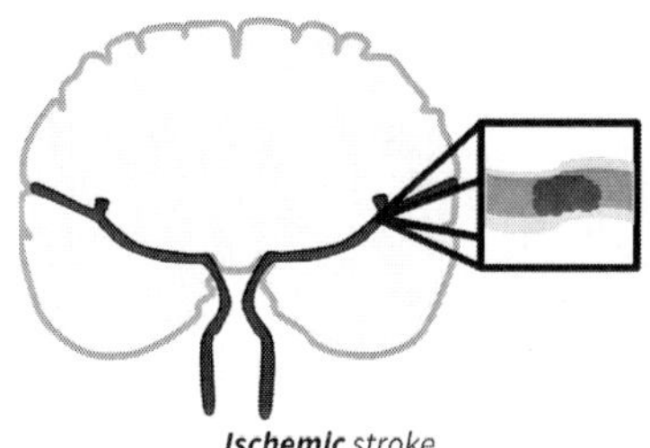

***Ischemic** stroke*

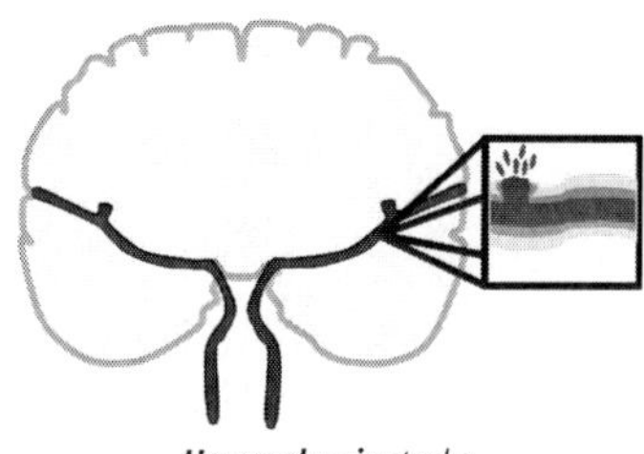

***Hemorrhagic** stroke*

DIAGNOSIS OF STROKES

Because specific arteries supply specific parts of the brain, the signs and symptoms of a stroke are largely dependent upon which areas have been damaged. For example, a stroke in the frontal lobe will have a completely different presentation than a stroke in the occipital lobe due to the distinct functions that each of these lobes perform. We will spend most of this chapter talking about how to localize strokes based on the specific signs and symptoms that the patient is presenting with.

However, as a starting place it's helpful to know that a few **general signs and symptoms** can be seen across *most* cases of strokes! These are encapsulated in the mnemonic **BE FAST** which stands for **B**alance issues, **E**ye or vision problems, **F**acial drooping, **A**rm or leg weakness, **S**peech impediments, and **T**iming (specifically a **sudden onset**, as the brain requires a constant supply of oxygen to keep running so a stroke will often produce these signs within a couple of minutes rather than with a slow onset as is seen in other neurologic disorders like autoimmune diseases or brain tumors). These six signs and symptoms are effective at identifying the majority of patients presenting with a stroke! However, it's important to note that many strokes do not cause any immediate signs or symptoms. These so-called "**silent strokes**" may not cause obvious damage right away, but they are still associated with permanent damage and place the patient at higher risk for more strokes in the future.

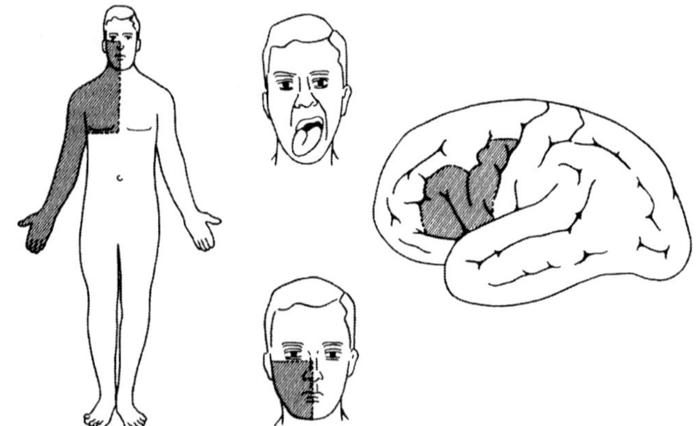

*Common **signs and symptoms of strokes**, including limb weakness and facial asymmetry.*

The most common **signs and symptoms** of a stroke are a **sudden onset** of **facial drooping**, **extremity weakness**, **speech difficulty**, and **visual loss**.

*If you recognize a **stroke**, you need to **BE FAST**:*
***B**alance issues*
***E**ye problems (loss of vision)*
***F**acial drooping*
***A**rm or leg weakness*
***S**peech difficulties*
***T**iming (sudden onset)*

By definition, any observed neurologic deficits must persist for **at least one day** to be classified as a stroke. (To be clear, there's nothing special about 24 hours! It was arbitrarily chosen as an easy-to-remember cut-off point.) Cases of focal neurologic deficits related to cerebral ischemia that resolve in *less than* 24 hours are classified instead as a **transient ischemic attack** (often abbreviated as TIA and occasionally called a "mini-stroke").

While clinical findings (such as those in the BE FAST mnemonic) can provide the initial clue that a stroke is happening, neuroimaging is almost always used as well, as this can help not only to localize the damage in the brain but also to distinguish between ischemic and hemorrhagic strokes. Due to its speed, CT is the most widely used imaging modality for strokes, but use of MRI is becoming more common.

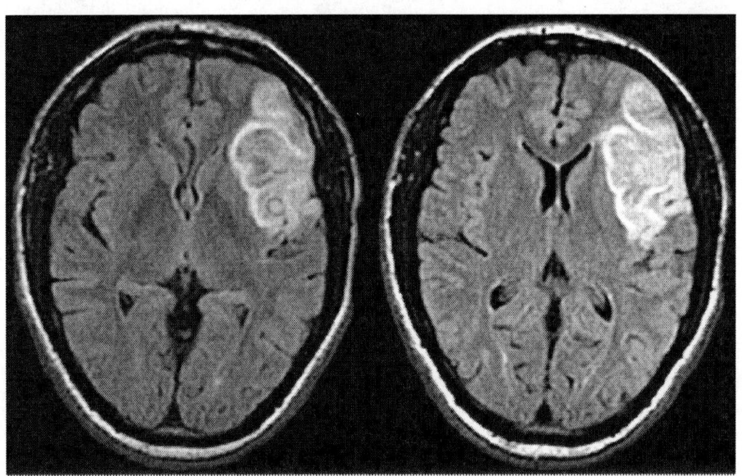

*An **MRI** showing an **ischemic stroke** in the territory of the **left middle cerebral artery**.*

TREATMENT OF STROKES

Treatment of a stroke consists of two things: **acute management** to prevent further damage to the brain and **long-term prevention** of future stroke episodes. Even with adequate treatment, strokes are a deadly disease, with around one-quarter of all patients presenting with a stroke dying within one month.

ACUTE MANAGEMENT

Immediate management of a stroke depends entirely on the type of stroke (ischemic or hemorrhagic). For *hemorrhagic* strokes, treatment is pretty limited, as once the blood has escaped its confines there is little you can do to put it back. For *ischemic* strokes, however, there is often more that can be done!

With an ischemic stroke, the goal is to get rid of the blockage as fast as possible. This is done with either medicine or surgery. A specific medication known as **tissue plasminogen activator** (or tPA) helps to break down blood clots by stimulating key enzymes in the body's fibrinolytic pathway. These medications go by various names that all end in –teplase (such as alteplase or reteplase). When given **within 3 hours** of the stroke, tPA can significantly reduce the amount of brain tissue lost and lead to better functional outcomes in the future. Because it acts to break down blood clots, tPA does carry a risk of *inducing* a hemorrhage, so make sure you know what kind of stroke you are dealing with before initiating treatment! To make some associations here, think of someone who is impatient because they have finished their meal at a restaurant and have been waiting for their server for nearly **three hours**. When another waiter walks by, they grab them and ask, "Hey, where's **te plase te pay**?!" This will help you associate drugs ending in –**teplase**, **tPA**, and the **three hour** time window in which it can be used.

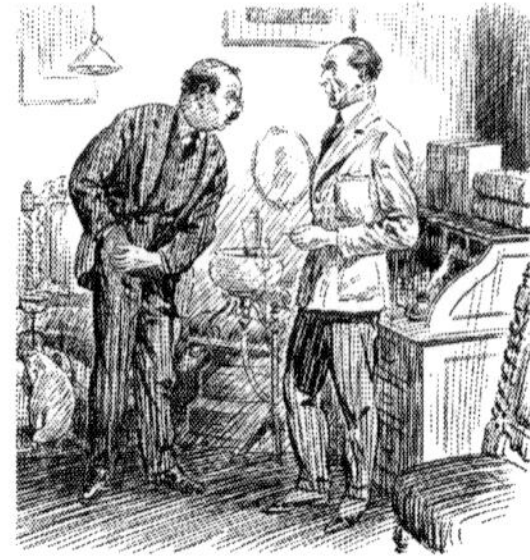

Tissue plasminogen activator (tPA) is used to **treat ischemic strokes** and can **improve functional outcomes** if given **within 3 hours of stroke onset**.

Think of someone who impatiently grabs a waiter and asks, "Hey, where's ***te plase te pay****?!" because they have been waiting to leave for nearly* ***three hours****.*

Surgical removal of blood clots (known as a **thrombectomy**) is generally only used when an ischemic stroke occurs in a large, easily accessible artery. If initiated within 12 hours of onset, thrombectomy appears to reduce the extent of brain death.

LONG-TERM PREVENTION

Given that strokes can be incredibly disabling and deadly, it is imperative to not only treat strokes when they occur but also to prevent them from happening in the first place. This can be done by understanding the specific risk factors that place someone at higher risk of having a stroke. By knowing these risk factors, we can try to modify them as much as possible.

Essentially, all stroke risk factors boil down to one of two mechanisms: either a **narrowing** of blood vessels (which makes blood clots more likely to get trapped in them) or a **weakening** of vessel walls (which makes them more likely to rupture). You can remember the key risk factors using the mnemonic **DASHCAM**:

D is for Diabetes. Diabetes is associated with a higher risk of stroke, as high blood sugars can lead to stiff and weak arterial walls that are prone to clogging or breaking.

A is for Atrial fibrillation. Atrial fibrillation is associated with an increased risk of a **thrombus**, or blood clot, forming in the left atrium. Parts of the blood clot may then break off and travel via the bloodstream to other parts of the body. A thrombus that goes on the lam like this is known as an **embolus**. (To be clear, a "thrombus" and an "embolus" are not the same thing even though you may sometimes hear them used interchangeably. It's more accurate to say that an embolus is a particular *type* of

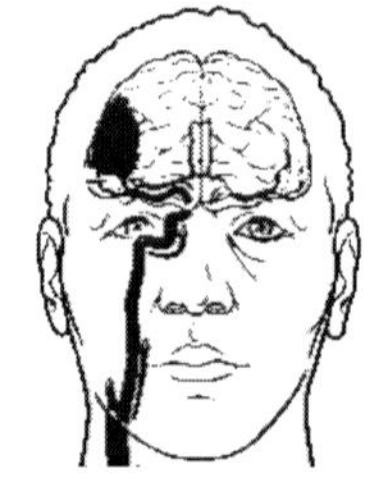

thrombus.) Because the size of the artery tends to narrow the farther into the brain you go, an embolus that was traveling freely in the larger arteries near the heart may become stuck in the narrower passageways in the brain, leading to an ischemic stroke.

S is for Smoking. Smoking even a single cigarette per day raises one's risk of a stroke significantly by damaging the integrity of arterial walls.

H is for Hypertension. High blood pressure is the **single largest risk factor** for both ischemic and hemorrhagic strokes, as the elevated pressure wears down arterial walls and makes them more likely to rupture and create a *hemorrhagic* stroke. The body then tries to strengthen the arterial walls again, but this tends to make the arteries more brittle and narrow, increasing the risk of an *ischemic* stroke.

C is for Cholesterol. High levels of cholesterol and other lipids increase the risk of forming atherosclerotic plaques that can both weaken and narrow arterial walls.

A is for Age. Old age is a major risk factor for strokes, with almost all strokes occurring in people over the age of 50.

M is for Male. Finally, men are 25% more likely to have a stroke compared to women.

Stroke risk factors include conditions that **narrow or weaken blood vessel walls**. Some of these factors can be modified to **reduce the risk of future strokes**.

DASHCAM:
***D**iabetes*
***A**trial fibrillation*
***S**moking*
***H**ypertension*
***C**holesterol*
***A**ge*
***M**ale*

While some of these factors (like age) cannot be changed, others can, and you should try to modify these as much as possible (such as helping someone to quit smoking, lower their blood pressure, or manage their blood sugar). Specific medications can be helpful as well. For people at high risk, **aspirin** is widely used to prevent strokes as it helps to prevent clot formation. It does not have a huge effect, but it has the advantage of being cheap, available, and easy to take. Oral **anticoagulants** such as warfarin and clopidogrel can also help to prevent formation of blood clots, especially in people who are prone to clotting (such as someone with atrial fibrillation). Finally, **surgical interventions** can be used as well, with carotid endarterectomy (or mechanical removal of atherosclerotic plaques from the walls of the carotid artery) being used to reduce the risk of another stroke significantly.

CORTICAL STROKES

Now that you have a broad overview of how to diagnose and treat strokes, we are going to shift our attention to the process of **stroke localization**, or how to determine the likely location of a stroke based on your clinical exam findings. To facilitate your learning, the clinical presentations used here are simplified to only show deficits related to a single area at a time. In real life, however, there is no "rule" that a stroke can affect only one artery at a time, so keep that in mind!

Let's start with strokes in the **cerebral cortex**. Because the cortex is responsible for higher-level functions, strokes in this region will produce characteristic deficits including **aphasia** (lack of speech), **agnosia** (lack of recognition), **neglect** (lack of awareness), **apraxia** (inability to plan movements), and **hemianopsia** (blindness in some or all of the visual field). These are known collectively as **cortical signs**. These general signs are then combined with additional specific motor and sensory deficits depending on which of the three arteries that supply the cerebral cortex have been affected (the anterior, middle, or posterior cerebral arteries) to produce more detailed syndromes, as we will see now!

ANTERIOR CEREBRAL ARTERY SYNDROME

Occlusions in the early parts of the **anterior cerebral arteries** don't tend to cause much damage due to the presence of collateral circulation through the various communicating arteries. However, occlusions farther down can lead to a stroke. If you refer back to the maps of the motor and sensory cortices on pages 23 and 24, you can think of the anterior cerebral artery as being "**down in the canyon**" where it will affect the lower half of the body, specifically causing both **paralysis** and **sensory loss** in the **contralateral lower limbs**. There can also be dysfunction of lower body organs such as the bladder, resulting in **urinary incontinence**. In addition, due to damage of the frontal lobe, difficulties in **executive functioning** (including loss of motivation and planning) can occur, and in some cases **primitive reflexes** can re-emerge. Overall, you can remember the association of the **anterior cerebral artery** with the lower body by drawing a stick figure where the legs form the letter **A** (for **A**nterior)!

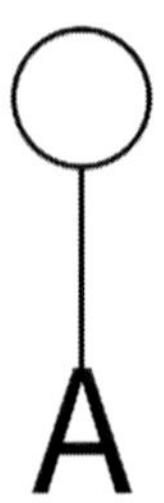

A stroke in the territory of the **anterior cerebral artery** can lead to **lower limb** hemiparesis and sensory deficits as well as **urinary incontinence**.

*Draw a stick figure using the letter **A** for the **lower half of the body**.*

MIDDLE CEREBRAL ARTERY SYNDROME

The **middle cerebral artery** is the **most common location** for a cortical stroke. (This is because the middle cerebral artery is the continuation of the internal carotid artery, so a traveling thrombus just needs to go straight to block the middle cerebral artery, as opposed to going left or right to enter the anterior or posterior cerebral arteries.) While the anterior cerebral artery hits "down in the canyon," the middle cerebral artery instead hits the sides of the brain, leading to both **paralysis** and **sensory loss** in the **contralateral *upper* limbs**. You can remember this association by continuing to add to the stick figure, this time using the letter **M** as their arms (as in someone doing the M part of the Y**MCA** dance)!

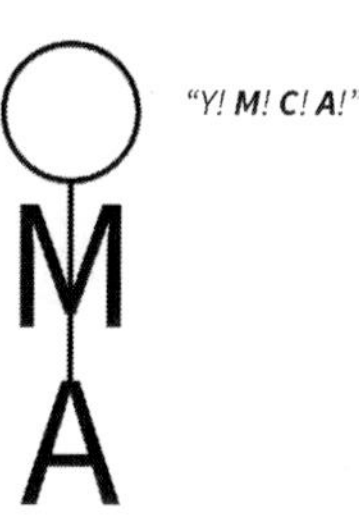

A stroke in the territory of the **middle cerebral artery** can lead to **upper limb** hemiparesis and sensory deficits.

*Draw a stick figure using the letter **M** for the **upper half of the body**.*

A middle cerebral artery stroke can have other effects depending on whether it has affected the dominant or non-dominant hemisphere. Ischemia in the *dominant* hemisphere can lead to various forms of **aphasia** (as the language centers lie in areas supplied by the middle cerebral artery). To help you remember the inclusion of the language centers, you can imagine the stick figure **yelling** out "Y! M! C! A!"

In comparison, ischemia in the *non*-dominant hemisphere can lead to a state of **contralateral hemineglect** in which the patient's awareness of the opposite half of their field of vision is completely ignored. (We talked about this back in Chapter 3, so go back if you need a reminder!) You can remember the association between the **N**on-dominant parietal lobe and hemi**N**eglect by focusing on the **N** in each.

Ischemia in the **middle cerebral artery** of the **dominant** hemisphere can lead to **aphasia**, while ischemia in the **non-dominant hemisphere** can lead to **hemineglect**.

*Picture a person **yelling** out "Y! **M**! **C**! **A**!"*
*The **N**on-dominant parietal lobe leads to hemi**N**eglect.*

POSTERIOR CEREBRAL ARTERY SYNDROME

Ischemic damage in the territory of the **posterior cerebral artery** is associated with various defects in the visual pathway. The most typical pattern seen is **contralateral homonymous hemianopsia with macular sparing**. (Remember that "damage to the back leads to sparing of the mac!") In cases of severe damage, complete **cortical blindness** can result. You can remember the association of the posterior cerebral artery with the visual cortex by drawing two **P**s like sunglasses on our stick figure.

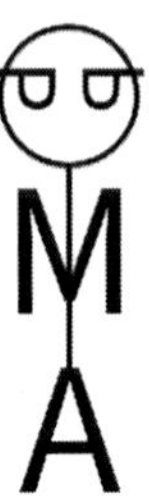

A stroke in the territory of the **posterior cerebral artery** leads to visual deficits, with **homonymous hemianopsia with macular sparing** being commonly seen.

*Draw a stick figure using two **P**s as sunglasses over the **eyes**.*

Of note, a stroke in the *left* posterior cerebral artery specifically can cause a finding known as **alexia without agraphia** in which someone is unable to read (owing to damage of both the visual cortex and a part of the corpus callosum) but can still engage in other forms of language including writing, speaking, and understanding speech. You can remember the association of this syndrome with the left **post**erior cerebral artery by thinking of someone who **cannot read letters** because the workers at the **post** office have **left** for the day.

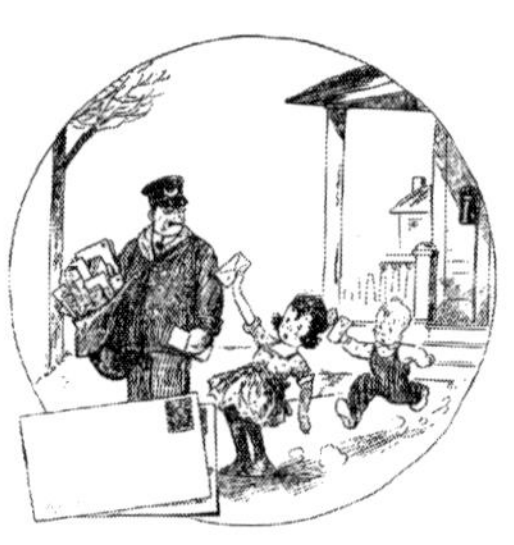

A **left posterior cerebral artery stroke** can lead to **alexia without agraphia** in which someone is **unable to read** but can still **write, speak, and listen**.

*Someone **cannot read letters** if the **post** office workers have **left** for the day.*

Finally, because the posterior cerebral artery lies near the arteries going to parts of the midbrain (such as the basilar artery and pontine arteries), a blockage here can produce various deficits that overlap with those seen in subcortical and midbrain strokes, which we will discuss in the next sections.

LACUNAR STROKES

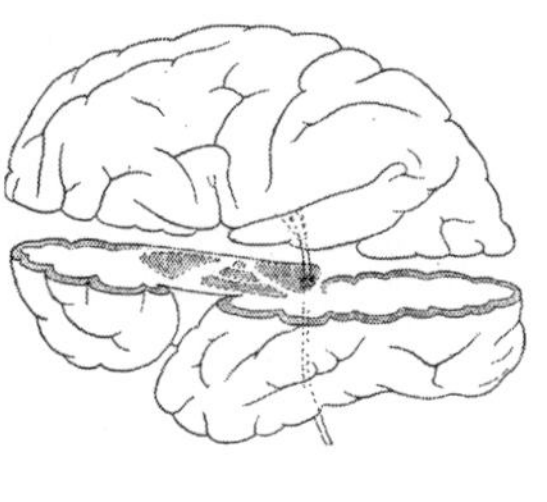

A **lacunar stroke** is one that occurs in the **subcortex** rather than the cortex. ("Lacunar" here comes from the Latin word for "lakes" or "empty spaces," a name that makes more sense when you consider that strokes in these areas have a tendency to leave *literal holes* in brain tissue as seen in the image below!) Patients with lacunar strokes often present with **motor deficits** and **loss of sensation**, but the **lack of cortical signs** helps to place us firmly in the region of the subcortex rather than the cortex.

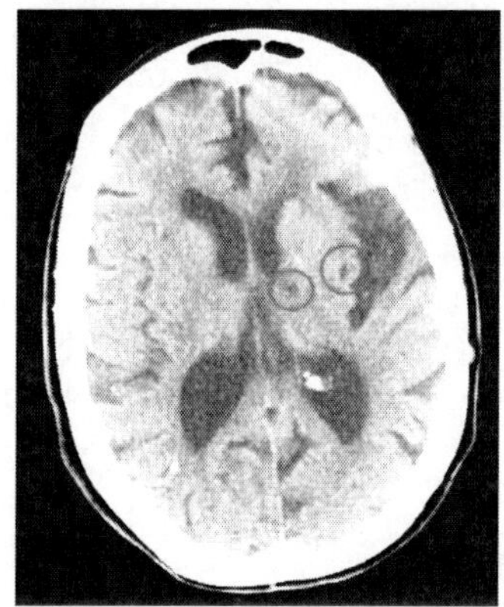

CT scan of ***lacunar strokes.***

There are three forms of lacunar strokes which we will go over now. Luckily, if you remember our discussion of the subcortex from Chapters 4 and 5, then there is no new information here that you will need to memorize!

PURE MOTOR STROKE

As its name implies, a **pure motor stroke** results in **hemiparesis of the contralateral face, arm, and leg** *without* any sensory deficits or associated cortical signs. This often results from ischemic damage to the **posterior limb of the internal capsule** which carries the corticospinal and corticobulbar tracts (remember the **PoLICe**-man!).

PURE SENSORY STROKE

A **pure sensory stroke** is also pretty straightforward and features **numbness of the contralateral face, arm, and leg** *without* any motor deficits or associated cortical signs. A pure sensory stroke results from ischemic damage to the **thalamus** (since the **th**alamus processes **th**en**th**ory information).

SENSORIMOTOR STROKE

Because the posterior limb of the internal capsule and thalamus are adjacent to each other, occasionally a stroke will produce ischemic damage in both of these regions at once, leading to **both hemiparesis and numbness** of the **contralateral face and extremities**. As with any lacunar stroke, cortical signs will be absent.

BRAINSTEM STROKES

As we move down from the subcortex to the brainstem, stroke localization becomes a bit more complicated. To make things as easy as possible, let's start with the basics: how do we know that we're dealing with a brainstem stroke in the first place? The pattern that should immediately make you think "It's in the brainstem!" is the presence of **crossed findings** where deficits in the *face* are on the *opposite* side as deficits in the *body* as seen below. (Note that this is different than Brown-Séquard syndrome which instead involves different *types of deficits* on the right side of the body compared to the left. That should instead have you thinking of a unilateral *spinal cord* lesion!)

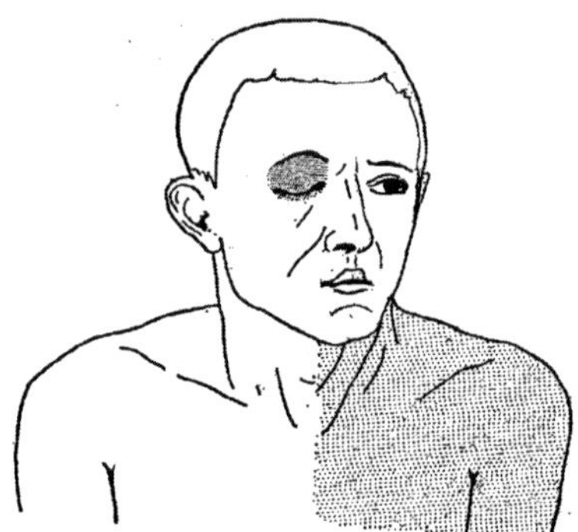

***Crossed findings** characteristic of a **brainstem stroke**.*

To remember the important fact that "**crossed findings = brainstem stroke**," think about what it means when someone has crossed their fingers when making a promise. It means that they are lying and the promise is **BS**! Similarly, crossed findings should also make you think of **BS** for **B**rain**S**tem.

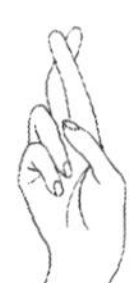

Brainstem strokes present with **crossed findings** of **ipsilateral facial deficits** and **contralateral body deficits.**

***Crossed fin**gers during a promise means the promise is **BS**, so **crossed fin**dings during a stroke means that the stroke is **BS** (**B**rain**S**tem)!*

Once you have a sense that the lesion is in the brainstem, your job then becomes to figure out exactly where. There are three questions to answer:

1. **Where** in the brainstem is the lesion (the midbrain, pons, or medulla)?
2. Is it more **medial or lateral** in this region?
3. Is the lesion on the **right or left** side?

To answer the first question, we'll need to use what we know about the **cranial nerves** in each region. Recall the "Rule of 4" which states that the first 4 cranial nerves exit from the brain and midbrain, the middle 4 exit from the pons, and the last 4 exit from the medulla. The presence or absence of dysfunction in these nerves serves as a helpful "map" of sorts to tell you what part of the brainstem has been affected on a **vertical** plane (the "latitude" of the lesion). For example, if someone presents with an oculomotor nerve palsy, the lesion is likely to be at the level of the midbrain. In contrast, someone presenting with facial nerve paralysis is likely to have a lesion at the level of the pons, while another patient presenting with an absent gag reflex is more likely to have a stroke in the medulla.

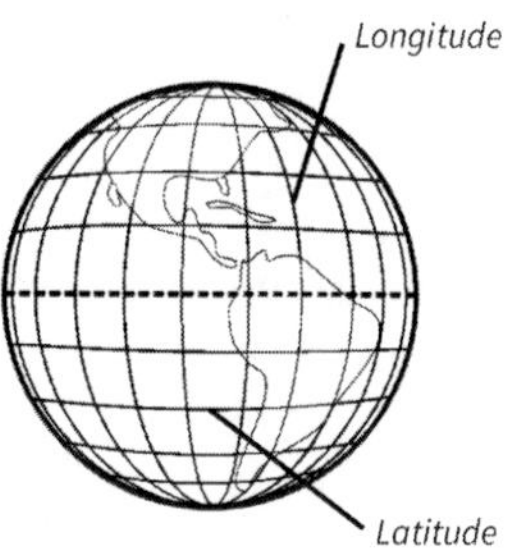

To answer the second question (whether the lesion is more medial or more lateral), it can be helpful to think about which structures are found medially in the brainstem and which are found laterally. There are 4 main **M**edial structures to think of: the **M**otor pathway (the corticospinal tract); the **M**edial lemniscus carrying fine touch, vibration, and proprioception; the **M**edial longitudinal fasciculus that controls movements of the eyes; and the **M**otor component of some (*but not all!*) cranial nerves, including those controlling extraocular movements and the tongue. In contrast, there are 4 main **S**ide structures to know: the **S**pinocerebellar pathway; the **S**pinothalamic tract carrying crude touch, temperature, and pain; the **S**ympathetic pathway traveling to the face; and the nuclei for the **S**ensory component of the trigeminal nerve. These structures can help you figure out the coordinates of the lesion on a **horizontal** plane (the "longitude" of the lesion).

Medial structures	**S**ide structures
Motor pathway (corticospinal tract)	**S**pinocerebellar pathway
Medial lemniscus	**S**pinothalamic tract
Medial longitudinal fasciculus	**S**ympathetic pathway
Motor part of some cranial nerves	**S**ensory nuclei for trigeminal nerve

The **medial and lateral brainstem** contain different structures.

*4 **M**edial structures = **M**otor pathway, **M**edial lemniscus, **MLF**, **M**otor cranial nerves.*
*4 **S**ide structures = **S**pinocerebellar pathway, **S**pinothalamic tract, **S**ympathetic pathway, **S**ensory nuclei for trigeminal nerve.*

Finally, to answer the third question (which side the lesion is on), in general you can expect that deficits in the *face* will be *ipsilateral* to the side of the lesion while deficits in the *body* will be *contralateral* to the side of the lesion. This is because the cranial nerves exit from the brainstem and innervate structures on the same side, while motor and sensory pathways traveling to the body all cross further down (at the very tail end of the medulla for the corticospinal tract and dorsal column—medial lemniscus pathway, and in the spinal cord for the spinothalamic tract).

And with that, you are now equipped to localize strokes in the brainstem! Let's walk through a few cases together, starting with the medulla at the bottom and working our way up.

MEDIAL MEDULLARY SYNDROME

As its name suggests, medial medullary syndrome involves a lesion in the medial medulla. This manifests through **contralateral hemiparesis** of the body (but not the face!), contralateral loss of **epicritic sensation** (but not protopathic!), and ipsilateral **tongue weakness**. How could we have predicted the location of this lesion based on the clinical findings? First, we know we are in the brainstem because of the presence of crossed findings (*ipsi*lateral tongue weakness in the face along with *contra*lateral hemiparesis in the body). Next, we can figure out the level of the lesion by determining what cranial nerves are involved. Given that tongue movement maps to the twelfth cranial nerve, we can feel confident saying that this lesion is localized to the medulla. To determine whether the lesion is medial or lateral, consider that the **M**otor pathway, **M**otor aspect of the hypoglossal nerve, and epicritic nerves traveling in the **M**edial lemniscus are all involved, while side structures such as the spinothalamic tract are not. Based on this information, we can localize the lesion to the medial medulla!

On test questions, you may sometimes get asked not only to identify *where* the stroke is but also *what artery* is involved. Medial medullary syndrome is typically caused by a stroke in the **anterior spinal artery**. There are some key words you want to associate here! You need to link **M**edial **M**edullary syndrome, the **A**nterior **S**pinal **A**rtery, and the clinical finding of tongue weakness and other motor findings. The best way to do that is by focusing on all the M's in the word **M**edial **M**edullary and thinking of the McDonald's arches. You use your tongue to eat the hamburgers and fries that McDonald's sells. The golden arches also resemble the anterior spinal artery itself! So when you hear medial medullary, think of the McDonald's arches to bring all these concepts together.

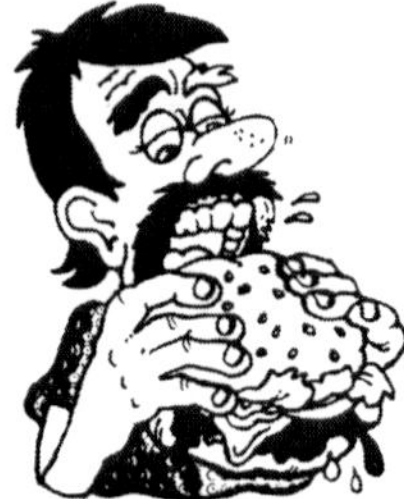

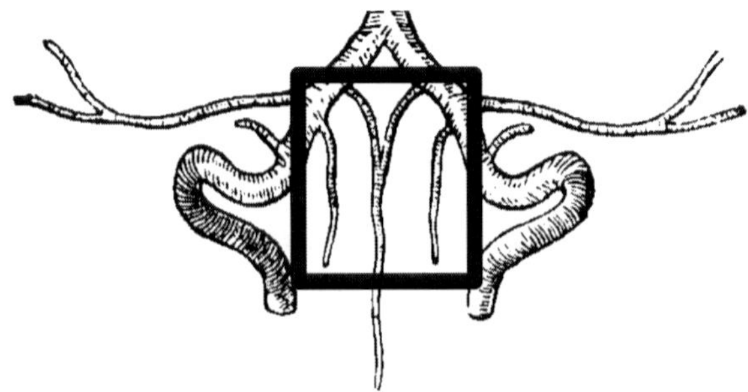

*The **anterior spinal artery**: your brain's version of the McDonald's arches!*

Medial medullary syndrome involves **contralateral hemiparesis**, **contralateral epicritic numbness**, and **ipsilateral tongue weakness**. It is caused by a stroke in the **anterior spinal artery**.

*When you see **M**edial **M**edullary syndrome, think of the **M**cDonald's arches to remind yourself of eating with your **tongue** as well as the arch-shaped **anterior spinal artery**!*

LATERAL MEDULLARY SYNDROME

Lateral medullary syndrome involves loss of **protopathic sensation** *contralaterally* in the limbs and *ipsilaterally* in the face, ipsilateral **Horner's syndrome**, problems with **balance** (including ataxia, vertigo, and nystagmus), and difficulty with both **speaking** (dysarthria) and **swallowing** (dysphagia). We can figure out that this is in the brainstem by the crossed findings (protopathic numbness on opposite sides in the face and limbs), then determine the "latitude" by looking at the cranial nerves involved. The presence of dysphagia and dysarthria strongly suggests involvement of the **glossopharyngeal and vagus nerves** which exit from the medulla. To determine the "longitude," let's look at whether the structures involved are found **M**edially or to the **S**ide. Given that there is involvement of the **S**pinothalamic tract (with protopathic numbness), the **S**ympathetic nervous system (with ipsilateral Horner's syndrome), the **S**pinocerebellar pathway (ataxia, vertigo, and nystagmus), and **S**ensory information from the trigeminal nerve (ipsilateral facial numbness), we can conclude that this involves the **S**ide of the medulla. (The involvement of motor dysfunction with speaking and swallowing is due to the involvement of the nucleus ambiguus rather than the motor pathways which are more medial!)

Lateral medullary syndrome is associated with a stroke in the **posterior inferior cerebellar artery**. You can remember this by thinking of the word **PICA-chew** to help you associate a stroke in the **P**osterior **I**nferior **C**erebellar **A**rtery with some of its most specific findings (in this case, difficulty with **chew**ing and speaking).

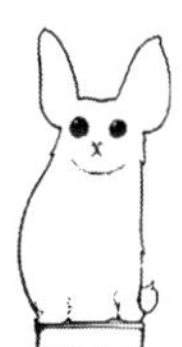

Lateral medullary syndrome involves loss of **protopathic sensation** in the **contralateral extremities** and **ipsilateral face**, **ipsilateral Horner's syndrome**, **cerebellar signs**, **dysarthria**, and **dysphagia**. It is caused by a stroke in the **posterior inferior cerebellar artery**.

***PICA-chew**: A **P**osterior **I**nferior **C**erebellar **A**rtery stroke makes it so you can't **chew**.*

LATERAL PONTINE SYNDROME

Lateral pontine syndrome is in many ways quite similar to lateral medullary syndrome. This is because the "longitude" of the lesion is the same, so many of the findings (loss of protopathic sensation contralaterally in the extremities and ipsilaterally in the face, ipsilateral Horner's syndrome, and ipsilateral cerebellar deficits) will still be present. Instead, only the "latitude" of the lesion has changed, meaning that different cranial nerves are going to be involved, with cranial nerves 5 through 8 now being implicated. As the trigeminal nerve involves facial sensation, **ipsilateral facial numbness** can appear. The sensory component of the facial nerve can result in **loss of taste** from the anterior part of the tongue. In addition, involvement of the vestibulocochlear nerve can result in **partial or complete deafness**. (In fact, lateral pontine syndrome is the only stroke that produces hearing loss!) The vestibular part of the vestibulocochlear nerve can be involved as well, causing nausea, vomiting, nystagmus, and vertigo.

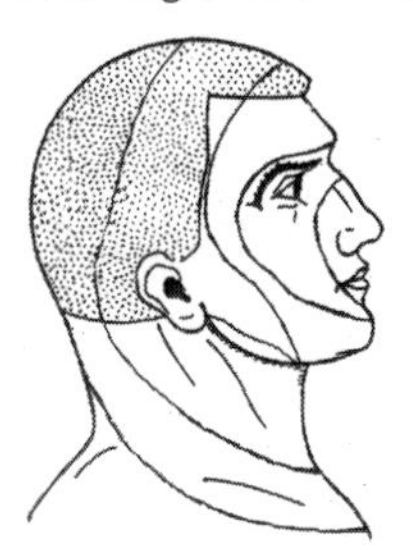

Lateral pontine syndrome is associated with a stroke in the **anterior inferior cerebellar artery**. Just as we can use **PICA-chew** to remember some of the more specific findings of lateral medullary syndrome, we can think of the **A**nterior **I**nferior **C**erebellar **A**rtery as causing problems in f**AICA**l sensation.

Lateral pontine syndrome is similar to lateral medullary syndrome but also involves **facial numbness** and **hearing loss**. It is caused by a stroke in the **anterior inferior cerebellar artery**.

A stroke in the ***A****nterior* ***I****nferior* ***C****erebellar* ***A****rtery messes up f****AICA****l sensation.*

MEDIAL PONTINE SYNDROME

Just as lateral pontine syndrome is very similar to lateral medullary syndrome, so too is **medial pontine syndrome** similar to medial medullary syndrome, with crossed findings and motor involvement both being prominent features. As before, the main distinction has to do with the cranial nerves involved! The motor component of cranial nerves 5 through 8 involve facial muscles and extraocular eye movements, so medial pontine syndrome can also lead to **facial asymmetry** and **horizontal gaze palsy**. However, there is also another **M**edial structure we need to account for in the pons that wasn't in the medulla: the **M**edial longitudinal fasciculus. This means that medial pontine syndrome can produce **internuclear ophthalmoplegia** (flip back to Chapter 10 if you need a refresher on what this would look like). Medial pontine syndrome is often related to an occlusion of a branch off of the **basilar artery**. You can remember this association by thinking of the phrase "Branches off the base lead to problems in the face" (specifically, facial asymmetry and internuclear ophthalmoplegia).

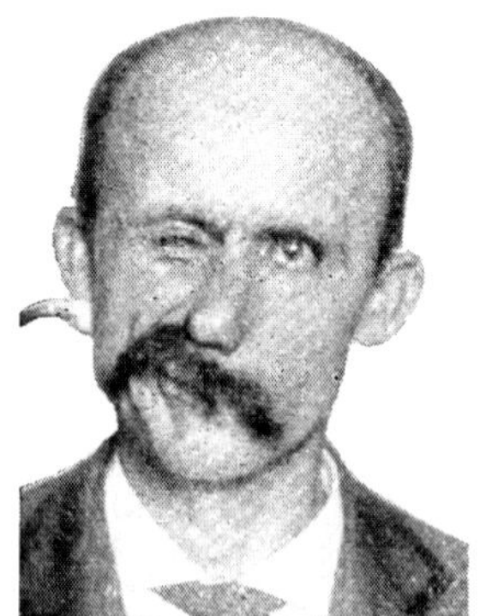

Facial asymmetry *as can be seen in* ***medial pontine syndrome****.*

Medial pontine syndrome resembles **medial medullary syndrome** but features **facial nerve palsy**, **horizontal gaze palsy**, and **internuclear ophthalmoplegia**. It is caused by a stroke in the **basilar artery**.

Branches off the ***base*** *lead to problems in the* ***face****!*

MIDBRAIN STROKES

Moving up from strokes in the medulla and the pons, we now hit midbrain strokes. Like all brainstem strokes we have talked about so far, midbrain strokes will produce crossed findings. However, because only two cranial nerves exit from the midbrain (the oculomotor and trochlear nerves), the crossed findings will tend to be more subtle, involving only eye paralysis rather than a more dramatic presentation like facial asymmetry. Your primary clue to a midbrain stroke will be an **oculomotor nerve palsy** (manifesting in ptosis, mydriasis, and a "down and out" position of the pupil) in addition to some form of **motor paralysis** in the body.

The condition most classically associated with a medial midbrain stroke is called **Weber's syndrome**. Weber's syndrome involves the combination of an **ipsilateral oculomotor nerve palsy** and a **contralateral hemiplegia** (there are those crossed findings so that you know it's in the brainstem!). How can we remember Weber's syndrome? Think about what happens when you're walking and suddenly get a spider **web** in your **eye**. You immediately try to close your eye (looking like ptosis) and you will likely try to use your *ipsilateral* arm to swat the spider web away, meaning that your *contralateral* side stays still (almost as if it's paralyzed!). Weber's syndrome results from a stroke in the **posterior cerebral artery** or the upper portion of the **basilar arteries**.

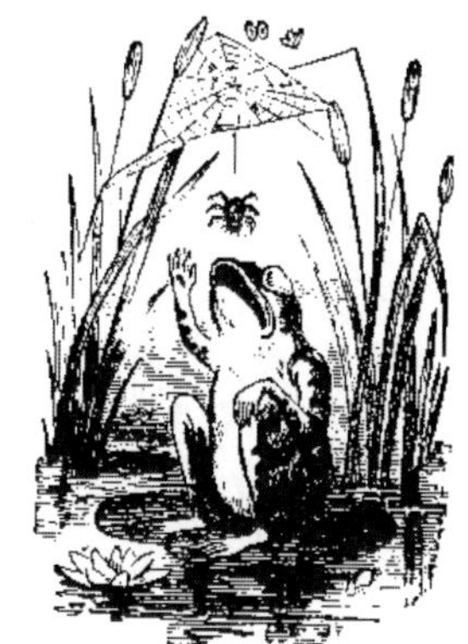

Weber's syndrome results from a **midbrain stroke** and presents as a combination of **ipsilateral oculomotor nerve palsy** and **contralateral hemiplegia**. It is caused by a stroke in either the **posterior cerebral artery** or the **basilar artery**.

When you get a spider ***web*** *in your* ***eye****, your eyelid will shut (like* ***ptosis****) and your will use your ipsilateral hand to swat it away (leaving your* ***contralateral extremities still****).*

LOCKED-IN SYNDROME

Finally, in cases of severe stroke, the blood supply to all three parts of the brainstem can be cut off simultaneously. This can result in **locked-in syndrome**, a tragic condition in which someone is almost completely paralyzed due to damage of the corticospinal tract as well as most of the cranial nerves. However, because cortical functions remain intact, the person is usually fully aware of their situation. Depending on the extent of the damage, higher cranial nerves may be spared, so someone with this condition may at times be taught to communicate using eye movements and blinks. Locked-in syndrome is most often related to occlusions of the **basilar artery** (compared to medial pontine syndrome which instead involves *branches off* the basilar artery). Overall, locked-in syndrome is a devastating reminder of just how important the brainstem is for our ability to function.

CEREBELLAR STROKES

While significantly less common than cerebral or brainstem strokes, cerebellar strokes can occur. However, it's important to clear up a few misconceptions about **cerebellar strokes** right off the bat. First, as you can see in the diagram below, arteries with "cerebellar" in the name do *not* necessarily affect the cerebellum! (Think of the anterior inferior cerebellar artery and its association with lateral pontine syndrome, or the posterior inferior cerebellar artery and its relationship to lateral medullary syndrome.) Second, the presence of cerebellar signs (such as vertigo, ataxia, nystagmus, and the rest of the "**dizzy AUNT with 3 dishes**" mnemonic from Chapter 6) is not automatically indicative of a stroke in the *cerebellum* itself! Because cerebellar pathways travel not only in the cerebellum but also in the cerebrum, brainstem, and spinal cord as well, lesions throughout the central nervous system can produce these signs. (Recall that cerebellar signs can be seen in lateral brainstem syndromes due to involvement of the spinocerebellar pathway.)

When they do occur, cerebellar strokes can be picked up by looking for the presence of the aforementioned cerebellar signs in combination with the general BE FAST pattern we talked about earlier (especially the "sudden onset" timing). Due to the fact that the arteries supplying the cerebellum also supply the brainstem, there will often be overlapping features with some of the brainstem syndromes we talked about earlier. Finally, remember from Chapter 6 that the ***cerebe◊um*** is a dirty **double crosser**! This means that a stroke in the cerebellum will lead to deficits that are *ipsilateral* to the lesion (rather than contralateral as is seen in cortical strokes).

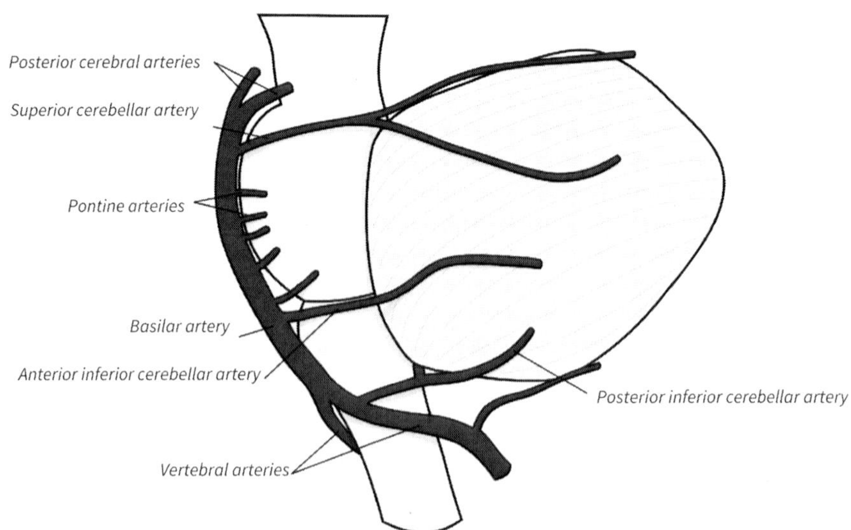

***Blood supply** to the **brainstem** and **cerebellum**.*

SPINAL CORD STROKES

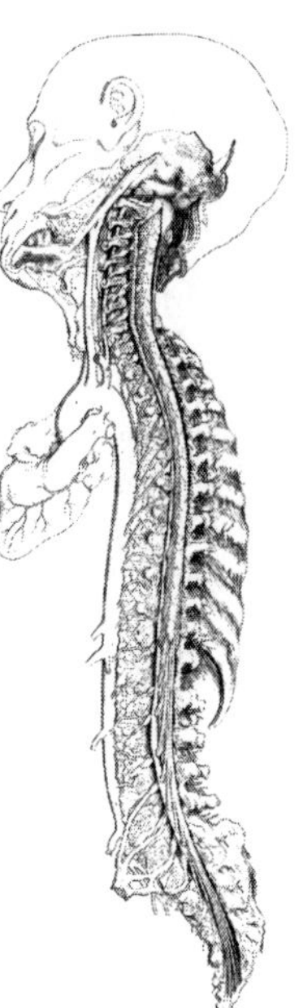

While most people associate strokes with the brain, strokes can occur in the spinal cord as well. Depending on the parts of the spinal cord that are involved, a variety of presentations can occur. By far the most common is an **anterior cord stroke** which, as you might guess, presents similarly to the anterior cord syndrome we talked about back in Chapter 8 (including loss of motor function as well as crude touch, temperature, and pain sensation below the level of the lesion, with sparing of fine touch, pressure, and proprioception). Ischemia in the anterior spinal artery occurs most commonly in the **thoracic cord**, as the anterior spinal artery receives collateral supply from additional arteries that come off of the aorta. These "booster" arteries are most pronounced in the cervical and lumbar cord, making the thoracic cord a **watershed area** that is particularly vulnerable to ischemia.

In contrast, **posterior cord strokes** are quite rare. This is because the posterior cord is supplied by the *two* **posterior spinal arteries** (as opposed to the single anterior spinal artery), making ischemia less likely. If a posterior cord stroke does occur, it tends to present as a posterior cord syndrome involving loss of fine touch, vibration, and proprioception in affected areas.

PUTTING IT ALL TOGETHER

Strokes are among the most devastating neurologic diseases, as they can occur with little warning and leave a trail of destruction in their wake. Because of the potential for irreversible neurologic deficits and even death, the ability to rapidly recognize and treat a stroke is crucial. The **BE FAST** mnemonic can help you to recognize the overall pattern of a stroke, while your neurological exam can assist in identifying the specific areas involved. Neuroimaging with CT or MRI is almost always used as well.

When it comes to stroke localization, being as systematic as possible when conducting your neurological exam and interpreting its findings is the key. Broadly, the presence of **cortical signs** should have you thinking of a stroke in the cerebral cortex, while the *absence* of cortical signs is more consistent with stroke lower down in the subcortex or brainstem. If you see **crossed findings** (facial deficits on one side and limb deficits on the other), you can be pretty sure you are working with a stroke in the brainstem. From there, look at the specific muscle groups and sensory modalities involved which should help you to pinpoint *where* in this area they are occurring. By using what we have already learned about the vascular supply of the central nervous system, you will likely be able to identify even the specific artery involved when asked (and you *will* be asked!). Use the practice questions on the next few pages to get comfortable with the process of stroke localization!

REVIEW QUESTIONS

1. A 61 y/o right-handed F with a history of diabetes mellitus, atrial fibrillation, hypertension, hyperlipidemia, and tobacco use is brought to the emergency department after she awoke and noticed that she could not move her left arm. Vital signs are HR 104, BP 184/108, RR 20, and T 98.8°F. The doctor reviewing her medical record notices that one year ago she underwent MRI angiography which showed narrowing in her cerebral circulation as seen below:

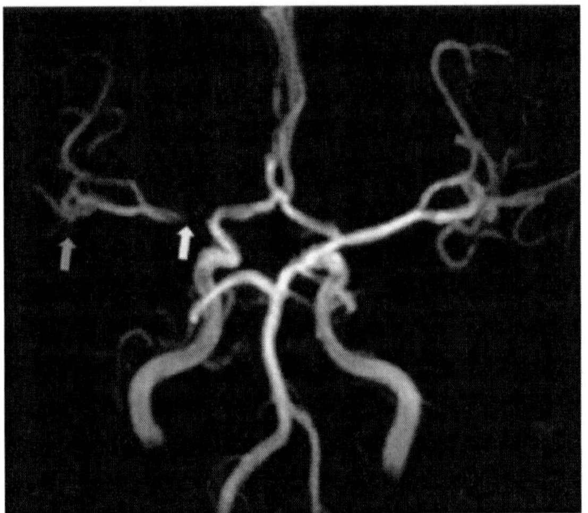

   Which of the following is most likely to be found on exam?
   A. Numbness to pain and temperature in the right arm
   B. Weakness of the left leg
   C. Not responding to activity in her left visual field
   D. Difficulty understanding what is being said
   E. Being able to only speak one or two words at a time with extreme difficulty

2. (Continued from previous question.) Which of the following is most likely to have prevented this outcome?
   A. Aggressive management of her blood pressure
   B. Anticoagulant medication
   C. Smoking cessation
   D. Use of a cholesterol-lowering medication
   E. Tight glycemic control

3. (Continued from previous question.) The doctor asks the patient how much time has passed since she last had full use of her left arm. She replies by saying that she went to bed around 10:30 last night. It is currently 11:00 in the morning. What is the most likely reason why the doctor asked this question?
    A. To localize the lesion more precisely
    B. To determine whether the stroke is ischemic or hemorrhagic
    C. To decide on the most appropriate medications to prescribe
    D. To assess her prognosis for functional recovery of her left arm
    E. To estimate her chance of mortality within the next 24 hours

4. An 83 y/o M comes to the hospital after noticing the sudden onset of weakness in his left face, left arm, and left leg. On exam, there is significant facial asymmetry. He has a widely dilated right pupil, with the right eye pointed inferiorly and laterally compared to the left eye as seen below:

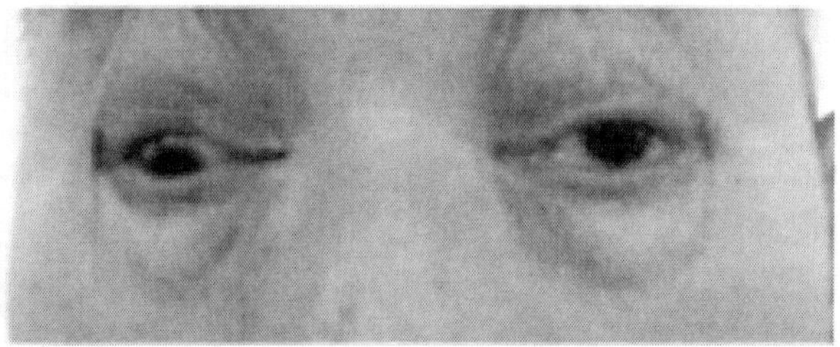

   Hearing is intact bilaterally. The gag reflex is present. There is no notable tongue deviation. Pain, temperature, vibration, and proprioception sensation are intact throughout. Which part of the midbrain has most likely sustained damage in this patient?
    A. Left medial midbrain
    B. Right medial midbrain
    C. Left lateral midbrain
    D. Right lateral midbrain
    E. Left medial pons
    F. Right medial pons
    G. Left lateral pons
    H. Right lateral pons
    I. Left medial medulla
    J. Right medial medulla
    K. Left lateral medulla
    L. Right lateral medulla

5. A 64 y/o M presents to the emergency department reporting a sudden onset of headache, dizziness, and difficulty walking. On exam, extraocular movements are intact, but the left pupil is significantly smaller than the right. There is drooping of the left eyelid, though all other muscles of facial expression are intact. There is numbness to pain and temperature on the left face as well as the right arm and leg, drooping of the left eyelid, and difficulty with heel-to-shin and finger-to-nose testing on the left side. His speech is mumbling and difficult to understand. Oral examination reveals the soft palate being pulled to the right side as seen below:

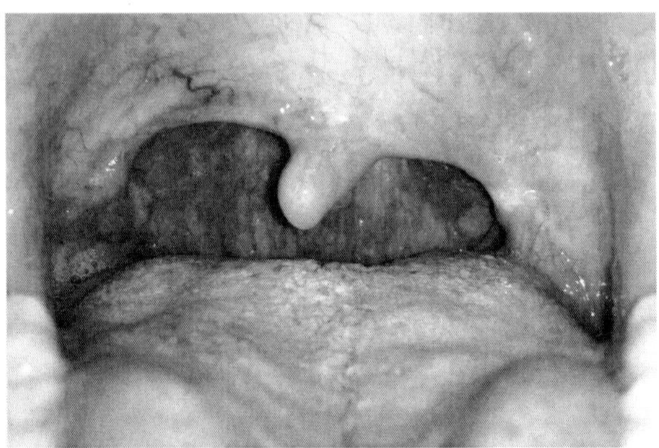

Vital signs are HR 78, BP 146/78, RR 18, and T 98.8°F. Neuroimaging is most likely to reveal an occlusion of which of the following arteries?

A. Left anterior cerebral artery
B. Right anterior cerebral artery
C. Left middle cerebral artery
D. Right middle cerebral artery
E. Left posterior cerebral artery
F. Right posterior cerebral artery
G. Left anterior inferior cerebellar artery
H. Right anterior inferior cerebellar artery
I. Left posterior inferior cerebellar artery
J. Right posterior inferior cerebellar artery
K. Anterior spinal artery

6. (Continued from previous question.) Which of the following is this patient at particularly high risk for?

A. Swallowing food into his airway while eating
B. Progressive hearing loss
C. Double vision related to weakness of extraocular muscles
D. Requiring a ventilator due to weakness of the diaphragm
E. Urinary incontinence

1. **The best answer is C.** The patient's presentation and medical history are both highly consistent with a stroke in the region of the right middle cerebral artery, and the available imaging shows significant stenosis in this region. As the patient is right-handed, we can be fairly certain that she has a left-dominant hemisphere. Therefore, a stroke in the non-dominant territory of her right middle cerebral artery is likely to lead to hemineglect, which would present as her ignoring things occurring to her left. A stroke in her non-dominant hemisphere is likely unlikely to lead to aphasia, as the language centers are most often found in the dominant hemisphere (answers D and E). Sensory deficits would be found on the contralateral arm, not the ipsilateral arm (answer A). Finally, weakness of the left leg would be expected in a right anterior cerebral artery stroke, not a middle cerebral artery stroke (answer B).

2. **The best answer is A.** All of the patient's comorbid conditions place her at higher risk for a stroke. However, in almost all cases, hypertension is the single largest risk factor, making aggressive management of elevated blood pressure a key step in stroke prevention.

3. **The best answer is C.** Knowing how long it has been since the onset of the stroke is crucial for determining whether tissue plasminogen activator can be given. Tissue plasminogen activator helps to improve functional outcomes but only when given within 3 hours of symptom onset. In cases where it has been longer than 3 hours since symptom onset, the risks of this treatment often outweigh the benefits. Knowing the amount of time that has passed since symptom onset may help to provide an estimate of functional and mortality prognosis, but this is not as immediate of a decision as whether or not to administer tissue plasminogen activator (answers D and E). Knowing time of symptom onset does not help to localize a stroke or determine its likely etiology (answers A and B).

4. **The best answer is B.** The combination of an oculomotor nerve palsy with contralateral weakness is known as Weber syndrome, which localizes to the medial midbrain. Weakness of the face and body is caused by involvement of the corticospinal and corticobulbar tracts, respectively, while the oculomotor nerve exits the brainstem at the level of the midbrain. In Weber syndrome, the oculomotor nerve palsy is ipsilateral while the weakness is contralateral, placing this on the right, not left (answer A). The involvement of the motor pathways places this medially in the midbrain, not laterally where deficits in pain and temperature sensation would be more likely (answers C and D). A lesion in the medial pons would likely involve the abducens nerve, not the oculomotor nerve (answers E and F). Further, intact hearing argues against lateral pontine syndrome (answers G and H), an intact gag reflex argues against lateral medullary syndrome (answers K and L), and lack of tongue deviation argues against medial medullary syndrome (answers I and J).

5. **The best answer is I.** Crossed findings (in this case, numbness on the left face and right extremities) are highly suggestive of a brainstem lesion rather than a stroke in the anterior, middle, or posterior cerebral arteries (answers A through F). To determine which part of the brainstem has been damaged, consider which cranial nerves are involved. The presence of palatal asymmetry and dysarthria both are suggestive of the 9th and 10th cranial nerves being involved, which localizes this to the medulla. To determine whether it is medial or lateral, consider that the spinothalamic tract (numbness to pain and temperature), sympathetic nervous system (Horner's syndrome), and spinocerebellar tracts (vertigo and ataxia) are involved, all of which travel laterally in the brainstem. Lateral medullary syndrome is often related to a stroke in the posterior inferior cerebellar artery. Facial deficits are ipsilateral while deficits in the extremities are contralateral, which localizes this to the left, not the right (answer J). Anterior inferior cerebellar artery strokes are more associated with lateral pontine syndrome which would present with facial weakness and/or asymmetry (answers G and H). A stroke in the anterior spinal artery is associated with medial medullary syndrome which would involve the corticospinal tract and the medial lemniscus, neither of which appear to be involved here (answer K).

6. **The best answer is A.** A stroke in the lateral medulla is likely to affect the nucleus ambiguus which is responsible for swallowing and speech. This patient already shows signs of dysarthria, so it is likely that his swallowing muscles may be impaired as well. Weakness of the glossopharyngeal and vagus nerves will also impair his gag reflex, putting him at even higher risk of aspiration. For this reason, care must be taken to prevent aspiration in patients admitted with lateral medullary syndrome. Extraocular muscles are controlled by cranial nerves exiting from the midbrain and pons, not the medulla (answer C). Hearing is controlled by the vestibulocochlear nerve which attaches to the brainstem at the level of the pons (answer B). The diaphragm is controlled at the level of the C3-C5 spinal nerves (answer D). Finally, urinary incontinence is more likely to be seen with an anterior cerebral artery stroke (answer E).

15 INTRACRANIAL HYPERTENSION

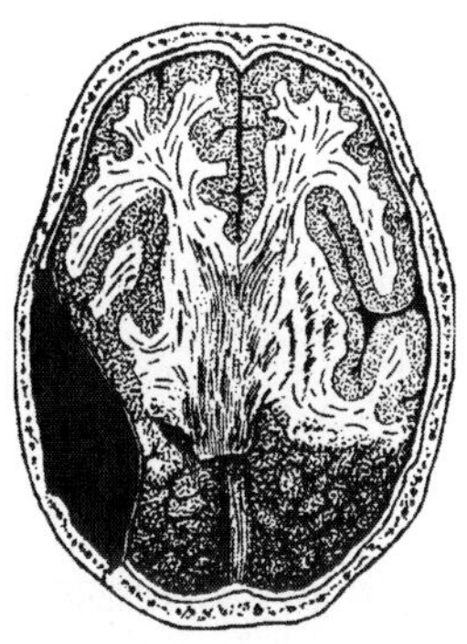

Gently knock on your head a few times with your fist. Pretty hard, right? It's not at all like the soft squishy texture that we normally associate with the brain. This is because the brain is kept safe within the hard and inflexible bones of the **skull**. For the most part, this is a good thing, as the skull helps to protect the brain from injury. However, in some cases the enclosed nature of the skull can actually be a liability. Because the skull cannot expand, any increase in the amount of matter inside the skull (whether that is an increase in **blood**, **cerebrospinal fluid**, or **nervous tissue** itself) must necessarily be accompanied by an increase in pressure, as there is no wiggle room for the volume of the intracranial space to increase. Therefore, a significant expansion of any of these components will lead to a state of **intracranial hypertension** (not to be confused with the high *blood* pressure that is often called simply "hypertension"). Intracranial hypertension can be damaging or even deadly to the brain, as it not only compresses the nervous tissue directly but also can impinge upon the arteries in the area, cutting off the supply of oxygen and vital nutrients.

There are many possible causes of intracranial hypertension. In this chapter, we will focus on two main forms in particular: **intracranial bleeds** and **hydrocephalus**. We will also discuss a dreaded complication of intracranial hypertension known as **brain herniation** in which the increased pressure pushes parts of the brain into places they don't belong. (It should be noted that this chapter should not be seen as an exhaustive list of all the potential causes of intracranial hypertension! We will talk about a few other types of neurologic diseases that can also raise intracranial pressure, such as brain tumors or infections, in later chapters.)

SIGNS AND SYMPTOMS OF INTRACRANIAL HYPERTENSION

Just like strokes, intracranial hypertension can result in various signs and symptoms depending on the specific brain regions affected. However, there are a few common manifestations that tend to be found most of the time, including **headaches**, **nausea**, **vomiting**, **changes in mental status** (such as sleepiness or confusion), **seizures**, and **focal neurologic signs** (including changes in vision and motor strength).

One particularly high-yield sign to know is swelling of the optic disc known as **papilledema** (as seen below). If left untreated, this pressure on the optic disc can even lead to progressive visual loss.

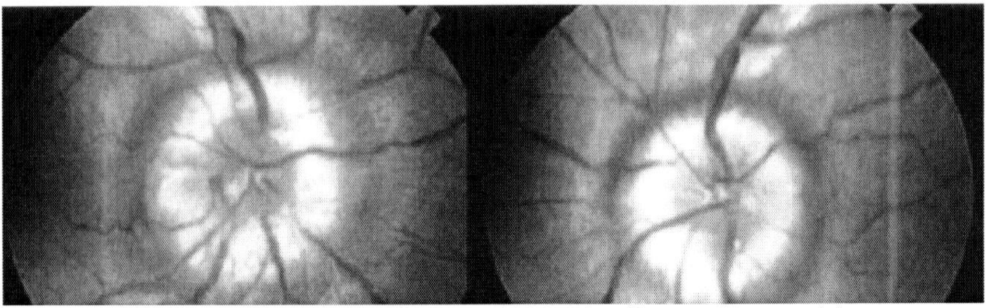

*Swelling of the optic disc known as **papilledema**, which is a sign of **increased intracranial pressure**.*

Autonomically, a sudden increase in intracranial pressure can lead to a trio of signs known as **Cushing's triad** which consists of irregular breathing, a slow heart rate, and increased blood pressure. You can link Cushing's triad to increased **I**ntra**C**ranial **P**ressure using the letters **ICP**: **I**nspirations, **C**ardiac, and **P**ressure. The presence of Cushing's triad is typically a *late* sign of increased intracranial pressure, so action must be taken immediately to prevent additional injury due to brain herniation!

A **sudden increase in intracranial pressure** can lead to **Cushing's triad** of **irregular breathing**, **bradycardia**, and **hypertension**.

*Increased **I**ntra**C**ranial **P**ressure leads to **I**rregular **I**nspirations, a **C**rawling **C**ardiac rate, and **P**ushed up blood **P**ressure.*

INTRACRANIAL BLEEDS

The first major cause of increased intracranial pressure that we will talk about is **intracranial bleeding**. In contrast to strokes (where most of the problems are caused by the *absence* of blood in places that it *should* be), with intracranial bleeding most of the problems are related to the *presence* of blood in places that it *shouldn't* be.

Intracranial bleeding can have several possible causes. **Mechanical head trauma** is by far the most common cause of most intracranial bleeds. However, as with strokes, **high blood pressure** is also a major risk factor. Uncontrolled hypertension also increases the risk of developing an **aneurysm** or a ballooning of an arterial wall. Aneurysms create a weak point in the artery, significantly increasing the risk of future rupture and subsequent hemorrhage.

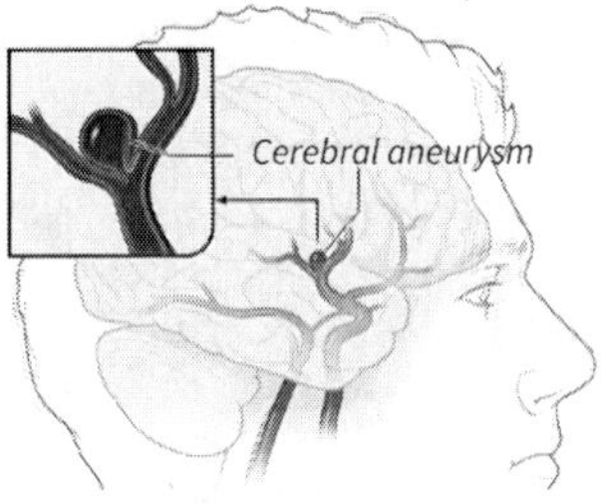

Prior to rupturing, aneurysms may cause focal neurologic signs and symptoms by compressing nearby structures. For example, an aneurysm of the **anterior communicating artery** can compress the optic chiasm (leading to bitemporal hemianopia), while an aneurysm of the **posterior communicating artery** can disrupt the **oculomotor nerve**.

There are four main types of intracranial bleeding depending on the location of bleeding in the skull as seen in the image below: **epidural hematomas**, **subdural hematomas**, **subarachnoid hemorrhages**, and **intracerebral hemorrhages**. (Just to make sure we are on the same page, the word "hematoma" is used to describe a *localized* collection of blood while "hemorrhage" is generally used to describe a *diffuse* bleed.) While all of these will result in the characteristic signs and symptoms of increased intracranial pressure, the specifics of the patient's history and clinical presentation will vary, making it possible for a diligent clinician to make a diagnosis based on what they are seeing. While learning about these, pay close attention to the differences in the clinical history, as this will often allow you to guess at what type of bleeding is present even before seeing the brain scan!

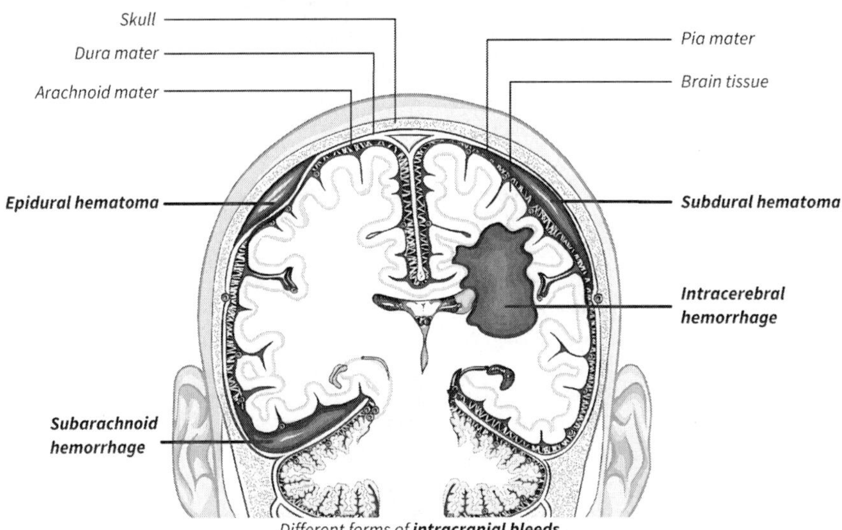

Different forms of ***intracranial bleeds****.*

EPIDURAL HEMATOMA

An **epidural hematoma** arises from bleeding in the space between the dura mater and the skull. The typical history involves **blunt head trauma** (such as being hit in the head during a mixed martial arts match) followed by a brief **loss of consciousness**. After regaining consciousness, the patient may appear totally fine, with no significant symptoms or neurologic deficits (this is known as a **lucid period**). However, despite benign outward appearances, the bleeding continues behind the scenes, leading to more and more blood in the fixed space of the skull. As the intracranial pressure rises, compression of the brainstem can again lead to unconsciousness, loss of function, and even death! If you ever see this characteristic history (blunt head trauma followed by a lucid period and subsequent re-emergence of neurologic dysfunction), think of an epidural hematoma!

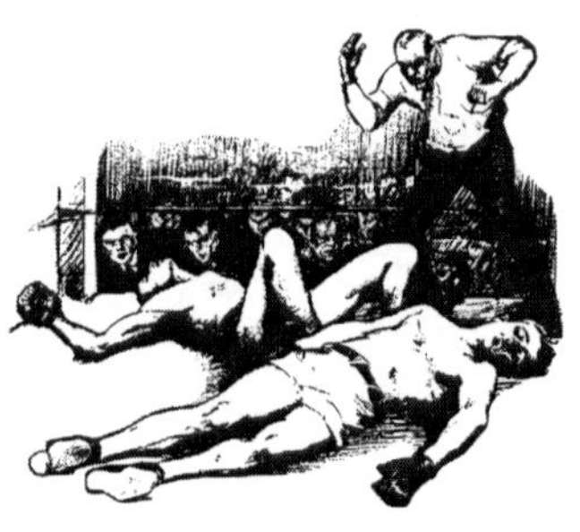

A CT scan of the head can confirm the presence of blood in the epidural space. Because the dura mater is attached to the skull, the expansion of blood is limited, leading to a characteristic **bulge-like appearance** on CT:

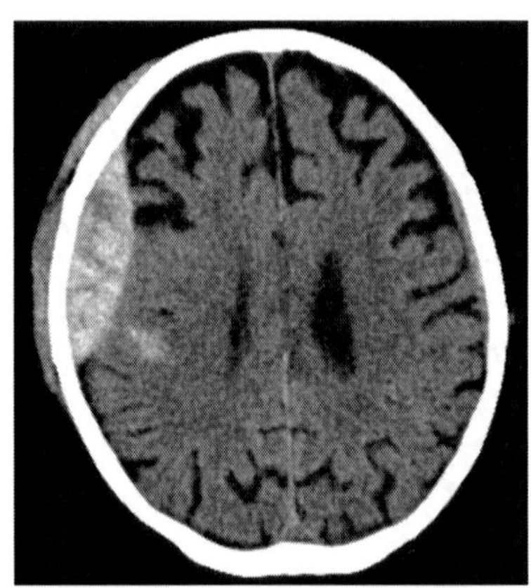

*An **epidural hematoma** as seen on a CT scan.*

Treatment of an epidural involves **surgical removal of the blood** through a burr hole to reduce intracranial pressure.

In most cases, an epidural hematoma is caused by bleeding from the **middle meningeal artery**. You can remember the association of an **epi**dural hematoma, **head trauma**, and the **M**iddle **M**eningeal **A**rtery by thinking of someone who passes out after getting punched during an **epi**c **M**ixed **M**artial **A**rts (**MMA**) match.

An **epidural hematoma** is caused by bleeding of the **middle meningeal artery**. A history involving **head trauma** and a **lucid period** is often diagnostic.

*Think of an **epi**c (**epi**dural) **M**ixed **M**artial **A**rts (**M**iddle **M**eningeal **A**rtery) match!*

SUBDURAL HEMATOMA

A **subdural hematoma** results from bleeding in the space below the dura mater. Like epidural hematomas, subdural hematomas are related to head trauma. However, subdural hematomas generally take **longer to develop** (in fact, some people can live with a subdural hematoma for months before it is discovered!). This is because subdural hematomas result from injuries of the **bridging veins** that cross the subdural space which have much lower pressure compared to the middle meningeal artery. For this reason, the classic clinical history associated with a subdural hematoma involves **gradually increasing headache with confusion**. Because the walls of veins are often quite weaker than those of arteries, the force required to break them is often less, making subdural hematomas more common than epidural hematomas.

Diagnosis is based on the classic history of (even minor) head trauma with a gradual build-up of symptoms. A head CT will show a characteristic **crescent shape** as seen below:

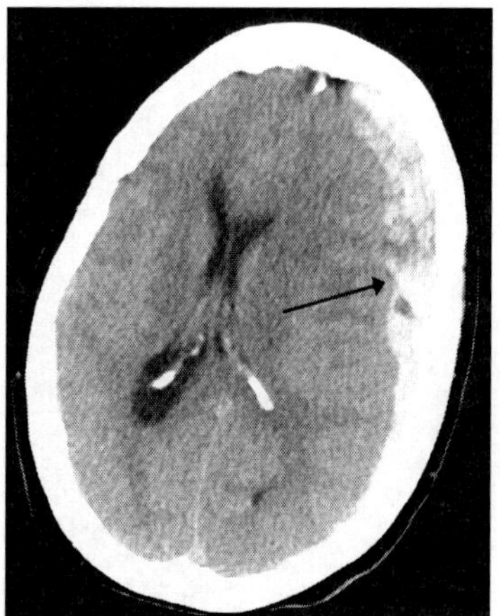

A ***subdural hematoma*** *as seen on a CT scan.*

In cases of a small or chronic hematoma, no treatment may be required. For more acute cases, neurosurgical intervention may be needed to control the bleeding and reduce intracranial pressure.

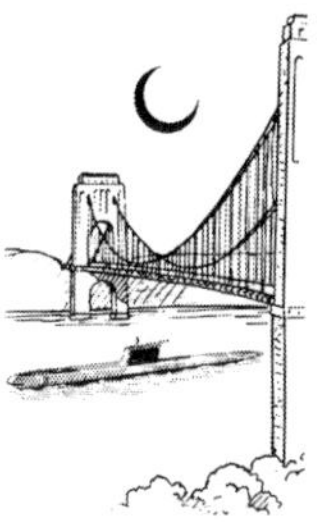

You can remember the association of a **sub**dural hematoma with **bridging** veins by picturing a **sub**marine going under the **bridge** at night under a **crescent** moon. Think about how **slowly** the submarine is going. However, because the sub sneaks up on you, it can still be **deadly**!

A **subdural hematoma** involves bleeding from the **bridging veins** after even minor **head trauma**. It often presents with **gradually increasing headache and confusion**.

Picture a ***sub****marine (****sub****dural) going under a* ***bridge*** *(****bridging*** *veins) at night under a* ***crescent*** *moon (its shape on CT) to* ***slowly sneak up*** *on its target.*

SUBARACHNOID HEMORRHAGE

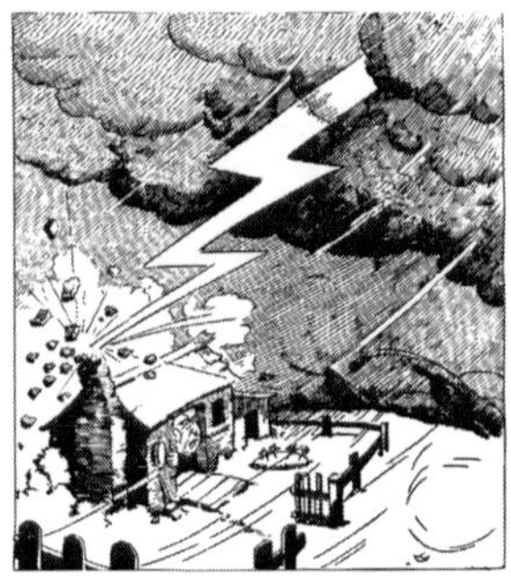

A **subarachnoid hemorrhage** involves bleeding into the subarachnoid space between the arachnoid mater and the pia mater. The classic presentation of a subarachnoid hemorrhage is a **thunderclap headache** or a severe headache with a sudden onset that is often described as "the worst headache of my life." Other signs and symptoms such as nausea, vomiting, changes in consciousness, and **neck stiffness or pain** (due to irritation of the meninges in the spinal cord) are common. As the intracranial pressure grows, various other signs may develop, including **seizures**.

A head CT will show blood localized to the subarachnoid cisterns which are small pockets filled with cerebrospinal fluid in specific parts of the brain (often radiating out from around the ventricles in an almost **spider-like shape**):

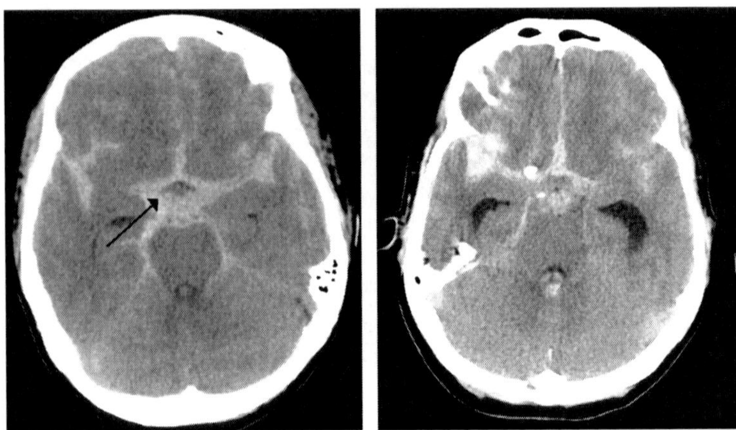

*A **subarachnoid hemorrhage** as seen on a CT scan.*

Because the subarachnoid space is where cerebrospinal fluid flows, a lumbar puncture may reveal an elevated number of **red blood cells**. In cases of suspected subarachnoid hemorrhage when a head CT is negative, a lumbar puncture is required.

A subarachnoid hemorrhage is no joke, with a one-month mortality rate around 50%! (Many patients don't even reach the hospital.) For this reason, it is important to keep this condition on your radar whenever someone presents with a sudden onset headache. While a sudden headache is associated with a subarachnoid hemorrhage, it is only a small minority of patients with headaches who *actually* have a subarachnoid hemorrhage and would require head imaging to rule this in or out. You can remember the factors that increase someone's risk of needing brain imaging when presenting with a headache using the convenient mnemonic **CT HEAD** which stands for **C**onsciousness loss, a **T**hunderclap quality to the headache, **H**urt neck, **E**xertional onset (many subarachnoid hemorrhages are brought about by physical exertion), patient **A**ge above 40 years, and **D**ecreased flexion of the neck.

A **subarachnoid hemorrhage** is a type of **hemorrhagic stroke** that is associated with a severe and sudden-onset **thunderclap headache.**

*Consider a **CT HEAD** to rule out a subarachnoid hemorrhage when there is:*
***C**onsciousness loss*
***T**hunderclap headache*
***H**urt neck*
***E**xertional onset*
***A**ge 40 years or older*
***D**ecreased neck flexion*

As with epidural and subdural hematomas, most cases of subarachnoid hemorrhage are associated with a history of trauma. Unlike epidural and subdural hematomas, however, a subarachnoid hemorrhage is not reliably associated with a break in any *particular* artery. Instead, because many arteries pass through the subarachnoid space, any of them can be affected by mechanical trauma. Spontaneous cases of subarachnoid hemorrhage (those not related to trauma) most often occur due to a **ruptured aneurysm**, typically in the circle of Willis.

INTRACEREBRAL HEMORRHAGE

While epidural hematomas, subdural hematomas, and subarachnoid hemorrhages all can cause problems in the brain due to compressive damage, it's important to remember that the site of bleeding is not actually in the *brain tissue itself* but rather in the meningeal pad *around* the brain. In contrast, cases of **intracerebral hemorrhage** *do* involve bleeding within the brain itself, allowing the blood to run amok and wreak havoc on nerves directly. Intracerebral hemorrhages can occur in either the nervous tissue (known as an **intraparenchymal hemorrhage**) or in the ventricular system (known as an **intraventricular hemorrhage**). Because intracerebral hemorrhages occur in the deepest part of the skull, they are by far the most difficult to treat.

The presentation of an intracerebral hemorrhage can resemble a subarachnoid hemorrhage, including a sudden onset of headache and other symptoms such as nausea and vomiting. Because intracerebral hemorrhages not only lead to ischemia but can also increase intracranial pressure, a wide variety of additional signs and symptoms can be seen depending on the specific areas involved. For example, putaminal hemorrhages (the most common type) often present with exclusively **m**otor deficits (remember to "**put an M** for **putamen**!") while **th**alamic hemorrhages (the second most common type) involve **th**en**th**ory deficits. **P**ontine hemorrhages often present with **p**in**p**oint **p**u**p**ils and an abrupt loss of consciousness, with a high associated mortality rate.

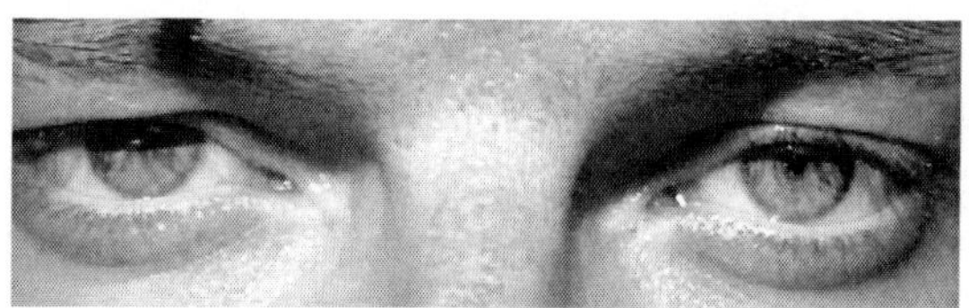

***Pinpoint pupils** can be seen in **pontine hemorrhages**.*

Pontine hemorrhages are associated with **bilateral pupillary constriction**.

***P**ontine hemorrhages present with **p**in**p**oint **p**u**p**ils.*

Due to the variations in presentation, an intracerebral hemorrhage is more often diagnosed by head imaging than by a neurological exam. An intraparenchymal hemorrhage will show focal areas of bleeding (called a "**spot sign**" as seen in the left image below), while an intraventricular hemorrhage will have signs of bleeding in the ventricular system (as seen on the right).

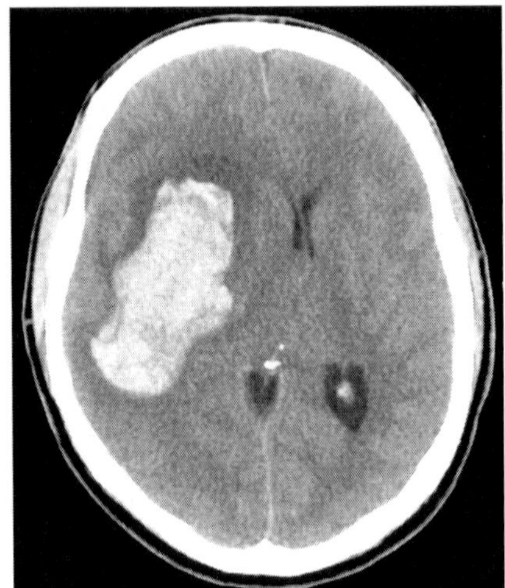

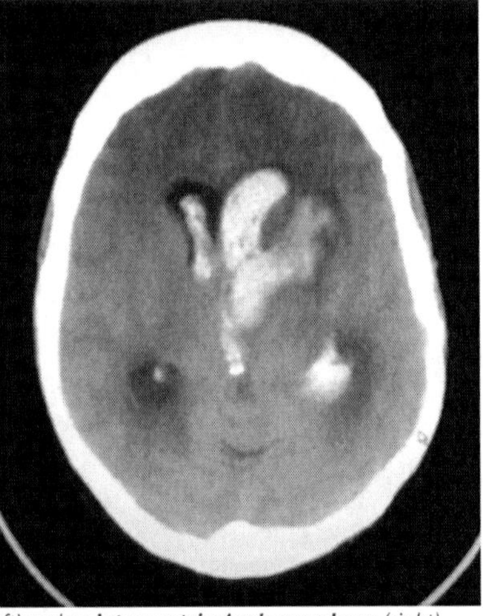

*CT imaging of an **intraparenchymal hemorrhage** (left) and an **intraventricular hemorrhage** (right).*

Like a subarachnoid hemorrhage, an intracerebral hemorrhage is a serious condition, with nearly half of patients dying within one month. Patients generally need to be managed in an intensive care unit. Treatment depends on the nature and size of the bleed, with medications, neurosurgery, and life support measures often being required.

HYDROCEPHALUS

While intracranial bleeds contribute to increased intracranial pressure by bringing too much *blood* into the enclosed space of the skull, you can also increase intracranial pressure by bringing in too much *cerebrospinal fluid* into the ventricular system. This is known as **hydrocephalus**. (The third mechanism—increasing the volume of the brain tissue directly—will be covered more in Chapter 21 when we talk about brain tumors.)

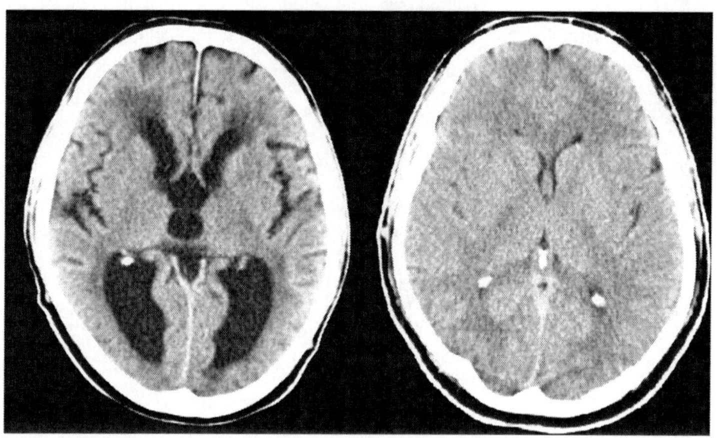

A CT scan of a patient with enlarged ventricles due to ***hydrocephalus*** *(left) compared to a* ***normal*** *scan (right).*

Hydrocephalus typically presents with all of the classic signs and symptoms of increased intracranial pressure including papilledema, headaches, nausea, vomiting, altered mental status, seizures, and focal neurologic signs. When it occurs in a developing fetus or infant, it may lead to growth in the size of the skull (as the bones are not yet set).

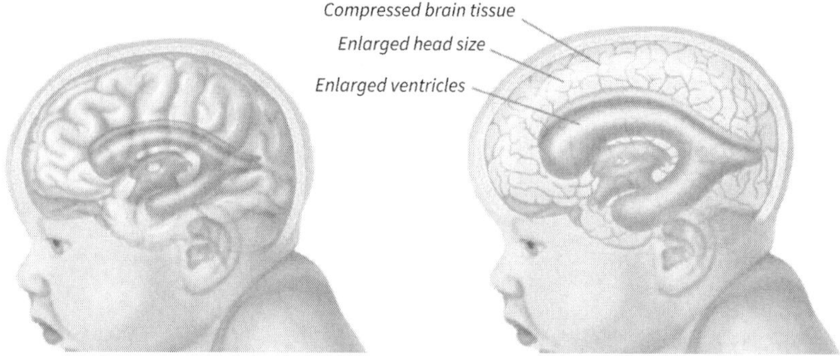

A ***normally developing*** *infant (left) compared to an infant with* ***hydrocephalus*** *(right).*

Hydrocephalus falls into four main categories. The first two forms (obstructive and communicating) are more common in **children** and *are* associated with increased intracranial pressure, while the second two forms (normal pressure hydrocephalus and hydrocephalus *ex vacuo*) are more common in **adults** and are *not* associated with increased intracranial pressure. We'll go over each of these four forms now.

OBSTRUCTIVE HYDROCEPHALUS

Obstructive (or non-communicating) hydrocephalus is caused by a **blockage in the flow** of cerebrospinal fluid anywhere in the ventricular system (but most often in the narrow foramina, aqueducts, and canals). These obstructions lead to the build-up of fluid in any ventricles "upstream." For example, narrowing of the cerebral aqueduct can lead to enlargement of both the lateral and third ventricles, while narrowing of the interventricular foramina would lead to obstruction of the lateral ventricles only. This is why it's so important to know the order in which cerebrospinal fluid travels through the ventricular system (remember "**C**SF is **LIT AF**" from Chapter 12)! Without that, you wouldn't be able to determine the likely effects of an obstruction.

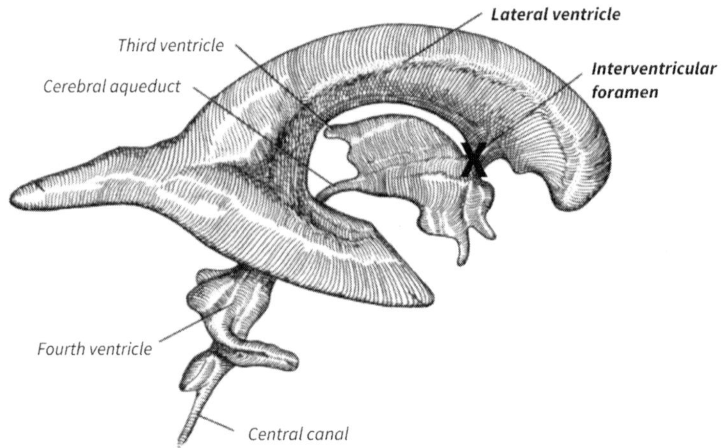

*Obstruction of the **interventricular foramen** will lead to dilation of the bolded structures in this drawing…*

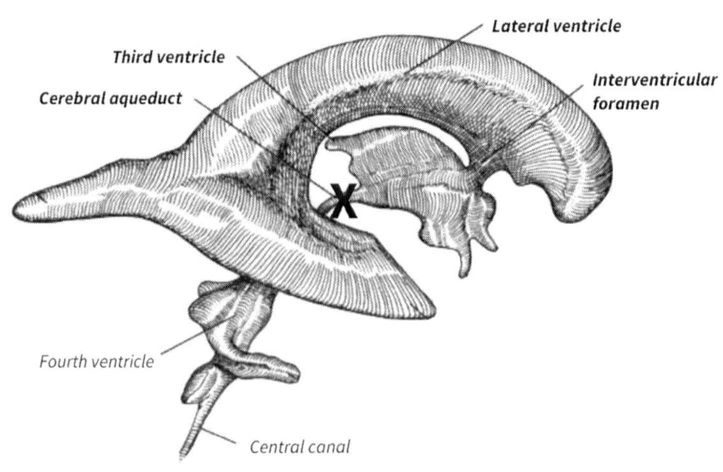

*… while obstruction of the **cerebral aqueduct** will lead to dilation of the bolded structures in this drawing.*

Obstructive hydrocephalus can also be caused by tumors, with **ependymomas** (tumors of cerebrospinal fluid-producing ependymal cells) being a common cause.

COMMUNICATING HYDROCEPHALUS

Communicating (or non-obstructive) hydrocephalus involves **impaired absorption** of cerebrospinal fluid due to dysfunction of the **arachnoid granulations**. Given that the function of the arachnoid granulations is to absorb cerebrospinal fluid back into the bloodstream, any damage here will cause an outflow obstruction, leading to build-up of cerebrospinal fluid in *all* of the ventricles as well as in the subarachnoid space. Communicating hydrocephalus can be caused by any condition that involves inflammation of or damage to the arachnoid granulations, with **meningitis** (or inflammation of the meninges, which we will talk about more in Chapter 22) being a particularly common cause.

NORMAL PRESSURE HYDROCEPHALUS

Normal pressure hydrocephalus (or NPH) sets itself apart from the first two forms of hydrocephalus in that it does *not* generally result in increased intracranial pressure (even though the pressure can be intermittently elevated). Instead, an **imbalance** between the amount of cerebrospinal fluid *produced* to the amount that is *absorbed* leads to dilated ventricles. Notably, the typical signs and symptoms of increased intracranial pressure (like headache or nausea) are often absent! Instead, cases of normal pressure hydrocephalus are characterized by a triad including **D**ementia, **I**ncontinence, and **G**ait instability (which you can remember using either the acronym **DIG** or the phrase "wet, wobbly, and wacky"). Of the three, gait instability tends to present first, with cognitive impairment and incontinence coming later. Normal pressure hydrocephalus is a **treatable condition**, with the first-line intervention being placement of a shunt that allows cerebrospinal fluid to drain into the abdomen.

Normal pressure hydrocephalus involves **dilation of the ventricular system** without necessarily increasing intracranial pressure, leading to **gait instability**, **cognitive impairment**, and **urinary incontinence**.

***DIG**: **D**ementia, **I**ncontinence, and **G**ait instability (or "wet, wobbly, and wacky").*

HYDROCEPHALUS EX VACUO

Finally, **hydrocephalus *ex vacuo*** is not a true form of hydrocephalus. Instead, it occurs when a generalized death of neurons in the brain (such as you might see in various forms of dementia or due to recurrent strokes) leads to loss of brain volume. The vacuum created by this atrophy leads to enlargement of the ventricles on brain imaging, giving the appearance of hydrocephalus without the actual increase in intracranial pressure. You can pick up on cases of hydrocephalus *ex vacuo* by looking at the brain tissue itself, as the overall volume will be decreased, giving it a shriveled or sunken appearance.

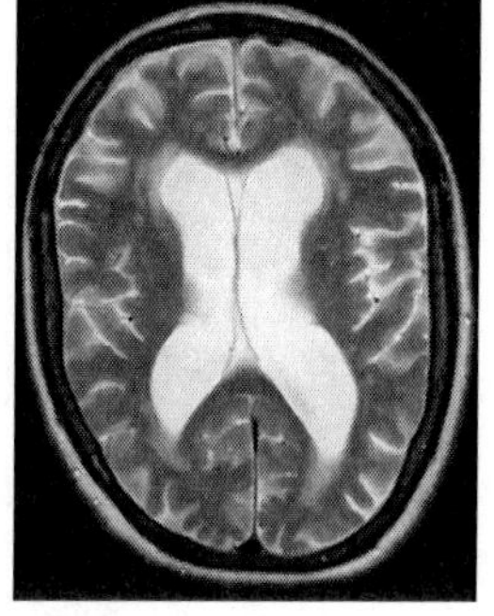

BRAIN HERNIATION

While the first two disease categories we talked about in this chapter can both *cause* increases in intracranial pressure, in this last section we will talk about a potential *consequence* of intracranial hypertension known as **brain herniation**. When intracranial pressure gets high enough, parts of the brain may get forced through the various holes leading into, out of, or between various compartments of the skull. (It's kind of like squeezing a water balloon with your hand: with enough pressure, the contents will squeeze out of whatever holes are available to them.)

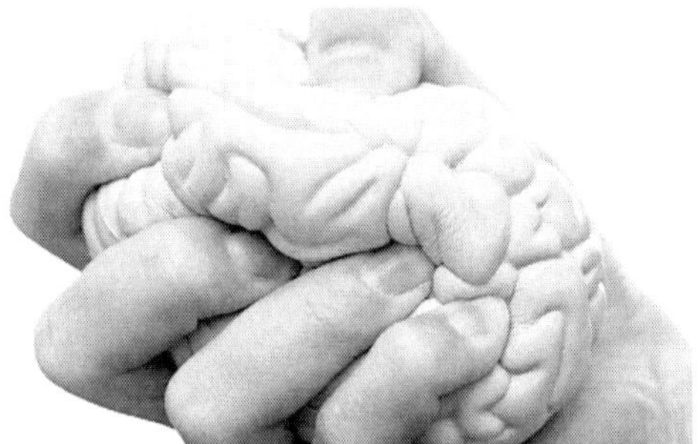

This is similar to what happens in ***brain herniation****.*

Because herniation often occurs suddenly and affects large parts of the brain, it tends to presents in a dramatic way, such as with **sudden loss of consciousness**. In cases of severe damage, the patient may show one of two forms of involuntary posturing. When upper parts of the brain such as the cerebral cortex and subcortex have been affected, the patient may display **decorticate posturing** which involves holding the arms inward towards the chest, almost like a mummy. In contrast, when structures in the brainstem have been affected, the patient may show **decerebrate posturing** which involves extension of the arms out to the side with rigidity across the entire body. (Other functions of the brain, such as sensory processing and hormone production, are often compromised as well, although these tend to be forgotten as they are not as immediately life-threatening as the other effects of central herniation.) You can remember the difference between decorticate and decerebrate posturing by thinking that de-**core**-ticate posturing involves bringing the arms towards the **core**.

Decorticate *posturing*

Decerebrate *posturing*

Brain herniation often presents with **sudden loss of consciousness**.
Decorticate or decerebrate posturing may be seen.

*De-**core**-ticate posturing involves bringing the arms towards the **core**.*

There are a few types of brain herniations to be aware of, each of which is illustrated visually in the drawing below. We will talk about each one in turn. Feel free to refer back to this image as needed to compare and contrast as you learn about each form of brain herniation!

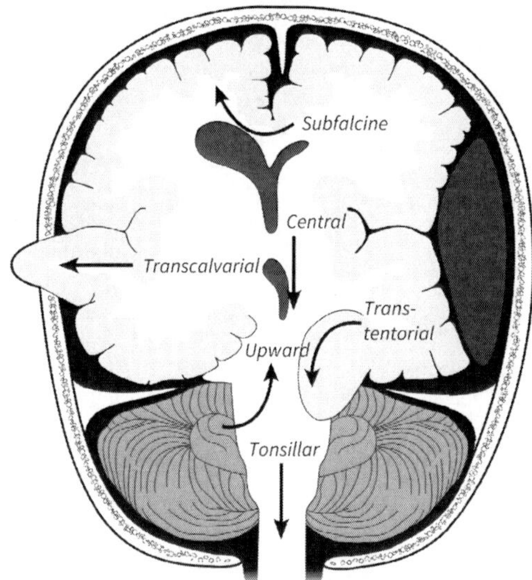

Various forms of ***brain herniation****.*

SUBFALCINE HERNIATION

As we learned in Chapter 12, the **falx cerebri** is the barrier separating the left and right cerebral hemispheres. With enough pressure on either side, the cerebrum can be forced under the falx cerebri into the other hemisphere (such as the right brain going into the left hemisphere). This is known as a **subfalcine herniation**. The particular part of the brain that is most often affected is the cingulate cortex of the **frontal lobe**. The anterior cerebral artery supplying this part of the brain may also get dragged in, creating an **anterior cerebral artery stroke**. Due to the involvement of these brain regions, a subfalcine herniation tends to cause **leg weakness** and **gait instability** from compression of the motor cortex deep within the longitudinal fissure.

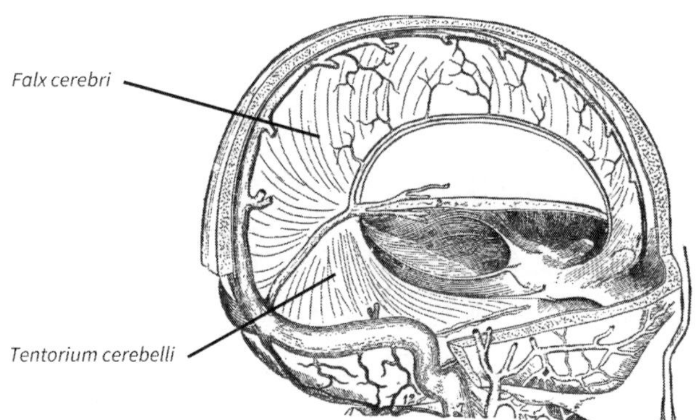

A ***subfalcine herniation*** *involves brain tissue crossing the* ***falx cerebri****.*

Subfalcine herniations are the **most common** form of brain herniation, as less pressure is generally needed to force brain tissue below the falx cerebri compared with the smaller holes we will discuss next. They also tend to be less damaging than the other types (although loss of consciousness and coma can occur in severe cases). However, subfalcine herniations can also be a "canary in a coal mine" by being the first herniation to occur when a source of increased intracranial pressure (such as a bleed or tumor) is present. For this reason, subfalcine herniations still require prompt attention to determine the cause of the increased intracranial pressure and fix it.

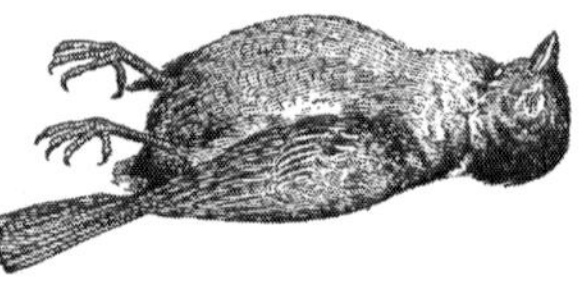

You can remember the association of a canary and subfalcine herniations by thinking of them as **sub-falcon** herniations, as a canary is generally agreed to be a lesser bird than a falcon (a "sub-falcon" bird, if you will). The word "**CAN**-ary" can also help to remind you of the involvement of the **C**ingulate cortex and **AN**terior cerebral artery strokes in cases of subfalcine herniation.

A **subfalcine herniation** involves the **cingulate cortex** being pushed under the **falx cerebri** and potentially compressing the **anterior cerebral artery**.

*A **sub-falcon herniation** is like a **CAN**-ary in a coal mine and is associated with compression of both the **C**ingulate cortex and the **AN**terior cerebral artery.*

TRANSTENTORIAL HERNIATION

Recall from Chapter 12 that the tentorium cerebelli forms a "hammock" of sorts separating the "upper" cerebrum from the "lower" cerebellum as seen below:

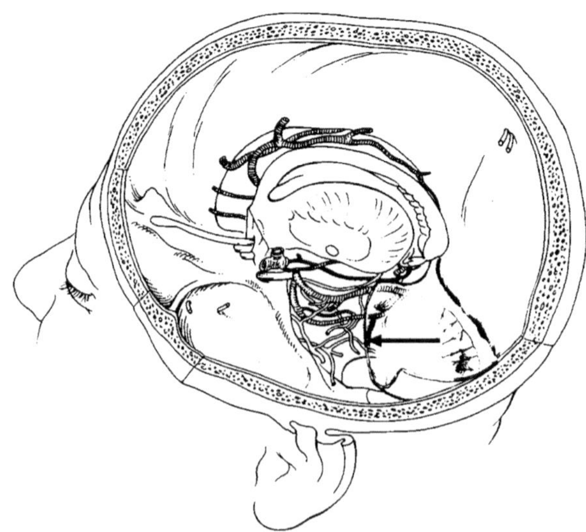

*The **tentorium cerebelli** indicated with an arrow.*

Naturally, a **transtentorial herniation** involves displacement of the brain down past this structure. The most common part of the brain affected by a transtentorial herniation is the **uncus** or the part of the temporal lobe that sits right above the tentorium cerebelli. Because of its location, the uncus is extra vulnerable to slipping through the tentorium if enough pressure is applied. To remember the key clinical signs and symptoms associated with an uncal herniation, think of someone named **Uncle CHIP the Third**. This should help you associate an **uncal** herniation with **C**ontralateral **H**emianopsia, **I**psilateral **P**aralysis, and a **Third** cranial nerve palsy. Let's go over these one by one:

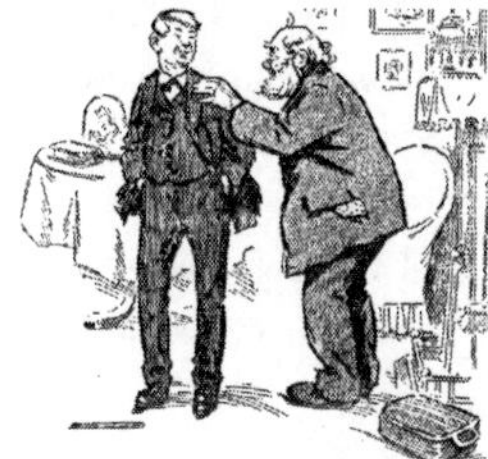

CH is for Contralateral Hemianopsia. Transtentorial herniation has a tendency to cause compression of the nearby posterior cerebral artery, leading to the usual visual field deficits related to occipital lobe strokes (specifically, contralateral homonymous hemianopsia with macular sparing).

IP is for Ipsilateral Paralysis. Transtentorial herniation is known to cause ipsilateral motor weakness in the body due to compression of the motor tracts running in the **cerebral peduncles** (remember the two "ears" of the midbrain's bear-like face!). Wait a minute... why are the motor deficits *ipsilateral* to the lesion? Shouldn't they be *contralateral* because the pyramidal decussation hasn't occurred yet? (That's good thinking, the kind that will get you far in neurology!) The reason that motor deficits are ipsilateral in an uncal herniation is because of a phenomenon known as **Kernohan-Woltman syndrome**. Essentially, what happens here is that if there is increased intracranial pressure and a resultant uncal hernia on *one* side of the brain, this can cause the cerebral peduncle on the *opposite* side to be pressed up into the tentorium there, causing an indentation (or "notch") that compresses and ultimately causes dysfunction of the motor neurons traveling in the corticospinal tract. By causing damage to the cerebral peduncles on the *opposite* side (which then crosses over in the medulla), an uncal herniation can result in *ipsilateral* paralysis. Because this phenomenon has a tendency to get clinicians to "call it" for the wrong side, it is sometimes called a **false localizing sign**.

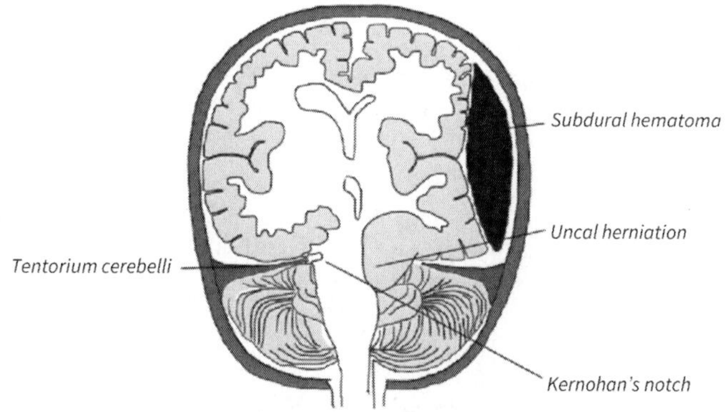

Mechanism of ***Kernohan's notch*** *in* ***transtentorial herniation****.*

The Third is for a Third cranial nerve palsy. A herniated uncus has a tendency to compress the **midbrain** (which makes sense, as it is the part of the brainstem that is closest to the tentorium cerebelli). In particular, dysfunction of the ipsilateral cranial nerves coming out of the midbrain are a reliable sign of this condition (with the **oculomotor nerves** being affected to a greater degree than the trochlear nerves). Damage to the oculomotor nerve first manifests through a **dilated pupil**, with a "**down and out**" deviation of the eye happening later. (The fact that pupillary dilation happens first makes sense if you remember **OOMMPP**: the **O**cul**O**motor nerve has **M**otor in the **M**iddle and **P**upils on the **P**eriphery, so a compressive force will affect the pupils first!) The presence of an oculomotor nerve palsy can help you to avoid falling for this "false localizing sign," as the side of the dilated pupil is the affected side in over 90% of cases!

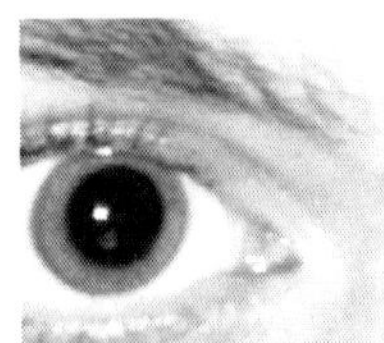
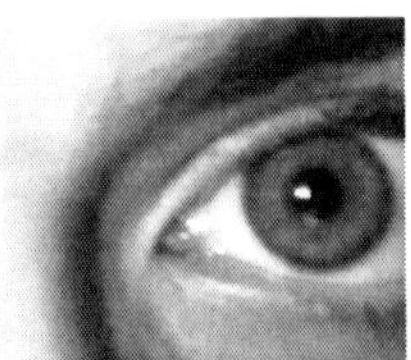

Transtentorial herniations *are a potential cause of* ***unilateral pupil dilation****.*

Transtentorial herniation involves the **uncus**, or the innermost part of the **temporal lobe**, moving past the **tentorium cerebelli** and putting pressure on the **midbrain**.

Uncle CHIP, the Third:

Uncal *herniation causes* ***C****ontralateral* ***H****emianopsia,* ***I****psilateral* ***P****aralysis (due to Kernohan's notch), and a* ***Third*** *nerve palsy.*

CENTRAL HERNIATION

Central herniation is similar in some ways to an uncal herniation, as it involves medial parts of the brain (including the inner parts of the temporal cortex) being displaced downward through the tentorium cerebelli. However, in central herniation, the lower parts of the cerebral *sub*cortex such as the **thalamus**, **epithalamus**, and **hypothalamus** are all dragged in as well! The involvement of the hypothalamus leads to hormone deficiencies, while involvement of the epithalamus leads to a weakness of upward eye movements with resultant downward displacement of the eyes (as in Parinaud's syndrome, which you'll remember from Chapter 4 is when you find someone's **peerin' odd**). This finding is sometimes called "**sunset eyes**" as the eyes cross the eyelids like a sun setting past the horizon. You can remember that all **th**ree of the "**th**alami" are involved by thinking of it as a **th**entral herniation.

Central herniation involves the **thalamus**, **epithalamus**, and **hypothalamus** moving downward through the tentorium cerebelli.

Th*entral herniation involves all* ***th****ree of the* ***th****alami!*

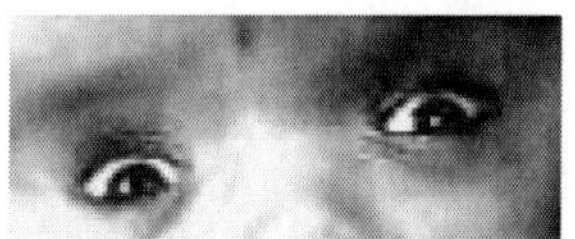 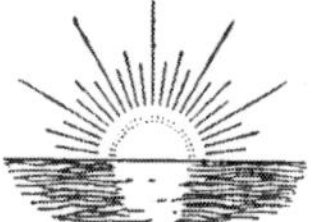

***Sunset eyes** are a common finding in **central herniation**.*

UPWARD HERNIATION

Upward herniation is the mechanical opposite of central herniation. Instead of the *cerebrum* coming *down* through the tentorium cerebelli, the *cerebellum* goes *up* through it. Despite the difference in direction, the same structures are affected, leading to an overall similar presentation (with both eye displacement and various pituitary hormone deficiencies being seen).

TONSILLAR HERNIATION

Tonsillar herniation involves parts of the **cerebellum** being pushed through the **foramen magnum** or the large hole at the bottom of the skull through which the medulla travels right before becoming the spinal cord. For this reason, tonsillar herniation can be **life-threatening**, as the medulla contains the vital cardiorespiratory centers. The upper cervical spinal cord can be affected as well. The primary signs and symptoms of a tonsillar herniation include headache, neck stiffness, changes in consciousness, and flaccid paralysis throughout the body.

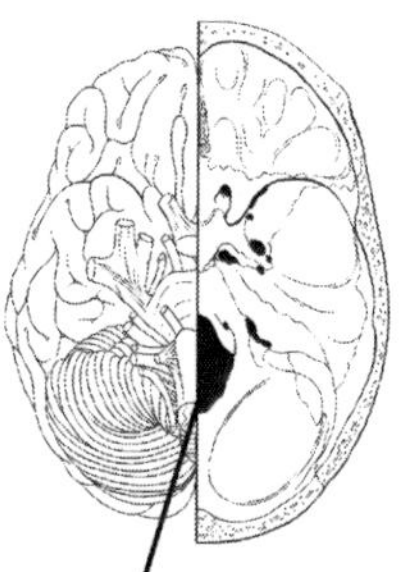

Foramen magnum

TRANSCALVARIAL HERNIATION

Finally, **transcalvarial herniation** is a rare form of brain herniation in which the brain is forced out through a hole in the **skull** itself. Under normal conditions, the skull is hard enough that a soft, squishy substance like the brain isn't able to force its way out. For this reason, transcalvarial herniation is really only a problem when the skull has been compromised somehow, whether that is a skull fracture related to a motor vehicle accident or a hole being made in the skull during neurosurgery.

PUTTING IT ALL TOGETHER

In this chapter, we've covered two different *causes* of increased intracranial pressure (**intracranial bleeds** and **hydrocephalus**) as well as a potential consequence of intracranial hypertension (**brain herniation**). Diagnosing these conditions relies upon recognizing the **classic pattern of symptoms** (including papilledema, headaches, nausea, vomiting, altered mental status, seizures, and focal neurologic signs) in the context of a **sudden onset** and/or a history of **head trauma** which are found in most cases. In addition, each disease has certain "clues" (like a lucid period in epidural hematomas or a thunderclap headache in subarachnoid hemorrhages) that will help you recognize them! Use these "buzz words" as a guide when encountering increased intracranial pressure both on tests and in clinical settings.

REVIEW QUESTIONS

1. A 55 y/o F undergoes a cerebral angiogram which shows an aneurysm in her right anterior communicating artery as seen below:

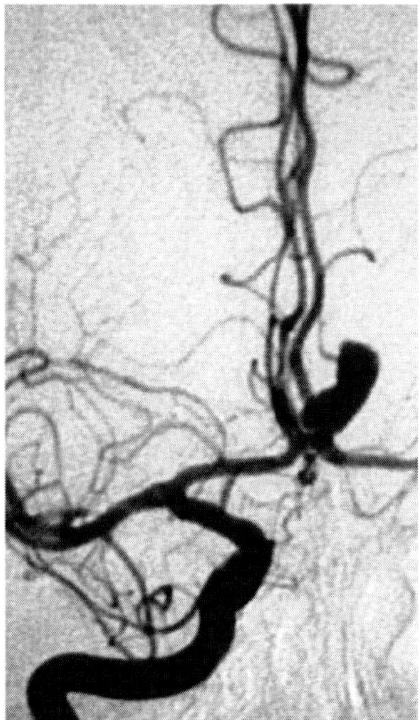

Which of the following conditions is she most at risk of developing first?

A. Intracerebral hemorrhage
B. Epidural hematoma
C. Subarachnoid hemorrhage
D. Subdural hematoma
E. Subfalcine herniation
F. Uncal herniation
G. Central herniation
H. Transcalvarial herniation
I. Upward herniation
J. Tonsillar herniation

2. (Continued from previous question.) If this aneurysm were to rupture, what is the most likely clinical presentation?
    A. An abrupt onset of motor and sensory deficits in the face, arms, and legs
    B. A brief loss of consciousness followed by regaining consciousness and then losing it again
    C. A slow onset of headache and confusion over weeks or months
    D. A sudden onset of "the worst headache of my life" with neck stiffness and pain
    E. Involuntary extension of the limbs with downward displacement of the eyes

3. A 25 y/o M is pitching in a baseball game without wearing a helmet. After one pitch, the batter accidentally loses his grip on the bat and sends it flying into the air, hitting the pitcher in the head. He loses consciousness for around 5 minutes but then awakens. He reports feeling dazed but "okay." Despite encouragement, he does not go to the hospital for evaluation. Several hours later, he suddenly experiences a severe headache with nausea and vomiting. Alarmed, his wife calls 911. On the way to the hospital, he becomes increasingly lethargic and confused, and he is unconscious by the time of arrival. Which of the following is the most likely blood vessel that has been injured?
    A. Anterior cerebral artery
    B. Anterior communicating artery
    C. Posterior communicating artery
    D. Middle meningeal artery
    E. Bridging veins

4. (Continued from previous question.) In the emergency department, the patient is noted to have a dilated left pupil and a "down and out" positioning of the left eye. Visual exam is notable for a right homonymous hemianopsia. There is complete motor weakness on his left side. Knowing that damage to the brain produces motor deficits on the opposite side, the clinical team diagnoses him with a right-sided hematoma and rushes him to the operating room for a craniotomy, a surgical procedure intended to control bleeding in the intracranial space. When the surgical team makes a hole in the right side, however, they find no bleeding. Surprised, they drill again on the left side and find a hematoma. Which of the following mechanisms most likely accounts for the unexpected findings in this patient?
    A. Developmental abnormality resulting in an absent decussation of the corticospinal tract in the medulla
    B. Damage to the cerebellum rather than the cerebrum
    C. Diagnosis of situs inversus, or a congenital condition in which all major organs are reversed on their left-right axis
    D. Sufficient compressive force to injure the opposite side of the brain
    E. Medical error on the part of the medical team accidentally confusing left for right

1. **The best answer is C.** While trauma is the most common cause of subarachnoid hemorrhage, a close second is the rupture of a cerebral aneurysm due to their propensity to bleed into the subarachnoid space. Intracerebral hemorrhage, epidural hematomas, and subdural hematomas are all associated with a history of head trauma as well, although they do not have the same link to cerebral aneurysms that a subarachnoid hemorrhage does (answers A, B, and D). On its own, an unruptured aneurysm is unlikely to increase intracranial pressure sufficiently to cause any form of herniation (answers E—J).

2. **The best answer is D.** The typical presentation of a subarachnoid hemorrhage involves a sudden onset "thunderclap" headache with neck stiffness and pain due to irritation of the meninges. Motor and sensory deficits in the face, arms, and legs are more consistent with a stroke in the region of the anterior or middle cerebral artery (answer A). The specific pattern of losing, regaining, and then losing consciousness again is more associated with an epidural hematoma (answer B), while a slow onset of headache and confusion is seen more often in a subdural hematoma (answer C). Finally, decerebrate posturing and "sunset eyes" are more often seen in central herniation.

3. **The best answer is D.** This case describes an epidural hematoma which is strongly associated with head trauma. The classic presentation is an initial loss of consciousness followed by a lucid period and a later lapse back into unconsciousness. Rupture of the middle meningeal artery, which supplies the dura mater, is a common cause of an epidural hematoma. Rupture of bridging veins is associated with a subdural hematoma (answer E), while a stroke in the anterior cerebral artery is associated with a subfalcine herniation (answer A). The anterior and posterior communicating arteries are both common sites of aneurysm formation in the circle of Willis which may then rupture and lead to a subarachnoid hemorrhage (answers B and C).

4. **The best answer is D.** As an epidural hematoma grows, it can increase intracranial pressure to the point of causing a transtentorial herniation. When there is sufficient compressive force, brain tissue on the *opposite* side of the bleeding can be compressed, a phenomenon known as Kernohan's notch. This can lead to motor weakness on the side *ipsilateral* to the bleeding. For this reason, in potential cases of uncal herniation, it is important to rely upon neuroimaging rather than observed motor deficits to localize the lesion. (The dilated pupil will also be ipsilateral to the lesion in the vast majority of all cases, which is another helpful clue.) The medical team mistaking the patient's left for his right would not account for the accurate representation of his ocular findings (answer E). Damage to the cerebellum would cause ataxia and other cerebellar signs but not the frank motor weakness observed in this case (answer B). Situs inversus does exist, but it would not account for the fact that the muscle weakness is generally contralateral to the side of the bleeding regardless of the positioning of the organs (answer C). Finally, there are no known cases of people being born without a pyramidal decussation (answer A).

16 MYOPATHY

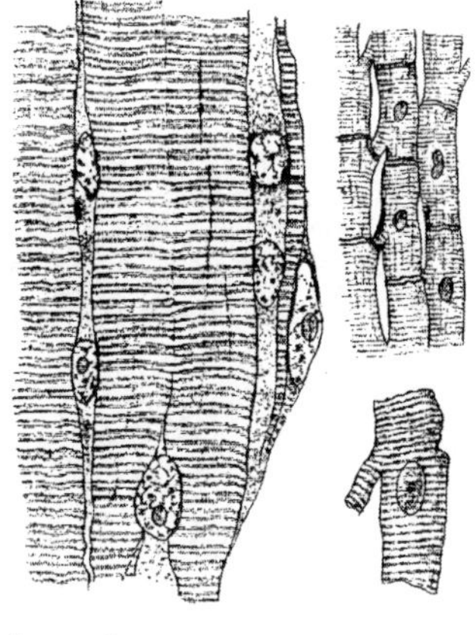

Starting here and continuing on for the next few chapters, we will pivot away from talking about the pathology of the central nervous system and begin a tour through diseases affecting the **motor system**. The term **neuromuscular disease** is used to refer broadly to the various forms of pathology that can all affect muscle function. These disorders can happen at any step along the way, including the **muscle itself** (as in myopathies like muscular dystrophy), the **nerves** supplying the muscles (as in motor neuron diseases such as amyotrophic lateral sclerosis), the **neuromuscular junction** connecting the two (as in neuromuscular junction diseases like myasthenia gravis), or in the regions of the **brain** controlling movement (as in movement disorders like Parkinson's disease).

We will begin our tour of neuromuscular diseases in this chapter by focusing on a group of disorders known as **myopathies** that all involve dysfunction of the muscles themselves (rather than being related to any "upstream" parts like the neuromuscular junction, motor neuron, or central nervous system). A variety of disease processes can cause dysfunction in the muscle, including muscle inflammation, degeneration of muscle tissues, and environmental injuries. We'll go over a few key diseases in each of these categories, with a particular focus on those that present with neurologic signs and symptoms.

MUSCULAR DYSTROPHIES

Muscular dystrophy refers to the loss, destruction, or degeneration of muscle in the body due to a **genetic condition**. While there are many possible causes of muscular dystrophy, we will focus on just three: **Duchenne muscular dystrophy** (which is the most common child-onset form of muscular dystrophy), its related condition **Becker's muscular dystrophy**, and finally **myotonic muscular dystrophy** (which is the most common adult-onset form).

DUCHENNE MUSCULAR DYSTROPHY

Duchenne muscular dystrophy is an **X-linked recessive** genetic disorder in which muscle tissue is progressively destroyed, leading to muscle atrophy and weakness. Duchenne muscular dystrophy affects **boys** more than girls. The telltale pattern of muscle weakness generally appears around the **age of 4**, although some signs (such as delayed motor milestones) may be apparent as early as the first two years.

The first muscles affected are generally those in **proximal** groups like the **hips and upper legs**, with more distal muscles like the calves generally spared. This leads to a characteristic way of getting up from the floor known as **Gower's sign** in which weakness of the hip and upper leg muscles leads to an overreliance on the calves and arms to move one's body off the ground, as seen below:

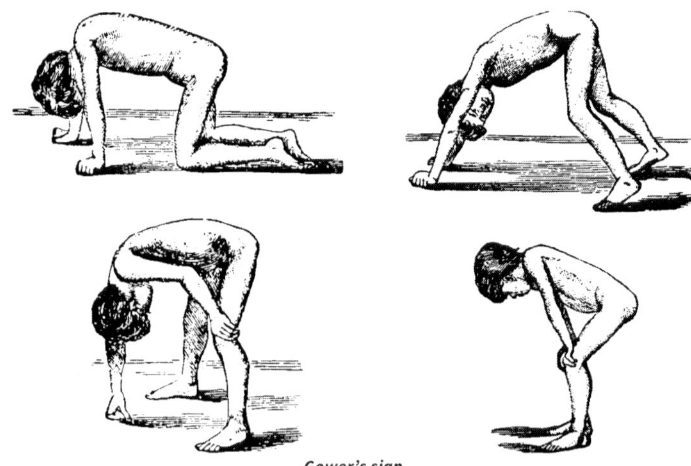

Gower's sign.

While wasting and atrophy of the affected muscles is often seen, hypertrophy of more distal muscles (like the calves) often occurs due to the compensatory overuse of these muscles. You can remember this by thinking that someone with **Duchenne's** muscular dystrophy will "**do shins**" more than most, leading to **hypertrophic calves**.

Duchenne muscular dystrophy is an **X-linked recessive disorder** that presents as **proximal weakness**, leading to overuse and hypertrophy of more distal muscles.

*If you always **do shins** (Duchenne's) in the gym, your **calves** will get **hypertrophic**.*

While the muscle weakness *begins* proximally, it often spreads distally as the disease progresses, and many people with this condition are unable to walk by adolescence. Life expectancy is often greatly reduced, and most patients die in their 20s or 30s (largely due to respiratory or cardiac failure, as the disease can progress to the point where the muscles of the heart and lungs fail as well).

Duchenne muscular dystrophy is caused by a mutation in the **dystrophin** gene which produces a protein responsible for stabilizing the cytoskeleton of muscle cells. Without dystrophin, the cell membrane becomes weak, leading to mitochondrial dysfunction and the eventual death of the cell. For this reason, laboratory markers of muscle damage such as **creatine kinase** (CK) are almost always high in patients with this condition.

BECKER'S MUSCULAR DYSTROPHY

Becker's muscular dystrophy is a related condition that is similar to Duchenne muscular dystrophy in almost every way. The major difference is that Becker's often has a better prognosis, with a longer life expectancy and a better quality of life.

MYOTONIC DYSTROPHY

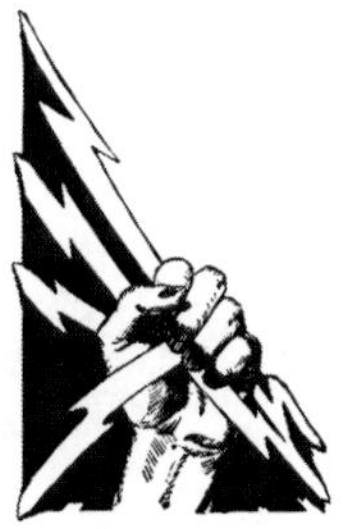

While Duchenne muscular dystrophy is the most common muscular dystrophy of *childhood*, **myotonic dystrophy** is the most common in *adults* (although it can begin during childhood as well). The term "myotonic" here refers to an **inability to relax a muscle once it has contracted**. (You can remember the association between myotonic dystrophy and an inability to relax a muscle by thinking of someone saying, "It's <u>*my*</u> otonic dystrophy!" and imagining that they *can't let go*.) This inability to relax is also combined with a generalized **muscle weakness**.

Myotonic dystrophy is not a single disease but rather a pair of diseases (type 1 and type 2). For this reason, it has considerable variation in its presentation, with some people having only mild disability while others are severely affected. Both forms of myotonic dystrophy feature prominent weakness of **distal muscles** such as the hands and feet, although type 2 can involve proximal weakness as well. Both forms of myotonic dystrophy are associated with an increased risk of developing specific other medical conditions including cataracts, insulin resistance, intellectual disability, and cardiac conduction abnormalities.

Both forms of myotonic dystrophy are **autosomal dominant** genetic disorders involving an expansion of the **trinucleotide repeat CTG**. While it typically does not appear until someone is in their adult years, in rare cases it may be present from birth. While there is no cure for myotonic dystrophy, physical therapy can help to improve the patient's quality of life.

Myotonic dystrophy is an **autosomal dominant genetic disorder** that presents as **distal weakness** and an **inability to relax muscles once contracted**.

*"It's **<u>my</u> otonic dystrophy**!" (This person is having trouble **letting go**.)*

INFLAMMATORY MYOPATHIES

Inflammation is a complex process in which the body attempts to respond to harmful or noxious stimuli by unleashing the power of the immune system, leading to the classic combination of **calor** (heat or warmth), **dolor** (pain), **rubor** (redness), and **tumor** (swelling). Inflammation is generally an uncomfortable state but, provided that it is helping to fight off infections and other threats to health, it can be functional. However, there are also times when inflammation occurs in the absence of an external threat or to such a great extent that it becomes maladaptive. When the immune system decides to attack muscle in particular, it leads to a state of muscle weakness and pain known as an **inflammatory myopathy** (also called **myositis**). Inflammatory myopathies come in a few different forms, three of which we will cover now.

POLYMYOSITIS

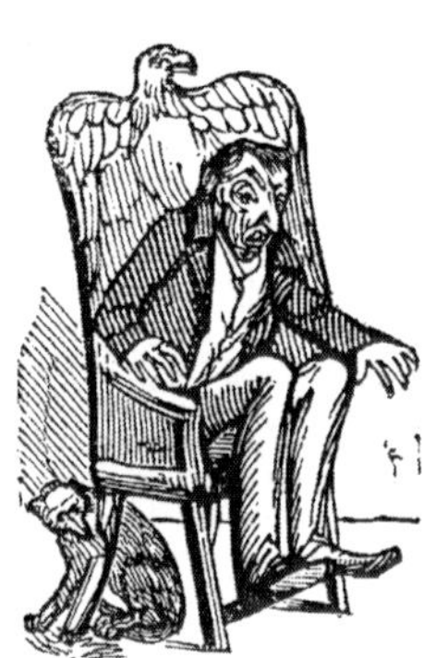

Polymyositis is an inflammatory myopathy in which **cytotoxic T cells** invade muscle tissues. This often presents as a slow onset of muscle weakness and atrophy over months or years. The clinical hallmark of polymyositis is **bilateral proximal weakness**, with the **hip extensors** often being affected first. This leads to difficulties in specific actions such as **rising from a chair**, which in many cases is the initial complaint that ultimately leads to a diagnosis of polymyositis. There is often **muscle pain** as well (remember "dolor!"). The extent and severity of muscle dysfunction increases as inflammation continues, making polymyositis a **progressive condition**. For unknown reasons, **women** are affected more often than men. The widespread inflammation seen in polymyositis can also cause problems in other organ systems as well, leading to heart failure, lung disease, and an increased risk of various forms of cancer.

A diagnosis of polymyositis is based on a characteristic history and neurological exam findings of proximal muscle weakness and atrophy. However, to definitively diagnose this disease, you must conduct a muscle biopsy which will show the invasion of T cells *within* the muscle fibers, as seen below. (Compare this to dermatomyositis, discussed next, in which the T cells are mostly found *outside* of the muscle fibers.)

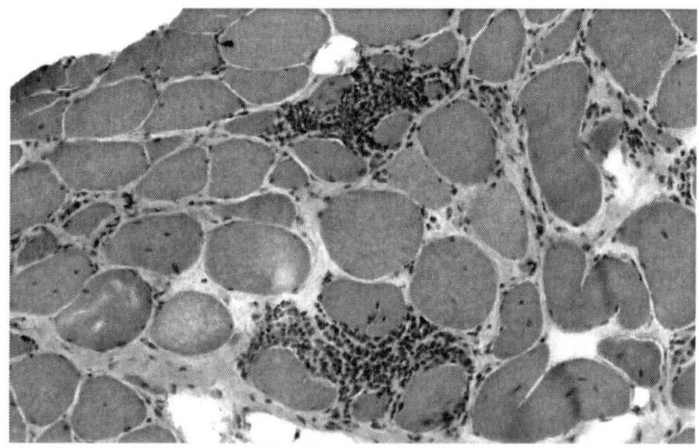

*Muscle biopsy in **polymyositis** will reveal immune cells within muscle fibers.*

Treatment of polymyositis involves **corticosteroids** to rapidly reduce the state of immune system hyperactivation. Steroids are highly effective treatments for this condition, and most patients improve dramatically. Interventions such as physical therapy are also a key component of helping patients to regain functional ability.

To remember the details of **poly**myositis, imagine a situation where **Polly** (an **adult woman**) wants a cracker but **can't get up from her chair** to get one. For this reason, she is stuck **inside**. This will help you remember the most common initial presenting complaint for polymyositis, its greater frequency in adults and females (as opposed to children or males), and the fact that the T cells are found *inside* of the muscle fibers on biopsy.

Polymyositis is an **inflammatory myopathy** characterized by **progressive bilateral proximal weakness**. It most often affects **adult women**. Muscle biopsy will show T cells **within muscle fibers**.

***Polly** wants a cracker but **can't get up from her chair**, so she is stuck **inside**.*

DERMATOMYOSITIS

Dermatomyositis is another inflammatory myopathy that is similar in many ways to polymyositis. Both present with **progressive bilateral proximal weakness** affecting the thighs and upper arms, leading to similar presenting complaints (such as difficulty getting up from a chair, climbing stairs, or lifting something above the head). Both begin in later adulthood (around 40 or 50 years old), are more common in women, and are associated with inflammatory changes in other parts of the body such as the heart and lungs. Like polymyositis, dermatomyositis can be treated with **steroids**.

Where dermatomyositis differentiates itself, however, is with its involvement of the **skin**, as this condition is associated with **rashes** in various parts of the body. These rashes are generally red in color, are very sensitive to sunlight, and may be itchy or painful. An example of a dermatomyositis-associated rash on the elbow is seen below:

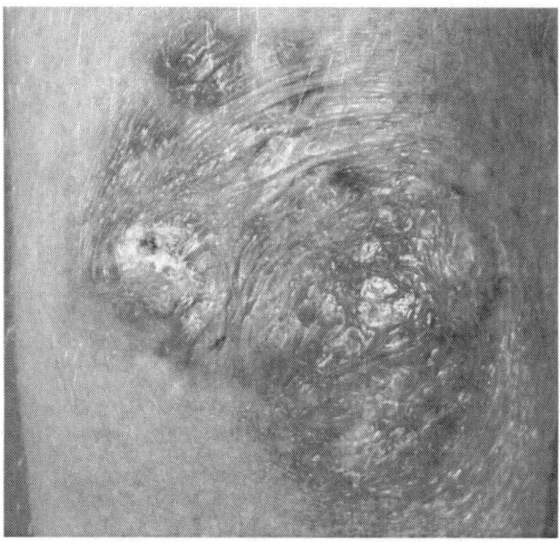

*A rash on the elbow related to **dermatomyositis**.*

Dermatomyositis also differentiates itself from polymyositis in its findings on muscle biopsy. While invasion of the muscle tissues by immune cells is seen in both, in dermatomyositis these cells are seen primarily around the *outside* of the muscle fibers (in contrast with polymyositis in which they are stuck *inside*). Compare the image below with the one from page 224:

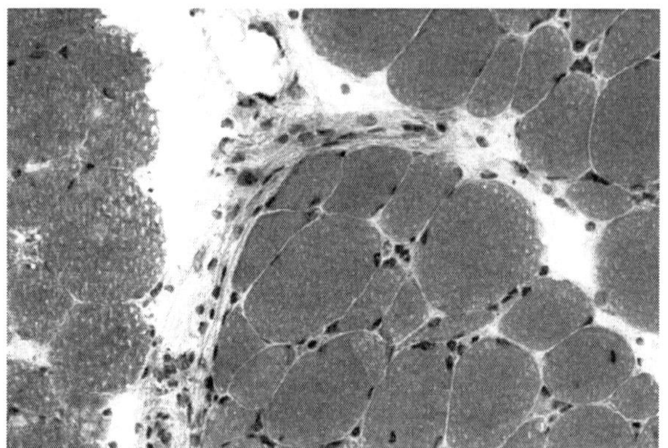

Muscle biopsy in ***dermatomyositis*** *will reveal immune cells outside of muscle fibers.*

Just as you associate polymyositis with the word *inside*, try to associate derm-**out**-omyositis with the word **out**-side. This should remind you of the rashes found on the *outside* of one's body and the presence of immune cells *outside* the muscle fibers.

Dermatomyositis is an **inflammatory myopathy** that is similar to polymyositis but also involves **skin rashes**. Muscle biopsy will show white blood cells in the space **surrounding muscle fibers**.

*Derm-**out**-omyositis is found **out**side:*
***out**side the body (on the skin) and **out**side the muscle fibers (on a biopsy).*

INCLUSION BODY MYOSITIS

The last of the inflammatory myopathies we will talk about is **inclusion body myositis**. Out of the three, inclusion body myositis is the odd one out. While it shares with polymyositis and dermatomyositis a tendency towards slowly progressive muscle weakness, it stands out in a few other ways. First, inclusion body myositis tends to affect **proximal and distal muscles** equally (including **finger flexors**, which aren't affected very often in polymyositis and dermatomyositis). Second, it often progresses **asymmetrically** (as opposed to bilaterally in the other two). Third, it primarily affects **elderly** adults, with **men** being affected more often than women. Fourth, it is not responsive to most forms of treatment (whereas both polymyositis and dermatomyositis respond well to immunosuppressive treatments such as steroids). In fact, the lack of a good response to treatment with steroids is sometimes used diagnostically to differentiate between inclusion body myositis and the other two inflammatory myopathies.

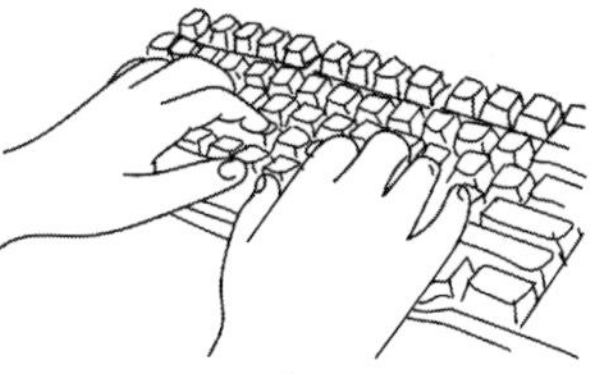

You can use the abbreviation **IBM** to remember the features of **I**nclusion **B**ody **M**yositis. The term IBM was often used synonymously with "computer" back in the 1980s and 1990s. This will help you remember the involvement of distal muscles like **finger flexors** (since you use your fingers for typing). Also, because use of the term "IBM" as a generic word for computer is not very common anymore, you will likely only hear **old men** say it.

Inclusion body myositis is an **inflammatory myopathy** that involves **asymmetric weakness of both proximal and distal muscles**. It primarily affects **older men** and is **not responsive to immunosuppressive treatment**.

*Think of an **older man** typing at an **IBM** using his **finger flexors**.*

PUTTING IT ALL TOGETHER

Myopathies are the first step along the way to understanding neuromuscular diseases, so make sure to learn them well by reviewing the mnemonics from this chapter (such as "do shins" and "derm-out-omyositis")! A major differentiating factor between these diseases is whether they impact proximal or distal muscles. **Proximal weakness** is the **most common pattern** (as it is seen in polymyositis, dermatomyositis, and both Duchenne and Becker's muscular dystrophy). In contrast, **distal weakness** is only seen in **myotonic dystrophy** and **inclusion body myositis**. If you see distal weakness in clinical settings or on tests, you're likely dealing with one of these two! Use the table below to summarize the most high-yield information about each of these diseases.

Disease	Distribution	Age/Gender	Features
Duchenne/Becker's	Proximal	Young boys	Calf hypertrophy, Gower's sign
Myotonic dystrophy	Distal	Adults	Inability to relax muscle
Polymyositis	Proximal	Adult women	T cells within muscle
Dermatomyositis	Proximal	Adult women	Rashes, T cells outside of muscles
Inclusion body myositis	Proximal and distal	Older men	Finger flexors involved

REVIEW QUESTIONS

1. A 28 y/o F has been seeing her neurologist since the age of 21. She was first seen in the clinic with concerns about her muscles tiring easily. She also noted at that time that her hand would "get stuck" on a door handle after opening it. During her initial evaluation, she had decreased motor strength in her hands and feet, with difficulty unclenching muscles once they had contracted. The patient was adopted and does not know her family's genetic history. She struggled with academics in her childhood but performed well enough to graduate from high school. She currently works as a grocery store bagger. At her visit today, the neurologist notes that when he shook her hand, she did not release his hand for several seconds. Her exam is notable for atrophy of several muscles in the face, decreased motor strength in all extremities, hypoactive reflexes in the arms, and absent reflexes in the legs. The patient informs the neurologist that she and her husband have been discussing the idea of having children. However, she is concerned about passing her disease on to her children. Her husband has no personal or family history of this disease. What is the most accurate response for the neurologist to give?
    A. "There is no chance of you passing this disease to your children."
    B. "There is a small chance of your children inheriting this disease, but it is remote enough that it shouldn't influence your decision making."
    C. "It is a definite possibility that you will pass it to your children, but it is still more unlikely than likely."
    D. "There is a good chance you will pass it to your children, especially if you have more than one child."
    E. "It is completely assured that your children will inherit this disease."

2. A 35 y/o M sees a neurologist with a chief complaint of increasing muscle weakness. On exam, there is marked weakness of muscles of the wrist extensors, finger flexors, hip abductors, and calves. Which of the following is the most likely diagnosis at this time?
    A. Duchenne muscular dystrophy
    B. Inclusion body myositis
    C. Polymyositis
    D. Dermatomyositis
    E. All of the above are equally likely

3. A 6 y/o M is seen by a pediatrician for an initial evaluation. His family immigrated to the United States recently, and due to prior societal instability he has not been in medical care for several years. His parents note that over the past year he has had difficulty engaging in physical activities at school and in the park. He sometimes trips while running, and after falling he often takes several moments to lift himself up by his hands. He has difficulty climbing the stairs up to his apartment. A picture of his legs is below:

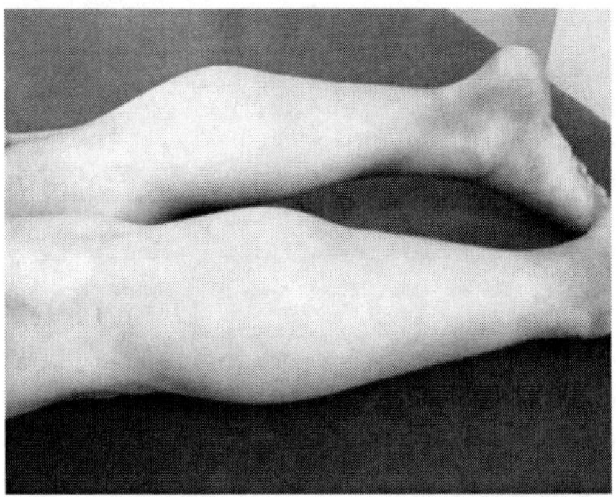

   Which of the following is most likely to be seen on further evaluation?
   A. Clouding of the lenses in the eyes
   B. High levels of muscle breakdown products in the blood
   C. A red itchy rash that is sensitive to sunlight
   D. Invasion of immune cells within muscle fibers
   E. Increased fasting glucose levels due to insulin resistance

4. A 39 y/o F presents to the emergency department reporting difficulty breathing. She has no history of asthma or any other medical condition. On interview, she reports severe "aching" pain in her neck, shoulders, and thighs over the past 2 months along with difficulty rising from a chair or walking, especially for long distances or up a flight of stairs. On exam, motor strength is decreased in her shoulders and hips but intact in her hands and feet. Deep tendon reflexes are intact throughout. A thorough skin exam is unremarkable. Labs are notable for increased creatine kinase levels. Which of the following is the most accurate statement about the patient's condition?
   A. "This condition is generally treatable with medication."
   B. "This condition is generally treatable with surgery."
   C. "There is no treatment for this condition, although physical therapy can help preserve function for longer."
   D. "There is no need for treatment, as this will likely get better on its own."
   E. None of the above are accurate

1. **The best answer is D.** This patient has myotonic dystrophy as evidenced by her motor weakness accompanied by delayed relaxation of muscles following voluntary contraction. Myotonic dystrophy is an autosomal dominant disease, meaning that there is a 50% chance of her child inheriting this condition. While the chance remains 50% for each individual child, her chance of having at least one child with the disorder goes up with every subsequent birth. Despite the high likelihood of passing this disease to her children, it is not completely assured that it will happen (answer E). However, the risk is still high enough that she should not be told that it is a small or unlikely risk (answers A—C).

2. **The best answer is B.** This patient is presenting with weakness involving both proximal and distal muscle groups. Notably, distal weakness is typically seen in only myotonic dystrophy and inclusion body myositis. All of the other conditions listed present primarily with weakness of *proximal* muscles such as the hips and legs in Duchenne muscular dystrophy (answer A), hip extensors in polymyositis (answer C), and thighs and upper arms in dermatomyositis (answer D). Duchenne muscular dystrophy is also unlikely to present for the first time in adulthood.

3. **The best answer is B.** The most likely diagnosis in this case is Duchenne muscular dystrophy given the onset of proximal muscle weakness during childhood, presence of calf hypertrophy, and positive Gower's sign. Duchenne muscular dystrophy is associated with high levels of creatine kinase, a muscle breakdown product, in the blood. Cataracts and insulin resistance are more characteristic of myotonic dystrophy (answers A and E). A red itchy rash is more often seen in dermatomyositis (answer C), while invasion of T cells within muscle fibers is characteristic of polymyositis (answer D).

4. **The best answer is A.** The most likely diagnosis in this case is polymyositis given the patient's age, female sex, and clinical presentation including proximal muscle weakness with preservation of distal motor function. Polymyositis is generally treated with medications, with corticosteroids being the first-line option. It is not appropriate to say that there is no treatment for the condition (answer C) even if physical therapy can be helpful as well. Surgery plays no role in management of polymyositis (answer B). Polymyositis is unlikely to resolve on its own, and with the presence of her breathing difficulties, neglecting to provide treatment is an unwise option (answer D).

17 NEUROMUSCULAR JUNCTION DISEASES

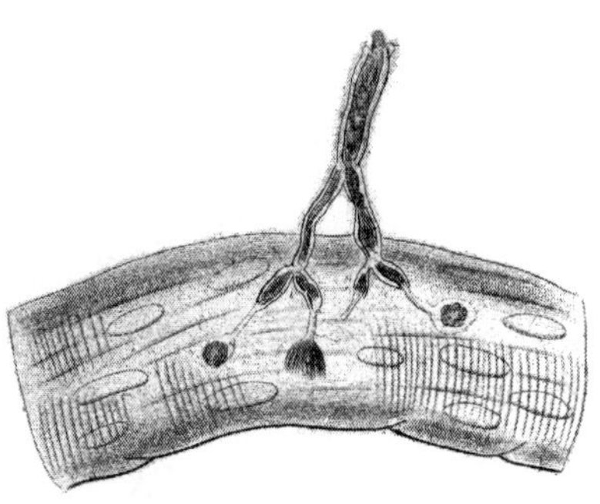

In the last chapter, we covered disorders involving the muscle itself. In this chapter, we will begin to work backwards and talk about diseases involving the connection between the muscle itself and the nerve supplying it: the neuromuscular junction. **Neuromuscular junction diseases** are a group of conditions that are united only by the fact that they all have an adverse effect on the transmission of a signal from the motor nerve to the muscle itself. However, within that loose framework lies an incredibly diverse group of diseases.

Before we begin, let's take a moment to review what we learned in Chapter 2 about what happens at the neuromuscular junction. The primary function of the neuromuscular junction is to take an action potential traveling on the axon of a motor neuron and translate it into a contraction of the muscle itself. When an action potential arrives at the end of an axon, it activates voltage-dependent calcium channels which allow calcium ions to enter the neuron. This influx of calcium activates a group of protein complexes known as **SNARE proteins** which then help synaptic vesicles to fuse with the cell membrane, releasing the **acetylcholine** inside. The released acetylcholine then diffuses across the neuromuscular junction and activates **nicotinic receptors** on the muscle cell. Binding of acetylcholine to the nicotinic receptors depolarizes the muscle cell and begins a cascade of events that results in muscle contraction.

Neuromuscular junction diseases can disrupt this process at various steps along the way, as we will see now! In this chapter, we will focus on four diseases in particular: **myasthenia gravis**, **Lambert-Eaton syndrome**, **botulism**, and **tetanus**.

MYASTHENIA GRAVIS

Myasthenia gravis is an **autoimmune disease** or one in which the immune system creates antibodies against its own body, with the muscles being particularly affected. There are several important associations to make with myasthenia **gravis** which all involve the letter **T**. To make this connection, think of it as **myasthenia gravi-T**:

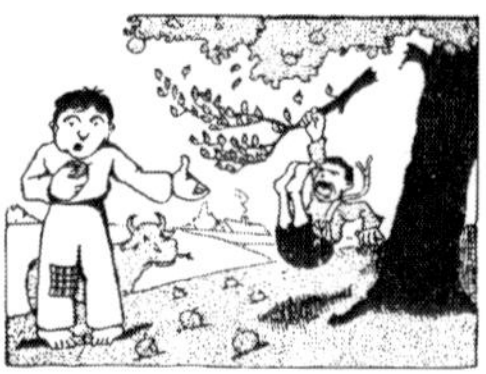

T is for nico-T-inic receptors. The antibodies seen in myasthenia gravis specifically target **nicotinic acetylcholine receptors**, effectively preventing acetylcholine from activating these receptors on the muscle and blocking the transmission of the signal across the neuromuscular junction. (Note that these antibodies are only directed against *nicotinic* acetylcholine receptors! For this reason, parasympathetic effects and other functions that rely on *muscarinic* acetylcholine receptors are spared.)

T is for Top down. Muscle weakness in myasthenia gravis affects multiple areas of the body but tends to **start at the top** and work its way down. Weakness is often first noted in the **eyes** (including both extraocular movements, resulting in double vision, and the eyelids, resulting in **ptosis** as seen in the picture below). The weakness then spreads to nearby parts of the body, including the muscles used for swallowing and speech, before spreading to distal parts of the body (such as the arms and legs) as the disease progresses further.

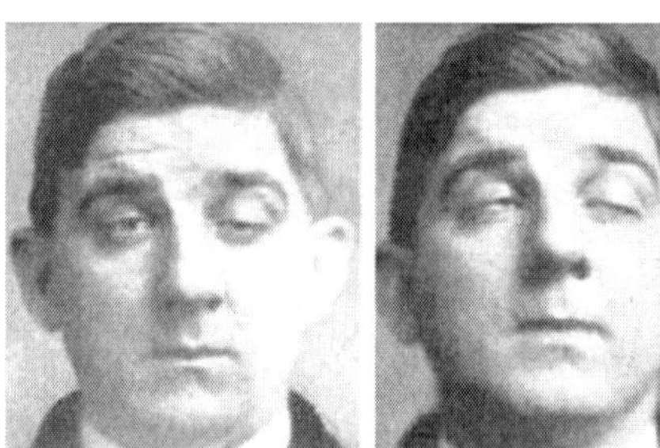

***Ptosis** in a patient with **myasthenia gravis**.*

T is for fa-T-iguing weakness. On a clinical level, you can look at the electrical activity of muscles using a technique known as **electromyography** (or EMG). In patients with myasthenia gravis, the electrical signal coming from the muscle is often strongest at the beginning but then slowly weakens with repeated stimulation of the muscle, a pattern known as "**fatiguing weakness**." This correlates with what is seen clinically, with muscle weakness usually getting worse the longer the activity goes on (with improvement following a period of rest). Fatiguing weakness also accumulates throughout the day such that patients are strongest in the morning but generally get weaker as the day progresses, with the **greatest weakness in the evening**.

T is for Tensilon test. A medication known as **edrophonium** (brand name Tensilon) has been used to differentiate between myasthenia gravis and other conditions that may present similarly. Edrophonium acts as an **inhibitor of acetylcholinesterase**

which is the enzyme that breaks down acetylcholine in the neuromuscular junction. By inhibiting the enzyme that breaks down acetylcholine, edrophonium *increases* the amount of this neurotransmitter that is active and available in the synapse, essentially giving the acetylcholine "army" more troops to fight the antibodies in the battle for nicotinic receptors. If someone's fatiguing weakness improves with edrophonium, a diagnosis of myasthenia gravis is more likely. This is known as a "Tensilon test."

T is for Thymoma. If antibodies against the nicotinic acetylcholine receptor are the problem here, where exactly did these errant antibodies come from in the first place? While the exact pathophysiology is not yet known, there does appear to be an association with abnormalities in the **thymus**, an organ in the immune system that "teaches" white blood cells how to recognize invading pathogens. In fact, over 10% of people with the condition will have a **thymoma** or a tumor of the thymus.

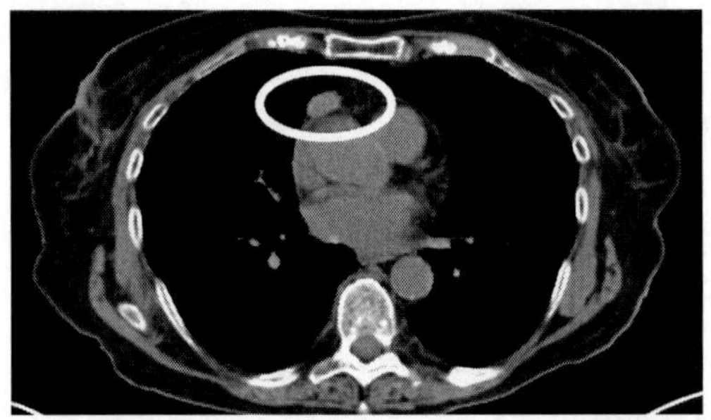

*A CT scan showing a **thymoma** (circled) in a patient with **myasthenia gravis**.*

T is for Treatable. Myasthenia gravis is a treatable condition. **Acetylcholinesterase inhibitors** are the mainstay of treatment (though make sure to use one that is longer lasting than edrophonium!). Screening for thymomas should be done, with surgical removal of the thymus performed if cancer is found. In cases where myasthenia gravis is severe enough that the muscles of respiration are involved (known as a **myasthenic crisis**), hospitalization with ventilator support may be necessary, with rapid removal of the offending antibodies from the bloodstream via **plasmapheresis** (in which the patient's blood is removed, filtered, and returned) or **intravenous immunoglobulins** (a mixture of antibodies donated by healthy people, often abbreviated IVIG).

Myasthenia gravis is an **autoimmune disease** in which the body produces antibodies against **nicotinic acetylcholine receptors**, resulting in a pattern of **fatiguing weakness**. It is associated with a **tumor in the thymus**.

*Myasthenia gravi-**T**:*
*Nico-**T**-inic receptors*
***T**op down*
*Fa-**T**-iguing weakness*
***T**ensilon test*
***T**hymoma*
***T**reatable*

LAMBERT-EATON SYNDROME

Like myasthenia gravis, **Lambert-Eaton syndrome** is an **autoimmune disease** in which antibodies attack the neuromuscular junction and prevent the transmission of motor signals. *Unlike* myasthenia gravis (in which the antibodies are attacking nicotinic acetylcholine receptors on the *post*-synaptic membrane), in Lambert-Eaton syndrome the auto-antibodies are directed against **voltage-gated calcium channels** on the *pre*-synaptic membrane, thus preventing the *release* of acetylcholine rather than its binding. (Recall from Chapter 2 that **call**-cium acts as the battle **call** to send neurotransmitters like acetylcholine marching out into the synapse.) Because Lambert-Eaton syndrome interferes with the release of acetylcholine throughout the entire body, **both nicotinic and muscarinic** receptors will be affected, resulting in not just **muscle weakness** but also **autonomic dysfunction** including constipation, dry mouth, and unstable blood pressure. Notably, the muscle weakness often begins in the legs (in comparison to the face in myasthenia gravis).

EMG findings in Lambert-Eaton syndrome are characterized by an **incremental response** in which repeated stimulation of the nerve causes a stronger contraction of the muscle, as more acetylcholine will be released. (Compare this to the fa-T-iguing pattern seen in myasthenia gravis in which repeated stimulation of the nerve will cause *less*, not more, muscle activity.) Like myasthenia gravis and thymoma, there is an association between Lambert-Eaton syndrome and cancer, in this case a type of lung cancer known as **small-cell lung cancer**.

Because Lambert-Eaton syndrome is caused by an overactive immune system, you can use **immunosuppressant** medications such as steroids or IVIG to help with symptomatic improvement. Notably, giving an acetylcholinesterase inhibitor (as in the edrophonium test) will *not* improve muscle weakness in Lambert-Eaton syndrome, as the problem isn't that there isn't enough acetylcholine to compete with antibodies on the post-synaptic membrane, it's that acetylcholine isn't even being released into the synapse in the first place!

You can remember the important associations here by renaming this as "Legbert eatin' syndrome." What is Legbert eatin'? Those small, dry pretzels (the kind they have at bars, not the large fresh kind they have at baseball games). "**Leg**bert **eatin' small, dry pre**tzels" will help you remember to associate paralysis in the **legs**, the connection with **small**-cell lung cancer, the presence of anticholinergic effects like **dry** mouth (which aren't present in myasthenia gravis), and the attack on **pre**-synaptic receptors (compared to post-synaptic receptors in myasthenia gravis).

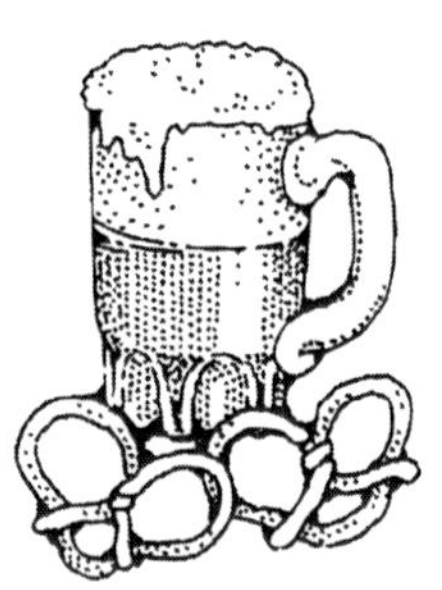

Lambert-Eaton syndrome is an **autoimmune disease** in which antibodies against **pre-synaptic voltage-gated calcium channels** cause **muscle weakness** and **anticholinergic signs and symptoms**. It is associated with **small-cell lung cancer**.

*What's **Leg**bert eatin'? Those **small, dry pre**tzels (**leg** paralysis, **small**-cell lung cancer, **dry** mouth and other anticholinergic symptoms, and **pre**-synaptic antibodies).*

BOTULISM

Botulism is a disease in which exposure to the **botulinum toxin** produced by the bacterium *Clostridium botulinum* leads to muscle weakness. Similar to Lambert-Eaton syndrome, the botulinum toxin interferes with the release of acetylcholine, although this time the mechanism is through interfering with the process of exocytosis by **damaging SNARE proteins**, thus preventing the vesicles from releasing their acetylcholine into the neuromuscular junction. This results in a blockade of **both nicotinic and muscarinic** receptors just like in Lambert-Eaton syndrome, leading to not only **muscle weakness** but also **anticholinergic** signs and symptoms like constipation. Botulism also features the same **incremental response** as seen in Lambert-Eaton syndrome, which makes sense as they are both *pre*-synaptic problems.

With so many areas of overlap with Lambert-Eaton syndrome, let's focus on the specific features that help to differentiate botulism from it and other neuromuscular junction diseases. Use the mnemonic **ROBOT** (as in "robot-ulism") to remember:

R is for Rapid onset. In contrast to both myasthenia gravis and Lambert-Eaton syndrome, botulism generally has an **rapid onset** rather than the insidious pattern seen with autoimmune diseases.

O is for Oxygen (absent). Because *C. botulinum* is an anaerobic organism that thrives in the absence of oxygen, **improperly canned foods** are a perfect medium for their growth.

B is for Babies. Botulism can develop in **infants given honey**, as *C. botulinum* toxins are commonly found in this food product. While older children and adults can eat honey without a problem, infants haven't yet developed the protective mechanisms against these spores, leading them to be at risk of widespread muscle paralysis if they ingest honey.

O is for Open wounds. *C. botulinum* also loves to grow in **open wounds** like the kinds that are created with recurrent injection of **intravenous drugs** like heroin.

T is for Top down. Like myasthenia gravis, the muscle weakness seen in botulism goes in a "top down" fashion beginning in the head with the cranial nerves and then descending down to the rest of the body.

Botulism presents as a **rapid onset** of **descending flaccid paralysis** in **babies** given honey or adults who eat **improperly canned foods** or have **open wounds**.

ROBOT*-ulism:*
R*apid onset*
O*xygen (absent)*
B*abies*
O*pen wounds*
T*op down*

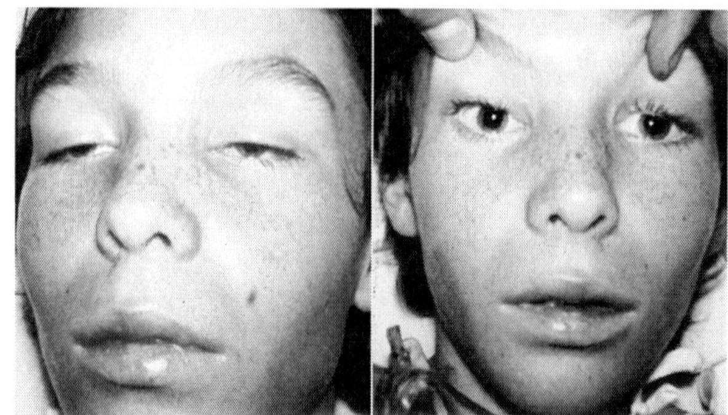

***Bilateral facial paralysis** and **fixed dilated pupils** in a patient with **botulism**.*

Because botulism is caused by a toxin, treatment should involve administration of an **antitoxin**. However, even with treatment, it can take time for the paralysis to reverse, so supportive care including respiratory support is often required during this time. Even with treatment, botulism can be fatal, with a 5 to 10% mortality rate. For this reason, the most important goal is to prevent botulism in the first place such as through proper canning of food or by avoiding giving honey to babies.

Finally, it's worth pointing out that botulinum isn't all bad news! The fact that this toxin causes muscle weakness and paralysis is actually used to positive effect in treating spasticity and other kinds of muscle overactivity. In addition, it can be used cosmetically as Botox to reduce facial wrinkles. So botulinum isn't necessarily your enemy as long as it's used in the right place, at the right time, and in the right amount!

TETANUS

Like botulism, **tetanus** occurs when a spore-forming bacterium produces a toxin that interferes with signal transmission across the neuromuscular junction. In this case, the bacterium is *Clostridium tetani*, and the toxin it produces is known as **tetanospasmin**. Unlike all of the diseases we have discussed so far, tetanus does not result in muscle *weakness*. Instead, the opposite happens: muscles begin contracting *too much*, often becoming so tight that they begin to **spasm** throughout the body. This tends to start at the top of the body (with **lockjaw** often being one of the earliest manifestations) and slowly spread downward. In this way, tetanus does the *opposite* of botulism and turns all the muscles in the body "**on**."

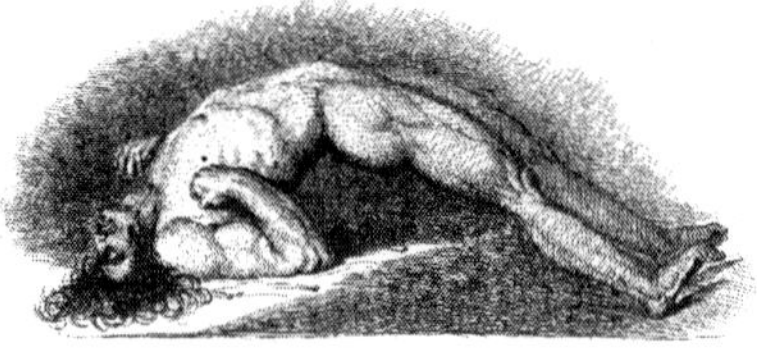

Like botulinum toxin, tetanospasmin interferes with the function of SNARE proteins and prevents vesicles from releasing their contents. While botulism prevents vesicles filled with *acetylcholine* from being released, tetanus interferes with vesicles containing two other neurotransmitters: **glycine** and **GABA**. Both glycine and GABA are **inhibitory** neurotransmitters that make neurons less likely to "fire." By *inhibiting* the release of *inhibitory* neurotransmitters, tetanus leads to the **widespread activation of muscles** that is characteristic of this disease.

While *C. tetani* is commonly found in soil, it can produce problems when it enters the body. The classic clinical scenario for tetanus is when someone steps on a rusty nail while working out in the yard, as breaking the skin allows this normally benign bacterium to bypass the body's defenses and wreak havoc in the wound. However, tetanus can be contracted in other ways as well, including during childbirth.

Treatment generally involves infusing an **antibody** against the tetanus toxin to remove it from the body. Supportive measures, such as giving benzodiazepines and muscle relaxants, can be used as well. Antibiotics are sometimes used to treat the *C. tetani* infection, although the evidence that this helps is not clear. Ultimately, the most effective treatment is prevention by **vaccination**.

To remember that both **B**otulism and **T**etanus block the release of neurotransmitters from vesicles in the neuromuscular junction by interfering with **SNARE** proteins, think of a **snare drum** on which someone is playing a **B**ea**T**, with tetanus on the **on beat** (since it turns all muscles "on") and botulism on the **off beat** (since it turns all muscles "off").

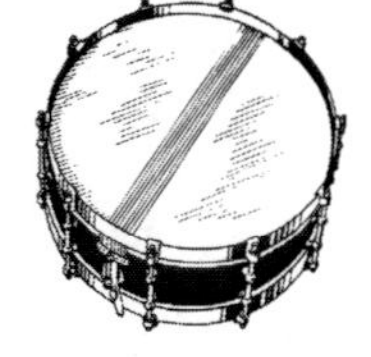

Both **botulism** and **tetanus** block **neurotransmitter release** by interfering with **SNARE proteins**. Botulism blocks the release of **acetylcholine**, leading to **weakness**. Tetanus blocks the release of **glycine** and **GABA**, leading to **spasms**.

*Play a **BeaT** (**B**otulism and **T**etanus) on a **SNARE** drum,*
*with **tetanus** on the **on beat** and **botulism** on the **off beat**.*

PUTTING IT ALL TOGETHER

While the four diseases in this chapter all disrupt signaling at the neuromuscular junction, they each do so in different ways that allow us to understand the process better. **Myasthenia gravis** results in the release of auto-antibodies that compete with acetylcholine for receptors on the muscle, **Lambert-Eaton syndrome** interferes with neurotransmitter release from the pre-synaptic neuron by blocking voltage-gated calcium channels, and **botulism** prevents exocytosis of acetylcholine from the pre-synaptic neuron, all of which lead to muscle weakness. In contrast, **tetanus** blocks the release of inhibitory neurotransmitters, leading to muscle spasms and sustained contractions. If you truly understand the mechanisms at play here, most of the other information will logically follow! Use the table below to make some key distinctions.

Disease	Target	Progression	Associations
Myasthenia gravis	Nicotinic receptors	Top down	Fatiguing weakness, thymoma
Lambert-Eaton	Calcium channels	Bottom up	Incremental response, small-cell lung ca.
Botulism	SNARE (↓ ACh)	Top down	Babies, open wounds, poorly canned foods
Tetanus	SNARE (↓ glycine, GABA)	Top down	Soil, rusty nails, childbirth

REVIEW QUESTIONS

1. A 66 y/o M sees his primary care doctor complaining of progressive weakness of his arms and legs. He first noticed weakness in his legs a few months ago, with arm weakness following around one month later. His legs are now weak to the point where he needs to walk with a cane. He denies any daily pattern to his muscle weakness, saying, "It's basically always there." Review of systems is positive for dry mouth and constipation, with his last bowel movement occurring three days ago. Exam is notable for decreased motor strength in proximal muscles and absent deep tendon reflexes in all extremities. Which of the following tests is most likely to reveal an abnormality?
   A. Radiographic imaging of the chest
   B. Edrophonium test
   C. Needle biopsy of the thymus
   D. Urine drug screen
   E. Physical exam for puncture wounds

2. A 55 y/o F schedules an intake appointment with a dermatologist after she is encouraged to go by a friend who says that this dermatologist made her look "decades younger." After a brief consultation, the dermatologist proceeds to inject a neurotoxin into various sites in her forehead, cheeks, and around her eyes as seen below:

   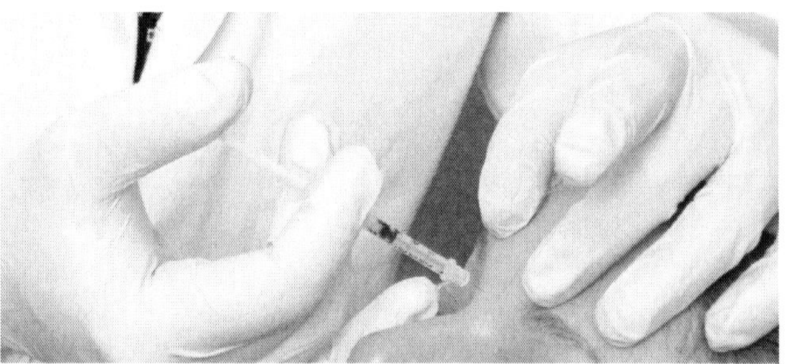

   Within several hours, she notices fewer wrinkles on her face. Which of the following mechanisms explains the effect of this neurotoxin?
   A. Demyelination of the pre-synaptic neuron
   B. Interference with acetylcholine binding with nicotinic receptors
   C. Inhibition of voltage-gated calcium channels
   D. Prevention of synaptic vesicle binding to the cell membrane
   E. Impedance of inhibitory neuron exocytosis

3. A 45 y/o F sees a neurologist saying, "It feels like my body is falling apart." She reports that around one year ago she began having episodes of double vision. She notices this the most when using her phone in bed at night, saying, "The letters on the screen get blurry and then separate." Around six months ago, she noticed that it felt like food was "getting stuck in my throat." She has had particular difficulty with hard foods such as apples and carrots, as she feels she "cannot chew them enough." These problems are particularly noticeable when eating dinner, as she says that breakfast usually doesn't cause her the same problems. She has lost 15 pounds over the past 3 months. During the interview, the neurologist notices that her speech is soft and difficult to understand at times. Vital signs are HR 88, BP 122/80, RR 16, and T 98.9°F. On exam, she is alert and oriented. There is drooping of her eyelid on the right as seen below:

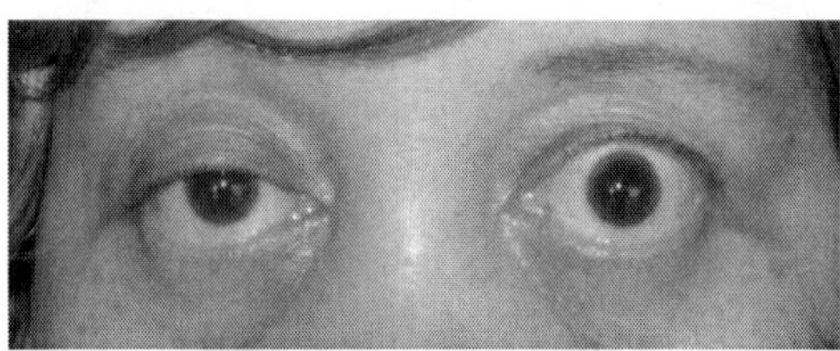

Her right eye shows weakness of lateral gaze. Her motor strength is decreased in both proximal and distal muscle groups in all four extremities, with greater levels of weakness the longer that the testing continues. The neurologist prescribes her an acetylcholinesterase inhibitor and sends her to radiology for a CT scan of the chest which shows no abnormalities. On a follow-up appointment several weeks later, he examines her eyes again and sees the following:

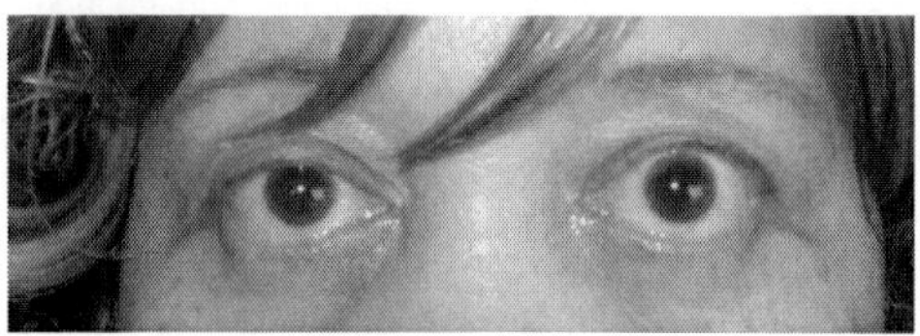

Which of the following is the best next step?

A. Stopping the acetylcholinesterase inhibitor as it is used for diagnostic purposes only
B. Continuing the acetylcholinesterase inhibitor
C. Surgical removal of the thymus
D. Mechanical filtration of the blood
E. Administration of donated antibodies

1. **The best answer is A.** The presence of muscle weakness with a gradual onset and anticholinergic signs and symptoms such as dry mouth and constipation is highly concerning for Lambert-Eaton syndrome. Lambert-Eaton syndrome is frequently related to the presence of a small-cell lung cancer, so ordering chest imaging is a high priority. Botulism can present similarly to Lambert-Eaton syndrome but tends to involve a much more rapid onset; it can be associated with use of certain intravenous drugs which would be picked up on a urine drug screen (answer D). An edrophonium test does not improve muscle weakness in Lambert-Eaton syndrome and is more specific for myasthenia gravis (answer B) which is associated with a thymoma (answer C). Myasthenia gravis is unlikely in this patient as his presentation lacks a fatiguing pattern but does include anticholinergic symptoms, which are absent in myasthenia gravis. Puncture wounds are more likely to be seen in cases of tetanus, though this would present with widespread muscle spasms, not weakness (answer E).

2. **The best answer is D.** Botulinum toxin can be dangerous under certain conditions, but when injected locally it can have beneficial effects by reducing muscle contraction. For this reason, it can be used cosmetically to reduce facial wrinkling. The mechanism by which botulinum toxin prevents muscle contraction is by interfering with SNARE proteins in the pre-synaptic neuron, preventing vesicular exocytosis and the release of acetylcholine into the synaptic cleft. Tetanospasmin also interferes with SNARE proteins, but it instead prevents the release of inhibitory neurotransmitters, thereby increasing muscle excitation (answer E). Interference with acetylcholine binding to nicotinic receptors describes myasthenia gravis (answer B), while inhibition of voltage-gated calcium channels describes Lambert-Eaton syndrome (answer C). Botulinum toxin does not affect the myelin sheath (answer A).

3. **The best answer is B.** Acetylcholinesterase inhibitors are the mainstay of treatment for myasthenia gravis and often help people achieve better functioning than they would without medications. While acetylcholinesterase inhibitors can be helpful diagnostically, they are used for long-term treatment as well (answer A). Surgical removal of the thymus should be pursued if there is evidence of a thymoma, but in this case the chest CT did not show evidence of cancer (answer C). Plasmapheresis (answer D) and intravenous immunoglobulins (answer E) are expensive and logistically complicated, so they are generally only used in cases of myasthenic crisis requiring admission to the hospital.

18 MOTOR NEURON DISEASES

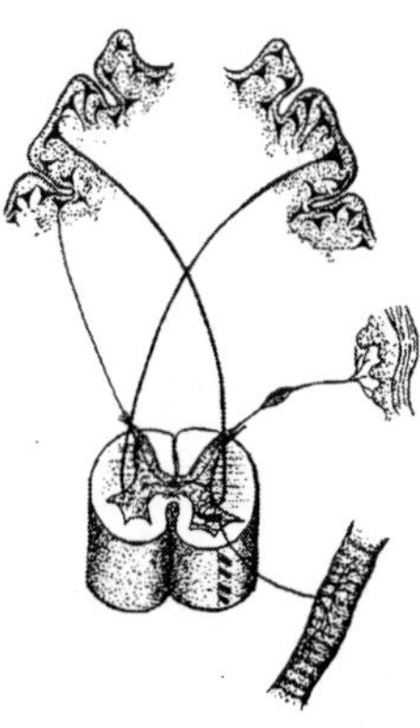

Let's continue our study of neuromuscular diseases by continuing to move up the neuronal "chain to the brain." We started with the muscle itself and then touched on the neuromuscular junction, and we will now go to diseases involving the **motor neurons** that connect muscles to the brain. Motor neurons can be damaged by a large variety of pathological processes, including various forms of peripheral neuropathy (which we will discuss further in Chapter 24). For the purposes of clarity, in this chapter we will limit our discussion to specifically those diseases that *only* affect motor neurons (while leaving other peripheral nerves, such as those responsible for transmitting sensory information, intact).

When learning about motor neuron diseases, it is crucial to understand the distinction between **upper and lower motor neurons**. Recall that there are **three neurons** between brain and muscle: the neuron connecting the brain to the anterior horn of the spinal cord, the interneuron in the anterior horn, and the peripheral nerve connecting the anterior horn with the muscle itself. In this way, the anterior horn acts as a "line in the sand" separating upper and lower motor neurons, as seen in the image on the next page. Lesions in the *first* neuron create **upper motor neuron signs**, while lesions in the *third* neuron instead create **lower motor neuron signs**. (It's worth pointing out that upper and lower motor neuron signs can occur simultaneously in the same person at the same time! For example, someone who sustains damage to their cervical spinal cord could develop a *lower* motor neuron syndrome in their *upper* limbs while showing signs of *upper* motor neuron syndrome in their *lower* limbs.)

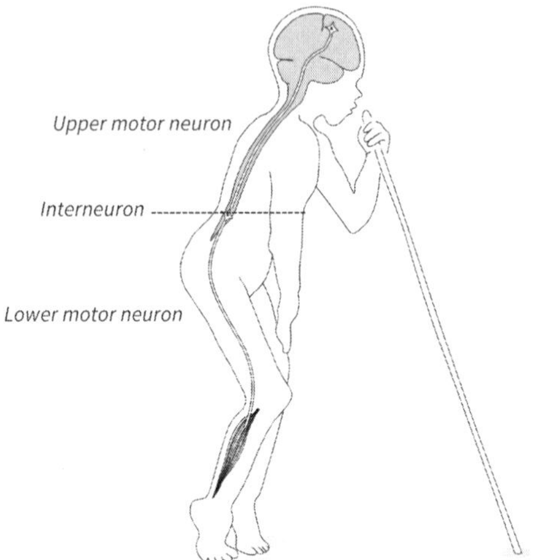

*The **anterior horn** marks the separation between **upper and lower motor neurons**.*

Each type of neuron produces a completely different set of signs when it is injured. In cases of *lower* motor neuron damage, the lack of innervation causes the muscle to wither and wilt like a flower without water, creating a state of **flaccid paralysis**. This causes the muscle to *lower* its output, producing weak reflexes, poor muscle tone, diminished power, decreased bulk, and a downgoing Babinski response. When using electromyography, you will see many small uncoordinated motor signals known as **fibrillations. Fasciculations**, or sudden twitches, are also seen as well.

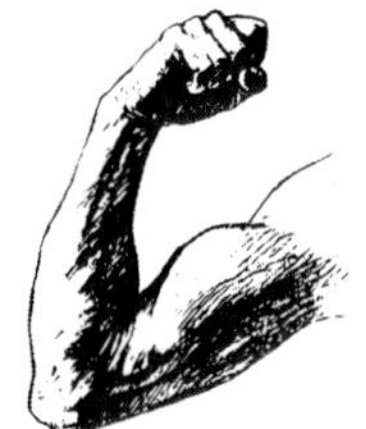

In contrast to lower motor neuron damage, *upper* motor neuron damage generally makes everything go *up*: muscle tone is increased, reflexes become spastic, and the Babinski is upgoing. This occurs because upper motor neurons are responsible not just for *initiating* movements but also for *inhibiting* them. When this inhibition is lost, the lower motor neurons become too strong. Unfortunately, upper motor neuron damage doesn't make you buffer! It only leads to a tightly-wound muscle that is ready to fly off the handle at any moment. Upper motor neuron damage also produces an inability to engage in **fine movements** requiring a high degree of dexterity (like playing the piano). This pattern of **spastic weakness** helps to distinguish upper motor neuron damage from the flaccid paralysis seen in lower motor neuron damage.

Lower motor neuron injuries lead to a state of **flaccid paralysis**,
while **upper motor neuron injuries** lead to a state of **spastic weakness**.

Lower *motor neuron damage* ***lowers*** *muscle output,*
while ***upper*** *motor neuron damage* ***ups*** *muscle output.*

With these basic principles in mind, let's talk about some of the most high-yield motor neuron diseases to know!

MOTOR NEURON DISEASES

The most common motor neuron disease is **amyotrophic lateral sclerosis**. (In fact, the term "motor neuron disease" is sometimes used synonymously with amyotrophic lateral sclerosis despite the fact that there are other diseases that also fall under this banner!) We will spend most of our time talking about this disease, followed by a brief discussion of a few other motor neuron diseases.

AMYOTROPHIC LATERAL SCLEROSIS

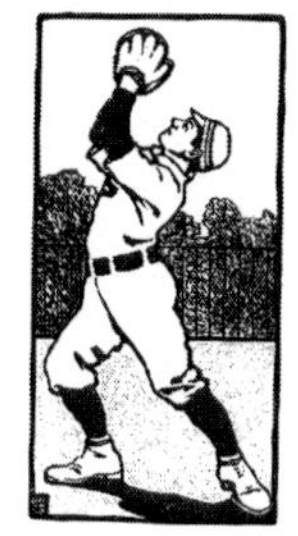

Amyotrophic lateral sclerosis (also called ALS or "Lou Gehrig's disease" after the baseball player who was diagnosed with this disease in the 1930s) is a condition in which degeneration of motor neurons leads to **progressive muscle weakness and atrophy**. Notably, amyotrophic lateral sclerosis affects **both upper and lower motor neurons** (in contrast to most other motor neuron diseases which tend to affect only one or the other). You can remember this by thinking that **A**myotrophic **L**atera**L** sclerosis wreaks havoc **ALL** over the place (both upper and lower motor neurons).

Signs and symptoms of amyotrophic lateral sclerosis generally begin in **middle age** between 40 and 60 years old. Muscle weakness and atrophy are usually **bilateral** (which helps to distinguish it from dysfunction in any one peripheral nerve). Unlike some of the other motor neuron diseases we will talk about later in this chapter, amyotrophic lateral sclerosis doesn't show a pattern of beginning in one part of the body or another. Instead, **any muscles** can be affected, including the arms and legs. (This is consistent with the idea that **A**myotrophic **L**atera**L** sclerosis wreaks havoc **ALL** over the place!) In some cases, the muscles of the mouth and throat are affected due to death of neurons in the medulla; these cases are said to have **bulbar** involvement. Notably, certain muscles (including those responsible for bowel function, bladder contraction, and eye movement) are often preserved until late in the disease.

Amyotrophic lateral sclerosis is a **progressive neurodegenerative disease** that affects **both upper and lower motor neurons** in muscles **throughout the body**.

__A__myotrophic __L__atera__L__ sclerosis wreaks havoc __ALL__ over the place.

Because amyotrophic lateral sclerosis involves all motor neurons, signs of *both* upper motor neuron damage (including spasticity, hyperreflexia, and re-emergence of primitive reflexes) *and* lower motor neuron damage (such as atrophy, poor muscle tone, hyporeflexia, and fibrillations) are present. **Fasciculations** are almost always seen when using electromyography. Weakness is often subtle at first but becomes more pronounced as the disease progresses. In later stages, the diaphragm begins to fail, and most people with amyotrophic lateral sclerosis will die from respiratory complications within 5 years of the initial diagnosis. While it was long thought that dementia was rare in this condition, some people with amyotrophic lateral sclerosis will exhibit **cognitive impairment**.

Most cases of amyotrophic lateral sclerosis are **sporadic** (occurring "out of the blue" with no known genetic or environmental triggers). However, inherited forms of the disease do exist. These tend to involve defects in the **superoxide dismutase 1** (SOD1) gene. You can remember this association by thinking of a baseball player (like Lou Gehrig) playing out on the **SOD** (or grass).

Most cases of **amyotrophic lateral sclerosis** are **sporadic**. Inherited versions of the disease tend to involve the **superoxide dismutase 1** (SOD1) gene.

Think of ***Lou Gehrig****, a baseball player who developed ALS, out on the* ***SOD*** *(grass).*

There is **no cure** for amyotrophic lateral sclerosis, and available treatments are often quite limited. Use of **physical, speech, and occupational therapy** can help to promote function and independence. When the diaphragm becomes affected, ventilator support is often required. Two medications have also been shown to help in amyotrophic lateral sclerosis. The first, **riluzole**, works by decreasing release of the neurotransmitter glutamate and can prolong life by around 2 or 3 months. The second, **edaravone**, can slow the rate of functional loss, though it is very expensive and requires daily intravenous infusions. Overall, amyotrophic lateral sclerosis is a tragic and deadly disease, although research efforts are ongoing to identify better treatments or even a cure.

PRIMARY LATERAL SCLEROSIS

The next two conditions we will talk about are similar to amyotrophic lateral sclerosis in many ways, and some have even argued that they should be seen as *variants* of amyotrophic lateral sclerosis rather than separate diseases. For the sake of clarity, we will treat them as separate conditions even though there is a significant degree of overlap between them and amyotrophic lateral sclerosis.

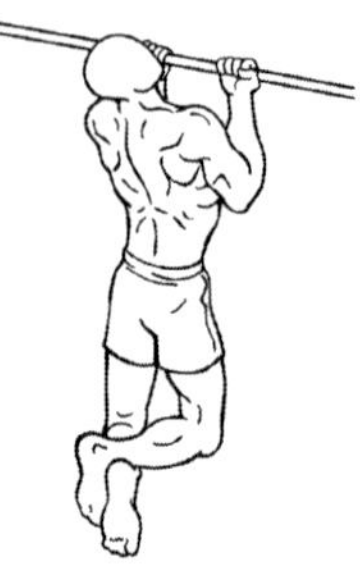

Primary lateral sclerosis is a progressive disease that exclusively damages **upper motor neurons**, resulting in muscle spasticity, hyperreflexia, and primitive reflexes. Notably, lower motor neuron signs will be *absent*! Signs of weakness tend to first be seen in the lower half of the body, with the disease affecting the legs before **moving up** into the trunk, the arms, and eventually the face. Compared to amyotrophic lateral sclerosis, primary lateral sclerosis has a **slower progression**, and many people with the condition have a **normal life span**. You can remember the key features of **P**rimary **L**atera**L** sclerosis by thinking of someone doing a **PuLL-up**, with the **up** reminding you of the presence of **upper** motor neuron signs and the fact that it often begins in the legs and moves **up**.

Primary lateral sclerosis is similar to amyotrophic lateral sclerosis except that it only involves **upper motor neurons** and has a **better prognosis**.

__P__rimary __L__atera__L__ sclerosis = ***PuLL-up*** *(__up__per motor neurons, moves __up__ the body).*

PROGRESSIVE MUSCULAR ATROPHY

Progressive muscular atrophy is the yin to primary lateral sclerosis's yang. Both are very similar to amyotrophic lateral sclerosis, but with **progressive muscular atrophy** only **lower motor neurons** are involved, leading to widespread flaccid paralysis across the entire body. Notably, upper motor neuron signs are conspicuously *absent* compared to the other two conditions! Progressive muscular atrophy is associated with a **better prognosis** than "textbook" amyotrophic lateral sclerosis.

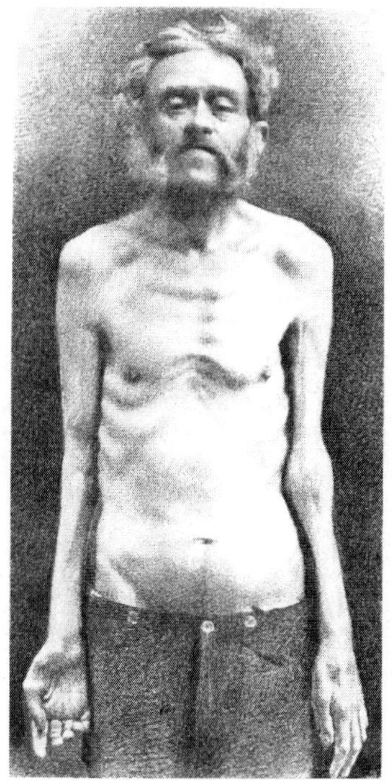

Diffuse loss of muscle bulk related to ***progressive muscular atrophy****.*

Just like we've turned **P**rimary **L**atera**L** sclerosis into "**P**u**LL**-**up**" to remember its association with **up**per motor neurons, let's turn **PR**ogr**ESS**ive muscular atrophy into "**PRESS-down**" to link it to **lower** motor neurons. Pull-up and press-down form a nice pair that will help you to link these in your mind!

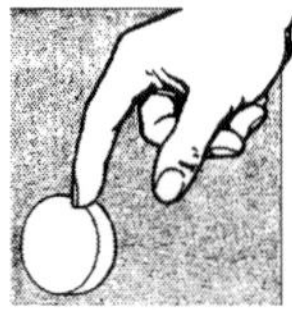

Progressive muscular atrophy is similar to amyotrophic lateral sclerosis except that it only involves **lower motor neurons** and has a **better prognosis**.

PR*ogr****ESS****ive muscular atrophy =* ***PRESS-down*** *(****lower*** *motor neuron).*

BULBAR PALSY AND PSEUDOBULBAR PALSY

If you remember that the term "bulbar" generally refers to the brainstem when used in neurology, it makes sense that **bulbar palsy** is a **lower motor neuron disease** that primarily affects the **brainstem** (the medulla in particular). Muscles responsible for speaking, chewing, and swallowing are often affected (recall that the nucleus ambig-"uh uh's" is located in the medulla!). Neurological exam will reveal tongue atrophy, fasciculations, and an absent gag reflex consistent with lower motor neuron damage.

Another condition known as **pseudobulbar palsy** is similar to bulbar palsy in some ways, as both involve dysarthria and dysphagia. However, pseudobulbar palsy is specifically an **upper motor neuron disease** and tends to present with specific signs (including spasticity of the tongue as well as exaggerated gag and jaw jerk reflexes) that aren't found in bulbar palsy. Pseudobulbar palsy also tends to produce a state known as **pseudobulbar affect** in which the "shuffle" button has been pressed on someone's emotions, leading to rapid switching between laughing, crying, and other emotional extremes that do not correlate with how the person is actually feeling (which is why pseudobulbar affect is sometimes referred to as "emotional incontinence"). You can remember these two distinctions by thinking that the **EU** of ps**EU**dobulbar adds the **E**motional incontinence and the **U**pper motor neuron involvement.

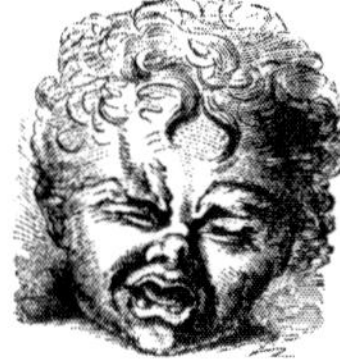

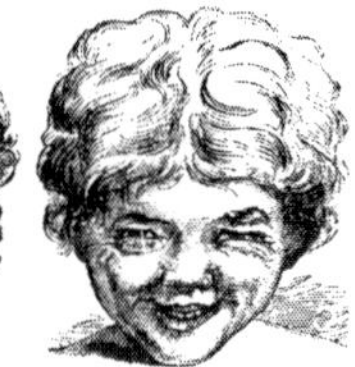

Both bulbar and pseudobulbar palsy can occur on their own, although they tend to occur more often as a result of a stroke in the brainstem or as a manifestation of another neurodegenerative disease. Most people with the condition are older (in their 70s or 80s), with men being affected more than women. Treatment primarily involves **speech therapy**, with medications to target individual symptoms (such as muscle relaxants to lower spasticity or anticholinergic drugs to reduce drooling).

Bulbar palsy involves damage to **lower motor neurons** in the **lower half of the brainstem**, leading to **dysarthria** and **dysphagia**. **Pseudobulbar palsy** affects **upper motor neurons** in the same area and can lead to **emotional incontinence**.

*The **EU** of ps**EU**dobulbar adds **E**motional incontinence and **U**pper motor neurons.*

POST-POLIO SYNDROME

Polio is a virus that targets the neurons in the **anterior horn** of the spinal cord, leading to **lower motor neuron** damage. While the availability of a polio vaccine has led to drastic reductions in the prevalence of this infection, someone who was infected with polio as a child may develop **post-polio syndrome** later in life (even decades after the initial illness!). Post-polio syndrome is like "polio's revenge," as the motor neurons in the anterior horn are attacked a second time, leading to widespread muscle weakness. You can remember the association of polio with motor weakness by thinking that someone with **pole**-io can't **pole** vault.

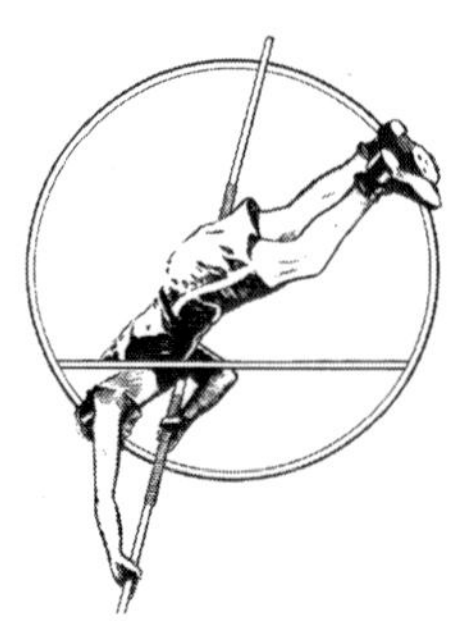

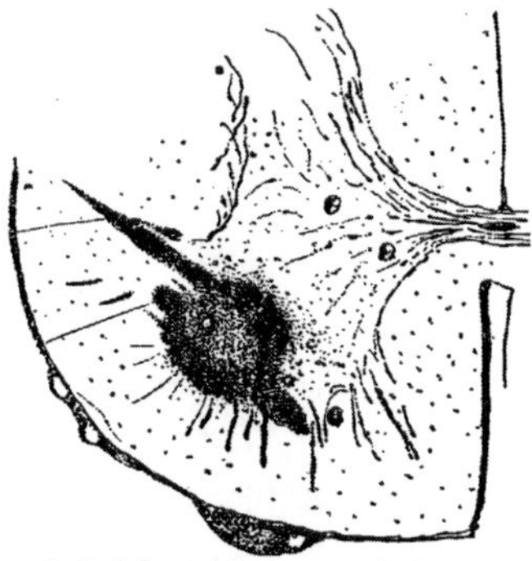

***Polio infection** in the **anterior horn**.*

Polio is a **viral infection** that targets the **anterior horn** of the spinal cord, leading to muscle weakness. **Post-polio syndrome** may develop later in life.

*Someone with **pole**-io can't **pole** vault.*

SPINAL MUSCULAR ATROPHY

Spinal muscular atrophy is a motor neuron disease affecting **lower motor neurons** exclusively (so upper motor neuron signs should be absent). There is a wide range of severity in this disease, although all but the most mild forms of the disorder will begin in **infancy and childhood**. This is because spinal muscular atrophy is an **autosomal recessive genetic disorder** in *all* cases (rather than only in some as with amyotrophic lateral sclerosis). You can remember these two key facts by adding two L's to the end of **S**pinal **M**uscular **A**trophy to form the word **SMALL**, with the L's standing for **L**ower motor neurons and **L**ittle ones (infants and children).

Spinal muscular atrophy is an **autosomal recessive** genetic disorder in which **lower motor neuron damage** leads to muscle weakness and wasting.

***SMALL**: **S**pinal **M**uscular **A**trophy affects **L**ower motor neurons in **L**ittle ones.*

The most severe form of the disorder, known as **Werdnig-Hoffmann disease** or "floppy baby syndrome," is the one you are most likely to be tested on. This presents in the first few months of life as a **sudden onset of complete paralysis** with areflexia and poor muscle tone (the "floppiness" mentioned earlier). It is rapidly progressive, and many infants die within the first year even with adequate treatment. You can remember the association between Werdnig-H**offmann** disease and floppy baby syndrome by thinking of one person asking another, "Hey, doesn't that baby look a little floppy to you?" and the other person responding, "Yeah, that baby looks **off, man**."

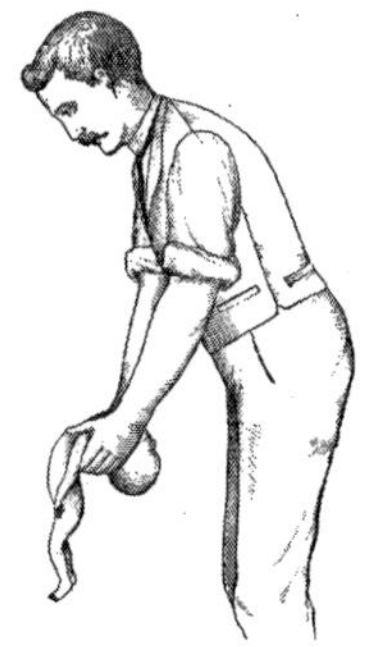

The **most severe form of spinal muscular atrophy** is known as **Werdnig-Hoffmann disease** and is **fatal in most cases.**

*Werdnig-H**offmann** disease:*
*"Doesn't that baby look a little **floppy** to you?" "Yeah, that baby looks **off, man.**"*

An initial diagnosis of spinal muscular atrophy is based on the characteristic history of muscular weakness in an infant. However, genetic testing is required for a definitive diagnosis. The specific gene involved is **SMN1** which codes for the **SMN** (or **S**urvival of **M**otor **N**euron) protein. When there is a defect in this gene, motor neurons become damaged and eventually die, leading directly to the loss of lower motor neurons that defines this condition. Interestingly, there is another gene (known as SMN2) which codes for the exact same protein, functionally acting as a "back-up" copy. People differ in the number of SMN2 gene copies that they have. People who develop a severe form of the condition as infants (Werdnig-Hoffmann disease) tend to have only 1 or 2 copies of the SMN2 gene, while those who don't develop the disease until adulthood often have 4 or more of these back-up copies. These additional copies of the SMN2 gene help to delay the onset of the disease and give it a better prognosis.

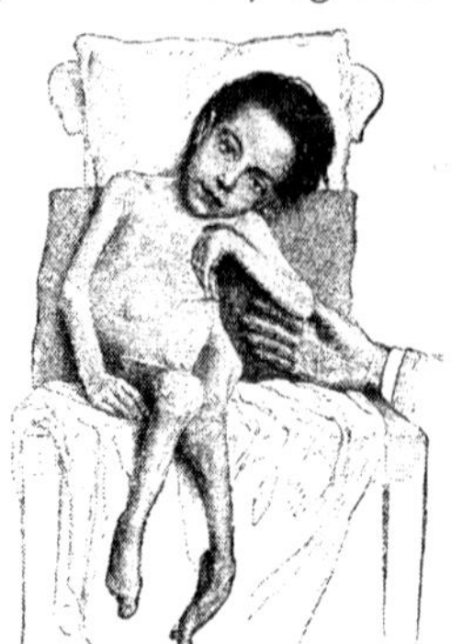

As with other forms of motor neuron disease, there is **no cure**. Treatment is primarily focused on improving quality of life through various forms of therapy, including **physical, occupational, speech, and nutritional therapy**. Assistive devices such as orthotics can be helpful as well. Pharmacologically, a medication known as **nusinersen** has been shown to halt progression of the disease when injected directly into the cerebrospinal fluid. Nusinersen acts by modifying the SMN2 gene in such a way that it is functionally converted into the SMN1 gene, effectively increasing the level of SMN protein in the central nervous system. While it has been shown to be effective, this medication is not without risk, including some pretty severe side effects. For this reason, a full exploration of the risks and benefits of treatment should be undertaken before beginning treatment with nusinersen. (It is also, as of the time of this book's publication, one of the most expensive drugs in the world, with the first year of treatment costing up to $750,000!)

PUTTING IT ALL TOGETHER

Motor neuron diseases are a diverse group of conditions that are unified by the fact that they all attack motor neurons preferentially over other types of nerve tissue. However, within that framework there is wide variation in what type of motor neurons are affected (upper, lower, or both) and in what parts of the body. **A**myotrophic **L**atera**L** sclerosis is the prototype motor neuron disease and attacks motor neurons **ALL** over the body. **Primary lateral sclerosis** and **progressive muscular atrophy** are two less severe variants of amyotrophic lateral sclerosis that only affect upper and lower motor neurons, respectively (remember **P**u**LL-up** and **PRESS-down**!). **Bulbar palsy** and **pseudobulbar palsy** each involve damage to the motor tracts of the medulla, with bulbar palsy affecting lower motor neuron and ps**EU**dobulbar palsy hitting **U**pper motor neurons as well as causing **E**motional incontinence. While **polio** is rare today due to vaccines, you may still encounter post-polio syndrome in people who had the infection earlier in life (in which case they wouldn't be able to **pole** vault). Finally, **S**pinal **M**uscular **A**trophy is a genetic disorder that tends to affect **L**ower motor neurons in **L**ittle ones (remember **SMALL**!) and with varying degree of severity. Use the table below to help you keep this straight!

Disease	UMN	LMN	Features
ALS	✓	✓	All over
PLS	✓		Starts in lower body and moves up
PMA		✓	Both upper and lower body
Bulbar palsy		✓	Speaking, chewing, and swallowing
Pseudobulbar palsy	✓		Tongue movement, emotional incontinence
Polio		✓	Occurs after initial infection
SMA		✓	Genetic, presents as paralysis in babies

REVIEW QUESTIONS

1. A 48 y/o F living in Manhattan notices that over the past year she is having increasing difficulty walking up the stairs to her apartment, so she decides to see her primary care doctor. In the meantime, she notices increasing difficulty with some everyday activities including squeezing shampoo out of the bottle and scooping ice cream out of the carton. On exam, she appears alert with no cognitive deficits. Her cranial nerves are intact. No sensory deficits are noted in any modality. Motor strength is decreased to 4/5 in all extremities, with particular difficulties in raising her arms past her shoulders. Deep tendon reflexes are intact throughout. Her gait is slowed but otherwise normal. Her Romberg sign is negative. On a follow-up visit several months later, her weakness has progressed to the point where she is unable to walk without assistance. There are signs of muscle atrophy in both arms and legs. Her deep tendon reflexes are exaggerated in her right arm and left leg but are absent in her left arm and right leg. The Babinski sign is positive bilaterally. An MRI is ordered which shows the following:

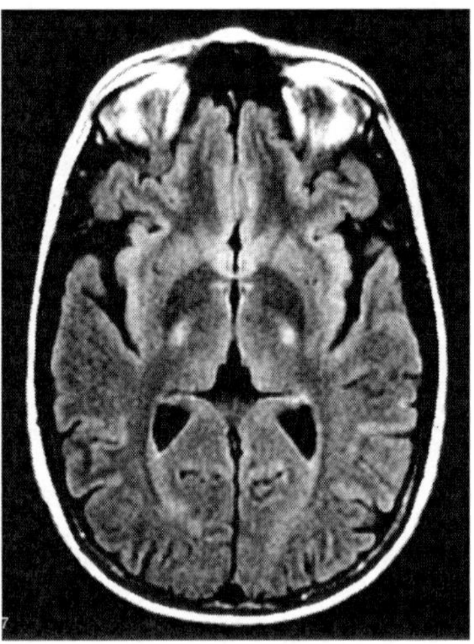

The patient wants to know about treatment. Which of the following is the most accurate statement?

   A. "No treatment is needed. This will get better on its own."
   B. "This is a treatable condition. As long as you stay on the medication you will likely make a full recovery."
   C. "Our goal is to help you live as long as possible, and only medications can help with that."
   D. "Medication can help with some of the symptoms, but really our focus should be on physical and speech therapy."
   E. "I'm very sorry, but there is no treatment for this disease."
   F. None of the above

2. (Continued from previous question.) The patient's disease continues to progress, and she passes away less than a year later. Which of the following is the most likely cause of death for this patient?
   A. Mechanical fall resulting in head trauma
   B. Aspiration of food into the airway
   C. Congestive heart failure
   D. Respiratory failure
   E. Systemic infection
   F. Malignancy

3. A 65 y/o F with no past medical history sees a neurologist out of concern that her arms are getting weaker. Exam reveals 4/5 weakness of the upper extremities bilaterally but full strength in the lower extremities. At a follow-up visit one month later, her arm strength has decreased to 3/5, and she now shows 4/5 weakness in both legs. Electromyography reveals fibrillations with occasional fasciculations. Over the course of the next several years, her muscle strength continued to deteriorate. A repeat exam 2 years later shows significant wasting of muscle tissues. Which of the following is most likely to be seen?
   A. Extension of the toes in response to stroking of the foot on exam
   B. Detectable mutation on genetic testing
   C. Neuronal loss in the anterior horns of the spinal cord on autopsy
   D. Degeneration of the corticospinal tract on autopsy
   E. Atrophy of the motor cortex on autopsy

4. A 4 m/o F is brought to the emergency department after 2 days of cough, fever, and difficulty breathing. Her mother notes that over the past month the patient has been less active than before, and for the past week she would go limp in her arms "like a doll" when picked up. On exam, the infant is in clear respiratory distress but shows little movement of intercostal muscles. There is generalized hypotonia throughout her body. Saliva is seen running down out of the corner of her mouth. The patient is admitted to the hospital but passes away from aspiration pneumonia several days later. Which of the following mechanisms explains the patient's presentation?
   A. Autosomal dominant mutation resulting in upper motor neuron damage
   B. Autosomal dominant mutation resulting in lower motor neuron damage
   C. Autosomal recessive mutation resulting in upper motor neuron damage
   D. Autosomal recessive mutation resulting in lower motor neuron damage
   E. Sporadic disease resulting in upper motor neuron damage
   F. Sporadic disease resulting in lower motor neuron damage

1. **The best answer is F.** The presence of both upper and lower motor neuron signs in this case are highly suggestive of amyotrophic lateral sclerosis, as is the rapidly progressive nature of the disease. The MRI shows abnormalities in both the motor cortex and basal ganglia which is consistent with upper motor neuron involvement. Amyotrophic lateral sclerosis is not curable, but treatment can be beneficial (answer E). In particular, a medication called riluzole can be helpful, with most guidelines suggesting that this medication should be started as soon as possible after an initial diagnosis. However, medications are not the only option that can prolong life, with non-invasive ventilation also being effective for this outcome (answer C). While physical and speech therapy is an important cornerstone of amyotrophic lateral sclerosis management and should be included as part of the treatment plan, it is not accurate to say that medication only helps with symptoms, as riluzole has been shown to prolong survival by several months (answer D). However, the benefits of the medication should not be oversold, as it will not enable patients to make a full recovery (answer B). Amyotrophic lateral sclerosis is not a self-limiting condition, and with or without treatment most patients will die from this disease (answer A). For these reasons, none of the listed statements would be appropriate at this time.

2. **The best answer is D.** The most common cause of death in amyotrophic lateral sclerosis is respiratory failure. While the diaphragm is often spared early in the disease, as amyotrophic lateral sclerosis progresses it often begins to involve respiratory muscles as well, necessitating respiratory support. Aspiration pneumonia can occur in amyotrophic lateral sclerosis as well, but it is not the most common cause of death (answer B).

3. **The best answer is C.** This vignette describes a case of progressive muscular atrophy, a motor neuron disease that primarily affects lower motor neurons. Due to sparing of upper motor neurons, the Babinski sign should be absent (answer A), and degeneration of upper motor neurons in regions including the motor cortex (answer E) and corticospinal tract (answer D) should not be observed. Instead, the primary areas of neuronal loss should be observed in peripheral motor nerves which have their cell bodies in the anterior horn of the spinal cord. Progressive muscular atrophy has not been shown to have a genetic component in the same way that some cases of amyotrophic lateral sclerosis do (answer B).

4. **The best answer is D.** This describes a case of spinal muscular atrophy type I (also known as Werdnig-Hoffman disease) which presents with a sudden onset of generalized hypotonia and other lower motor neuron signs in an infant. Upper motor neurons are not involved in spinal muscular atrophy (answers A and C). Spinal muscular atrophy is an autosomal recessive disease, not an autosomal dominant disease (answers A and B) or a sporadic disease (answers E and F).

19 MOVEMENT DISORDERS

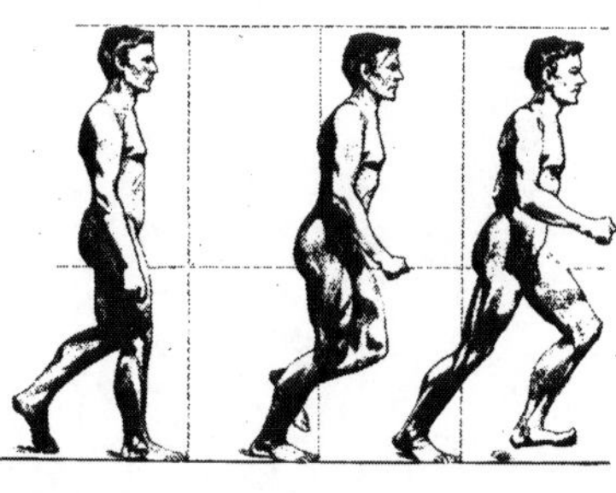

Now that we have looked at diseases of the muscle, the neuromuscular junction, and the motor neuron, it is time to examine diseases of the upper-most part of the motor pathway: the **brain** itself. As we learned in our study of neuroanatomy, the part of the brain that is most involved in movement is the **basal ganglia**, and indeed many of the conditions we will talk about in this chapter involve one or more parts of the basal ganglia directly!

Movement disorders are a **highly heterogeneous** group of conditions, and at first there can seem to be few unifying principles connecting one movement disorder to another. However, at their core all movement disorders boil down to one of two problems: either they involve difficulty *initiating* movement (resulting in ***hypo*kinetic movement disorders**) or they present as trouble with *stopping* movement (leading to ***hyper*kinetic movement disorders**).

We will start off by discussing hypokinetic movement disorders, the prototype of which is **Parkinson's disease**. From there, we will move on to hyperkinetic movement disorders, including both broad categories like **tremors** and **dystonias** as well as a few specific conditions like **Huntington's disease** and **Wilson's disease**.

PARKINSONISM

Any discussion of hypokinetic movement disorders needs to start with **Parkinson's disease**, as it is the prototypical disorder involving difficulty initiating movement (and the one you will need to know best for both boards and wards!). However, we'll also cover a few other **Parkinson-plus syndromes** that feature many of the same signs and symptoms of Parkinson's disease but with their own unique twists.

PARKINSON'S DISEASE

Parkinson's disease is a **neurodegenerative disorder** that primarily affects the motor system. Specifically, Parkinson's disease involves the death of dopaminergic neurons in the **substantia nigra**, leading to a general **dopamine deficit** in the brain. (Recall from Chapter 7 that the substantia nigra is located in the midbrain and is a major site of dopamine production.) A subregion of the substantia nigra known as the **pars compacta** appears to be hit the hardest in Parkinson's disease.

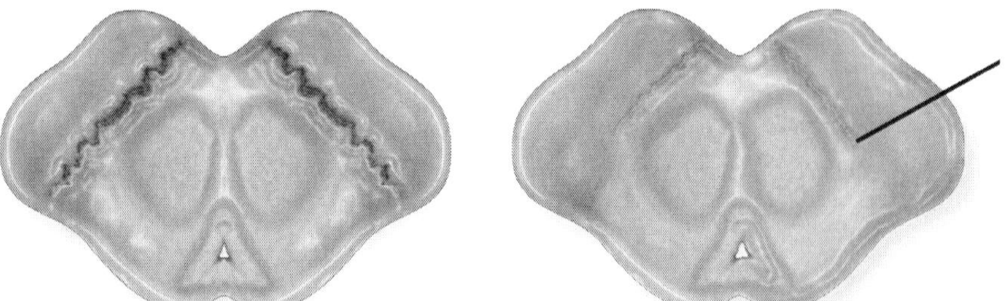

*Comparison between a **healthy control** (left) and a patient with **Parkinson's disease** (right) showing neuronal loss in the **substantia nigra** (solid line).*

As we talked about previously in Chapter 5, dopamine plays an interesting role in movement. It doesn't *cause* motion per se but rather makes movement *more likely to happen* (like adding grease to a hinge). When dopamine-producing cells begin to die, it is as if all the joints in the body lose their grease, and movements start to become difficult to initiate. You can remember the role of dopamine in this condition by thinking that **Pa**rkinson's **D**isease is what happens when do**Pa**mine is **D**epleted.

Parkinson's disease involves the death of **dopamine-producing neurons** in the **substantia nigra**, particularly **the pars compacta.**

__Pa__rkinson's __D__isease is what happens when do__Pa__mine is __D__epleted.

This loss of dopamine results in a specific combination of signs and symptoms known as **Parkinsonism**. There are four key signs of Parkinsonism: slowed or absent movement (known as **bradykinesia** and **akinesia**, respectively), **tremor**, **rigidity**, and **postural instability**. You can remember these using the word **TRAP**, which you can link to Parkinsonism by thinking of someone who is immobile because they have been **TRAP**ped inside of a statue:

T is for Tremor. Hold on, hold on… aren't we talking about disorders involving by too *little* movement? Then what is tremor doing here? This is our first clue that the pathophysiology of Parkinson's disease is much more complex than it appears at first, as the tremor seen in this condition does not appear to result directly from dopamine depletion. Regardless of the mechanism behind it, tremor is a common finding in this disease, and it is often one of the first signs to appear. A classic Parkinsonian tremor has a few distinctive characteristics. First, it is typically a **resting tremor**, meaning that it is there most of the time but will disappear when someone initiates a voluntary movement. Second, it is a **slow tremor** (around 5 shakes per second). Third, it is often described as a "**pill-rolling**" tremor, as it almost looks as if the patient is continuously rolling a pill between their thumb and index finger.

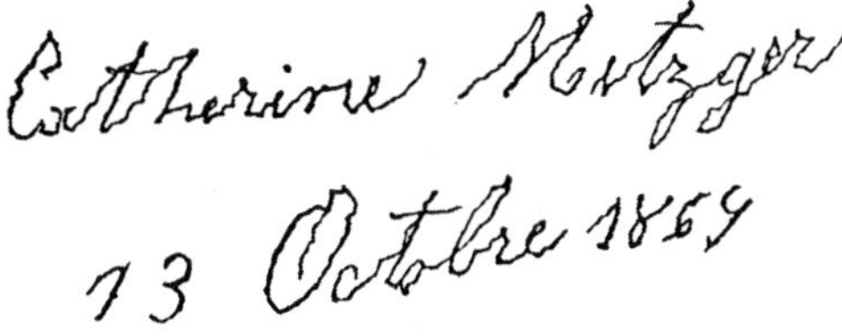

Writing by a patient with ***Parkinson's disease*** *showing evidence of a* ***tremor***.

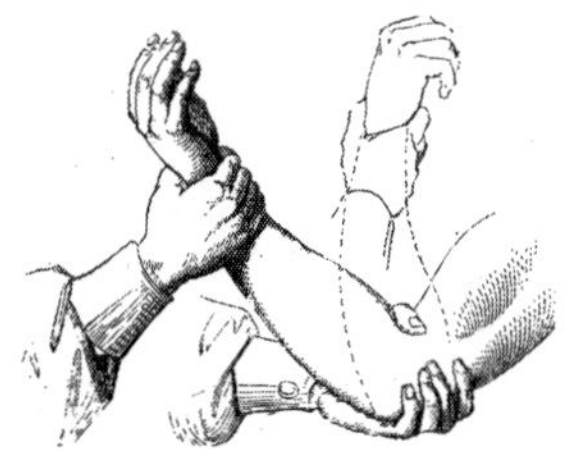

R is for Rigidity. Someone with Parkinson's disease looks, well, *stiff*. Not only is movement slowed, but the disease seems to give the appearance of *actively resisting* movement due to the presence of increased muscle tone at rest. When you ask a patient to relax and then try to move their arms for them, you will often be met with some degree of resistance, either in a sustained way known as **lead-pipe rigidity** or in a ratchety *click-click-click* manner known as **cogwheel rigidity** (as it resembles the clicking of cogwheels or gears). Rigidity is often progressive in Parkinson's disease, showing up in just a few areas at first and then slowly taking over more of the body. Rigidity also encompasses the muscles of the face, leading to a "frozen" or **mask-like face** that is devoid of emotional expression (as seen in the image below):

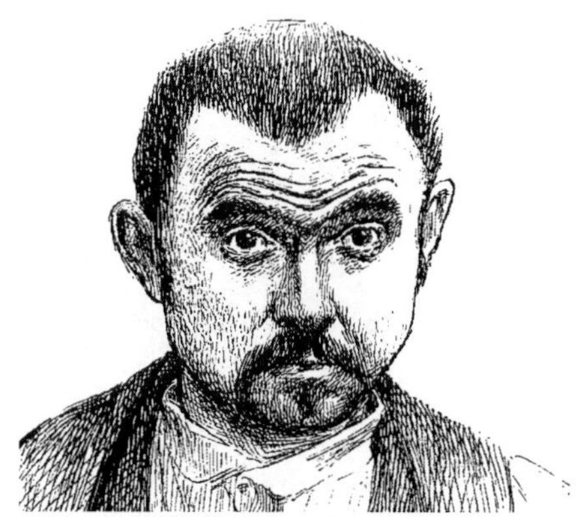

Mask-like face *in* ***Parkinson's disease***.

A is for Akinesia and bradykinesia. Slowness of movement, known as **bradykinesia**, is the **hallmark sign** of Parkinson's disease and is found in every case. The slowness involves all stages of a movement, including planning it, starting it, and completing it. When slowness becomes particularly severe, it can even lead to a total lack of movement known as **akinesia**. Slowness is particularly noticeable in the distinctive way that people with the disease walk, as they tend to walk slowly with their body flexed forward, barely bringing their feet off of the ground. Turning is often done slowly in small increments, almost like a heavy statue being turned through much effort. All of this gives a "shuffling" appearance to the patient's walk which is known as a **Parkinsonian gait** or **festination**. Notably, **arm swinging** is generally absent in one arm, almost as if the patient is walking around with one hand in an invisible pocket. Decreased arm swing is generally **unilateral** and **asymmetrical** at the beginning of the disease (although it may progress to being bilateral as the disease advances).

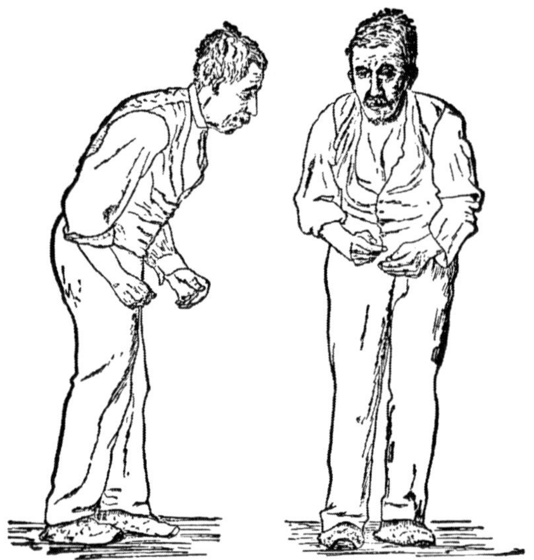

*A **Parkinsonian gait** with forward flexion of the body.*

P is for Postural instability. The final cardinal sign of Parkinson's disease is a distinct **lack of balance** which tends to emerge late in the disease. Indeed, the number of falls that someone experiences is often a marker of how severe their condition is.

The **four cardinal signs of Parkinson's disease** are **bradykinesia**, **tremor**, **rigidity**, and **postural instability**.

*Someone with **Parkinson's disease** becomes **TRAP**ped inside of a statue:*
***T**remor*
***R**igidity*
***A**kinesia and bradykinesia*
***P**ostural instability*

Outside of the four cardinal signs, Parkinson's disease can also present with a variety of **neuropsychiatric phenomena**. These include **cognitive changes** ranging from mild impairment to outright dementia; a high rate of comorbid psychiatric symptoms such as **depression** and **anxiety**; **psychotic symptoms** including paranoid delusions and auditory hallucinations; and **sleep changes** such as fatigue and insomnia. While it was long thought that Parkinson's disease primarily affected only the voluntary motor aspect of the efferent nervous system, some patients can develop **autonomic instability** as well, including changes in blood pressure, gastrointestinal motility, bladder function, and sweat production.

Parkinson's disease tends to affect **older people**, with an average age at diagnosis of over 60 years. While it is known that Parkinson's disease results from the death of dopaminergic neurons in the substantia nigra, it's *not* known why these neurons start dying in the first place (although a history of head injury or exposure to specific chemicals does appear to raise the risk of developing the disease slightly). Diagnosis is typically made on the basis of clinical signs and symptoms, although head imaging can help to support the diagnosis.

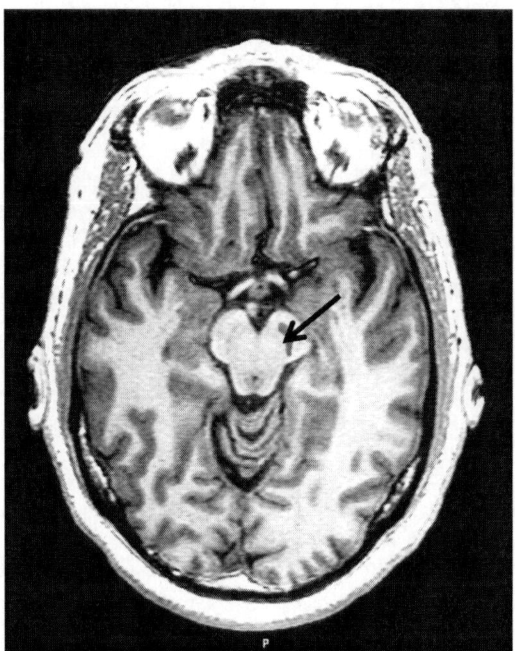

MRI showing degeneration of the ***substantia nigra*** *in a patient with* ***Parkinson's disease****.*

There is **no cure** for Parkinson's disease, so treatment is targeted towards reducing the symptom severity and increasing one's quality of life. **Exercise** as well as **physical, occupational, and speech therapy** all can have beneficial effects. The most widely used medication for treating Parkinson's disease is a combination drug known as **carbidopa-levodopa**. Levodopa is a precursor to dopamine which is able to cross the blood-brain barrier and be converted into dopamine, effectively helping to replace some of the dopamine that has been lost. Carbidopa, which makes up the other half of the drug, does not turn into dopamine itself but instead plays a supporting role by inhibiting the conversion of levodopa into dopamine in places *outside* the central nervous system. This not only helps more of the levodopa get into the brain but also prevents the extra dopamine from causing unpleasant side effects (like nausea and vomiting) in the rest of the body. You can remember the function of each component of carbidopa-levodopa by thinking that **car**bidopa is the **car** that drives levodopa to its destination.

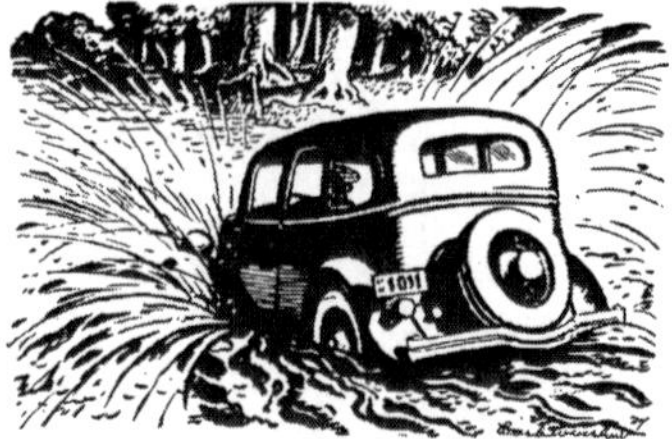

Carbidopa-levodopa is used to treat **Parkinson's disease. Levodopa** is the **active ingredient**, while **carbidopa** helps to **prevent peripheral conversion** of levodopa.

Car*bidopa is the* ***car*** *that drives levodopa to its destination (the brain).*

Even with carbidopa around, carbidopa-levodopa can still cause some pretty obnoxious side effects. For this reason, a different class of drugs known as **dopamine agonists** (which are less effective than carbidopa-levodopa but also tend to cause less severe side effects) can be preferred in some cases, especially early on in the disease when symptoms are not as severe. In rare cases, a **deep brain stimulator** may be surgically implanted into the basal ganglia to help improve symptoms. Even with treatment, however, Parkinson's disease remains a stubbornly progressive disease, with more dopaminergic neurons being lost as time passes, leading to increasingly severe symptoms and greater functional impairment. Many patients end up entirely dependent upon others, and life expectancy is significantly reduced.

MULTISYSTEM ATROPHY

Now that we have a good sense of "textbook" Parkinson's disease, let's talk about a few **Parkinson-plus syndromes** that feature the core pathology of Parkinsonism *plus* a few unique features. The first of these syndromes is **multisystem atrophy** (also known as Shy-Drager syndrome) which can best be described as "Parkinson's *plus* autonomic and cerebellar dysfunction." In contrast to Parkinson's disease (where autonomic dysfunction is either absent or plays a small role), multisystem atrophy *prominently* features **autonomic nervous system dysfunction**, including signs and symptoms such as abnormal blood pressure, excessive sweating, dry mouth, urinary incontinence, and loss of sexual function. Ataxia and other **cerebellar signs** are often present as well. You can remember this by thinking that patients with **M**ulti**S**ystem **A**trophy are **M**issing **S**table **A**utonomics.

Multisystem atrophy is a Parkinson-plus syndrome that features prominent dysfunction of the **autonomic nervous system**.

*Multi**S**ystem **A**trophy = **M**issing **S**table **A**utonomics.*

PROGRESSIVE SUPRANUCLEAR PALSY

Progressive supranuclear palsy is another Parkinson-plus syndrome. This time, it can be thought of as "Parkinson's *plus* abnormal eye movements." It shares with "textbook" Parkinson's disease both motor deficits (including abnormal gait, loss of balance, and frequently bumping into other people or objects) and dementia-like deficits in memory and cognition. However, progressive supranuclear palsy uniquely involves a **downward gaze palsy** or an inability for the extraocular muscles to point the eyes down. To remember the association of **P**rogressive **S**upranuclear **P**alsy with a downward gaze palsy, think of someone who is asked to **P**lease **S**top **P**eering. What is the first thing they do? Try to avert their gaze by looking down.

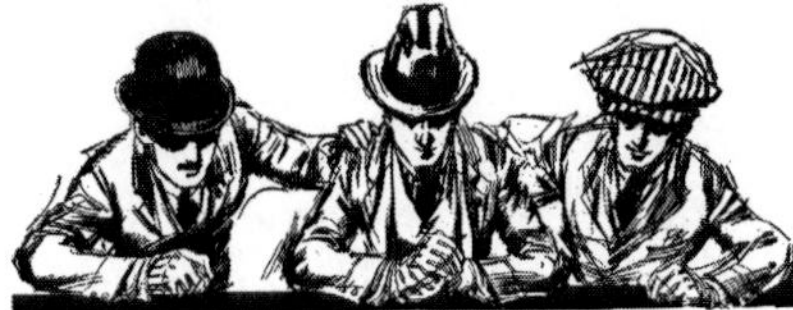

> **Progressive supranuclear palsy** is a Parkinson-plus syndrome resulting in **movement deficits**, **cognitive impairment**, and **downward gaze palsy**.
>
> *Someone who is asked to **P**lease **S**top **P**eering immediately tries to **look down**.*

CORTICOBASAL DEGENERATION

The final Parkinson-plus syndrome we will talk about is **corticobasal degeneration** which affects both the cerebral cortex and the basal ganglia (hence its name). This results in both **cognitive and motor deficits** including slowed movement, difficulty walking, and memory loss. The "plus" in the case of corticobasal degeneration is a bizarre finding known as **alien hand syndrome** in which patients feel unable to move their hand due to a sensation that their limbs are foreign to them. This is typically **asymmetric**, affecting only one hand. Alien hand syndrome is seen in about 60% of cases, making it a unique marker of this disease. You can remember this association by linking **C**ortico**B**asilar **D**egeneration to a feeling that your arm is **C**ontrolled **B**y aliens in **D**eep space.

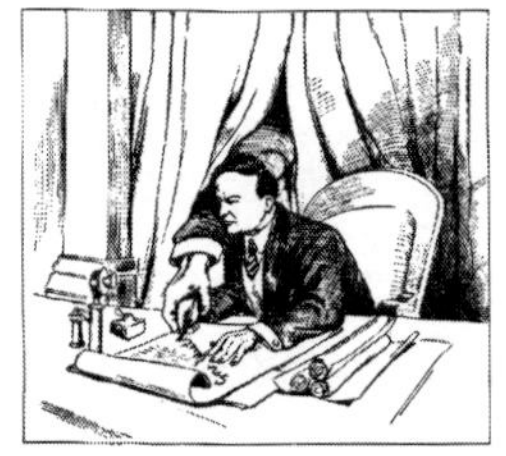

> **Corticobasal degeneration** is a Parkinson-plus syndrome that features **alien hand syndrome** in the majority of cases.
>
> ***C**ortico**B**asilar **D**egeneration = **C**ontrolled **B**y **D**eep space.*

Overall, you should consider one of these Parkinson-plus syndrome when the core **TRAP** signs of Parkinson's disease are there *plus* a few that don't quite match (whether that is autonomic dysfunction and cerebellar signs in multisystem atrophy, downward gaze palsy in progressive supranuclear palsy, or alien hand syndrome in corticobasal degeneration). Compared to people with "textbook" Parkinson's disease, patients with Parkinson-plus syndromes tend to have a **worse prognosis** and see less benefit from treatments like carbidopa-levodopa.

HUNTINGTON'S DISEASE

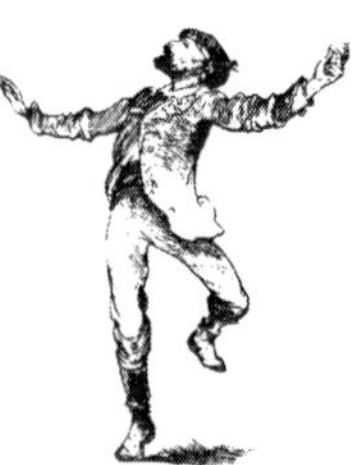

For the remainder of this chapter, we will shift our focus from *hypo*kinetic movement disorders like Parkinson's disease towards *hyper*kinetic movement disorders. These conditions are all unified by the presence of *too much* movement, whether that takes the form of large dance-like movements as in **chorea**, involuntary shaking as in **tremors**, or a sustained muscle contraction as in **dystonias**. We'll focus on chorea first, the prototype of which is seen in Huntington's disease.

Huntington's disease is a hyperkinetic movement disorder that involves the onset of progressively worsening **movement and behavioral problems**. The hallmark movement abnormality seen in Huntington's disease is **chorea** which is a series of quick, jerky, flailing movements that resemble dancing (in fact, the word is Greek for "dance," as in "*chore*ography"). The movements of chorea are not under voluntary control, and they occur without any effort on the part of the patient.

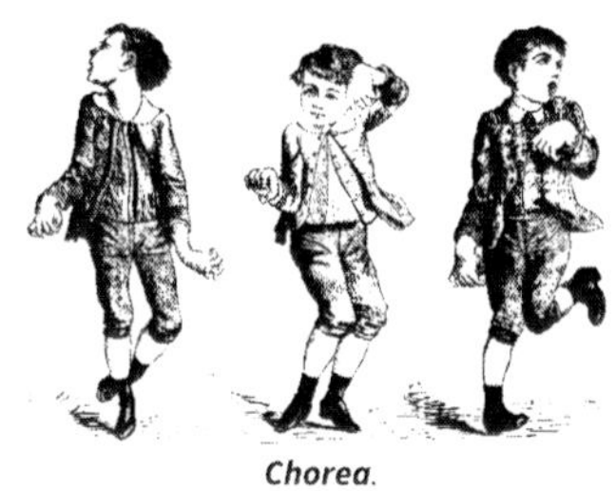

Chorea.

While chorea is typically the first sign to appear, other **motor deficits** (such as difficulty walking, talking, chewing, and swallowing) soon appear as well. These will often progress to the point where the patient can no longer engage in coordinated movement. **Cognitive disabilities**, including memory loss, begin to appear and slowly become more prominent so that, by the time of death, most patients meet criteria for clinical dementia. On a behavioral level, both **impulsive and compulsive behaviors** can emerge, including aggression, substance abuse, gambling, and uninhibited sexual behavior. While chorea is the hallmark sign of Huntington's disease, it is these latter changes that are often *most* disabling to the patient and distressing to their families.

The **hallmark sign of Huntington's disease** is a dance-like movement known as **chorea**, although other **motor and neuropsychiatric deficits** are seen as well.

*Think "**chorea**" like in "**choreography**" or the art of designing a dance.*

The first signs of the disorder often begin in **adulthood** between the ages of 30 and 50, with most patients dying within 20 years of diagnosis (often due to aspiration pneumonia, as the ability to swallow becomes increasingly impaired). However, up to a quarter of patients will attempt suicide (which highlights both the frequency and severity of psychiatric symptoms in this disease).

Huntington's disease is an **autosomal dominant genetic disorder** involving mutations in the **huntingtin gene** on **chromosome 4**. A significant portion of this gene is made up of the **trinucleotide repeat CAG**. It is normal to have some amount of this repeat sequence. However, in people who have too many CAG repeats (more than 35), the gene becomes dysfunctional and begins to produce a mutant version of the huntingtin protein that damages the brain and leads to neuronal death, particularly in the **caudate** (which explains the presence of **cau**gnitive deficits in this disease). The number of CAG repeats is directly correlated with the severity of the disease, with people who have 36 to 39 copies often showing a later onset and slower progression than people with more than 40 (who may show signs of the disease as early as age 20, with subsequent rapid progression).

However, when passing the gene on to one's offspring, the number of CAG repeats may spontaneously increase. This means that people with few or no symptoms (who may have less than 36 copies) can still end up passing a more severe version of the disease on to their children if the number of CAG repeats increases. This steady increase in the number of repeats resulting in greater disease severity over successive generations is known as **anticipation**. It is more likely for CAG repeats to increase during spermatogenesis than oogenesis, so fathers are more likely to pass on a mutated version of the gene to their children than mothers.

These concepts are key to understanding Huntington's disease, so let's try to link them all together using a mnemonic. Imagine a young man who sees a beautiful girl on the first day of school and develops a crush. A few days later, he tells one of his new friends about his new love interest. His friend reacts with horror, saying, "You **caun't date** Huntington's **daughter**! Her **father** is very **dominant**. If he finds out, he'll hunt **4** you and put you in a **CAG**e." This mnemonic ties together the primary location of cell damage (the **caudate**), the concept of anticipation (with **fathers** being more likely to pass a severe version of their disease on to their children), the autosomal **dominant** pattern of inheritance, and the location of the **CAG** repeats on chromosome **4**.

Huntington's disease involves a **CAG trinucleotide repeat** on **chromosome 4**, leading to a **mutated huntingtin protein** that damages neurons in the **caudate**.

*"You **caun't date** (caudate) **Huntington's daughter**! Her **father** is very (autosomal) **dominant**. He'll hunt **4** you and put you in a **CAGe** (CAG repeat on chromosome 4)."*

As with most movement disorders, there is **no cure** for Huntington's disease. Instead, treatment is directed towards improving the patient's quality of life using **physical and occupational therapy** (such as preparing foods to be easier to swallow). A drug known as **tetrabenazine** can reduce the severity of chorea. Genetic counseling can be offered to patients who are considering having children. However, because the first signs of the disease often do not appear until after the age of 30, some patients may have had children already.

TREMOR

A **tremor** is an **involuntary rhythmic movement** in which muscles alternate between contraction and relaxation, producing an **oscillating or twitching motion**. We've talked about tremors already as a specific sign of Parkinson's disease, but let's take a step back and look at tremors in a more general sense!

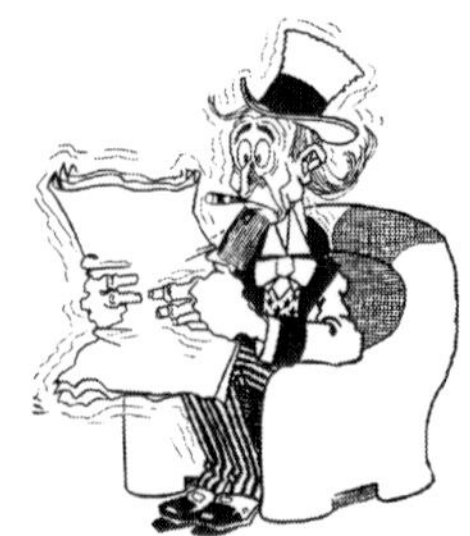

First off, it's worth pointing out that tremors are not always a sign of pathology! For example, most people will shiver when they are cold to help generate body heat. In other cases, tremor can be a manifestation of anxiety, agitation, or other emotional states. Certain substances, including both prescription and recreational drugs, can cause tremor (like drinking too much caffeine in a single sitting). In other cases, tremor can be a manifestation of another disease (like we talked about with Parkinson's disease). Finally, tremor can occur on its own in a way that is unrelated to any other condition at which point it can be considered a hyperkinetic movement disorder all by itself.

Because of the many possible causes of tremors, it can be helpful to break them down into a few distinct categories. There are **four main forms of tremor** that we will cover here which you can remember using the word **PAIR** (as in a tremulous pair of hands):

P is for Physiologic tremor. Many people have some degree of tremor that is barely noticeable and generally doesn't lead to any distress or disability. This is known as a **physiologic tremor**. A physiologic tremor tends to occur most when a particular body part is held upright against gravity for a prolonged period of time (such as a child raising their hand to go to the bathroom). In many cases, the tremor is so slight as to be barely noticeable. You can see your own tremor better by taking a piece of paper in your hand and holding your arm straight out in front of you. You should be able to see small twitches in the paper, especially if you hold it long enough!

A is for Action tremor. An **action tremor** is one that worsens when you try to use that particular part of the body. For example, if you place a pencil in the hand of a patient with an action tremor, it will initially remain still. However, as soon as they try to write with the pencil, their hand will begin to shake.

The most common cause of an action tremor is an idiopathic condition known as an **essential tremor**. Essential tremor is the most common movement disorder, with up to 5% of the population having it. It generally affects the hands and upper extremities, although less often it can affect other parts of the body as well. There is no known cause, although genes appear to be involved in around half of all cases, with transmission generally following an **autosomal dominant** pattern. Essential tremor is a progressive condition, with most cases being relatively mild at the beginning and then becoming more and more severe as time passes. Because an essential tremor interferes with one's ability to carry out intentional actions such as writing, it can be quite disabling in severe forms.

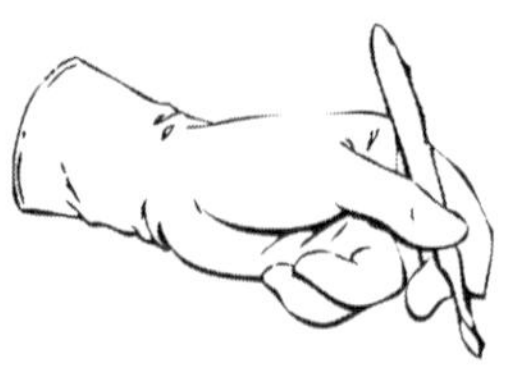

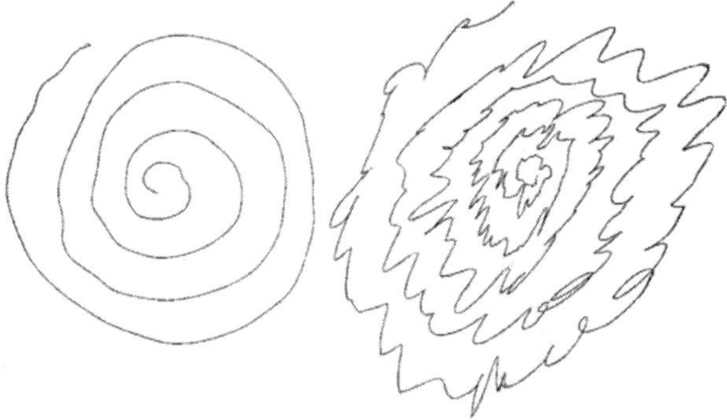

*An attempt by a patient with an **essential tremor** to copy the figure on the left.*

Treatment of essential tremor involves use of **beta-blockers** which are effective at reducing the severity of the tremor (and luckily have few side effects!). Interestingly, **alcohol** is quite effective at reducing essential tremors as well, and a patient's report that their tremor improves after drinking is highly suggestive of this form of tremor! However, alcohol is not an appropriate form of long-term treatment for essential tremor due to its brief duration of action and the risk of alcohol addiction.

I is for Intention tremor. An **intention tremor** (also known as a **cerebellar tremor**) is one that tends to occur at the *end* of an intentional action. For example, if someone is reaching their hand out to press a button, the beginning of this action may be smooth, but by the end (with their arm completely outstretched) a tremor will appear. (This is in contrast to an action tremor in which the tremor would be present *throughout* the duration of the action, including its beginning). An intention tremor is associated with damage to the **cerebellum** and is commonly seen alongside the other cerebellar signs as captured in the "**dizzy AUNT with 3 dishes**" mnemonic.

R is for Resting tremor. Finally, a **resting tremor** occurs even when the body is not actively moving. While there are other possible causes of a resting tremor, as a general rule of thumb the presence of a resting tremor should make you immediately think of **Parkinson's disease**, especially if it is accompanied by other signs such as muscle rigidity or bradykinesia. Other causes of Parkinsonism (such as use of dopamine-blocking medications) can lead to a resting tremor as well.

There are **four main forms of tremors**, each of which has its own causes.

*Think of a **PAIR** of tremulous hands:*
***P**hysiologic (normal)*
***A**ction (essential tremor)*
***I**ntention (cerebellar dysfunction)*
***R**esting (Parkinsonism)*

DYSTONIA

The next type of hyperkinetic movement disorder that we will talk about is **dystonias** which are **involuntary sustained muscle contractions** that will generally make the patient adopt a specific posture. They are often quite painful as well (as most people know from having experienced a dead leg or Charley horse!). Like tremors, dystonias can either be a manifestation of another pathological process, a side effect of particular substances, or a disease in and of itself. For that reason, the presence of a dystonia often requires further evaluation.

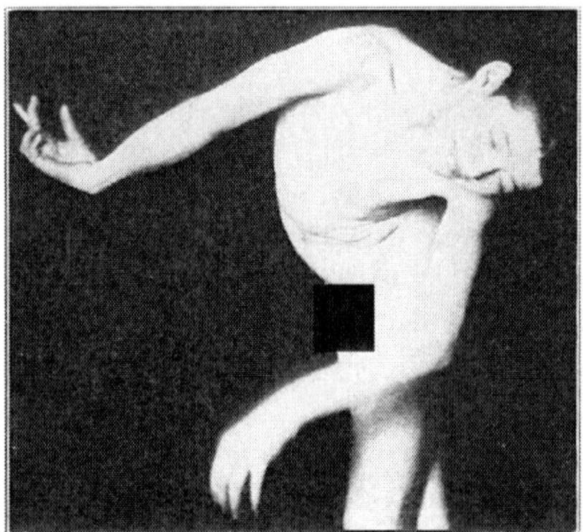

*A case of **dystonia**.*

When a dystonia happens recurrently without any clear cause, it is known as a **primary focal dystonia** ("primary" because they are not happening secondary to another cause and "focal" because they affect one part of the body in particular). These are generally named by their location, such as **blepharospasm** (dystonia of the eyelids), **cervical dystonia** (dystonia of the neck), and **writer's cramp** (dystonia of the hand). Dystonias can be incredibly impairing, and people have been forced to give up careers as musicians, engineers, or other occupations due to the onset of a dystonia. Treatment of primary focal dystonias involves turning an old enemy into a new friend by using injections of **botulinum toxin** to help relax the muscle! To link "**robot**-ulism" with **dysto**nias, think of how **robot**s are often associated with **dysto**pian futures!

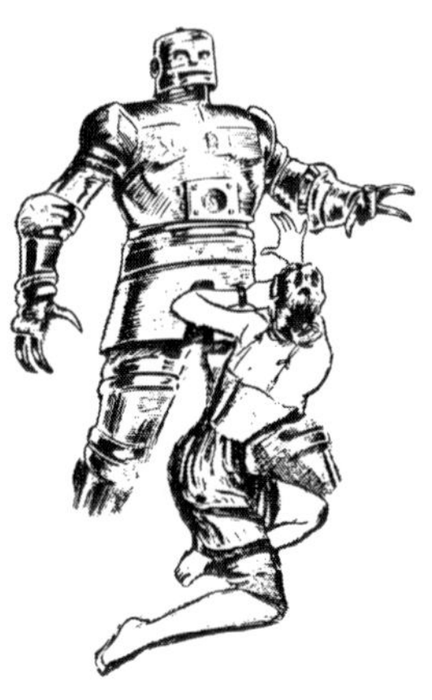

Primary focal dystonias can be treated with **botulinum toxin**.

*"**Robot**-ulism" can be used in **dysto**nian futures!*

WILSON'S DISEASE

The final movement disorder we will talk about is **Wilson's disease**. Wilson's disease occurs when a **defect of copper metabolism** results in copper deposits accumulating throughout the body. While a certain amount of copper in the body is normal, when it collects in excessive amounts, it can cause damage to various organ systems. Let's use the word **WILSON** itself to remember the key clinical features of this disease:

W is for Wilson's disease. This is just to remind us what disease we're talking about!

I is for Inherited. Wilson's disease is an **autosomal recessive genetic disorder** that occurs when the ATP7B gene, which codes for an enzyme that transports copper into bile, becomes mutated and produces a defective enzyme. The affected gene is on **chromosome 13**. To remember the association of Wilson's disease and chromosome 13, write it as **ω1**lson's disease so that the W looks like a 3 turned on its side!

Wilson's disease is an **inherited defect of copper metabolism** that is localized to **chromosome 13**.

*Write it as **ω1**lson's disease to remember chromosome **13**!*

L is for Liver. The liver is particularly sensitive to copper, and a variety of liver-related conditions (including cirrhosis, ascites, and hepatic encephalopathy) are common in people who have Wilson's disease.

S is for Serum abnormalities. Laboratory testing of the serum will show evidence of abnormalities, including **increased copper** and **decreased ceruloplasmin** (which is the major copper-carrying protein in the blood).

O is for Ocular findings. When levels of copper become high enough, it can deposit into various tissues in a way that is even visible to the naked eye. In particular, copper has a tendency to deposit in the cornea of the eye, leading to the appearance of **Kayser-Fleischer rings** that are pathognomonic for Wilson's disease (meaning that if you see these, you can be 100% confident in your diagnosis of Wilson's disease!).

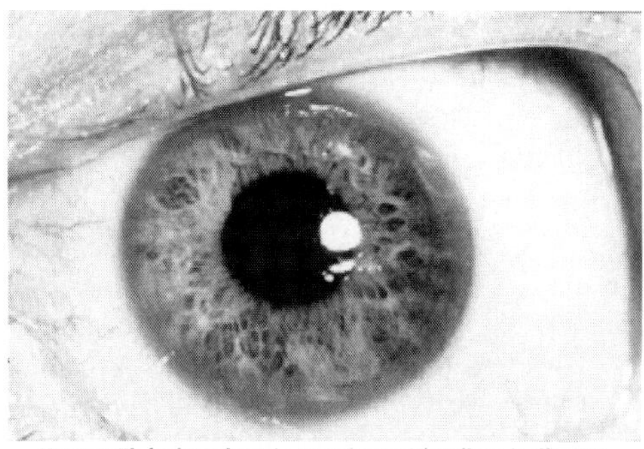

***Kayser-Fleischer rings** in a patient with **Wilson's disease**.*

N is for Neurologic deficits. Similar to the liver, the brain is quite sensitive to excess copper, with the **putamen and basal ganglia** being particularly affected. For this reason, **all types of movement disorders** can be seen in Wilson's disease, including ataxia, bradykinesia, chorea, dysarthria, and tremor. Given the involvement of so many types of abnormal movement, Wilson's disease resists easy classification as either a hypokinetic or hyperkinetic movement disorder.

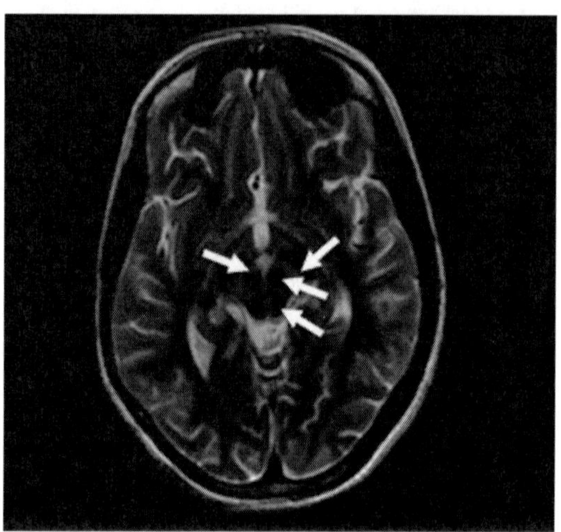

*MRI of the brain in a patient with **Wilson's disease** showing **copper deposits** in the **basal ganglia**.*

The **defective copper metabolism** in **Wilson's disease** manifests as **liver failure** and **abnormal movement**.

WILSON:
W*ilson's disease*
I*nherited (autosomal recessive)*
L*iver disease*
S*erum abnormalities (↑ copper, ↓ ceruloplasmin)*
O*cular findings (Kayser-Fleischer rings)*
N*eurologic signs (movement disorders)*

Because the disease is genetic, it tends to begin in **childhood or adolescence**. Given that most movement disorders affect older adults, any movement disorder in a *young* patient should immediately put Wilson's disease high on the differential!

There is **no cure** for Wilson's disease. However, people with the disease can lead relatively normal lives by adhering to a **low-copper diet**. Medication treatments include **penicillamine** which reduces copper levels in the body by binding to copper in the blood and causing it to be excreted in the urine. **Zinc acetate** can also be used to keep copper levels low by preventing the absorption of copper in the gastrointestinal tract. As with other movement disorders, **physical and occupational therapy** can be helpful for managing the neurologic effects.

PUTTING IT ALL TOGETHER

When evaluating a patient with a movement disorder, your first priority should be to determine whether it is *hypo*kinetic or *hyper*kinetic. If it's hypokinetic, you are likely in the realm of **Parkinson's disease** or one of its related conditions. In contrast, if it's hyperkinetic, you are probably looking at **chorea**, a **tremor**, or a **dystonia**. Wilson's disease straddles both worlds and may present with *either* hypo- or hyperkinetic signs.

When diagnosing a hyperkinetic movement disorder, look at what kind of movement is in excess. Is it a constant shaking? A sudden sustained contraction? A dance-like swinging of the arms? While all these would be united under the banner of "hyperkinetic movement disorders," on a clinical level they will present quite differently. As with any neurologic condition, use the neurologic exam to conduct a structured assessment, then combine your findings with what you know about the patient's history to come up with a clinical diagnosis! The table below will help to summarize the key features of each disorder.

Disease	Hypokinetic	Hyperkinetic	Features
Parkinson's	✓		TRAP (Tremor, Rigidity, Akinesia, and Postural instability)
MSA	✓		TRAP + autonomic dysfunction
PSP	✓		TRAP + downward gaze palsy
CBD	✓		TRAP + alien hand syndrome
Huntington's		✓	Chorea, weakness, dementia, psychiatric symptoms
Tremor		✓	PAIR (Physiologic, Action, Intention, or Resting)
Dystonia		✓	Involuntary sustained muscle contractions
Wilson's	✓	✓	Movement disorders in a young patient

REVIEW QUESTIONS

1. A 30 y/o F comes to see her neurologist for a follow-up visit. One year ago she began having abnormal movements of the arms and face that she describes as "jerky" and "writhing." These movements began in a mild form but have progressively worsened over time. During the interview, she is seen constantly moving her head and hands in fluid motions with no detectable purpose to an outside observer. When asked, she is unable to stop these movements and stay completely still. Her speech is slurred and difficult to understand at times. She is currently married and has two children aged 3 and 5. Her husband accompanies her to the visit, although they are currently separated. The husband says that she is "a totally different person now" and wonders if she has "bipolar" because of her "constant mood swings." Which of the following is *least* likely to be present?
    A. Positive family history of the disease
    B. Deficits in executive functioning on cognitive testing
    C. Difficulty completing heel-to-toe walking
    D. Atrophy in the region of the basal ganglia on MRI
    E. All of the above are likely to be present

2. (Continued from previous question.) Which of the following is most predictive of her prognosis?
    A. Number of trinucleotide repeats on genetic testing
    B. Extent of atrophy seen on neuroimaging
    C. Number of affected family members
    D. Severity of motor weakness in the limbs
    E. Age of onset at 29 years
    F. None of the above are predictive of prognosis for this disease

3. A 61 y/o M is brought to the doctor by his wife who reports that he "looks depressed." He previously worked as an elementary school teacher and won several awards for his work with children. However, over the past 6 months his wife reports that "it's like he's stopped existing." During the interview, he rarely responds with more than one or two words at a time, saying he feels "fine" and that he "dunno" why he is here. He is diagnosed with major depressive disorder and started on an antidepressant. When he returns for a follow-up visit one month later, his presentation is largely unchanged. His wife says, "The drugs you prescribed didn't do much. If anything, they made things worse." The patient now rarely takes care of himself and will only eat if food is put in front of him. On exam, the patient has a tremor in his right hand that goes away when the doctor asks him to shake hands. There is cogwheel rigidity in the right arm. Rapid alternating movements are intact but slowed. When asked to walk, his gait is slow and unsteady, with a forward-leaning posture as seen in the following image:

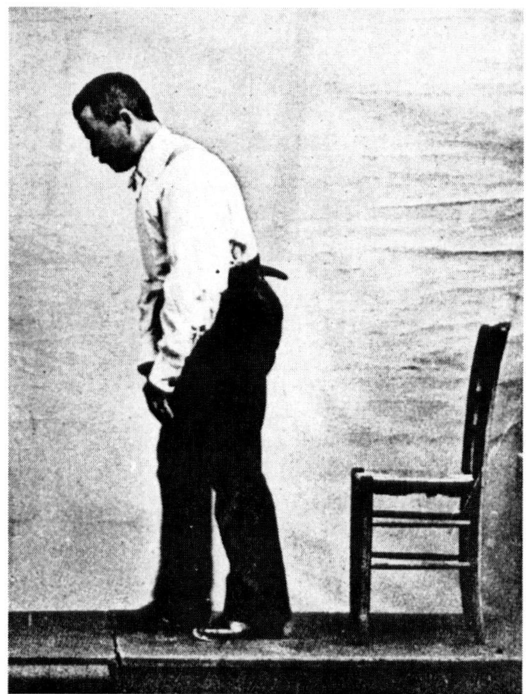

Which of the following regions is most likely affected?

A. Motor cortex
B. Caudate nuclei
C. Internal capsule
D. Substantia nigra
E. Red nuclei
F. Periaqueductal grey

4. (Continued from previous question.) The patient is started on pramipexole, a dopamine agonist. However, after several months with little benefit from this drug, he is switched to carbidopa-levodopa. What is the function of carbidopa?

A. Stimulating dopamine receptors in the central nervous system
B. Stimulating the release of dopamine in the central nervous system
C. Inhibiting dopamine receptors in the central nervous system
D. Stimulating peripheral conversion of levodopa to dopamine
E. Inhibiting peripheral conversion of levodopa to dopamine
F. Inhibiting dopamine receptors in the peripheral nervous system
G. Inhibiting the release of dopamine in the peripheral nervous system
H. None of the above

1. **The best answer is E.** This patient likely has Huntington's disease as evidenced by the presence of chorea and other characteristic signs and symptoms including mood changes. While chorea is often the initial and most noticeable sign of the disorder, Huntington's disease does not only affect movement but can also cause cognitive impairment (answer B) and unsteady gait (answer C). As an autosomal dominant disease, there is often a positive family history (answer A). Atrophy of the caudate nuclei occurs and can be seen on MRI (answer D).

2. **The best answer is A.** The number of CAG repeats in the huntingtin gene on chromosome 4 is directly correlated with the severity of Huntington's disease, as people who have more than 40 repeats are often more severely affected than those with 36 or fewer repeats. The extent of brain atrophy and the age at onset are best seen as manifestations, rather than predictors, of a more severe disease (answers B and E). The number of affected family members is driven more by genetics and chance than disease severity (answer C). Motor weakness is not a predictive factor in this disease (answer D).

3. **The best answer is D.** This vignette describes a classic presentation of Parkinson's disease including bradykinesia, muscle rigidity, a resting tremor, a mask-like face, and a festinating gait. Parkinson's disease is associated with loss of dopaminergic neurons in the substantia nigra of the midbrain. Disorders related to the motor cortex or the internal capsule would instead present with motor weakness (answers A and C). Damage to the caudate nuclei is seen in Huntington's disease (answer B). The red nuclei is also found in the midbrain but plays a relatively small role in movement in humans (answer E). The periaqueductal grey, another resident of the midbrain, is largely involved in pain perception (answer F).

4. **The best answer is E.** Levodopa is the active ingredient in carbidopa-levodopa. It crosses the blood-brain barrier and is converted to dopamine which helps to offset the loss of dopaminergic neurons. However, levodopa is also converted to dopamine in the rest of the body as well where it can cause side effects including nausea and vomiting. Carbidopa acts as an inhibitor of peripheral conversion to dopamine and thereby helps to reduce these side effects. Stimulating peripheral conversion to dopamine would have the opposite effect and would likely *increase* side effect burden (answer D). Carbidopa does not act in the central nervous system (answers A—C), nor does it act on peripheral dopamine release (answer G) or on receptors directly (answer F).

20 SEIZURES

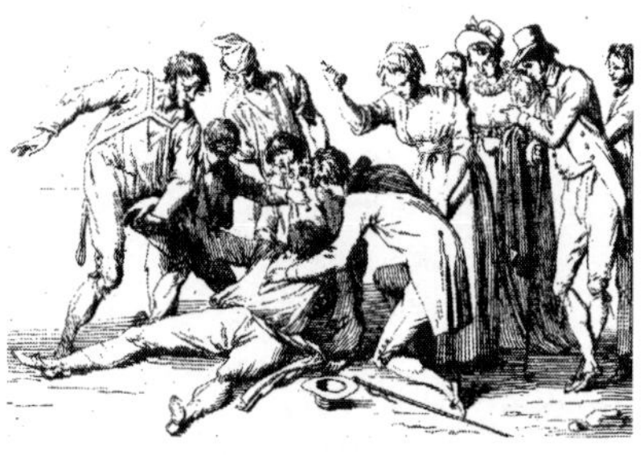

A **seizure** (also known as a convulsion or fit) is a period of **excessive neural activity in the brain**, like an "explosion" of neurons all firing in unison. Seizures can have dramatic effects throughout the body and brain, including muscle contractions and changes in consciousness. They can occur as a result of specific stresses on the body (such as a fever, infection, or electrolyte imbalance), be related to the effects of psychoactive substances (such as alcohol withdrawal), or occur completely on their own. When seizures occur repeatedly with no clear cause, they are diagnosed as **epilepsy**.

Seizures can occur in a variety of different "flavors," and the key to correctly diagnosing and treating epilepsy is to be able to distinguish between the various forms that you will see. For this reason, our first priority will be to learn some new vocabulary so that we can communicate clearly about what we are observing when a patient presents with a seizure. We can then use these differences in presentation to come to a more specific diagnosis and be able to match that to the best treatment. It's worth pointing out that the vocabulary used to describe seizures has changed over time, so you may see different words used to describe the same thing (for example, a "complex partial" seizure is now called a "focal-onset impaired-awareness" seizure). In this book, we will try to adhere to the updated terminology whenever possible. However, the fact remains that the older terms are simpler to use and understand, so you are likely to still encounter them on a regular basis!

SIGNS AND SYMPTOMS OF SEIZURES

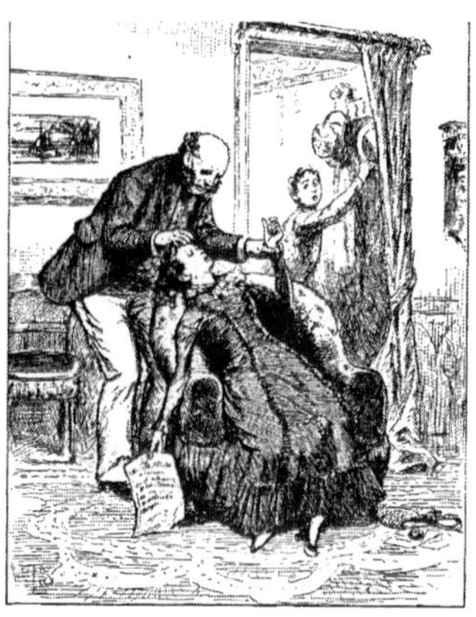

Similar to a stroke, a seizure can take on many forms depending on which parts of the brain are affected. A **generalized seizure** is one that involves both the left *and* right hemispheres of the brain. On a clinical level, the key sign that a seizure has become generalized is when the patient develops **loss of consciousness** (as the entire brain is seizing and is thus unable to normally process conscious information). In contrast, seizures that affect only particular parts of the brain are known as **focal** or **focal-onset seizures** (previously called "partial" seizures). Because a focal seizure is localized to a *single* hemisphere, the patient generally remains conscious throughout the episode.

Focal seizures can at times turn into generalized ones, like a small fire that blazes out of control and begins spreading throughout the entire forest. This is known as a **focal to bilateral seizure** (formerly a "secondarily generalized" seizure). In fact, focal to bilateral seizures are the rule rather than the exception, as around two-thirds of generalized seizures begin as focal seizures and then secondarily generalize.

The majority of seizures are **convulsive seizures**, meaning that they affect the motor system and lead to **uncontrollable muscle contractions**. Convulsive seizures themselves come in a few types, including tonic, clonic, and myoclonic (each of which we will talk about soon). In contrast, **non-convulsive** seizures spare the muscles but cause abnormalities in other areas such as **sensation** or **attention**.

All seizures consist of a period of excessive neuronal activity known as the **ictal phase**. The ictal phase generally lasts anywhere from a few seconds to a few minutes. Seizure activity lasting for more than 5 minutes is known as **status epilepticus** and can represent a life-threatening emergency. Following certain forms of seizures, some people enter into a **postictal state** characterized by drowsiness, confusion, and disorientation. The postictal state usually lasts between 10 and 15 minutes.

Seizures can be either **provoked** (occurring as the direct result of a particular physiologic stress) or **unprovoked** (striking "out of the blue" with no clear cause). People who *only* have seizures in response to specific stimuli (for example, seeing flashing lights or hearing specific sounds) are said to have **reflex seizures**.

Some people experience certain phenomena that clue them into the fact that a seizure is about to occur. This is known as an **aura** and is more common with focal seizures than generalized ones. The specific clues that make up an aura vary from person to person. For some, it may take the form of seeing bright lights; for others, it may involve a distinct odor; for still others, an aura isn't a specific thing but rather a vague premonition (like a "Spidey sense") that a seizure is about to occur.

Okay! That's a lot of new words. Now that we have a vocabulary with which to describe seizures, let's talk about the most common forms of seizures that you will encounter in clinical practice, beginning with generalized seizures.

GENERALIZED SEIZURES

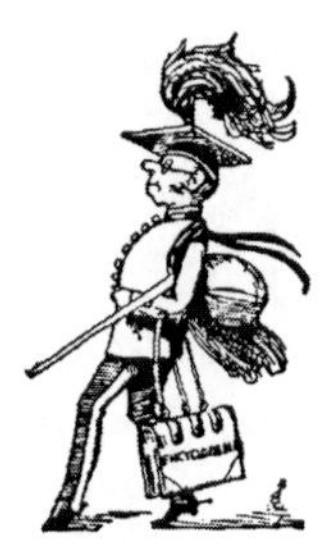

Generalized seizures, or those that involve a **complete loss of consciousness**, come in a variety of forms. These can be hard to keep straight, as many of the words sound similar even if they refer to completely different things. To keep the different ways that generalized seizures can present clear in your mind, think of a man named **General McTATA** whose name stands for all the forms that a **General**-ized seizure can take: **M**yo**c**lonic, **T**onic-clonic, **A**tonic, **T**onic, and **A**bsence. We will go over each of them now (although not in mnemonic order).

The **primary forms of generalized seizures** are **tonic-clonic**, **tonic**, **atonic**, **myoclonic**, and **absence seizures**.

General McTATA:
__M__yo__c__lonic
__T__onic-clonic
__A__tonic
__T__onic
__A__bsence

TONIC-CLONIC SEIZURES

The most common and severe form of a generalized seizure is known as a **tonic-clonic seizure** (formerly known as a "grand mal" seizure). This form of seizure begins with a change in consciousness and evolves into a widespread sustained contraction of muscles (the **tonic phase**) that causes the body to contort into odd or seemingly uncomfortable positions, as seen below. The tonic phase of a seizure is short (lasting only 10 or 20 seconds) but may cause the patient to fall if they are standing up.

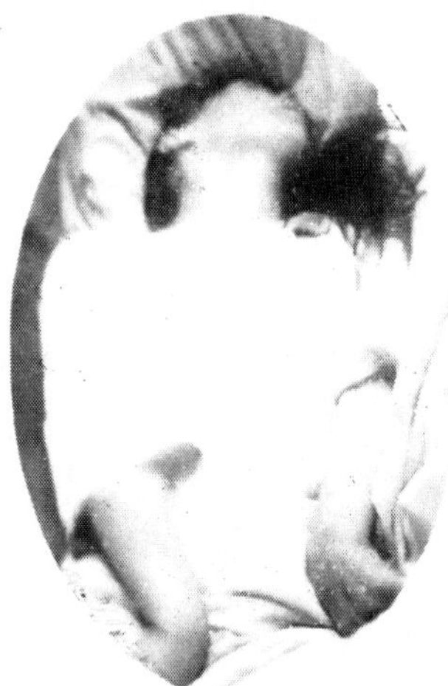

*Widespread muscle contraction seen in the **tonic phase** of a **tonic-clonic seizure**.*

The rest of the seizure consists of the **clonic phase** which is characterized by rapid alternation between contraction and relaxation across the entire body. This is the characteristic **shaking** that most people think about when they hear the word "seizure." The clonic phase is longer than the tonic phase, often lasting 1 to 2 minutes.

To remember the difference between the tonic and clonic phases, think of them as the "town-ic" and "clown-ic" phases. In the "town-ic" phase, the body is completely *rigid* like the brick buildings of an old medieval town, whereas in the "clown-ic" phase it is *shaking* like a hyperactive clown.

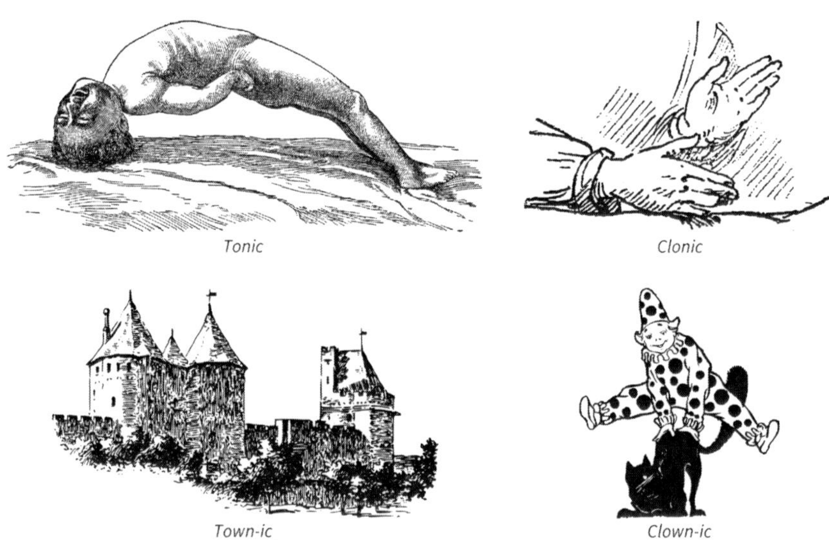

Tonic *Clonic*

Town-ic *Clown-ic*

A **generalized tonic-clonic seizure** involves an initial **loss of consciousness** accompanied by **widespread sustained contraction** (the **tonic phase**) followed by **rapid alternation between contraction and relaxation** (the **clonic phase**).

*During the **town**-ic phase the body is **stiff and rigid** like the walls of a town, while in the **clown**-ic phase the body is **shaking** like a hyperactive clown.*

Since generalized seizures cause excessive neuronal activity in all areas of the brain, muscles throughout the body are activated which can potentially lead to injury (such as biting of the tongue related to muscle contraction in the jaw). Urinary and fecal incontinence may also occur. Given how the entirety of both the brain and body are involved, generalized tonic-clonic seizures are almost always followed by a profound **postictal state**.

Some people may develop neurologic deficits following a seizure, including weakness or paralysis in the arms, legs, vocal cords, or eyes. This is known as **postictal paresis** (or Todd's paresis) and occurs in over 10% of seizure cases. These deficits are transient, lasting only a day or two at most.

TONIC SEIZURES

Some people have seizures involving only the tonic phase *without* an accompanying clonic phase. These are known as **tonic seizures.** (Interestingly, while *tonic* seizures without a *clonic* phase exist, *clonic* seizures without a *tonic* phase are exceedingly rare and are not considered to be a subtype of generalized seizures.) Tonic seizures are generally shorter than a tonic-clonic seizure (lasting less than 20 seconds), and there is not always a postictal period. However, due to the widespread muscle contraction and loss of consciousness, patients may still injure themselves if they fall.

MYOCLONIC SEIZURES

A **myoclonic seizure** involves a series of **repeated and uncontrollable jerks** in specific muscles. To understand better what this means, consider that hiccups are a good example of *non*-pathologic myoclonus! (It's also worth pointing out that myoclonus is *not* the same thing as clonus! *Clonus* is a series of repetitive *rhythmic* contractions alternating with relaxation that leads to shaking, while *myo*clonus is an *irregular* contraction of a muscle that appears as a jerk or a spasm.) To remember the definition of a myoclonic seizure, think of them as "my-old-clinic seizures." Why did you leave your old clinic and find a new one? Because the people there were a **bunch of jerks**!

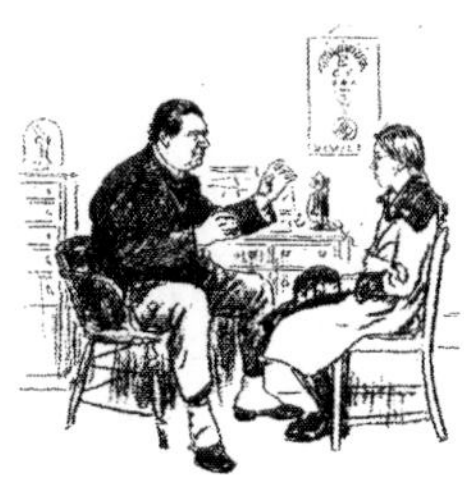

As with other forms of generalized seizures, myoclonic seizures are generally accompanied by a loss of consciousness, although given how quickly myoclonic seizures can pass, the loss of consciousness is not always noticed by others.

A **myoclonic seizure** involves a **series of uncontrollable jerks** in specific muscles.

I left ***my-old-clinic*** *because the people there were a* ***bunch of jerks****.*

ATONIC SEIZURES

In contrast to tonic, tonic-clonic, and myoclonic seizures (all of which involve *too much* muscle contraction), **atonic seizures** result in a sudden *loss* of muscle tone, leading the patient to pass out and fall (they are sometimes called "**drop attacks**" for this reason). Drop attacks are usually brief (lasting no more than a few seconds) but can occur without warning, resulting in injury. Because of how they present, atonic seizures can easily be confused for fainting. To remember the meaning of **ate**-onic seizures, think of the phrase "**ate** it" which is used to describe someone who fell (as in, "Dude, that guy totally **ate** it!")

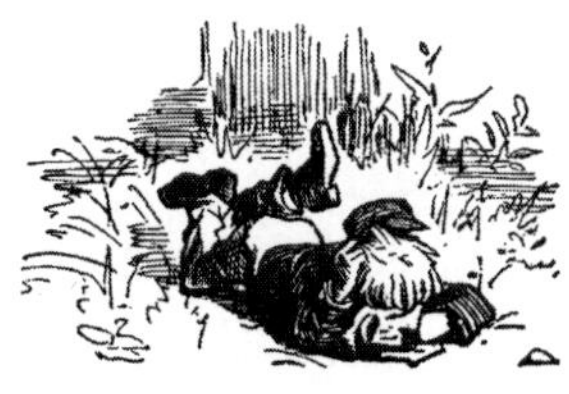

An **atonic seizure** involves a **sudden loss of muscle tone** which can lead to a fall.

*The phrase "****ate*** *it" describes someone who fell, so* ***ate****-onic seizures refer to the same.*

ABSENCE SEIZURES

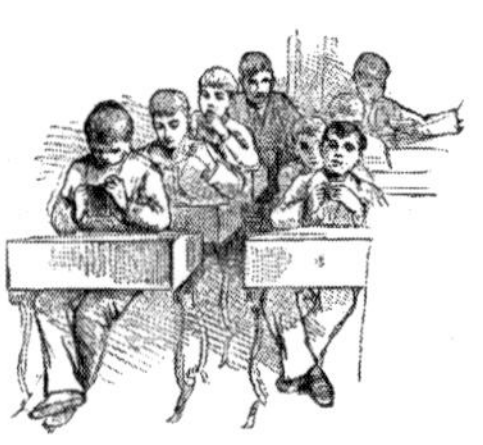

The last type of generalized seizure we will talk about is an **absence seizure** (formerly called a "petit mal" seizure). Like any generalized seizure, absence seizures involve a **sudden loss of consciousness**. However, unlike the other seizure types we have talked about so far, they are generally *not* associated with significant motor abnormalities. Instead, the only outward sign of an absence seizure may be a sudden change in the patient's level of consciousness. This may appear to others as a **blank stare**, a sudden break in the activity that they are doing, and/or a lack of responding to stimuli. Notably, absence seizures are also *not* associated with a postictal period. Really, absence seizures are **all about absence**: *absence* of mind, *absence* of a motor component, and *absence* of postictal period.

An **absence seizure** involves a **sudden loss of consciousness** with **no corresponding changes in muscle tone.**

Absence *seizures are* ***all about absence:***
Absence of ***mind,*** *absence of* ***motor component,*** *and absence of* ***postictal period.***

FOCAL SEIZURES

Focal (or focal-onset) seizures involve excessive activity in the brain leading to motor and other abnormalities. Unlike generalized seizures, however, they do *not* involve a loss of consciousness. While significantly less dramatic to witness, **focal seizures** are actually more common than generalized seizures, accounting for around 80% of seizures in people with epilepsy.

While focal seizures do not result in a total loss of consciousness, that is not to say that consciousness remains fully intact during an episode. This is because focal seizures can result in an *alteration* in consciousness even if they do not involve a complete *loss* of consciousness like in a generalized seizure. Seizures in which consciousness is altered but not completely lost are known as **focal-onset impaired-awareness seizures** (or "complex partial" seizures) and tend to manifest as a momentary change in memory or awareness. In contrast, seizures that do not result in *any* change in consciousness are known as **focal-onset aware seizures** (or "simple partial" seizures). We'll now go over both of these in more detail.

FOCAL-ONSET AWARE SEIZURES (SIMPLE PARTIAL)

Compared to generalized seizures, focal-onset aware seizures are much more variable in their presentation. This is because the specific location of the seizure activity in the brain can differ from person to person and even from seizure to seizure. For example, a seizure in the parietal lobe may cause sensory abnormalities such as numbness or tingling, while a seizure in the occipital lobe may instead lead to visual warping or even hallucinations. When seizure activity occurs in the motor cortex, it can cause movements ranging from slight twitching all the way to full-on muscle contractions. Even during a single seizure episode, the site of excessive activity can move within the brain. Abnormal movements often begin in one's extremities and then make their way up the arm and into the neck and face. This is known as a **Jacksonian march** (named after the neurologist who discovered them) and reflects the spreading wave of seizure activity in the brain. Unlike generalized tonic-clonic seizures, the patient remains fully awake and aware of what is happening to them. In addition, there is **no postictal period**, and the person typically has complete awareness and memory of the event.

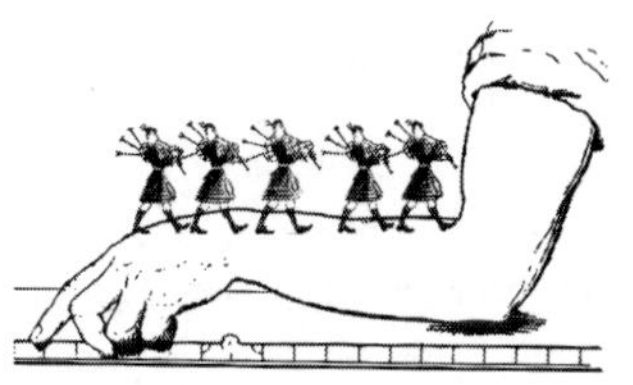

FOCAL-ONSET IMPAIRED-AWARENESS SEIZURES (COMPLEX PARTIAL)

While "focal-onset impaired-awareness seizure" is a mouthful to say, it really does describe what is going on during this type of seizure (although the older terminology of "complex partial seizure" is still used frequently as well). Like focal-onset aware seizures, focal-onset impaired-awareness seizures only involve a part of the brain, with the presenting signs and symptoms varying depending on what parts have been hit. Where focal-onset impaired-awareness seizures differentiate themselves is that they *impair* one's consciousness without fully *eliminating* it. The borderland between awareness and unconsciousness can be difficult to describe, but the patient often appears awake but does not respond to stimuli or engage in purposeful activities. Instead, their behavior often involves **automatisms** or pre-set motor "tasks" such as eye rolling, teeth clenching, lip smacking, or chewing that are more elaborate than a simple twitching or contraction of a single muscle but still fall short of fully purposeful behavior.

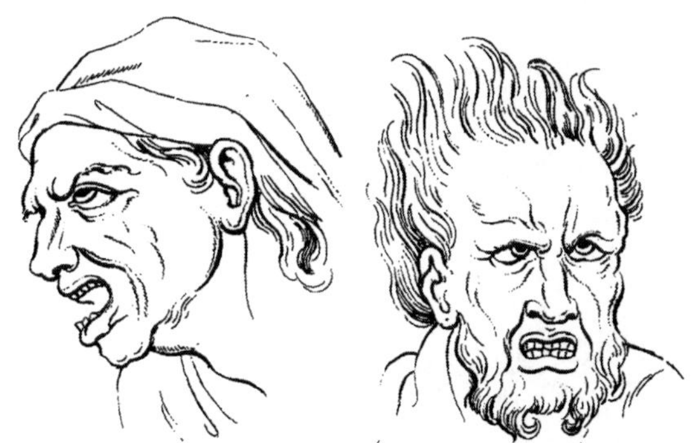

Automatisms *as seen during a* ***focal-onset impaired-awareness seizure****.*

Focal-onset impaired-awareness seizures tend to be **brief**, lasting only a minute or two. Because the behaviors involved appear normal (even if they are a bit odd for the situation, such as someone engaging in a chewing automatism with no food in their mouth), these seizures can at times be misdiagnosed as a psychiatric condition, especially when the patient appears confused during or after these events.

DIAGNOSIS AND TREATMENT OF SEIZURES

Now that we have built up a sizeable vocabulary with which we can describe seizures, we are ready to learn about how to diagnose and treat them. Seizures are **common**, with around 10% of people having had a seizure at some point in their lifetime. For those who have had at least one seizure, the chance of having another seizure increases to around 50%.

Seizures are not necessarily a disease in and of themselves, as the vast majority of seizures occur as the result of another condition. These are known as **symptomatic seizures**, and they do not necessarily require long-term treatment. (For example, most infants who have seizures as the result of a fever are not at risk of worse health outcomes, and treatment of the seizures themselves is generally not recommended.) The full list of medical conditions that can cause seizures is extensive and could likely fill a book of its own, but it includes everything from brain tumors and infections to drug intoxication and poor diet. (We'll cover a few of these in later chapters.)

Around a quarter of all people who have recurrent seizures appear to experience them with no clear cause. These people are said to have **epilepsy**. Someone with epilepsy can have multiple different seizure types or even switch from one to another over time. (For example, someone who first presents with focal-onset aware seizures may later develop generalized tonic-clonic seizures.) An initial diagnosis of epilepsy is often based on the clinical history, with a particular focus on ruling out potential causes such as infections or tumors that could be provoking them. A **seizure calendar** can be used to track the timing and location of seizures. An **electroencephalogram** (EEG) is often performed to provide an objective measure of brain activity, which can help to distinguish between different seizure types.

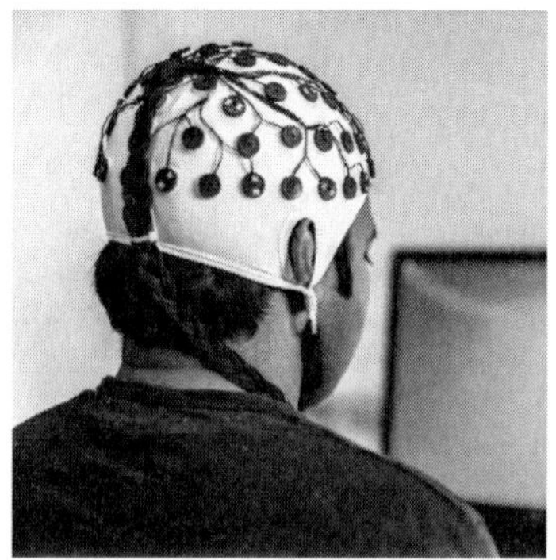

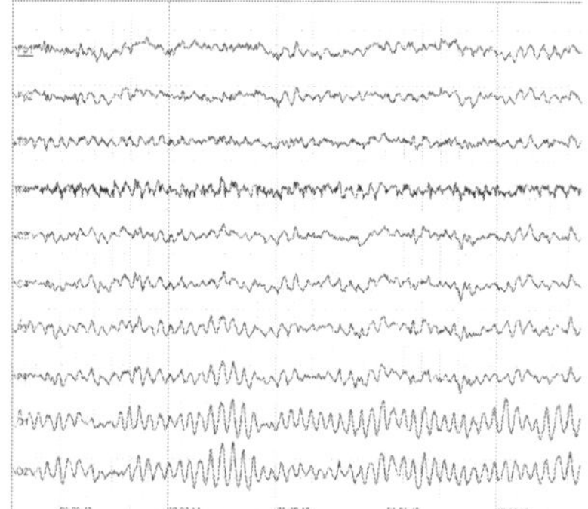

Someone undergoing ***electroencephalography*** *(left) with* ***normal resting state activity*** *seen (right).*

Treatment of epilepsy involves not only **acute management** of seizure activity but also **long-term prevention** of future episodes. Because most seizures are self-limited (lasting only a few minutes), immediate management of a seizure mostly involves simple safety measures such as placing the patient on their side to prevent aspiration. In cases of status epilepticus (where seizure activity continues for more than 5 minutes), pharmacologic interventions may be needed as well. The first-line treatment for status epilepticus is to use a **benzodiazepine**, a class of central nervous system depressants that helps to rapidly abort a seizure episode.

For long-term prevention of seizures, a class of drugs known as **anticonvulsants** is used. Many anticonvulsants work by either directly or indirectly inhibiting the ion channels that help neurons to fire, reducing their ability to generate and transmit an electrical signal (kind of like throwing water on dry brush to make it less likely to catch fire). Anticonvulsants are generally effective, with around 70% of people becoming seizure-free as long as they stay on the medication. There are many anticonvulsant medications available, with some of the most common ones being valproate, levetiracetam, carbamazepine, oxcarbazepine, lamotrigine, phenytoin, ethosuximide, lacosamide, gabapentin, pregabalin, topiramate, and zonisamide. Choosing between these drugs depends on a lot of factors, including which types of seizures are present. As a general rule, **valproate** is the most broad-spectrum anticonvulsant available, so if you are unsure of what to pick, this is a reasonable guess! (A major exception to this is if the patient is pregnant, as valproate is a known teratogen and can cause spinal cord defects in the fetus.)

Outside of medications, make sure to consider **psychosocial interventions** as well, including stress reduction, sleep hygiene, and both psychological and behavioral therapies. In addition, consider whether someone who has had a seizure should be engaging in driving or other activities where a sudden loss of consciousness could lead to major harm.

EPILEPSY SYNDROMES

Once the pattern of seizure activity is clear, the next step in diagnosing epilepsy is to determine whether the recurrent seizures fit any known patterns that might help to differentiate them from other forms of epilepsy. Cases that involve specific and consistent combinations of signs and symptoms are known as **epilepsy syndromes**. Diagnosing an epilepsy syndrome has important implications for both prognosis and treatment. While there are dozens of epilepsy syndromes, we will limit our discussion to the most high-yield ones that you are most likely to encounter on boards and on wards. Most epilepsy syndromes begin in childhood, although we will cover some that begin in adulthood as well.

TEMPORAL LOBE EPILEPSY

The most common syndrome leading to recurrent focal seizures is **temporal lobe epilepsy**. Of note, the *medial* temporal lobe (near the amygdala, hippocampus, and other parts of limbic system) is most often affected, with only 20% of cases involving the outer cortex. For this reason, seizures in the temporal lobe often present as **memory or mood changes**, including amnesia, sudden feelings of fear, rapid swings in emotion, flashbacks to old memories, and/or feelings of *déjà vu*. Hallucinations can occur, although they are rarely auditory (which makes sense, as hearing takes place in the *outer* cortex while temporal lobe epilepsy tends to hit more *medial* structures). Instead, hallucinations generally take the form of distinct odors and smells (known as **olfactory hallucinations**). Because the motor strip in the frontal lobe is not involved, there is no tonic-clonic component unless if the seizure secondarily generalizes.

For those with onset of temporal lobe seizures in childhood, many will stop having them by adulthood. People who continue to experience temporal lobe seizures may have **mesial temporal sclerosis** or damage in their temporal lobe that is identifiable on neuroimaging as seen below:

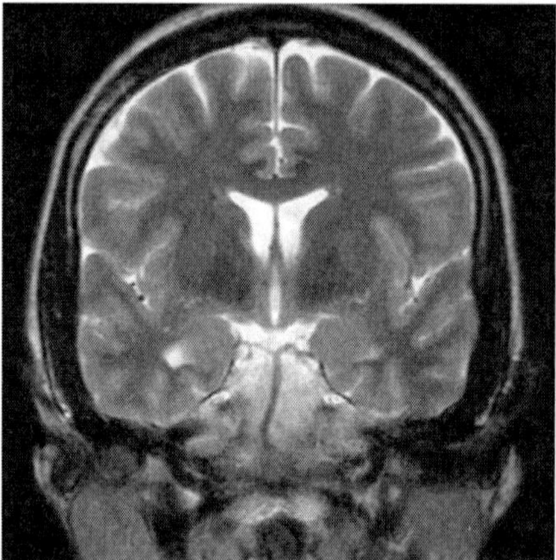

*MRI showing **mesial temporal sclerosis**.*

FRONTAL LOBE EPILEPSY

The frontal lobe is the second most common site of recurrent focal seizures. Because you know the function of this lobe already, you can predict what sorts of signs and symptoms you might see! Due to the location of the motor cortex in the frontal lobe, frontal lobe seizures tend to involve **abnormal movements** including twisting, turning, grimacing, tics, body posturing, and rocking. In around one-third of cases, a tumor in the frontal lobe is the culprit.

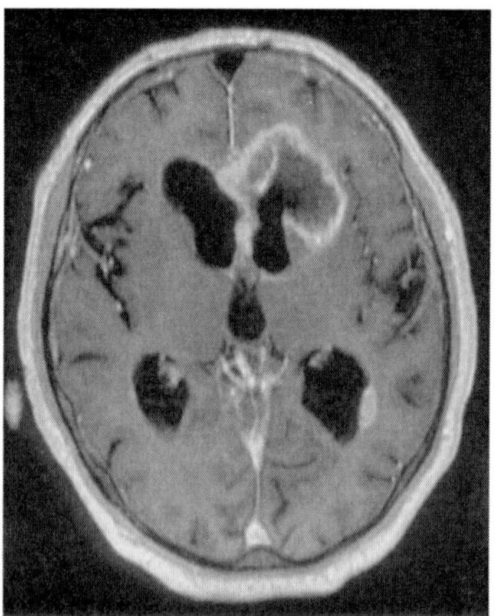

*A **brain tumor** is a common cause of **frontal lobe epilepsy**.*

BENIGN ROLANDIC EPILEPSY

Benign Rolandic epilepsy is the most common epilepsy syndrome in **childhood**, affecting 15% of all children with epilepsy. Benign Rolandic epilepsy is characterized by infrequent **focal aware seizures** that manifest as a wide variety of experiences, including tingling sensations, grunting noises, and impaired speech. These seizures tend to last only a minute or two at most, although they may at times secondarily generalize to a full tonic-clonic seizure. Seizures typically occur at night without interrupting the child's ability to function (as suggested by the "benign" in the name).

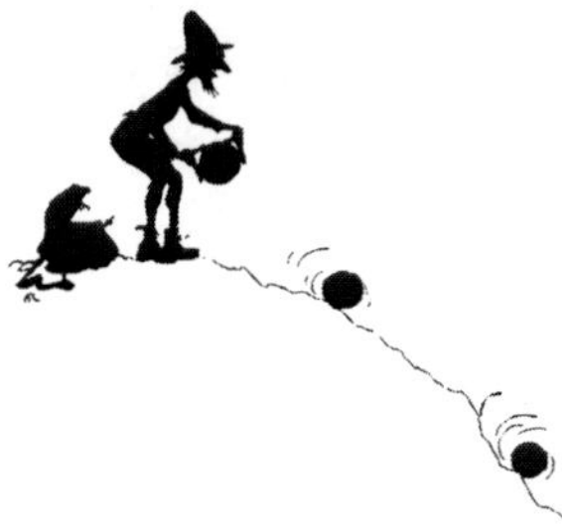

EEG will show **centrotemporal spikes** which are characteristic of this syndrome. Due to the infrequent and non-impairing nature of these seizures, treatment is often not necessary, and many children will outgrow it by adolescence. You can remember benign **Roll**-andic epilepsy by thinking of the acronym **FAST ROLL** which stands for **F**ocal **A**ware **S**eizures **T**hat **R**arely **O**utlast **L**ater **L**ife. The **Roll** of **Roll**-andic can also help you to remember the centrotempo-**Roll** spikes that are seen on EEG.

Benign Rolandic epilepsy is the most common form of epilepsy in **childhood**. It involves **focal aware seizures** and generally **does not require treatment**.

***FAST ROLL**: **F**ocal **A**ware **S**eizures **T**hat **R**arely **O**utlast **L**ater **L**ife.*

*Benign **Roll**-andic epilepsy should remind you of centrotempo-**Roll** spikes on EEG.*

JUVENILE MYOCLONIC EPILEPSY

Juvenile myoclonic epilepsy is a common epilepsy syndrome that involves **sudden involuntary irregular muscle contractions** (remember that "my-old-clinic was a bunch of jerks") beginning in late childhood or adolescence. These contractions tend to involve the arms and occur in the transition between sleep and wakefulness, although other triggers may include flashing lights or loud sounds. Many people who have juvenile myoclonic epilepsy also have other seizure forms as well, including absence seizures and generalized tonic-clonic seizures. **Valproate** is the most commonly used medication treatment (remember: if you're ever unsure about which anticonvulsant to pick, valproate is probably your best bet!).

CHILDHOOD ABSENCE EPILEPSY

Childhood absence epilepsy is another common form of epilepsy (accounting for around 10% of childhood cases) that is characterized by the presence of **recurrent absence seizures**. Absence seizures can occur several or even dozens of times per day. However, because the sudden losses of consciousness come and go so quickly, it is often diagnosed as mere inattention or even attention deficit hyperactivity disorder (ADHD). For this reason, thorough history taking is key for correctly identifying this condition.

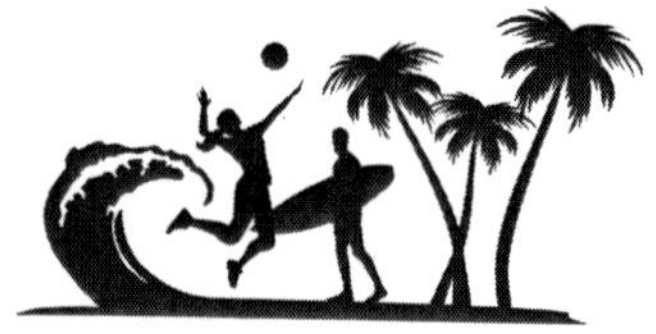

Absence seizures can often be provoked through **hyperventilation**, which can be a useful diagnostic test. Another key finding supporting a diagnosis of absence seizures is the presence of a fast (3 Hz) **spike-and-wave** pattern on EEG. You can remember this by thinking of some students who decide to skip school (resulting in their **absence**) and go to the beach to play volleyball ("**Spike**!") and surf the **waves**.

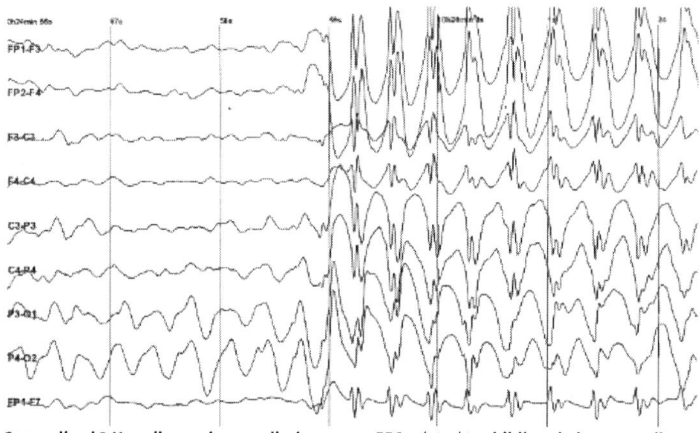

***Generalized 3 Hz spike-and-wave discharges** on EEG related to **childhood absence epilepsy**.*

Childhood absence epilepsy presents as **recurrent brief losses of consciousness.** EEG will show a **3 Hz spike-and-wave** pattern.

*Think of some students who decide to be **absent** from school so they can go to the beach to play volleyball ("**Spike!**") and surf the **waves**.*

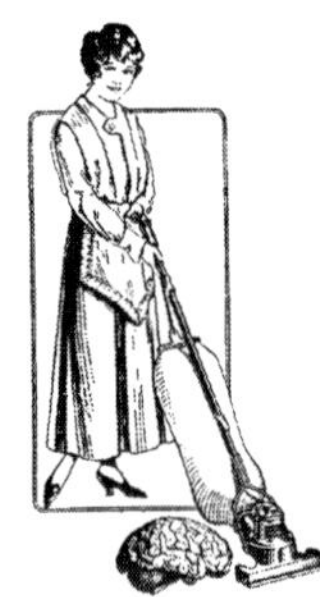

A specific anticonvulsant known as **ethosuximide** is very effective for treating absence seizures (although unfortunately not as good for other kinds of seizures). You can remember the association of absence seizures with ethosuximide by thinking of it as etho-**sucks-the-mind**, as an absence seizure *sucks* thoughts out of the mind like a vacuum, leading to the blank mind and blank stare that are characteristic of these episodes. With etho-**sucks-the-mind**, absence seizures can't do that anymore. In cases where someone has both absence *and* other forms of seizures, you could consider a more broad-spectrum anticonvulsant like valproate.

Absence seizures can be treated with **ethosuximide** or **valproate**.

*With etho-**sucks-the-mind**, absence seizures won't **suck the mind** anymore.*

LENNOX-GASTAUT SYNDROME

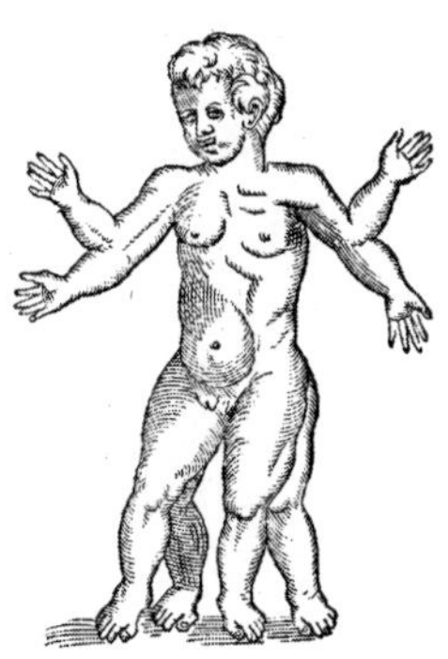

Lennox-Gastaut syndrome is a rare but severe form of epilepsy that is characterized by a core triad of **seizures**, **intellectual disability**, and **specific EEG findings**. Almost all cases of Lennox-Gastaut syndrome begin in **early childhood** (before the age of 5), although the vast majority of patients continue to have seizures into adulthood. Most cases occur as a direct result of damage to the brain (such as brain infections, tumors, and trauma), although one-third occur with no known trigger. You can remember the key clinical features of this disease using the mnemonic "**LeGS & ARMS**" to remember that **Le**nnox-**G**astaut **S**yndrome causes:

A is for All types of seizures. Seizures in Lennox-Gastaut syndrome can take many different forms, with the most common being **tonic-only seizures** (which are normally quite rare). These seizures often occur on a daily basis.

R is for Resistant to treatment. Seizures related to Lennox-Gastaut syndrome are incredibly difficult to treat, with anticonvulsants being much less effective than in other forms of epilepsy.

M is for Mental disabilities. Patients with Lennox-Gastaut syndrome have intellectual disabilities which can limit their ability to function.

S is for Slow spike-and-wave discharges. EEG will show characteristic **spike-and-wave discharges**. (Remember that spike-and-wave discharges are also seen in absence seizures! While the pattern is the same, it tends to be slower in Lennox-Gastaut syndrome, typically less than 3 Hz.)

Many patients with Lennox-Gastaut syndrome don't show all of these features immediately, with the full pattern often emerging only a few years after the first seizure. Lennox-Gastaut syndrome is associated with a poor prognosis, with around 5% of patients dying within 10 years of the diagnosis.

Lennox-Gastaut syndrome is a rare form of epilepsy characterized by **multiple seizure types**, **intellectual disability**, and **slow spike-and-wave discharges** on EEG.

__LeGS__ & __ARMS__:
__Le__nnox-__G__astaut __S__yndrome
__A__ll types of seizures
__R__esistant to treatment
__M__ental disabilities
__S__low (<3 Hz) spike-and-wave discharges on EEG

PSYCHOGENIC NON-EPILEPTIC SEIZURES

It is estimated that up to 20% of all patients who come to clinics reporting seizures do not have epilepsy but instead have **psychogenic non-epileptic seizures** (PNES). This term is used to describe seizure-like episodes that are *not* linked to any abnormal electrical activity in the brain. The name "psychogenic" underscores that many of these cases occur in the context of severe life stress, maladaptive patterns, and other findings that suggest a psychological origin.

A few signs are common in PNES but very *un*common in generalized tonic-clonic seizures and are therefore high-yield to know! You can remember these using the mnemonic **2 minute RAGES**:

2 minutes. Psychogenic non-epileptic seizures often last more than 2 minutes, which is rare in epilepsy outside of the context of status epilepticus.

R is for Recall. Being able to recall events that happened during an episode is unusual in generalized tonic-clonic seizures due to the loss of consciousness that occurs.

A is for Asynchronous movements. Movements involving different muscle groups moving in different directions (like someone bicycling) are uncommon in epilepsy.

G is for Gradual. Given that most epileptic seizures occur suddenly, a gradual onset of seizure activity is more characteristic of PNES.

E is for Eyes. Eyes generally remain open during an epileptic seizure, so eyes that are closed or crying should clue you in to PNES.

S is for Side-to-side head shaking. This is common in PNES but rare in epilepsy.

Most patients with this condition do not intentionally "fake" seizures and may even be unaware that these episodes are non-epileptic. If you suspect that a patient is experiencing PNES, take their impairment and distress seriously while trying to avoid anticonvulsants, many of which are associated with some pretty major side effects (remember to "do no harm"). Instead, consider a referral to more helpful forms of treatment including **psychological and behavioral therapies**.

Psychogenic non-epileptic seizures are episodes of shaking that are related to **psychosocial factors** rather than excessive electrical activity in the brain.

2 minute RAGES:
2 minutes *or more*
R*ecall of events*
A*synchronous movements*
G*radual onset*
E*yes (closed or crying)*
S*ide-to-side head shaking*

PUTTING IT ALL TOGETHER

Even for an experienced clinician, seizures can be complicated to diagnose and treat. Rather than get lost in the complexity, take a systematic approach to evaluating seizures both on tests and when seeing patients in a clinical setting! The mnemonic **CAPPELLA** can help to clue you in to the right diagnosis:

C is for Consciousness. Whether the patient loses consciousness, has impaired consciousness, or retains full consciousness helps to distinguish between generalized, focal-onset impaired-awareness, and focal-onset aware seizures, respectively.

A is for Activity. Look at the specific kinds of motor activity present (tonic, clonic, myoclonic, or atonic). A lack of motor activity suggests absence or focal seizures.

P is for Postictal state. Most generalized tonic-clonic seizures are followed by a postictal state. If there is no postictal period, it may suggest a different etiology.

P is for Provoked. Whether the seizure was provoked by a medical condition, an external trigger (such as loud sounds or flashing lights), or came entirely out of the blue matters for the final diagnosis.

E is for EEG findings. Specific findings on EEG are suggestive of specific types of seizures (such as 3 Hz spike-and-wave patterns being suggestive of an absence seizure or centrotemporal spikes being characteristic of Benign Rolandic epilepsy).

L is for Localizing symptoms. Specific symptoms that occur around the time of a seizure can help to localize the precise location of seizure activity in the brain (like olfactory hallucinations suggesting temporal lobe epilepsy).

L is for Labs and imaging. While not required in every case, labs and brain imaging can help to rule out brain tumors, infections, or other possible causes of seizures.

A is for Age of onset. While most causes of epilepsy begin in childhood, some (such as temporal lobe epilepsy) are also seen in adults.

A **systematic approach** to evaluating **seizures** leads to a more accurate diagnosis.

***CAPPELLA**:*
***C**onsciousness*
***A**ctivity*
***P**ostictal state*
***P**rovoked*
***E**EG findings*
***L**ocalizing symptoms*
***L**abs and imaging*
***A**ge of onset*

REVIEW QUESTIONS

1. An 18 y/o M is brought to the emergency department after falling in a grocery store. His mother reports that while they were out shopping he suddenly began to look "distant." She then saw his eyes roll back in his head before he fell to the ground. Initially his back was arched, with outward rolling of his wrists. However, within several seconds he began shaking across his entire body. His mother called 911, and an ambulance arrived 5 minutes later. At the time of arrival to the hospital, he continues to convulse. Vital signs are HR 138, BP 132/88, RR 24, and T 100.1°F. His oxygen saturation is 97%. Which of the following is the best next step in management?
   A. Ordering a 24-hour electroencephalography
   B. Ordering a CT scan of the brain
   C. Ordering an MRI of the brain
   D. Administering valproate, an anticonvulsant
   E. Administering lorazepam, a benzodiazepine
   F. Immediate endotracheal intubation

2. A 23 y/o M presents to a neurology clinic for "staring spells" that have gradually worsened over the past few months. He describes these episodes as "blacking out" with no memory of what happens during the spell. Friends who have observed these episodes report that he will smack his lips and pull at his shirt repeatedly. Prior to each episode he experiences a "rising feeling" along with an "odd smell, kind of like burnt rubber." He also describes having a sense of *déjà vu* before each episode, saying, "I get this overwhelming feeling that this has all somehow happened before. I can't explain it any better than that." Following these episodes he typically is "confused and out of it" for up to half an hour. Seizure activity is most likely to be localized to which of the following structures?

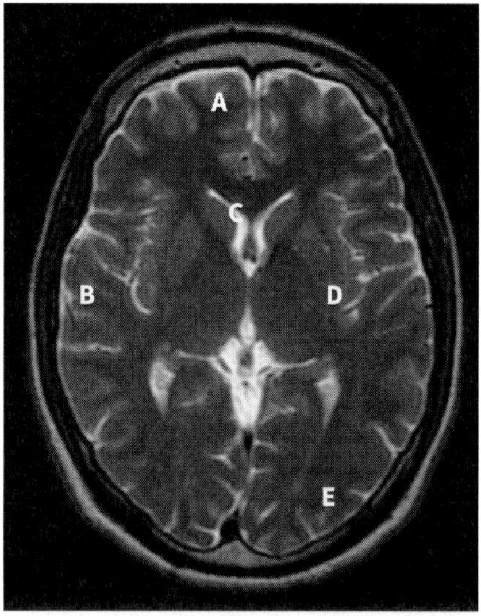

3. A 7 y/o F is brought to a child psychiatrist for evaluation of possible attention deficit hyperactivity disorder. Over the past 6 months, she has been struggling at school, and her teacher has requested that she undergo a full psychiatric evaluation. Her teacher's report notes that she regularly "spaces out" during class and has difficulty paying attention to the subject matter. These episodes last for around 10 seconds at a time and happen dozens of times a day. There is no loss of consciousness or abnormal movements observed before, during, or after these episodes. Electroencephalography demonstrates generalized spike-and-wave discharges at 3 Hz. Which of the following is the best next step in management?
    A. Starting methylphenidate, a stimulant used to treat ADHD
    B. Starting amphetamine salts, a stimulant used to treat ADHD
    C. Starting clonazepam, a benzodiazepine used to treat seizures
    D. Starting lamotrigine, an anticonvulsant used to treat seizures
    E. Starting ethosuximide, an anticonvulsant used to treat seizures
    F. None of the above

4. A 22 y/o F is brought to the hospital after a seizure that was witnessed by her husband. She has a history of epilepsy beginning in her teenage years for which she is taking valproate. Since starting this medication 5 years ago, she has not had any further seizures until today. Upon arriving to the emergency department, she has another seizure lasting for 10 minutes. During this time, her body is seen shaking. Her fists are clenched, and her toes are curled. Her eyes are shut tight, and she is shaking her head back and forth. After the episode ends, she is unresponsive to questions for 90 minutes, though she does withdraw from deep pressure applied to her fingernail beds. Physical exam reveals no injuries to the inside of her mouth or evidence of incontinence. Laboratory analysis is unrevealing except for a positive urine pregnancy test. A 24-hour EEG shows no abnormal activity. Which of the following is the best next step?
    A. Stopping valproate
    B. Adding a second anticonvulsant
    C. Adding a benzodiazepine
    D. Discharging the patient immediately
    E. Increasing the dose of valproate

1. **The best answer is E.** This patient is in a state of status epilepticus, as he has been having continuous seizure activity for more than 5 minutes. The first-line treatment for status epilepticus is use of a benzodiazepine, as these medications are effective at rapidly lowering neuronal activity and quickly aborting a seizure. Valproate may be indicated in the future for prevention of additional seizures but does not have a role in immediate management of status epilepticus (answer D). Additional diagnostic studies such as electroencephalography or neuroimaging are important but do not take precedence over treating status epilepticus, which is a medical emergency (answers A—C). Endotracheal intubation is needed in some cases of status epilepticus, but this patient's intact oxygenation level shows good circulatory function at this time (answer F).

2. **The best answer is D.** This vignette describes a prototypical case of temporal lobe seizures with automatisms and olfactory hallucinations. The presence of *déjà vu* also suggests involvement of the hippocampus, which is located on the inner aspect of the temporal lobe. Less than 20% of temporal lobe seizures involve the outer cortex, so cortical structures are less likely to be involved (answers A, B, and E). The lateral ventricles are not made of nervous tissue and therefore cannot be the origin of abnormal electrical activity (answer C).

3. **The best answer is E.** Absence seizures are characterized by the absence of several features that are commonly seen in tonic-clonic seizures such as noticeable convulsions or a postictal period. They are instead defined by recurrent brief episodes of lapsed consciousness and a characteristic spike-and-wave pattern on electroencephalography. The primary treatment for absence seizures is an anticonvulsant that has efficacy at T-type calcium channels, including ethosuximide and valproate. Other anticonvulsants, such as lamotrigine, that do not interact with this type of calcium channel will not be effective (answer D). Benzodiazepines are primarily used for treating an ongoing seizure rather than as prophylaxis (answer C). Starting a stimulant when there is no clear evidence of attention deficit hyperactivity disorder is unlikely to help (answers A and B).

4. **The best answer is A.** Several features of this patient's presentation are highly suggestive of psychogenic non-epileptic seizures, including a seizure duration greater than 2 minutes, head shaking, and lack of incontinence or unintentional injury. While she may have a history of epileptic seizures as well, it is not uncommon for someone presenting with psychogenic non-epileptic seizures to also have a history of epileptic seizures. The first priority should be stopping valproate given valproate's teratogenic effects, not increasing the dose (answer E). Adding another medication in the absence of clear seizure activity is not indicated (answers B and C). In cases of suspected psychogenic non-epileptic seizures, arranging for immediate discharge of a patient is not helpful (answer D). Instead, a discussion should be had regarding the diagnosis and the reasons why the treatment team feels that other forms of treatment such as psychological or behaviorally therapy may be more necessary at this time.

21 NEOPLASMS

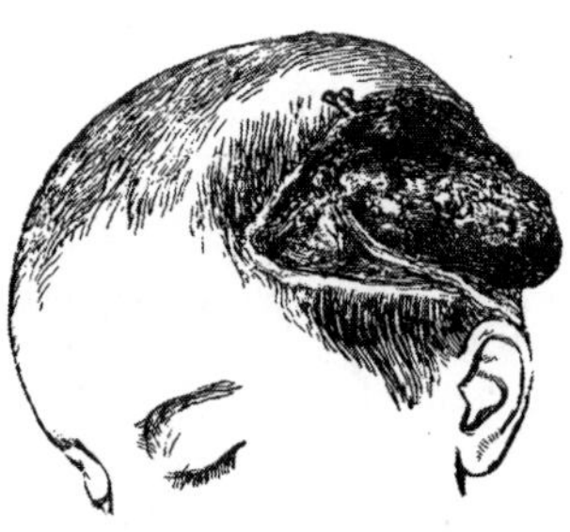

A **neoplasm** refers to any abnormal and excessive growth of tissue, including various forms of **cancer**. Neoplasms can occur in organs all across the body, and the nervous system is no exception. While any tumor can be frightening, when it grows in a vital organ like the brain, it can be particularly devastating. Cancers of the nervous system are also notoriously difficult to treat, as it is much harder to remove cancerous tissue from the brain than it is to excise it from a more peripheral organ.

When discussing neoplasms of the nervous system, it is helpful to first review some vocabulary. Most central nervous system cancers present as a **tumor** or a focal area of unregulated cell growth. However, it's important to point out that not all tumors are necessarily cancerous! Some tumors are **benign**, meaning that they are growing only within a localized area and have not invaded surrounding tissues. In contrast, **malignant** tumors have begun to spread outside of their initial area and are now invading nearby tissues. Only *malignant* tumors are considered to be **cancer**. A malignant tumor that spreads to another distal location (such as a liver tumor that spreads to the brain) is said to have **metastasized**.

It's also worth specifically pointing out that just because a tumor is *in* the brain doesn't mean it's *from* the brain! Tumors in the nervous system can either be **primary** (originating from nervous tissue) or **secondary** (a metastasis from a tumor originating in a different organ). In fact, secondary tumors make up around 50% of all tumors in the brain, so they are far from a rare entity! On the other hand, primary brain tumors themselves rarely metastasize to other organs.

DIAGNOSIS AND TREATMENT OF BRAIN TUMORS

The signs and symptoms associated with nervous system tumors can be divided into **focal and generalized symptoms**. Focal symptoms are related to the tumor's **mass effect** or its ability cause damage by impinging upon nearby structures. Luckily, your existing knowledge of neuroanatomy can help to guide you here! For example, a tumor in the frontal lobe may cause disinhibited behavior, a tumor in the parietal lobe may cause sensory abnormalities, a tumor in the occipital lobe may lead to changes in vision, and so on.

Aside from these focal findings, brain tumors can also cause generalized signs and symptoms as well. Recall from Chapter 15 that there are three ways to increase intracranial pressure: increasing the amount of blood, increasing the amount of cerebrospinal fluid, or increasing the amount of nervous tissue. A tumor in the brain does the third thing, so signs and symptoms of **intracranial hypertension** are often seen. **Headaches** are the most common presenting symptom, with **seizures** coming in second place (especially in an older adult who has never had a seizure before). **Papilledema** can often be seen on exam as well.

In addition to a full neurological exam, diagnosing a brain tumor generally relies upon **neuroimaging** to definitively demonstrate the presence of a tumor. In fact, in some cases brain tumors do not cause signs and symptoms at all, so the only way they get diagnosed is as an incidental finding when imaging is ordered for another reason (such as someone who is in a car accident and gets a CT scan done which reveals a previously undiscovered brain tumor).

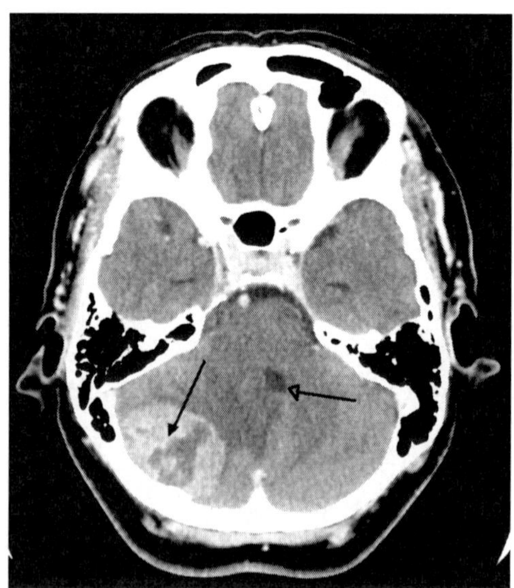

***Mass effect** caused by a tumor in the **posterior fossa**.*

Once the presence of a tumor has been established, a **biopsy** (or a sample of brain tissue that has been surgically removed for examination under a microscope) is needed to determine if the tumor is primary or secondary, benign or malignant, and other characteristics which have important implications for prognosis and treatment.

As with other forms of cancer, there is no single "correct" treatment for a brain tumor. The three mainstays of cancer treatment are **surgery**, **radiation**, and/or **chemotherapy**. The decision on which type of treatment to use is informed by the specific kind of neoplasm present and whether it is localized or metastasized (with surgery often being more effective when the tumor has not yet metastasized and is still largely confined to one place).

With these principles in mind, we are ready to look at the specific types of tumors that can occur in the brain. We will first talk about adult-onset tumors before moving on to discuss childhood-onset tumors. To keep our focus squarely on what is the most high-yield, we will limit our discussion to the **five most common tumors** in each age group.

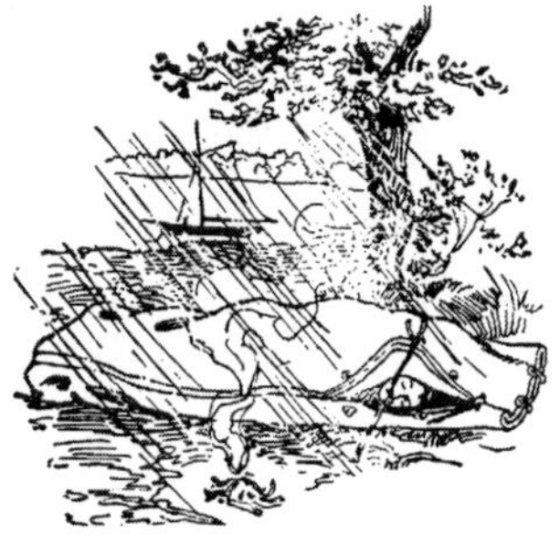

As a general rule of thumb, brain tumors in children are often **infratentorial** (meaning that they grow *below* the "hammock-like" tentorium cerebelli separating the cerebellum from the cerebral cortex that we talked about back in Chapter 12). In contrast, brain tumors in adults tend to be **supratentorial**. This is not a hard and fast rule, but it is accurate enough to provide some guidance! To remember this, think about what would happen if a storm struck while a family was out camping. The adults will try to protect the children by getting them *under* the tent (*infra*-**tent**-orial) while bravely staying *outside* of the tent themselves to weather the storm (*supra*-**tent**-orial).

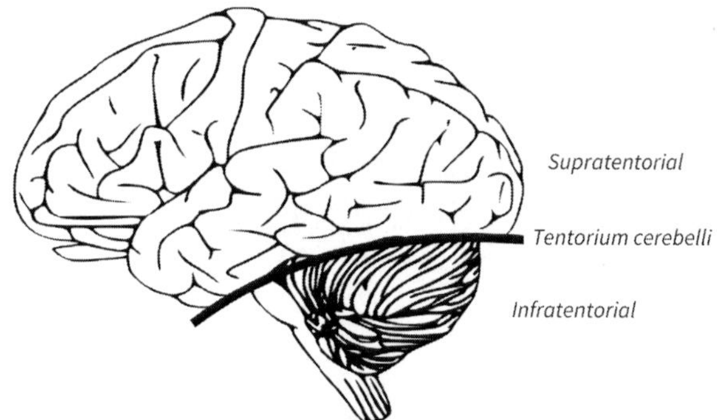

***Supratentorial tumors** are more common in **adults**, while **infratentorial tumors** are more common in **children**.*

As a general rule of thumb, **brain tumors** in **adults** tend to be **supratentorial** while those in **children** tend to be **infratentorial**.

*If a storm hits while a family is out camping, the adults will try to protect the **children** by getting them **under the tent** (infra-**tent**-orial).*

ADULT-ONSET BRAIN TUMORS

In this section, we will cover five adult-onset brain tumors in order from most common to least common. As we go through the rest of this chapter, pay attention to specific **buzzwords** that you would do well to associate with each tumor type!

GLIOBLASTOMA MULTIFORME

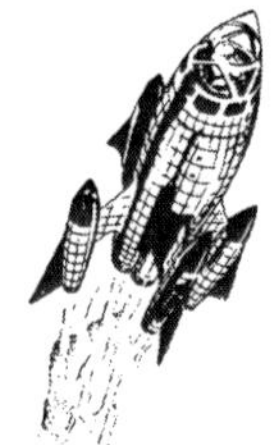

Glioblastoma multiforme (often abbreviated GBM) is the **most common** primary brain tumor in adults, making up 15% of all cases. As with most brain tumors, there are no signs or symptoms that are specific to glioblastoma multiforme. Instead, many patients present with vague or non-specific symptoms like headaches, nausea, seizures, unexplained focal neurologic deficits, or even no symptoms at all. Once symptoms do appear, they tend to progress quickly in severity, as glioblastoma multiforme is a very **fast-growing cancer**. Accordingly, it often has a **poor prognosis**, and most patients who are diagnosed with this disease will live only around one year. You can remember the rapidly-growing nature of glio**blast**oma multiforme by thinking of a speedy rocket **blast**ing off into space.

Glioblastoma multiforme is a **rapidly-growing tumor** with a **poor prognosis**.

*Glio**blast**oma is fast like a rocket **blast**ing off into space.*

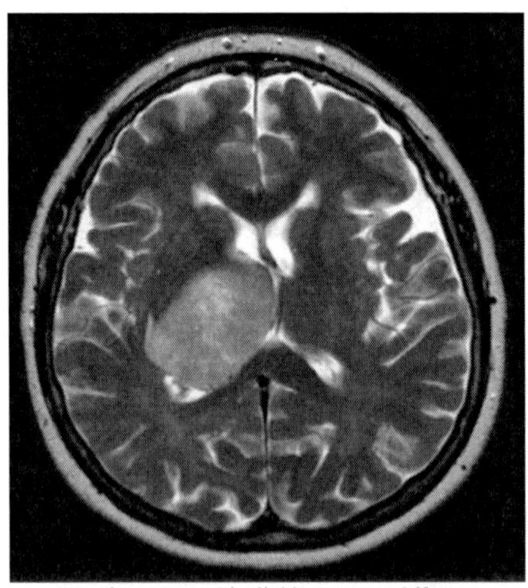

*MRI of a patient with **glioblastoma multiforme**.*

Glioblastoma multiforme is diagnosed more often in **men** than women, with an average age of 65 years. Cases of glioblastoma multiforme can either occur "out of the blue" (a **primary** glioblastoma) or can grow from a pre-cancerous lesion (a **secondary** glioblastoma). Primary and secondary glioblastomas have very different prognoses and treatment responses, so making this distinction via biopsy is important.

To recognize glioblastoma multiforme on test questions, you should be on the lookout for a few buzzwords. First, serum levels of a specific protein known as **G**lial **F**ibrillary **A**cidic **P**rotein (or **GFAP**) are often elevated in patients with glioblastoma multiforme, making this a helpful diagnostic marker with very high specificity. Second, when looked at under a microscope, glioblastoma multiforme appears as areas of **pseudopalisading necrosis** in which tumor cells surround central areas of necrosis. Finally, if the tumor grows large enough that it crosses the corpus callosum, it can have a symmetrical butterfly-like appearance on brain imaging (sometimes called a "**butterfly glioma**"). To associate **G**lio**B**lastoma **M**ultiforme with elevated serum levels of **G**FAP, a **B**utterfly glioma appearance on neuroimaging, and a predilection for older **M**en, pack those three ideas into the initials **GBM** themselves!

Glioblastoma multiforme is diagnosed most often in **older men**. Serum levels of **GFAP** are typically **elevated**. Neuroimaging can show a "**butterfly glioma**" pattern.

__G__lio__B__lastoma __M__ultiforme = __G__FAP + __B__utterfly glioma + __M__ale predominance.

MENINGIOMA

A **meningioma** is a tumor that arises from the **meninges** wrapping around the brain. It is the second most common form of brain tumor in adults. It often grows either in the central falx cerebri or along the surface the brain between the brain and the skull. On imaging, the tumor is usually **well circumscribed** with clearly demarcated borders as in the image below:

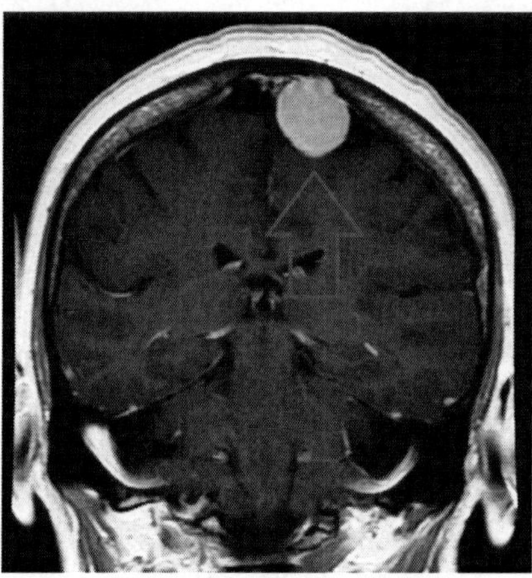

MRI of a patient with a __meningioma__.

Meningiomas are diagnosed twice as often in **women** than men. This is because many meningiomas express **estrogen receptors**, so the higher levels of circulating estrogen in women put them at higher risk. In contrast to the aggressive nature of glioblastoma multiforme, meningiomas are often **benign** and slow-growing. In fact, most cases don't even need to be treated unless if they become symptomatic! Meningiomas that grow large enough to be bothersome can be effectively treated with

surgery, as they are a highly **resectable** tumor with a low recurrence rate. While most meningiomas are relatively benign, a small percentage (roughly 10%) are more invasive and aggressive.

As with glioblastoma multiforme, there are a few buzzwords to know here. First, meningiomas have a **whorled appearance** when viewed under a microscope:

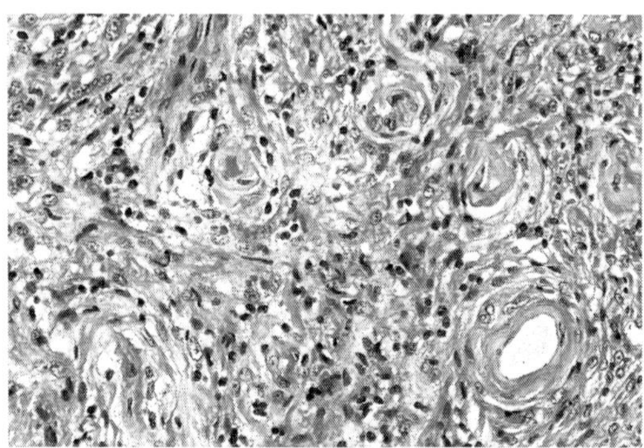

Microscope image of a ***meningioma*** *showing a* ***whorled appearance****.*

Meningiomas also have a tendency to calcify and form **psammoma bodies** or rounded collections of calcified tissue. (Notably, psammoma bodies are *not* specific to meningiomas and can be found in a variety of other conditions as well!)

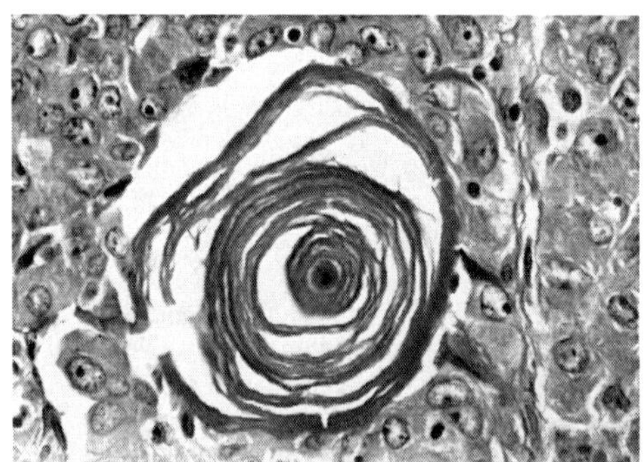

Microscope image of a ***meningioma*** *showing a* ***psammoma body****.*

You can remember the important associations with **men**ingiomas by thinking of some **men**'s names: **Sam** (for "p**sam**moma bodies") and **Ben** (for **ben**ign prognosis). Most men have a romantic predilection for women, so it shouldn't surprise us that **men**ingiomas have a preference for women as well!

Meningiomas are **slow-growing tumors** of the **meninges** with a relatively **good prognosis**. Due to **estrogen sensitivity**, they are more common in **women** than men.

*When you see "**men**ingioma," think of **men**'s names (**Sam** for "p**sam**moma bodies" and **Ben** for **ben**ign prognosis). Men also have a **preference for women**!*

SCHWANNOMA

Schwannomas are neoplasms of **Schwann cells** or the support cells that myelinate peripheral nerves. Schwannomas are generally slow-growing and **benign**, with only 1% becoming malignant. However, they can still cause problems in the nerve that is being myelinated!

The most common location for schwannomas is in the **vestibulocochlear nerve** where they can cause unilateral **sensorineural hearing loss**, tinnitus, poor balance, and vertigo. As the tumor grows, it may begin to impact the nearby **facial and trigeminal nerves** (causing loss of motor function and/or sensation in the face) as well as the **cerebellum** (resulting in ipsilateral ataxia).

Schwannomas are **highly resectable**, and surgery is generally quite successful at removing the tumor. This is because schwannomas tend to "stay in their lane" rather than messily mixing in with surrounding tissues, making surgical removal relatively simple (well, as simple as brain surgery can be, anyway!).

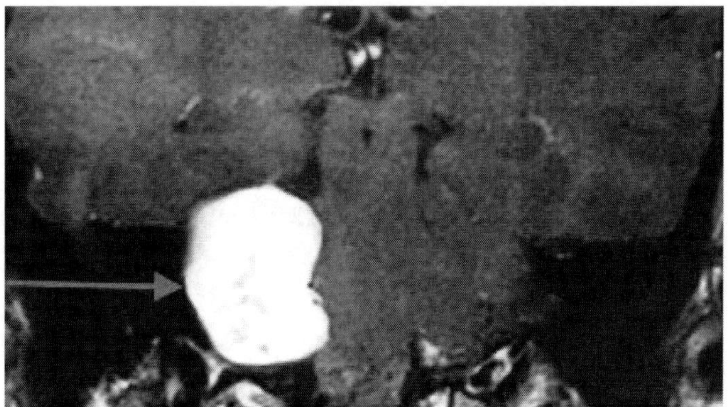

*MRI of a **schwannoma** showing well-demarcated boundaries.*

Time for some more buzzwords! Schwannomas produce **S-100 proteins** which are found in multiple cell types derived from the neural crest, meaning that they are found in all cases of schwannomas (making them very sensitive) even if they are found in other tumors as well (they are not specific). You can remember this by expanding our mnemonic from earlier: **Schw-one cells** (which myelinate only **one** neuron at a time) are **Schw-one-hundred positive**.

Schwannomas are **slow-growing tumors** of **Schwann cells**. They most commonly occur in the **vestibulocochlear nerve**. **S-100 protein** is a very sensitive marker.

***Schw-one**-omas are **Schw-one-hundred** (S-100) positive.*

As a final note, schwannomas tend to occur sporadically on one side of the brain or the other. However, if a patient has *bilateral* schwannomas, this is highly suggestive of a genetic disease known as **neurofibromatosis type II** (which we will cover in more detail in Chapter 27).

OLIGODENDROGLIOMA

The fourth most common type of adult-onset brain tumor is an **oligodendroglioma** which is a neoplasm of **oligodendrocytes** or the support cells that myelinate neurons in the *central* nervous system (as opposed to the Schwann cells in the *peripheral* nervous system). Oligodendrogliomas are **slow-growing** tumors with an overall **good prognosis**. However, because they tend to set up shop in the **frontal lobe**, they can be bothersome to patients, causing **headaches** (due to increased intracranial pressure) and **seizures** (which are often the first sign of the disease).

Like most brain tumors, an initial clinical diagnosis can be supported by head imaging, although definitive diagnosis generally requires a biopsy. There is no cure for oligodendrogliomas, but many people with the disease live for years or even decades following the diagnosis due to its slow-growing nature.

We learned in Chapter 2 that ol-**egg**-odendrocytes often have a "**fried egg**" appearance under the microscope, and this feature can help us to identify the tumor on biopsy! A proliferation of fried egg cells surrounded by branching blood vessels (sometimes described as "**chicken wire**" capillaries) is the characteristic finding on microscopic examination, as seen in the image below. Thinking of **chickens** and **eggs** is the easiest way to remember the key buzzwords for an ol-**egg**-odendroglioma: the **fried egg** cells, the **chicken wire** capillaries, and the **fried brain** (seizures) that can result from an oligodendroglioma in the frontal lobe.

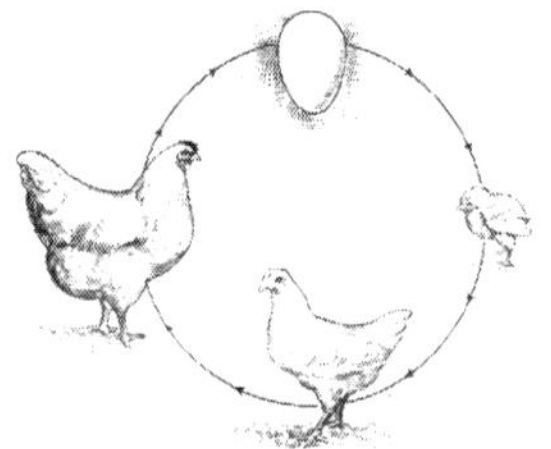

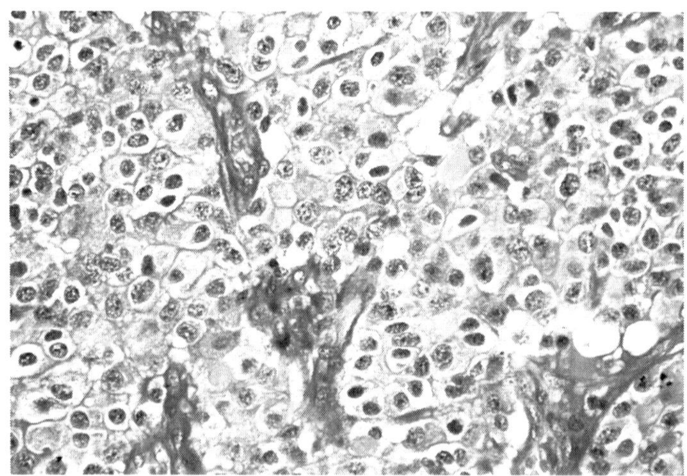

*Microscope image of an **oligodendroglioma** showing the characteristic "**fried egg**" appearance.*

Oligodendrogliomas are **slow-growing tumors** of **oligodendrocytes**.
They often grow in the **frontal lobe** where they can cause **seizures**.

*Think of **chickens and eggs:** ol-**egg**-odendrocytes, **fried egg** cells,
chicken wire capillaries, and **fried brain** (seizures).*

PITUITARY ADENOMA

The last adult-onset brain tumor we will talk about is a **pituitary adenoma** or a tumor of the pituitary gland. Most pituitary adenomas are **benign** (so benign, in fact, that most cases never become symptomatic, with the tumor only being found incidentally when imaging the brain for other reasons!). These **incidentalomas** are common, with up to a quarter of the population having one. In contrast, *clinically significant* pituitary adenomas are more rare. The specific signs and symptoms of a pituitary adenoma relate both to its **anatomical location** in the brain as well as its **specific physiologic functions**. Let's look at each part separately.

Anatomically, the pituitary gland sits right above the optic chiasm, so a tumor here can compress this part of the visual tract, leading to **bitemporal hemianopsia**.

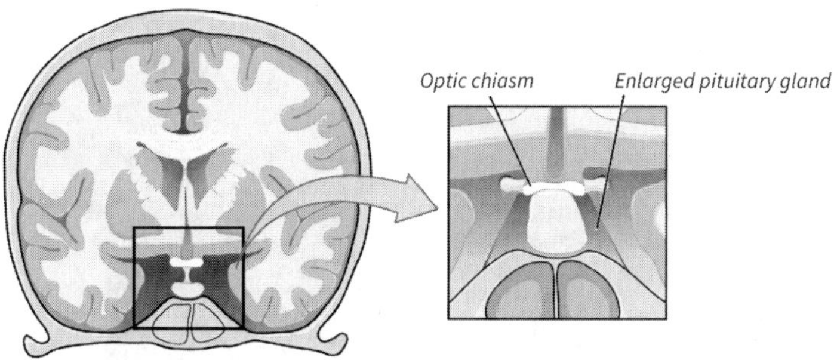

***Pituitary adenomas** can compress the **optic chiasm**, leading to **bitemporal hemianopsia**.*

On a functional level, the anterior pituitary gland is responsible for releasing the six hormones found in the **FLAT PiG** mnemonic, so an adenoma can result either in too *many* of these hormones being released or too *few*. (Recall that the hormones released by the *posterior* pituitary gland are actually produced in the *hypothalamus*, so a pituitary adenoma wouldn't necessarily change production of either vasopressin or oxytocin.) Around 75% of all pituitary adenomas tend to "specialize" in secreting a single hormone, with the most common being adenomas that secrete either **prolactin** or **growth hormone** (30% of all cases). ACTH- and FSH-producing adenomas are less common (5 to 10%), while TSH- and LH-producing adenomas are the most rare (<1%).

In contrast, the remaining quarter of pituitary adenomas are **non-secreting**, meaning that they produce the same amount of hormones or can even lead to *decreased* hormone production. Each hormone is affected to different degrees, with some (like growth hormone) being lost very quickly and others (like prolactin) going missing only in severe cases. You can remember the order of sensitivity using the phrase "**G**o **L**ook **F**or **T**he **A**denoma **P**lease" to remind yourself that hormones tend to be lost in this order: **G**H > **L**H > **F**SH > **T**SH > **A**CTH > **P**rolactin.

Non-secreting pituitary adenomas can reduce hormone secretion by **mass effect**, with release of some hormones being affected more than others.

Go Look For The Adenoma Please:
GH > LH > FSH > TSH > ACTH > Prolactin.

PEDIATRIC BRAIN TUMORS

Let's now move onto brain tumors that typically have their onset in childhood and adolescence. Recall that most of these will be *infra*tentorial (in contrast to the supratentorial location of most adult-onset brain tumors). As with the adult-onset tumors, pay attention the buzzwords for each!

PILOCYTIC ASTROCYTOMA

Pilocytic astrocytomas are the most common type of brain tumor in people under 20, accounting for about half of all cases. Astrocytomas are tumors of **astrocytes** or the support cells of the central nervous system. While astrocytes are found throughout the brain, astrocytomas tend to arise near the cerebellum, brainstem, hypothalamus, and other infratentorial regions. Luckily, pilocytic astrocytomas are often slow-growing and have a **good prognosis**.

The primary signs and symptoms of a pilocytic astrocytoma include headache, nausea, visual abnormalities, and poor balance. Head imaging will reveal a **well-circumscribed** mass in the lower part of the brain, as in the image below:

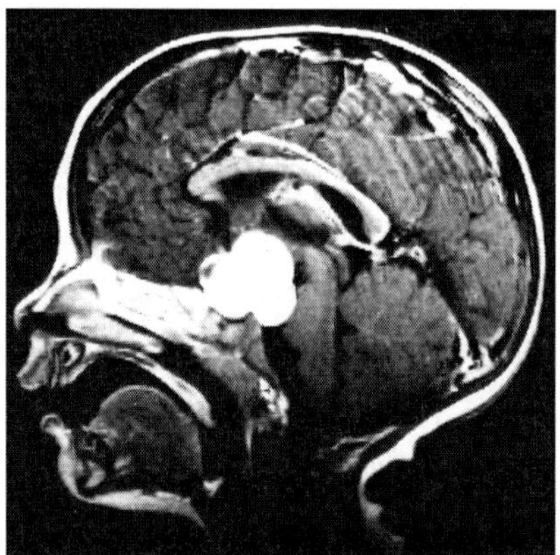

*MRI of a **pilocytic astrocytoma** in the region of the hypothalamus.*

Given how well-defined the tumor is, **surgical resection** is often the treatment of choice. However, because the tumors are located deep in the brain, resection is not always possible. In these cases, chemotherapy and/or radiation are considered.

As with other brain tumors, definitive diagnosis relies upon a brain biopsy. When looking at a pilocytic astrocytoma under a microscope, you can observe long thin hair-like processes (giving this disease its name, as "pilocytic" means that the cells look like fibers). These fibers are **GFAP positive** (see if you can remember which type of adult-onset brain tumor is GFAP positive as well!). In addition, thick worm-like bundles known as **Rosenthal fibers** are often seen as well, as in the following image. You can remember these associations by using the phrase "a **pile o' roses enthralls children**" to link **pilo**cytic astrocytoma, **Rosenthal** fibers, and **children**.

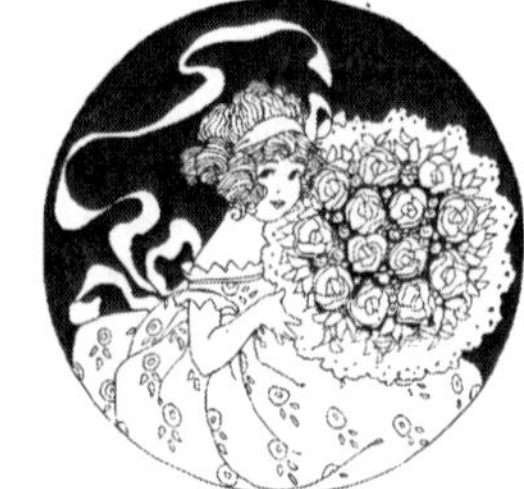

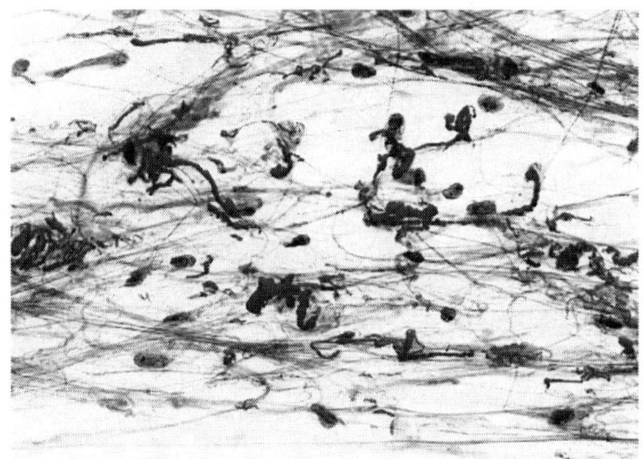

*Microscope image of a **pilocytic astrocytoma** showing intracytoplasmic Rosenthal fibers.*

Pilocytic astrocytomas are **slow-growing brain tumor** often seen in children. Biopsy will reveal **GFAP-positive processes** and **Rosenthal fibers.**

*Think of the phrase "a **pile o' roses enthralls children**" to associate **pilo**cytic astrocytoma, **Rosenthal** fibers, and **pediatric** brain tumors.*

MEDULLOBLASTOMA

A **medulloblastoma** is a tumor of **cerebellar stem cells** that arises near the fourth ventricle between the brainstem and the cerebellum. It is the second most common pediatric brain tumor (accounting for about 25% of all cases) and tends to occur in the first decade of life. It is usually **well-circumscribed**, with a stone-like appearance on head imaging as seen below:

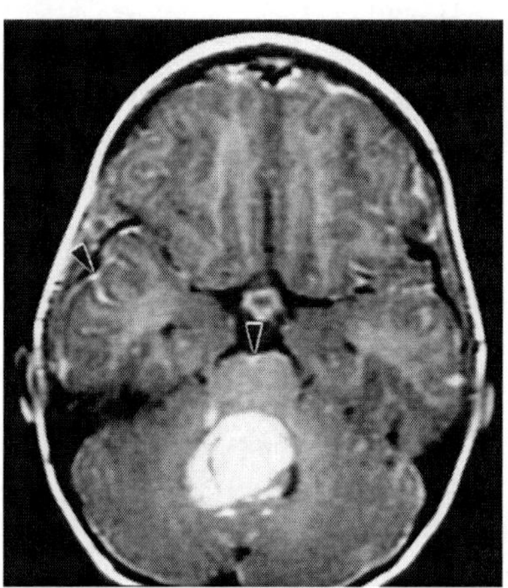

*MRI of a **medulloblastoma** in the cerebellar vermis.*

Because medulloblastomas are typically located around the brainstem and cerebellum, their growth can compress the fourth ventricle, leading to **intracranial hypertension** and **obstructive hydrocephalus**. This causes the distressing (but also frustratingly non-specific) signs and symptoms that are so classic of brain tumors, including fatigue, headache, vomiting, and papilledema. If the tumor continues to grow, **cerebellar signs** may appear as well, including ataxia and frequent falling.

Unlike slow-growing pilocytic astrocytomas, medulloblastomas are often **highly malignant**, growing rapidly and even metastasizing into other areas of the central nervous system (unlike most brain tumors). The term "**drop metastasis**" is used to describe cases that travel all the way down to the cauda equina. Because of their aggressive nature, medulloblastomas have a **high mortality rate**, with less than half of patients surviving 10 years after the diagnosis.

Treatment generally involves **surgery** aimed at removing as much of the tumor as quickly as possible. However, given their rapidly spreading nature, radiation and/or chemotherapy must often be used as well to target areas away from the initial tumor.

Under a microscope, the cells of a medulloblastoma are usually solid and well-circumscribed. They are often said to form **rosettes** or a pattern of cells surrounding an empty central hub (like the rose windows found on many gothic cathedrals).

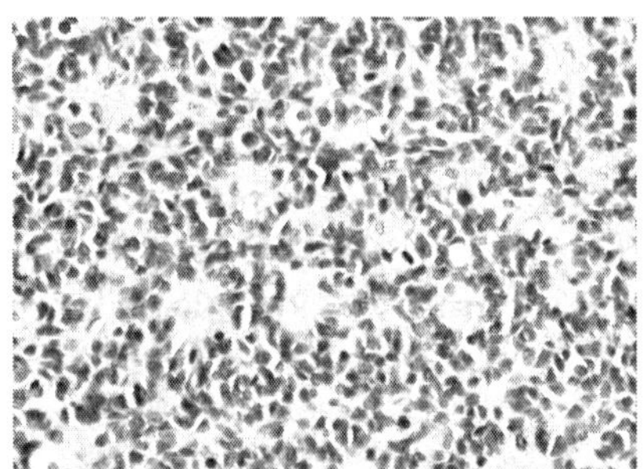

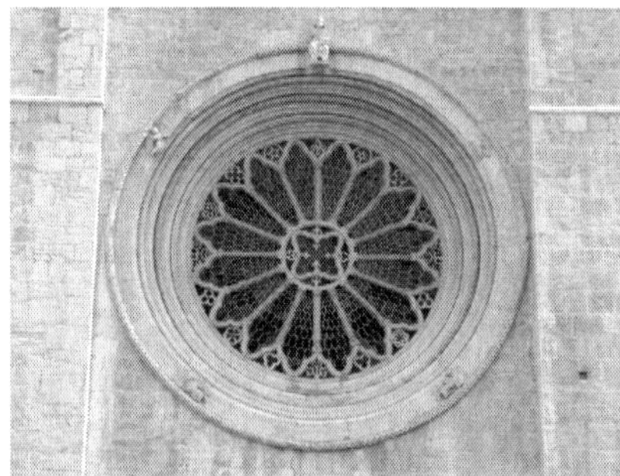

*Microscope image of a **medulloblastoma** featuring **rosettes**. Apparently these resemble each other?*

How can we remember all of this? When you hear "**medu**lloblastoma," think of **Medusa**, the mythological Greek monster with living snakes for hair. Medusa had the ability to turn humans to **stone**, just as a **Medusa**-blastoma has the ability to put a "stone" in someone's head (the well-circumscribed solid mass). Stones are heavy and want to drop down to the lowest part of the brain (the posterior fossa) or even all the way down into the cauda equina of the spinal cord (as in a "drop metastasis"). Like Medusa, Medusa-blastoma is a **highly deadly** monster that should be cut open as soon as possible (with a sword in ancient Greece and a scalpel in modern medicine).

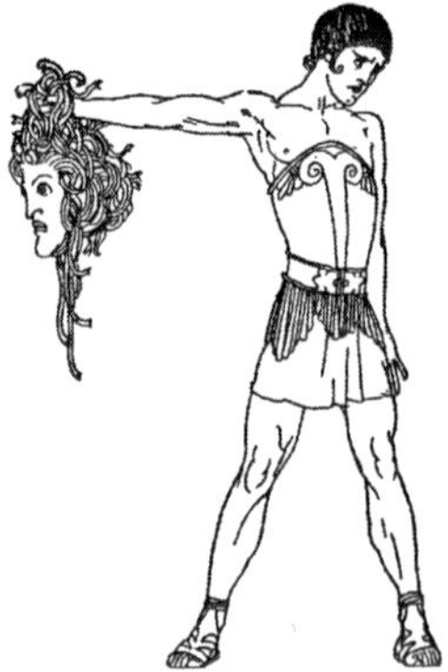

Medulloblastomas are **aggressive tumors** that often grow **near the fourth ventricle** in the **posterior fossa**.

***Medusa**-blastomas can create a **stone** in the brain (a **solid tumor** that can do a "**drop metastasis**"). They are **dangerous** and should be **cut open quickly**.*

EPENDYMOMA

An **ependymoma** is a tumor of ependymal cells which (as you'll recall from Chapter 2) form a lining on the inside of the ventricular system and are responsible for producing, circulating, and absorbing cerebrospinal fluid. While an ependymoma can technically form anywhere in the ventricular system, it has a tendency to form most often in the **fourth ventricle** where it can lead to **obstructive hydrocephalus** in upstream areas. Signs and symptoms of intracranial hypertension are common, including headaches, papilledema, visual changes, nausea, poor balance, and altered mental status.

An ependymoma is a **fast-growing** tumor with a **poor prognosis**. Treatment generally consists of **surgical removal** of the tumor followed by radiation. In general, chemotherapy is not very helpful for treating ependymomas.

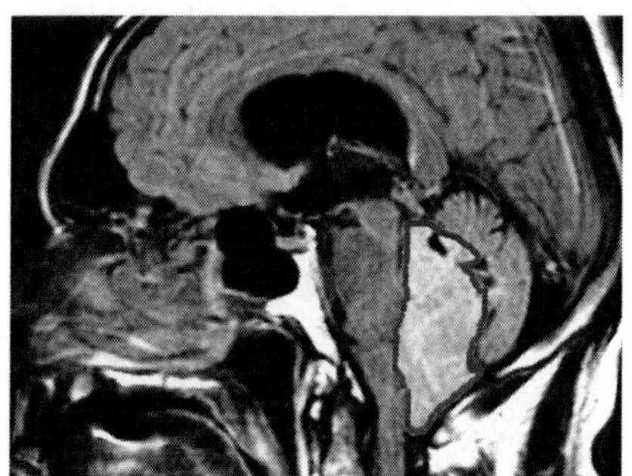

*MRI of an **ependymoma** between the brainstem and cerebellum.*

It may seem like every brain tumor has its own buzzword, and ependymomas are no exception! The word you are looking for is **perivascular pseudorosettes** (or just "pseudorosettes"). The reason they are called *pseudo*rosettes is because "true" rosettes surround the tumor itself, whereas pseudorosettes are found around blood vessels. Perivascular pseudorosettes are found in almost all cases of ependymoma, making them very sensitive markers of this condition. To remember this important association, use the rhyming phrase "ependymomas have **pretendy-rosas**!"

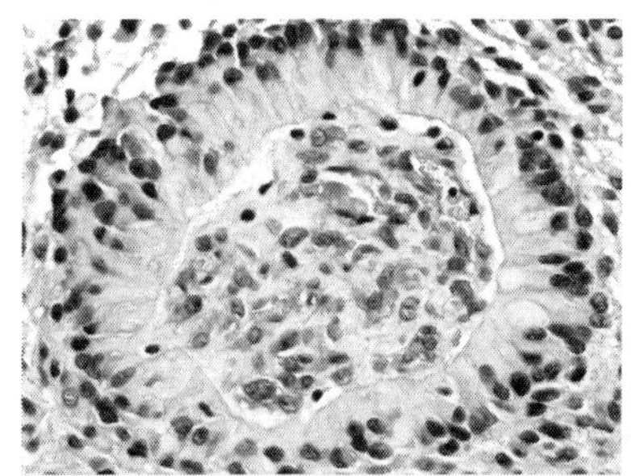

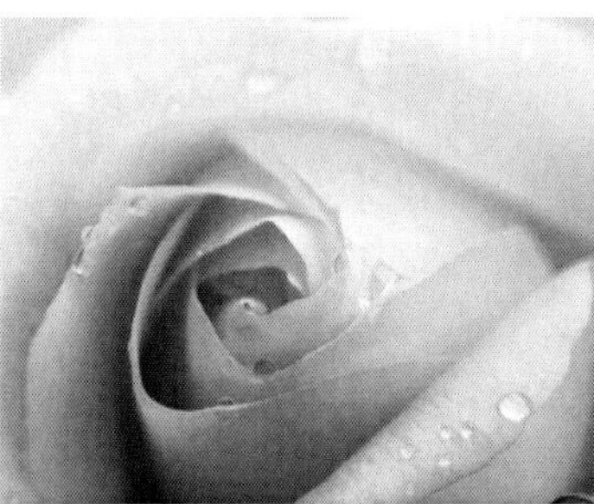

*Microscope image of an **ependymoma** showing a **pseudorosette**. Apparently these resemble each other as well?*

Ependymomas will show **perivascular pseudorosettes** under the microscope.

*Ependymomas have **pretendy-rosas (pseudo-rosettes)**.*

HEMANGIOBLASTOMA

Hemangioblastomas are intracranial tumors that originate not from the *nerves* of the brain but from the **vasculature** supplying it. Their classification as a pediatric brain tumor is somewhat dubious, as they are actually more common in adults! However, for patients with a specific genetic disorder known as **von Hippel-Lindau disease** (which we will talk about in Chapter 27), they may show up in childhood.

Hemangioblastomas are often found in the posterior fossa and in particular seem to enjoy popping up in the **cerebellum**. They are typically **slow-growing** and can often be successfully removed with **surgery**, with an overall **good prognosis**. (However, people who develop hemangioblastomas as a result of von Hippel-Lindau disease often have multiple tumors and therefore have a worse prognosis.)

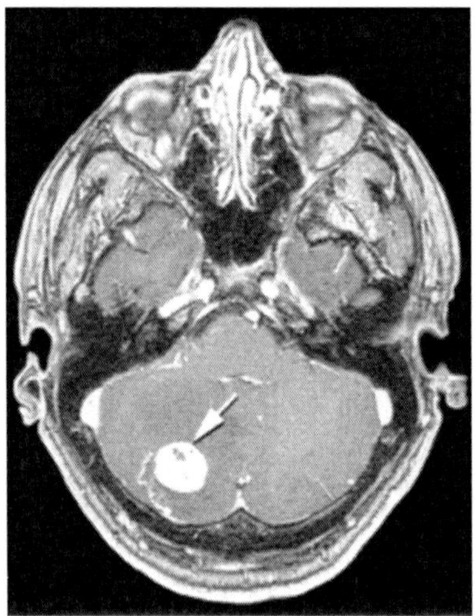

*MRI of a **hemangioblastoma** in the cerebellum.*

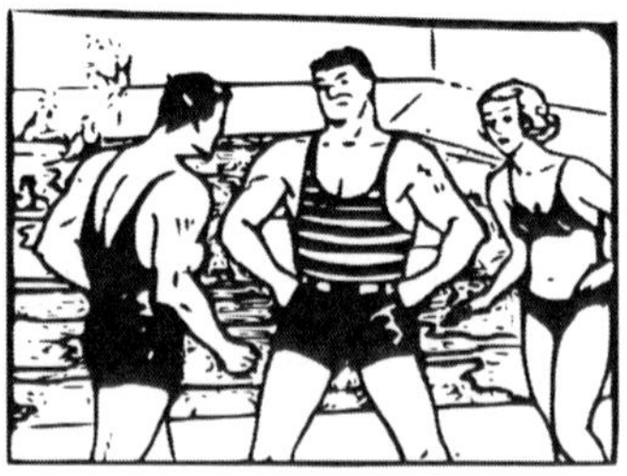

A unique feature of hemangioblastomas is that they can produce **erythropoietin** which is the hormone that stimulates production of red blood cells. This can cause a secondary **polycythemia** or an excessive amount of red blood cells in the bloodstream. This will not necessarily present with any signs or symptoms on a clinical level, although it may be picked up when doing lab tests. To make this association, think of this tumor as a **He-Man**(glioblastoma) and form a mental image of a buff dude who considers himself a **red-blooded** male.

Hemangioblastomas are brain tumors derived from the **vasculature of the brain**. They can produce **erythropoietin** and cause a **secondary polycythemia**.

*A **He-Man**(glioblastoma) is a burly dude who considers himself a **red-blooded** male.*

CRANIOPHARYNGIOMA

Finally, the fifth most common pediatric brain tumor is a **craniopharyngioma** or a tumor of embryonic cells in the **pituitary gland**. (Of note, craniopharyngiomas are the only one of the five pediatric brain tumors we will discuss that are *supra*tentorial!) Craniopharyngiomas are derived from remnants of **Rathke's pouch**, an embryonic structure that gives rise to the anterior pituitary. This means that, while they are found in the pituitary, they are not made of pituitary tissue, so these tumors don't result in hypersecretion of hormones. (In fact, they may even *suppress* hormone secretion!) Craniopharyngiomas can often be confused with pituitary tumors, as both are located near the optic chiasm and can cause **bitemporal hemianopsia**. Interestingly, because craniopharyngiomas arise from the same embryonic cells that form teeth, they have a tendency to **calcify**, leading to a bright appearance on head imaging as seen below:

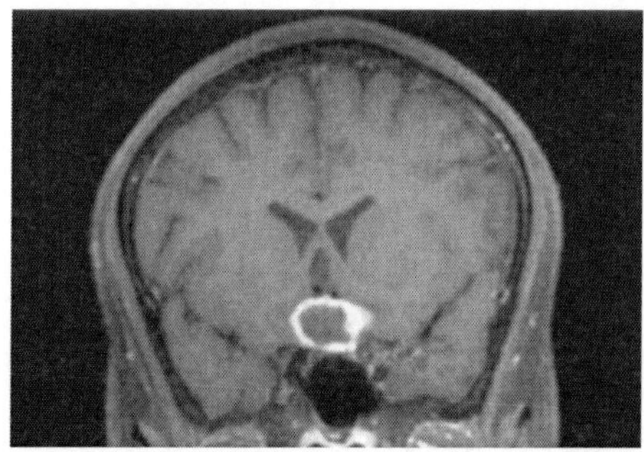

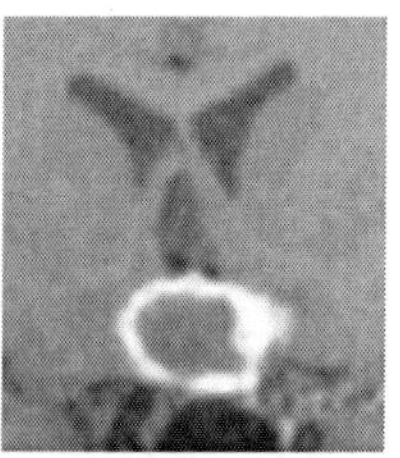

*MRI of a **craniopharyngioma**, with a close up of the calcified mass on the right. (It kind of looks like a mouth!)*

Craniopharyngiomas are often slow-growing and **benign**. Nevertheless, because they have the ability to turn malignant in rare cases, it is generally worth pursuing **surgical removal** with additional radiation and/or chemotherapy.

You can remember the important associations here by thinking of a **child standing on a chair to get away from a rat**. This should help you think of **children** (the population most affected by craniopharyngiomas), the **supra**tentorial nature of this tumor (since the child is standing **above** the chair), **Rat**hke's pouch (from which a craniopharyngioma derives), the **calcified** nature of both rat teeth and craniopharyngiomas, and a **bite**-temporal hemianopsia (which is caused compression of the optic chiasm). In addition, if you use your imagination, the calcified tumor above almost looks like the mouth of an evil rat! Rat bites, while painful, are **rarely deadly**, reflecting the benign nature of this tumor.

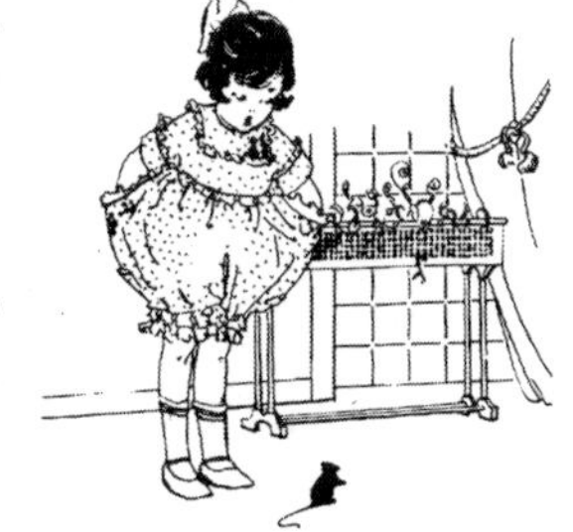

Craniopharyngiomas are **benign brain tumors** derived from **Rathke's pouch**, They can compress the optic chiasm and lead to **bitemporal hemianopsia**.

*Think of a **child afraid of a rat bite** to associate this with **children, Rat**hke's pouch, **bite**-temporal hemianopsia, **calcified** teeth, and a **rarely deadly** prognosis.*

BRAIN METASTASES

As pointed out earlier, just because a tumor is *in* the brain doesn't mean it's *from* the brain. In fact, secondary brain tumors are actually just as common as primary brain tumors! **Brain metastases** often set up shop in multiple locations and can therefore present with diffuse neurologic findings (in contrast to a primary brain tumor which is more often localized to a single area). However, this pattern is not consistent enough to rely on, so diagnosis ultimately relies on head imaging and a brain biopsy. As a general rule, any patient with a known history of cancer who presents **with new-onset neurological or behavioral changes** should be evaluated immediately for possible brain metastases.

Different forms of cancer have varying tendencies for metastasizing to the brain. **Lung cancer** is far and away the most common, accounting for nearly half of all cases. However, **breast cancer** is not far behind. Rounding out the top five are **melanoma**, **colon cancer**, and **kidney cancer**. You can remember this order using the phrase "**L**otsa **B**ad **S**tuff **C**an **K**ill" which stands for **L**ung, **B**reast, **S**kin, **C**olon, and **K**idney.

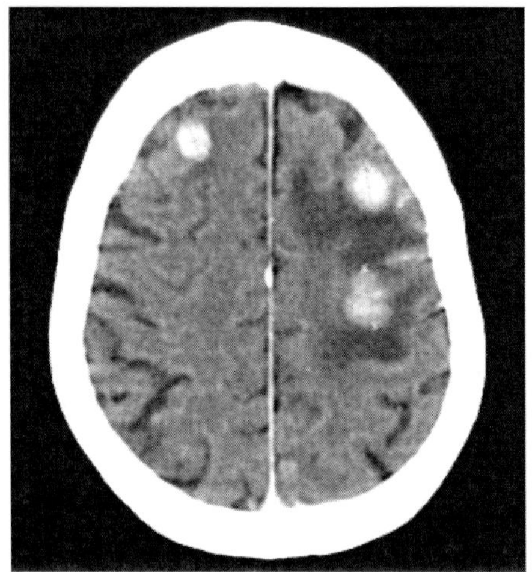

Multifocal ***brain metastases*** *from a primary* ***breast cancer***.

The **most common types of cancer** that **metastasize to the brain** are **lung** and **breast** followed by **melanoma**, **colon**, and **kidney**.

__L__otsa __B__ad __S__tuff __C__an __K__ill: __L__ung > __B__reast > __S__kin > __C__olon > __K__idney.

The presence of a brain metastasis often involves a **poor prognosis**, as it shows just how aggressive the cancer is (as it has not only escaped from its original location but has managed to infiltrate one of the hardest-to-reach parts of the body). For this reason, treatment generally tends to be **palliative** rather than curative, although patients who are younger or who have only a single site of metastasis may benefit from more aggressive treatment. All in all, though, brain metastases are generally nothing but bad news.

PUTTING IT ALL TOGETHER

Brain tumors can be difficult to diagnose, as they often present with **non-specific signs and symptoms** like headaches (although focal deficits can be seen as well depending on the specific parts of the brain involved). They also tend to come on very **slowly** (reflecting the slow growth of the tumor itself) which is often less dramatic and noticeable compared to the sudden-onset nature of, say, a stroke. Accordingly, you should always keep brain tumors on your differential, especially when the clinical presentation is unusual in any regard! For example, someone with a known history of headaches who presents with another headache is unlikely to need brain imaging to rule out a tumor. In contrast, someone who has *no* history of prior headaches who now presents with a severe headache that awakens them from sleep at night and is associated with dizziness and confusion would absolutely warrant an immediate investigation for a brain tumor. Keep an eye out for any **atypical patterns**, especially when they appear to have come on slowly in a patient with no prior history.

When diagnosing brain tumors, the first helpful distinction to make is between *supra*tentorial tumors (which are more common in adults) and *infra*tentorial tumors (which are more common in children). Use the image of adults ushering the children **under the tent** when it is raining to make this association. From there, be familiar with the most common types of tumors in both children and adults. All of these tumors come with various **buzzwords** that should immediately make you think of them (such as psammoma bodies in meningiomas, S-100 in schwannomas, and so on). For whatever reason, many of the childhood-onset brain tumors have buzzwords related to "roses" (such as **Rose**nthal fibers in pilocytic astrocytomas, pseudo**rose**ttes in medulloblastomas, and perivascular pseudo**rose**ttes in ependymomas), but don't let this confuse you! Do your best to keep these straight in your mind using the provided mnemonics as summarized in the table below:

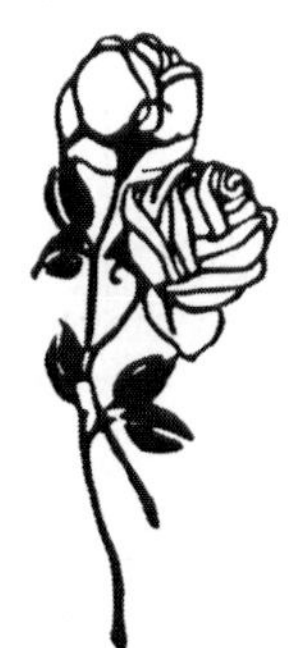

Disease	Age	Prognosis	Buzzwords
GBM	Adults	☹ Poor	GFAP+, pseudopalisading necrosis, butterfly glioma
Meningioma	Adults	☺ Good	Whorled appearance, psammoma bodies
Schwannoma	Adults	☺ Good	S-100, sensorineural hearing loss
Oligodendroglioma	Adults	☺ Good	"Fried egg" cells, "chicken wire" capillaries
Pituitary adenoma	Adults	☺ Good	Bitemporal hemianopsia
Pilocytic astrocytoma	Children	☺ Good	GFAP+, Rosenthal fibers
Medulloblastoma	Children	☹ Poor	Rosettes, "drop metastasis"
Ependymoma	Children	☹ Poor	Perivascular pseudorosettes
Hemangioblastoma	Both	☺ Good	Secondary polycythemia
Craniopharyngioma	Children	☺ Good	Rathke's pouch, bitemporal hemianopsia

REVIEW QUESTIONS

1. A 48 y/o M makes an appointment with a primary care doctor. He is wary of seeking medical care and has not seen a health care provider in over 20 years. However, he decided to make an appointment after experiencing increasingly severe headaches with nausea and occasional vomiting over the past 3 months. A full physical and neurological exam reveals no significant abnormalities. His vital signs are within normal limits. A CT scan reveals a lesion in his right temporal lobe with surrounding edema and compression of the right lateral ventricle. A tissue biopsy confirms the diagnosis. When discussing the case with the patient, the doctor says, "This is a very difficult condition to treat, and while we should never lose hope, it is important to prepare for all possible outcomes." Which of the following is the most likely diagnosis?
    - A. Pilocytic astrocytoma
    - B. Glioblastoma multiforme
    - C. Oligodendroglioma
    - D. Hemangioblastoma
    - E. Meningioma
    - F. Schwannoma

2. A 6 y/o F is brought to the pediatrician for refusing to eat for the past several days, with vomiting this morning. The patient is visibly upset and refuses to answer the doctor's questions. When asked if she is having any pain, she points to the back of her head. Neurological exam reveals bilateral papilledema and an unsteady gait. She is unable to name the animal when shown a picture of a dog. MRI reveals a cystic tumor in the right cerebellum. She is diagnosed with the most common primary brain tumor in children and is scheduled for surgery. During the surgery, a sample of the tumor is sent for microscopic analysis. Which of the following is most likely to be seen?
    - A. Rosenthal fibers
    - B. Rosettes
    - C. Perivascular pseudorosettes
    - D. Pseudopalisading necrosis
    - E. None of the above

3. A 3 y/o M with a history of delayed motor development is seen by his pediatrician after he becomes increasingly irritable over the past month, with frequent crying. His mother notes that she has seen him falling while walking several times in the past week. He had previously been toilet trained, but he has had several episodes of both bowel and bladder incontinence in the past 3 days. On exam, his cranial nerves are intact including pupillary response and extraocular muscles, though some nystagmus is noted. Moderate papilledema is seen bilaterally. His upper extremities are at full motor strength, but there is significantly decreased strength in his lower extremities bilaterally, with absent patellar and ankle jerk reflexes. Anal sphincter tone is absent. Which of the following is the most likely explanation for these findings?

A. Supratentorial tumor in the cerebellar cortex
B. Infratentorial tumor in the cerebellum
C. Spinal cord tumor in the cervical cord
D. Spinal cord tumor in the thoracic cord
E. Spinal cord tumor in the lumbar cord
F. Spinal cord tumor in the cauda equina
G. More than one of the above
H. None of the above

4. A 45 y/o M is brought to the hospital by his wife after he appeared drowsy and confused this morning. On exam, he is stuporous and does not respond to questions, though he does flinch when painful stimuli is applied. His wife reports that he has been complaining of increasingly severe headaches for the past 2 weeks, with vomiting over the past 3 days. While the doctor is talking with his wife, the nurse runs out of the room and yells, "He's having a seizure!" The doctor observes a generalized tonic-clonic seizure lasting approximately 90 seconds. A CT scan is obtained which shows a space-occupying lesion in the right frontal lobe. Surgical excision is scheduled. Biopsy of the tumor is diagnostic for oligodendroglioma. Which of the following images is most likely to be seen by the pathologist examining the excised tissue?

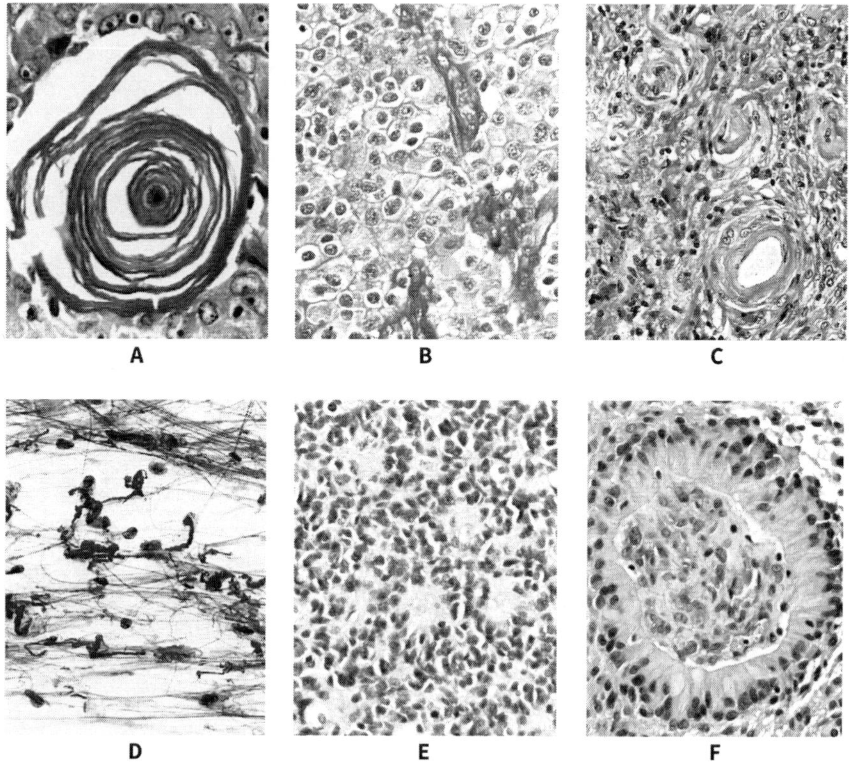

1. **The best answer is B.** Of the listed brain tumors, glioblastoma multiforme is the one with the worst prognosis, and many patients do not live more than one or two years after their initial diagnosis. Oligodendrogliomas, meningiomas, and schwannomas are all slow-growing or highly resectable (answers C, E, and F). Pilocytic astrocytomas and hemangioblastomas are both diagnosed more often in children than adults and are each associated with a good prognosis (answers A and D).

2. **The best answer is A.** The most common primary brain tumor in children is a pilocytic astrocytoma, accounting for about half of all cases. Microscopic analysis of the tumor will often reveal Rosenthal fibers as well as characteristic cells with long hair-like GFAP-positive processes. Rosettes are seen in medulloblastomas (answer B), perivascular pseudorosettes are seen in ependymomas (answer C), and pseudopalisading necrosis is seen in glioblastoma multiforme (answer D).

3. **The best answer is G.** This vignette describes a case of medulloblastoma with a drop metastasis causing a cauda equina syndrome. A cerebellar lesion on its own could explain the presence of ataxia and nystagmus. However, it could not also explain the additional presence of motor weakness in the lower extremities as well as the presence of bowel and bladder dysfunction (answer B). These findings strongly suggest the involvement of the spinal cord and in particular the cauda equina given the reduced anal sphincter tone (answers C—F). However, a tumor in just the cauda equina would not explain the ataxia and nystagmus, so it is most likely that there is both a primary tumor in the cerebellum and a secondary "drop metastasis" in the cauda equina (answer F). Supratentorial tumors are rare in children and would not explain these findings (answer A).

4. **The best answer is B.** Oligodendrocytes have a highly characteristic "fried egg" appearance when examined under a microscope, so it should not come as a surprise that oligodendrogliomas have this feature this as well. Whorling (answer A) and psammoma bodies (answer C) are seen in meningiomas, Rosenthal fibers (answer D) are seen in pilocytic astrocytomas, rosettes (answer E) are seen in medulloblastomas, and finally perivascular pseudorosettes (answer F) are seen in ependymomas.

22 MENINGITIS

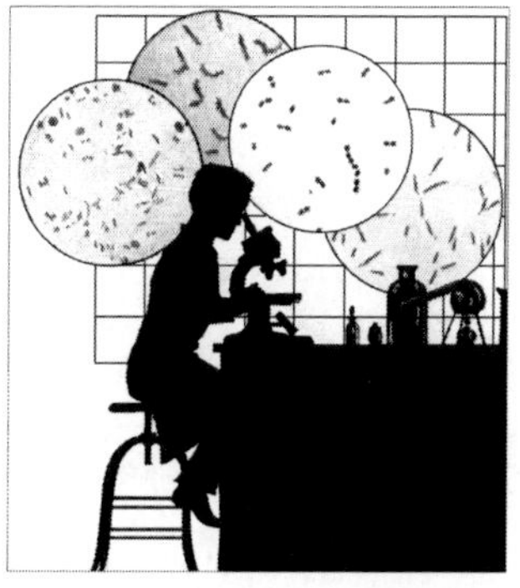

A variety of **infectious diseases** are known to target the nervous system, resulting in various forms of neurologic damage. While sometimes the neural dysfunction is due to specific effects of the bugs themselves, in other cases some of the harm comes from the process of **inflammation** which is the body's way of using the immune system to fight off potential threats from the environment (remember "calor, dolor, rubor, and tumor" from Chapter 16!). Indeed, at times the body's innate response can end up causing as many problems as the infection itself (as we'll see in future chapters).

With hundreds of infectious diseases in the world, there is no way to cover every single bug that could potentially interact with the nervous system in a short amount of time. Instead, in the next few chapters, we will focus primarily on the infectious diseases that have a *particular* tendency to attack the nervous system. There are two ways to "slice the bread" here. We can either divide up the diseases by the **specific parts of the nervous system** that they affect (either the brain, spinal cord, meninges, and/or peripheral nerves), or we can group the diseases based on their **causative agents** (the specific viral, bacterial, and fungal organisms creating the mess in the first place). We will take the former approach, as that is the one that is most clinically relevant (as the patient's presenting signs and symptoms generally match the part of the body that is affected moreso than the specific bug that is involved). In this chapter, we will talk specifically about **meningitis** or inflammation of the meninges, while in the next chapter we will talk about **encephalitis** of inflammation of the brain. We will also cover a few infections that can affect the peripheral nervous system when we talk about peripheral neuropathy in the chapter after that!

DIAGNOSIS OF MENINGITIS

Meningitis often presents with a classic triad of symptoms including **fever**, **headache**, and **neck stiffness** that is severe enough that it results in an inability to flex the neck forward (known as "nuchal rigidity"). Additional signs and symptoms including confusion, headache, nausea, seizures, and photophobia (extreme discomfort from looking at lights) can occur as well. Like most infectious illnesses, these symptoms often come on **acutely** over several hours or days.

There are two physical exam maneuvers that can help to support the diagnosis. The first is to bend both the hip and the knee to a 90° angle (as seen in the image below). If the patient shows signs of severe pain when you try to extend the knee back out, there is likely to be inflammation of the meninges. This is known as **Kernig's sign**.

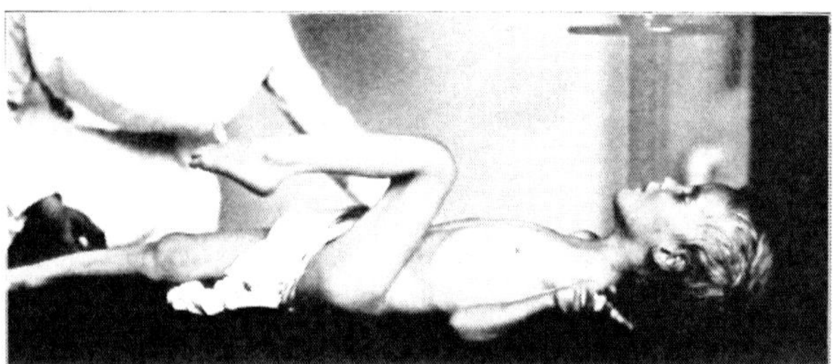

Pain upon extension of the knee is known as ***Kernig's sign****.*

The second exam maneuver you can do is to have the patient lie flat on their back while you gently flex their neck by raising their head up with your hand. If they reflexively draw in their legs towards their chest due to pain, this is also consistent with meningitis. This finding is known as **Brudzinski's sign**. You can remember the difference between Kernig's sign and Brudzinski's sign by thinking that **K**ernig involves extending the **K**nee while **B**rudzinski involves flexing the **B**rain.

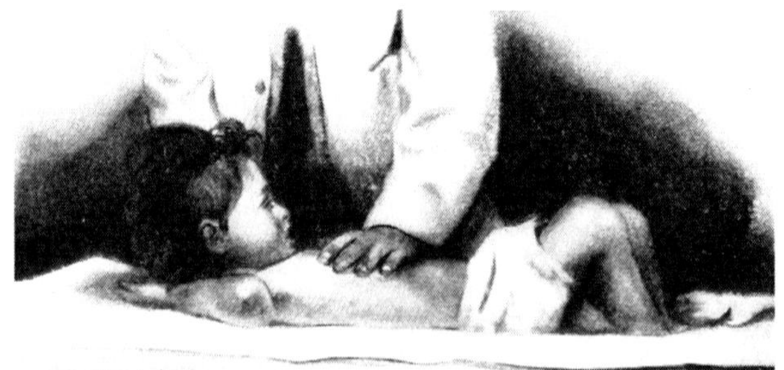

Reflexively drawing the legs inward upon flexion of the neck is known as ***Brudzinski's sign****.*

Kernig's sign and **Brudzinski's sign** are two exam maneuvers that suggest **inflammation of the meninges.**

K**ernig involves extending the* ***K*nee, while* ***B****rudzinski involves flexing the* ***B****rain.*

Most cases of meningitis are caused by an infection, although cases of non-infectious meningitis (related to drugs or other conditions) do exist. **Viral meningitis** (also called aseptic meningitis due to the lack of living organisms in the meninges) is the most common infectious cause, although it is thankfully also the least debilitating and deadly. **Bacterial meningitis** is less common, but it is much deadlier. **Fungal meningitis** can be lethal as well, although this form of meningitis is less common as it primarily affects those who are immunocompromised.

Determining the cause of a meningeal infection almost always requires doing a **lumbar puncture**, as viral, bacterial, and fungal forms of meningitis each present with a distinct pattern of findings. These are summarized in the table below:

	Appearance	Pressure	Glucose	Protein	Cells
Viral	Clear	Normal or slightly ↑	Normal	Normal	Lymphocytes
Bacterial	Cloudy	↑	↓	↑	Neutrophils
Fungal	Cloudy	↑	↓	↑	Lymphocytes

What patterns can we tease out of this? First, notice that findings in viral meningitis are all pretty normal, while those in bacterial and fungal meningitis are distinctly *abnormal*. Second, notice that the abnormal findings in bacterial and fungal meningitis are largely the same, with a cloudy appearance, high opening pressure, low glucose, and high protein. Given that both bacterial and fungal cases of meningitis are **strong** (high protein) infections, it makes sense that this is a **high pressure** situation (increased opening pressure) that is **not sweet** (low glucose) in any way!

Bacterial and fungal meningitis show specific findings on lumbar puncture, including a **high opening pressure**, **low glucose**, and **high protein**.

*Both are **strong** infections, making for a **high pressure** situation that is **not sweet**!*

There is, however, one big difference between bacterial and fungal meningitis: the type of cells present! **Bac**terial meningitis causes an increase in **N**eutrophils, while **fun**gal meningitis causes an increase in **lym**ph**o**cytes. You can use the phrase "**Bac**k i**N** the **Fun Limo**" to tell them apart!

Bacterial meningitis shows a predominance of **neutrophils**, while **fungal meningitis** is associated with a predominance of **lymphocytes**.

***Bac**k i**N** the **Fun Limo**:*
***Bac**terial = **N**eutrophils, **Fun**gal = **Lym**ph**o**cytes.*

Now that we have a sense of how to differentiate between bacterial, fungal, and viral meningitis, let's look at each type in more detail.

BACTERIAL MENINGITIS

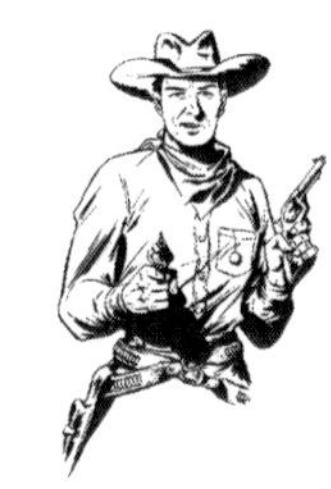

Cases of bacterial meningitis must be taken seriously. While a lumbar puncture is helpful for identifying the causative organisms in bacterial meningitis, you shouldn't necessarily wait for the test results to return before starting treatment! Because delays in treatment are associated with worse outcomes, you should generally take a "**shoot first and ask questions later**" approach with bacterial meningitis by starting antibiotics right away. Even with prompt treatment, there is a **high mortality rate** (around 10%), and some patients who survive are left with lasting repercussions including seizures, ataxia, and other neurologic deficits.

To help guide your choice of antibiotic, it is useful to **make assumptions based on age** about what the most likely causative organisms will be (as different organisms are more or less common in different age groups). For this reason, we will spend the next few sections going over not only how meningitis presents in each age group but also the causative organisms that are most commonly found.

INFANTS

Meningitis in infants requires some unique considerations. First, infants are not able to report their symptoms, so you may need to rely on some additional clinical signs that can be suggestive of meningitis, including **fever**, **inconsolable crying**, **bulging of the fontanelles** (or the soft openings in the skull where the bones have not yet fused), and an arched back and neck known as the **opisthotonus position**.

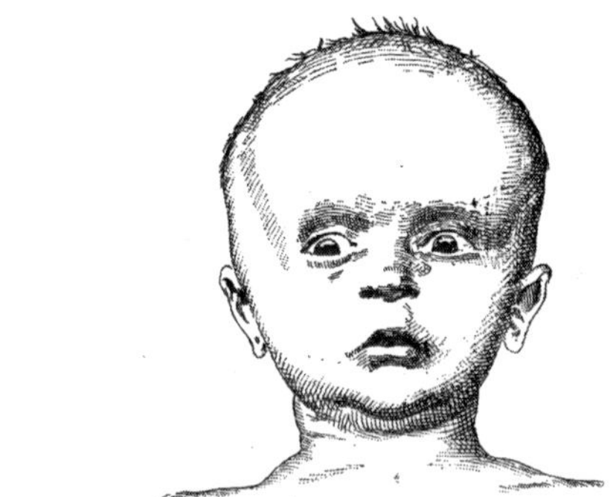

*An infant with **bulging fontanelles**.*

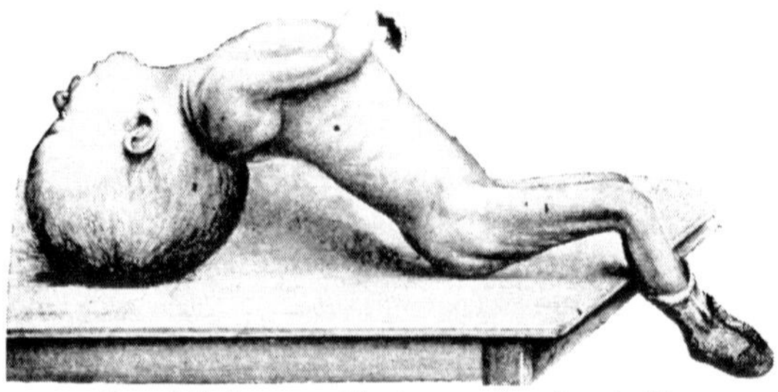

*The **opisthotonus position** is suggestive of meningitis.*

The causative organisms in infant meningitis are very different from those seen in children and adults. You can remember the most common bugs using the acronym **GEL**:

G is for Group B streptococcus. Group B streptococcus is a Gram-positive coccus that is the **most common cause of neonatal meningitis**. It is often picked up from the mother's vaginal canal during childbirth. Because group B streptococcal meningitis does not always present with because the classic signs of meningitis, it should be on the differential for **all infants presenting with a high fever**! You can remember the association of **G**roup **B S**treptococcus with neonatal meningitis by thinking of it as the mother **G**iving **B**aby an unpleasant **S**urprise.

Group B streptococcus is the most common cause of meningitis in **neonates**. It is picked up from the mother's vaginal canal during **childbirth**.

*Group **B S**treptococcus **G**ives **B**aby an unpleasant **S**urprise.*

E is for *Escherichia coli*. *E. coli* is a Gram-negative rod that is the second most common cause of meningitis in neonates. Like Group B streptococcus, it is often picked up from the mother during childbirth. Strains of *E. coli* that have the **K1 capsular antigen** appear to be particularly able to infect the meninges. You can remember this by thinking of **K-one heads** (as *E. coli* with K1 are more likely to go to the head).

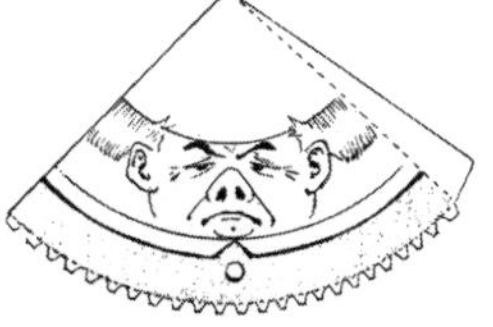

Escherichia coli is the second most common cause of meningitis in **neonates**. *E. coli* possessing the **K1 capsular antigen** are most likely to result in meningitis.

K-one heads: E. coli *with **K-one** are more likely to go to the head.*

L is for *Listeria monocytogenes*. Listeria is a Gram-positive rod that is a common cause of meningitis in newborns (as well as the **elderly** and other people with **compromised immune systems**, including those with AIDS, severe diabetes, or conditions that require them to take steroids).

The most common causes of **infant meningitis** are **Group B streptococcus**, ***E. coli***, and ***Listeria***.

Bulging fontanelles *(a sign of infant meningitis) are filled with **GEL**: **G**roup B streptococcus, **E**. coli, and **L**isteria.*

CHILDREN AND ADULTS

Cases of meningitis in children and adults involve a different set of organisms compared to infants. You can remember the most common bugs using the mnemonic **HeNS** (as **hens** are **grown-up** chickens):

H is for *Haemophilus influenzae*. *H. influenzae* is a Gram-negative rod that causes meningitis primarily in children under the age of 5. It is a common resident in the sinuses of children and can either spread to the meninges directly or by seeping into the bloodstream. Treatment consists of a cephalosporin. Even with treatment, up to a third of all patients are left with permanent damage, including deafness in some cases. In recent years, the availability of a vaccine has decreased rates significantly.

N is for *Neisseria meningitidis*. This Gram-negative diplococci, also referred to as **meningococcus**, is the most common cause of bacterial meningitis among children and teenagers (between 2 and 18). There are a three key points to know here!

First, it is often accompanied by a **purpuric rash** that is **non-blanching** (meaning that it does not lose its color when pressure is applied). The combination of classic meningitis symptoms plus a non-blanching rash should immediately have you thinking of meningococcus, although it's important to note that some patients may develop the rash without showing any of the classic signs of meningitis!

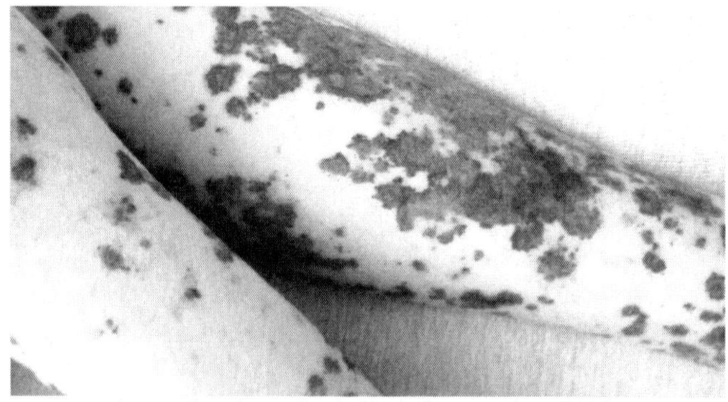

*A **purpuric rash** associated with **meningococcal meningitis**.*

Second, *N. meningitidis* often spreads among people living in **close quarters** such as college students or military recruits. For this reason, once a case is identified, close contacts should be treated as well to prevent the spread of infection.

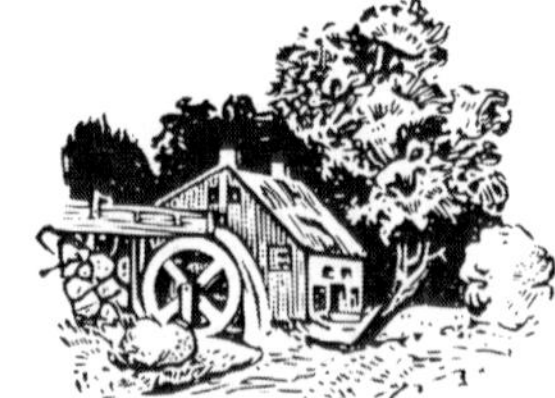

Third, meningococcal meningitis can be associated with a complication known as **Waterhouse-Friderichsen syndrome** in which bleeding into the adrenal glands occurs, leading to **adrenal insufficiency**. Any patient presenting with a combination of meningitis symptoms, petechial rash, and/or sudden-onset hypotension and tachycardia should have you thinking of Waterhouse-Friderichsen syndrome! To recognize this syndrome, focus on the "water" part of **Water**house-Friderichsen syndrome to link it to changes in **fluid balance** (such as a rapid drop in blood pressure and changes in electrolyte levels).

Waterhouse-Friderichsen syndrome is a severe complication of meningococcal disease that leads to **adrenal insufficiency**.

__Water__house-Friderichsen syndrome involves changes in __fluid balance__.

S is for *Streptococcus pneumonia*. This Gram-positive diplococcus is the single **most common cause of bacterial meningitis in children and adults** over the age of 18. Part of the reason it is so common is because it is a resident of most people's upper respiratory tract, where it generally lives in peace with its host. However, under certain conditions, it can grow out of control and lead to infection. Treatment involves a cephalosporin, though prevention via immunization is the best option.

The most common causes of **bacterial meningitis in children and adults** are ***Streptococcus pneumoniae***, ***Neisseria meningitidis***, and ***Haemophilus influenzae***.

__HeNS__ (__grown-up__ chickens) can remind us of the causes of meningitis in __grown-ups__:
__H__. influenzae
__N__eisseria meningitides
__S__treptococcus pneumoniae

All bacterial meningitis treatment regimens should include a **cephalosporin**. These are not only effective against the most common causes of adult meningitis but are also able to cross the blood–brain barrier into the central nervous system.

Cephalosporins are effective against the **most common causes of meningitis**.

__Cephalo__sporins can cross the blood–brain barrier to get into the __head__.

While cephalosporins are great, they don't cover all causes of meningitis. This is really **LAME**! Let's use the word **LAME** to remember the organisms against which cephalosporins do *not* have activity, including ***L**isteria*, **A**typicals bugs like *Mycoplasma* and *Chlamydia*, **M**ethicillin-resistant *Staphylococcus aureus*, and ***E**nterococci*. Because these bugs would escape unharmed if only a cephalosporin was used, additional drugs (like ampicillin or vancomycin) should be added for complete coverage.

Additional antibiotics are needed for **complete coverage** in meningitis treatment.

It's really __LAME__ that cephalosporins do not cover all possible causes of meningitis:
__L__isteria
__A__typicals organisms
__M__ethicillin-resistant Staphylococcus aureus
__E__nterococci

FUNGAL MENINGITIS

Fungal infections are a rare cause of meningitis, although they are more common in patients who are **immunocompromised**. Fungal meningitis presents with similar signs and symptoms as bacterial meningitis but tends to have a poorer prognosis and higher mortality rates. Fungal meningitis should be treated with **antifungals** such as amphotericin or fluconazole.

There are a few species of fungus that are able to infect the central nervous system, with most of these also being able to cause other types of infections as well (such as pneumonia). Each of these species is found in specific **geographic distributions** which are commonly included as clues on test questions.

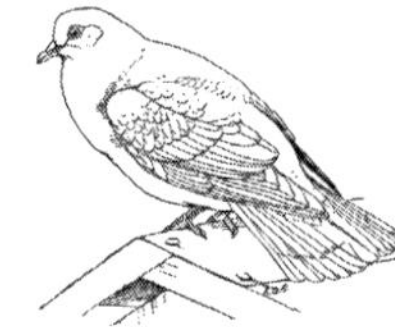

Cryptococcus neoformans is the most common cause of fungal meningitis and is found **worldwide**. It has a tendency to be found in soil that has been fouled (or should we say "fowled"?) by droppings from pigeons and other birds. You can remember this association by thinking of it as *Crypto-**caca** neoformans* to associate it with pigeon poop. Use of a special stain known as **India ink** is helpful for visualizing this fungus under a microscope.

Cryptococcus neoformans is the **most common cause of fungal meningitis** worldwide. It is found in soil that has been infested with **bird droppings**.

*Crypto-**caca** neoformans is found in pigeon **poop**.*

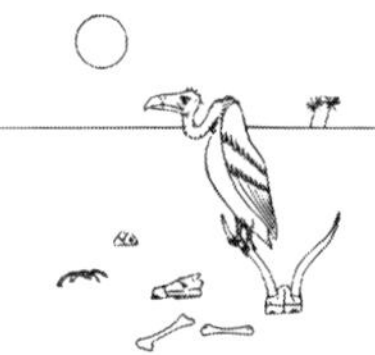

Coccidioides immitis is another potential cause of fungal meningitis that is found in the **soil** of the **southwestern United States** as well as parts of Central and South America. It most often is associated with a **lung infection** producing flu-like symptoms (known as "Valley fever" for the Central Valley of California), but in some cases it may develop into meningitis.

Histoplasma is a genus of fungus that can infect the central nervous system and cause meningitis. It is found worldwide but is particularly prevalent in the **Midwestern United States** near the Ohio and Mississippi Rivers, most often in places like the insides of caves that have been contaminated by bird or bat droppings. You can remember this association by sticking an **O** in front of it to make ***OHI**st**O**plasma*.

Histoplasma is a potential cause of **fungal meningitis** that is endemic to the **Midwestern United States**. It is associated with **bird and bat droppings**.

***OHI**st**O**plasma is found in **OHIO** and nearby places.*

The last potential cause of fungal meningitis we will talk about is ***Blastomyces dermatitidis***. Like *Histoplasma*, *Blastomyces* is found primarily in the **Midwestern United States** east of the Mississippi River. This time, however, it is associated with **wet and damp places** such as near lakes and rivers or in moldy wood.

VIRAL MENINGITIS

Finally, viruses are a common cause of meningitis in adults and may even represent a majority of cases in the United States. **Enteroviruses** are the most common cause, although **herpes simplex** often occurs as well. As a reminder, viral meningitis tends to present with relatively "bland" findings on lumbar puncture, with the main clue being a predominance of **lymphocytes**.

Compared to bacterial meningitis, viral meningitis is generally more benign, with less severe symptoms, a slower progression, and a more rapid resolution (patients generally feel better within a week). In contrast to both bacterial and fungal meningitis, most cases of viral meningitis do not require specific treatment outside of **supportive care**, although if herpes simplex meningitis is suspected an antiviral medication known as **acyclovir** can be used.

PUTTING IT ALL TOGETHER

While it can seem like you're just memorizing trivia when it comes to remembering the most common causes of meningitis in each age group, there are direct clinical implications of this information that make it worthwhile. Because you need to act quickly when treating meningitis (both to save the patient's life and to spare them lasting dysfunction down the road), you really are "playing the odds" a lot of the time. For this reason, having some "shortcuts" to identify the most common causes based on the patient's baseline demographic information (such as their age or geographic location) group is essential! Use the **GEL** and **HeNS** mnemonic to remember bacterial causes based on age, and use the **geographic information** for fungal meningitis! A summary of these bugs is found in the two tables below.

Bacteria	Infants	Children/Adults	Features
GBS	✓		Passed during childbirth
E. coli	✓		K1 antigen associated with meningitis
Listeria	✓		Also in elderly and immunocompromised adults
H. influenzae		✓	Common resident in sinuses
N. meningitidis		✓	Purpuric rash, Waterhouse-Friderichsen syndrome
S. pneumoniae		✓	Common resident in respiratory tract

Fungus	Geographic Location	Source
C. neoformans	Worldwide	Bird droppings
C. immitis	Southwest US	Soil
Histoplasma	Midwestern US	Bird/bat droppings (caves)
Blastomyces	Midwestern US	Wet/damp places (rivers)

REVIEW QUESTIONS

1. A 10 y/o M is brought to the hospital after a generalized tonic-clonic seizure. He is awake but poorly responsive. Vital signs are HR 112, BP 104/60, RR 20, and T 102.0°F. Per his parents, he recently returned from a camping trip in the woods near the Appalachian Mountains. Since his return, he has been complaining of chills and headache, with an episode of vomiting this morning. On exam, he is not able to follow instructions. However, he does cry out when his neck is flexed and when the doctor attempts to examine his pupils with a pen light. Sensing the patient's pain, the doctor does not examine his optic discs. He is placed on his side in preparation for a lumbar puncture. He again cries out when his legs are drawn up towards his chest prior to the needle being inserted into his back. A lumbar puncture is performed which shows an elevated opening pressure, a cloudy appearance, decreased glucose, elevated protein, and a high lymphocyte count. Which of the following causative organisms is most likely to be seen in his cerebrospinal fluid?
    A. *Neisseria meningitidis*
    B. *Streptococcus pneumoniae*
    C. *Haemophilus influenza*
    D. *Herpes simplex virus*
    E. *Coccidioides immitis*
    F. *Blastomyces dermatitidis*

2. A 19 y/o M college student comes to the emergency department complaining of chills and a worsening headache over the past 3 days. He continued to go to class on the first day, but since then he has been in his room unable to get up or attend to his studies. Vital signs are HR 112, BP 118/78, RR 20, and T 101.3°F. On exam, there is significant pain when asked to bend his neck forward. He is unable to tolerate a test of his pupillary light reflexes and yells when a penlight is used. Lumbar puncture shows a dusty appearance of the cerebrospinal fluid, with an elevated opening pressure, increased protein, decreased glucose, and a predominance of polymorphonuclear neutrophils. Which of the following is the best next step in management?
    A. Ordering a CT of the head
    B. Ordering an MRI of the head
    C. Administering an antibiotic drug
    D. Administering an antiviral drug
    E. Administering an antifungal drug
    F. Providing immunizations to the patient
    G. Providing immunizations to the patient's close contacts
    H. Discharging with ibuprofen and a follow-up appointment in 1 week
    I. None of the above

3. (Continued from previous question.) The remainder of the exam is notable for several patches of punctate red dots over the abdomen and chest as seen below:

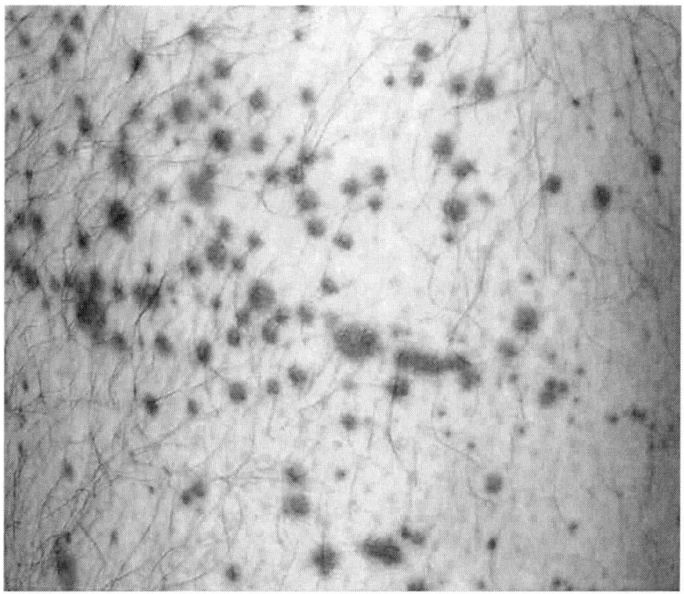

These patches do not lose their color when pressure is applied. Several hours after his initial presentation to the hospital, the patient begins to appear lethargic and has trouble answering questions. Repeat vital signs are HR 144, BP 70/32, RR 6, and T 101.8°F. He is seen coughing up blood, and his hands have turned a blue tint. Repeat labs are notable for hypoglycemia, hyponatremia, hyperkalemia, and thrombocytopenia. Which of the following is the most likely causative organism?

A. *Escherichia coli*
B. *Listeria monocytogenes*
C. *Streptococcus pneumonia*
D. *Neisseria meningitidis*
E. *Haemophilus influenza*
F. Herpes simplex
G. Herpes zoster
H. *Cryptococcus neoformans*
I. *Coccidioides immitis*
J. *Histoplasma*
K. *Blastomyces dermatitidis*

1. **The best answer is F.** Fever, headache, photophobia, a positive Brudzinski's sign, and a positive Kernig's sign are all highly suggestive of meningitis. The attributes of the cerebrospinal fluid on lumbar puncture can help to narrow down the possible infectious agents that could be causing his presentation. The presence of significant abnormalities in opening pressure, the elevated protein concentration, and the low glucose help to rule out an aseptic or viral meningitis (answer D). Fungal and bacterial meningitis both have these findings, so the best way of differentiating between them is to look at the cell predominance. Bacterial meningitis presents with a neutrophilic predominance while fungal meningitis presents with a lymphocytic predominance. In this case, the high number of lymphocytes argues against a bacterial cause of meningitis (answers A—C). The two fungi listed have different geographic distributions, with *Coccidioides* being found in the American southwest and *Blastomyces* being seen more in the eastern United States. In this case, the patient recently went camping in the Appalachian mountains, making *Blastomyces* more likely than *Coccidioides* (answer E).

2. **The best answer is C.** The patient's clinical presentation of headache, fever, nuchal rigidity, and photophobia is highly suggestive of meningitis, and his cerebrospinal fluid analysis makes bacterial infection the most likely cause. For this reason, administering an antibiotic should be the highest priority. His cerebrospinal fluid findings do not support a diagnosis of viral meningitis which would either be treated with antivirals or supportive care (answers D and H). Fungal meningitis would present with a predominance of lymphocytes, not neutrophils (answer E). Given the classic presentation of meningitis, there is no need for urgently ordering head imaging, especially if this would delay starting an antibiotic (answers A and B). Immunizing the patient would be of little benefit now (answer F). Depending on the specific organism causing the infection, immunizing close contacts should be done, but this is not the highest priority compared with treating the patient (answer G).

3. **The best answer is D.** The presence of a petechial rash as well as the patient's age range should both put *Neisseria meningitidis* high on your differential at this point. However, the strongest evidence is the development of Waterhouse-Friderichsen syndrome, or acute adrenal failure related to bleeding into the adrenal glands. Waterhouse-Friderichsen syndrome is strongly associated with meningococcal meningitis and is considered to be one of the most tragic outcomes, with a high mortality rate even with treatment. *Escherichia coli* and *Listeria monocytogenes* are both more common in infants than a young adult (answers A and B). The patient is in the correct age range for meningitis from *Streptococcus pneumonia* and *Haemophilus influenza*, though the presence of petechial rash and Waterhouse-Friderichsen syndrome make these much less likely (answers C and E). There is little evidence of viral meningitis (answers F and G) or fungal meningitis (answers H—K).

23 ENCEPHALITIS

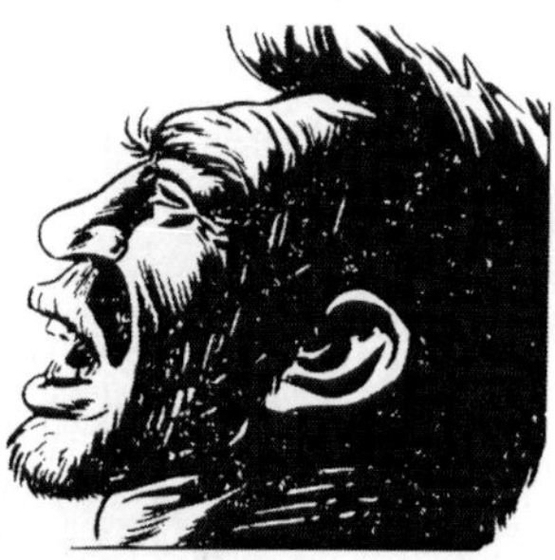

While meningitis involves inflammation in the layers covering the brain, **encephalitis** refers to a state of inflammation in the brain itself. This can occur as the result of an infection, an autoimmune reaction (where the immune system attacks its own body), or without a clear cause. In contrast to the "**neck symptoms**" such as nuchal rigidity, Kernig's sign, and Brudzinski's sign that are seen in meningitis, cases of encephalitis will often present with "**head symptoms**" such as headache, confusion, changes in cognition, and focal neurologic deficits (in addition to **non-specific symptoms** including fever and nausea). In some cases, meningitis and encephalitis can occur at the same time, such as when an infection spreads to both regions (this is known as **meningoencephalitis**).

Evaluation of patients suspected on having encephalitis typically involves a complete history and physical, neuroimaging, and lab testing of both blood and cerebrospinal fluid. If an infectious cause is found, treatment should be provided (such as **antibiotics** for a bacterial encephalitis or **antivirals** for a viral encephalitis). **Steroids** can be used to reduce swelling in the brain, while other medications can be used to increase the patient's comfort (like using NSAIDs for fever or sedatives for restlessness).

With that broad overview under our belts, we will now look at some of the most high-yield organisms with a tendency to infect the central nervous system!

VIRAL ENCEPHALITIS

Viruses are the most common cause of encephalitis, with bacterial, fungal, and parasitic causes being less common (though they are often more severe). Let's look at a few major causes of viral encephalitis.

HERPESVIRAL ENCEPHALITIS

Herpes simplex is the most common cause of viral encephalitis, with HSV-1 (the form of the virus that causes oral herpes or "cold sores") being much more common than HSV-2 (the form that causes genital herpes). Herpes simplex has a particular affinity for the **temporal lobe**, including the hippocampus and other parts of the limbic system. Inflammation in these areas can even show up on neuroimaging, as in the following MRI:

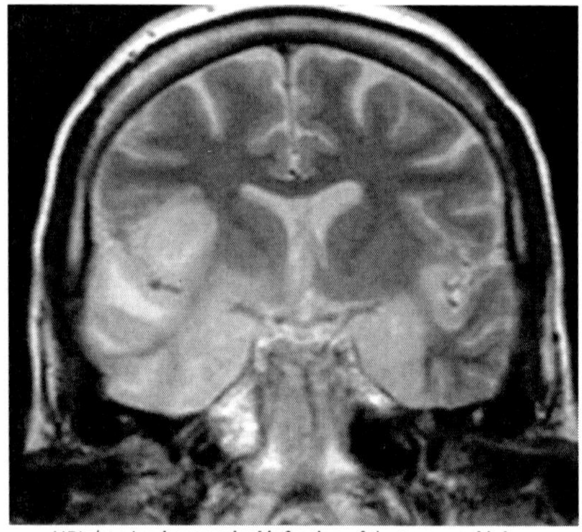

*MRI showing **herpesviral infection** of the **temporal lobes**.*

The fact that herpes infects the temporal lobe can be seen in the way it presents clinically, with **temporal lobe seizures** being common (in addition to the classic signs and symptoms of encephalitis including fever, headache, and altered mental status). Treatment involves the antiviral medication **acyclovir** which should be administered quickly and at high doses. Without treatment, herpes simplex encephalitis is almost uniformly fatal. Even with treatment, there is a high mortality rate. People who survive are often left with long-term neurologic deficits including **memory loss** (which makes sense considering that the hippocampus is often affected). You can remember the predilection of herpes for the hippocampus and other areas in the temporal lobe by thinking of it as the **herpe**-campus!

Herpes simplex is the most common cause of **viral encephalitis**.
It has a particular affinity for the **temporal lobe** and can cause **seizures**.

__Herpe__s tends to hit the __herpe-campus__ and other parts of the temporal lobe.

RABIES

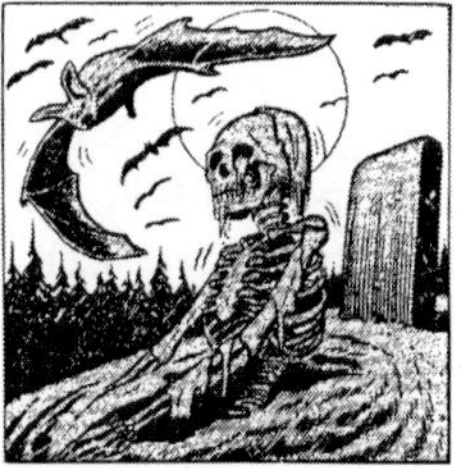

Rabies is an infection of the central nervous system involving various ***lyssaviruses***. It is most often caused by a bite from an infected animal. While dog bites are the most frequent source of rabies worldwide, in the United States **bat bites** are the most common. There are several unique features of rabies that you should be on the lookout for on boards and on wards! Let's use the acronym **FINISH** to keep these grouped together:

F is for Fatal without treatment. By the time a patient is showing symptoms, rabies is almost always fatal. If treatment has not been provided by this time, most patients will die within a week of diagnosis.

I is for Incubation period. Luckily, most people with rabies do not show signs and symptoms right away! Between the time of the bite and the disease presenting clinically is an **incubation period** lasting 1 to 3 months during which time the virus replicates. Once it has gathered sufficient numbers, it marches along motor neurons towards the central nervous system, essentially using the "streets" of the peripheral nervous system and the "highway" of the spinal cord to reach the "headquarters" of the brain in a process known as **retrograde transport**. Once there, it continues to replicate in the brain before sending additional viruses back out into the peripheral nervous system. This incubation period buys us some time to intervene and save the patient, as we will discuss shortly.

N is for Negri bodies. A diagnosis of rabies can be confirmed on autopsy, with a particular microscopic finding known as **Negri bodies** being found in motor neurons. These distinctive inclusion bodies are pathognomonic for rabies!

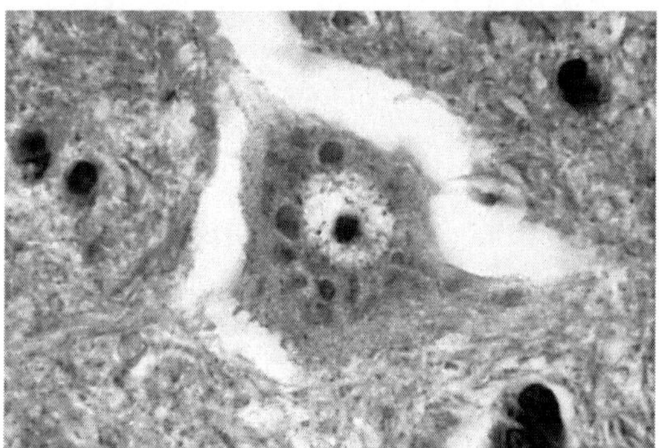

*Microscope image of brain tissue in a patient with **rabies** showing **Negri bodies**.*

I is for Immunization. The cornerstone of rabies treatment is to prevent symptoms from happening in the first place using **post-exposure prophylaxis**. This involves giving the rabies vaccine to anyone with a known or suspected bite from a rabid animal. Provided the vaccine is given within 10 days of exposure, it is **100% effective** for preventing progression to rabies!

S is for Salivary glands. Rabies uses the salivary glands as a base of operations to replicate, which explains why bites are the main form of viral transmission.

H is for Hydrophobia. One particularly notable sign that is specific for rabies is **hydrophobia** ("fear of water") which is found in the vast majority of cases. Someone infected with rabies may give a panicked response when presented with water even though they are extremely thirsty, and attempting to drink water will induce incredibly painful spasms of muscles in the throat. Hydrophobia is likely due to the tendency of the rabies virus to thrive in the salivary glands, as preventing water ingestion helps the virus to self-preserve and thereby increase its chances of transmission through a bite.

Overall, rabies is a tragic disease if it is not caught quickly, but luckily in the age of modern medicine the worst outcomes are usually preventable!

Rabies is a **viral disease** that infects the **central nervous system** after an **incubation period**, leading to **hydrophobia** and signs of **meningoencephalitis**.

FINISH:
Fatal without treatment
Incubation period
Negri bodies
Immunization
Salivary glands
Hydrophobia

SUBACUTE SCLEROSING PANENCEPHALITIS

Subacute sclerosing panencephalitis (or SSPE) is a rare but often fatal condition that is characterized by **widespread inflammation in the brain**. It is caused by the **measles virus**. It is unique among the forms of infectious encephalitis we have talked about so far in that it does *not* occur at the time of an acute infection. Instead, it can develop *years* after the patient has recovered from the initial illness.

While the vast majority of people who get measles will recover completely, a minority (0.01%) will go on to develop subacute sclerosing panencephalitis, with an average delay of 7 years. During this period, the patient is completely asymptomatic. However, over time some signs and symptoms begin to emerge, including changes in personality, cognitive deficits, muscle spasms, visual changes, and seizures. These abnormalities progressively accumulate to the point where vital functions such as breathing and heart rate are compromised, leading to death. Unfortunately, there is **no cure** for subacute sclerosing panencephalitis, so management is largely directed towards preventing infection with measles in the first place by use of a **vaccine**.

You can remember the typical course of SSPE by thinking of it as a comic book-like onomatopoeia for the sound of a bomb fuse slowly burning (SSssssssssssss) and then, after a long build-up, exploding (PppppEeeeee!). This will help you to remember the long delay between infection and onset as well as the catastrophic outcome!

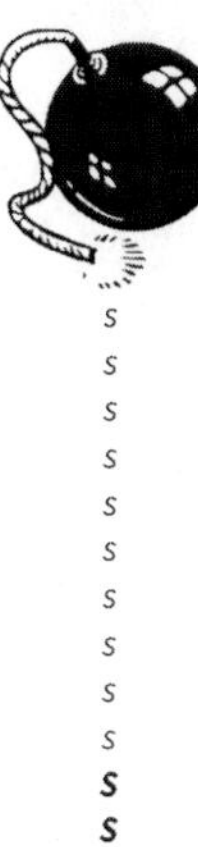

***P**ppppppppppppppppp**E**eeeeeeeeeee!*

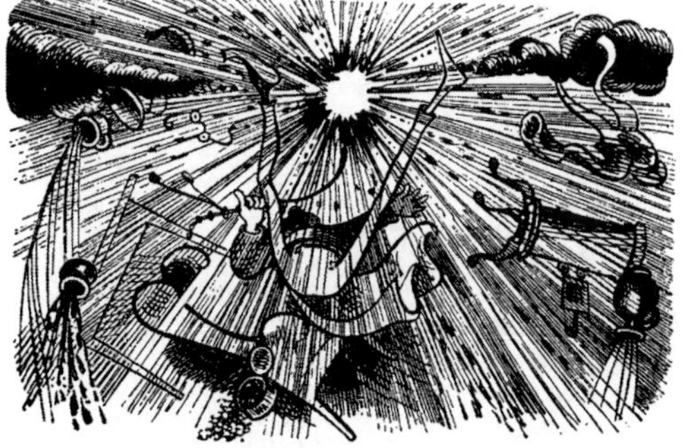

Subacute sclerosing panencephalitis (SSPE) is a disease involving **widespread inflammation in the brain** that occurs years after an initial **measles viral infection**.

*Think of **SSPE** as an onomatopoeia for a **bomb fuse** slowing burning (**SS**sssssss...) and then exploding (**P**pppppp**E**eeeeee!) after a long build-up.*

ARBOVIRUS ENCEPHALITIS

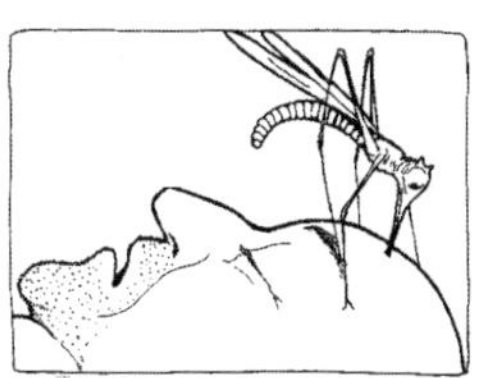

The final cause of viral encephalitis we will talk about are **arboviruses** which are carried by arthropods such as **mosquitos**. (In fact, the name arbovirus is a direct nod to this: **ar**thropod-**bo**rne **virus**.) Arboviruses are another leading cause of encephalitis, spanning a wide array of different syndromes that include such fanciful names as eastern equine encephalitis, western equine encephalitis, St. Louis encephalitis, and West Nile fever. The severity of these infections can vary significantly, with some cases producing only minimal symptoms and others resulting in life-threatening illness. The prevalence of arboviral encephalitis varies from region to region and even from season to season, with late summer (the period of highest mosquito activity, naturally) being the highest risk.

BACTERIAL ENCEPHALITIS

Bacterial infections of the brain are relatively rare compared to viral cases. While the clinical presentation is generally similar to viral encephalitis, it can also produce more **focal signs and symptoms** as well. This is because bacterial infections are more prone to creating a **brain abscess** which is a localized collection of pus that can affect nearby nervous tissue through **mass effect**. In this way, brain abscesses can at times present similarly to brain tumors, although abscesses tend to come on faster and present with other signs of infection such as fever.

Neuroimaging is almost always indicated if a brain abscess is suspected. If present, it can appear as a hole or "bubble" if it gets large enough (as seen in the following image). A lumbar puncture is generally not helpful, as abscesses are by definition localized meaning that organisms *won't* be found in the cerebrospinal fluid.

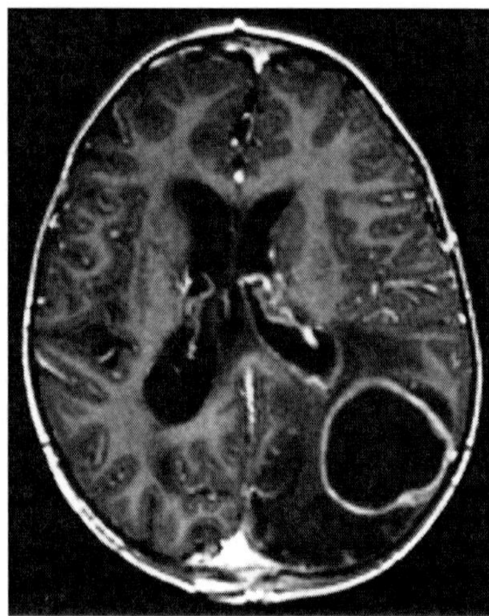

MRI of a ***brain abscess****.*

Most brain abscesses are caused by the spread of bacteria from the sinuses following a sinus infection, although a minority of cases are due to spread across the blood–brain barrier. Common organisms include *Streptococcus*, anaerobic organisms (such as *Bacteroides*), and *Staphylococcus aureus*. Treatment involves **antibiotics** tailored to the organisms present, with **surgery** being used if the abscess is at high risk of spreading to other areas.

NEUROSYPHILIS

Syphilis is a sexually transmitted infection caused by ***Treponema pallidum***, a corkscrew-shaped bacterium. While it doesn't often present with active inflammation of the brain, syphilis can affect the nervous system so it is worth talking about here.

Syphilis is notorious for being able to affect nearly every part of the body, making it one of the "great imitators" of medicine. However, it is particularly known for affecting the nervous system in later stages of the disease, often 5 to 10 years after the initial infection. Collectively, the neurologic manifestations of late-stage syphilis infection are called **neurosyphilis** (also known as **paresis** or **tertiary syphilis**). We can use the word **PARESIS** itself to remember the core signs and symptoms of the disease which include changes in **P**ersonality, changes in **A**ffect or emotion, hyperactive **R**eflexes due to upper motor neuron damage, **E**ye abnormalities (in particular the Argyll Robertson pupils that we talked about back in Chapter 10 where pupils will accommodate but not react), changes in **S**ensorium, **I**ntellectual and cognitive impairment related to atrophy of the brain (particularly in the frontal and temporal lobes) that can even lead to a state of full-blown dementia, and finally slurred **S**peech.

Neurosyphilis is a late-stage presentation of **syphilis infection** that involves the **nervous system**.

PARESIS:
P*ersonality changes*
A*ffective instability*
R*eflexes (hyperactive)*
E*ye abnormalities (Argyll Robertson pupils)*
S*ensorium changes*
I*ntellectual impairment*
S*peech slurring*

Neurosyphilis can take several different forms depending on where the infection is. When it affects the brain, it produces a syndrome known as **general paresis** which involves a variety of **psychiatric phenomena**. In contrast, when it attacks the spinal cord, it can lead to a particular syndrome known as **tabes dorsalis** (also known as syphilitic myelopathy). Tabes *dorsal*is involves demyelination of the *dorsal* columns, leading to loss of **F**ine touch, **V**ibration, and **P**roprioception (remember "**F**eeling **V**ery **P**atient!") with preservation of crude touch, pain, and temperature.

Neurosyphilis is relatively rare in the age of antibiotics. When it occurs, it can be quickly treated using **penicillin** (although any neuronal damage that has already taken place can usually not be reversed).

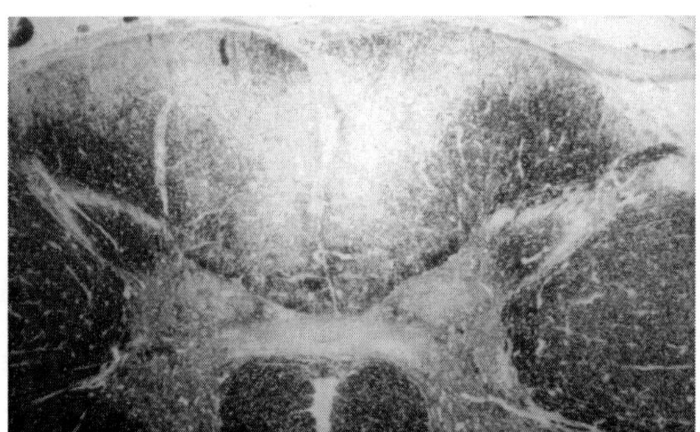

Cross-section of the spinal cord showing ***dorsal column demyelination*** *related to* ***tabes dorsalis****.*

PARASITIC ENCEPHALITIS

Unlike with meningitis (where most cases are attributed to either viruses, bacteria, or fungi), some cases of encephalitis are caused by **parasites** as well.

NEUROCYSTICERCOSIS

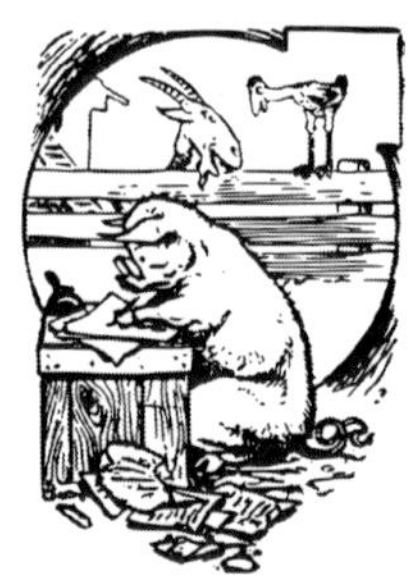

Cysticercosis is caused by an infection with ***Taenia solium***, a **parasitic tapeworm** found in **pigs**. When its larvae attack the central nervous system, it can lead to **neurocysticercosis**, with various signs and symptoms including headaches, confusion, blindness, and seizures. The "cysts" of neuro**cyst**icercosis refer to the cavitary lesions that occur in this condition which are visible on neuroimaging (as seen below). Due to its prevalence, neurocysticercosis is one of the leading causes of seizures worldwide, especially in parts of the world with poor sanitation. Treatment involves use of an **antiparasitic** medication such as albendazole or praziquantel as well as an **anticonvulsant** to help control seizures.

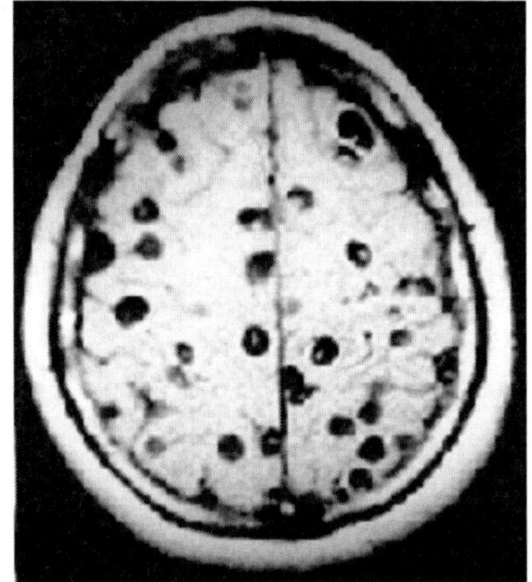

*MRI of **neurocysticercosis** showing multiple cysts within the brain.*

TOXOPLASMOSIS

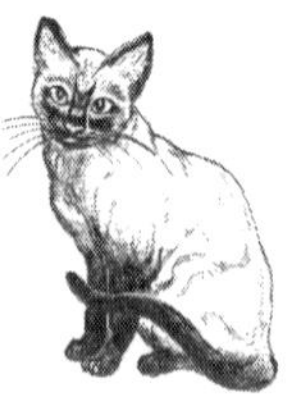

One particularly high-yield cause of parasitic encephalitis to know about is ***Toxoplasma gondii***, a single-celled protozoan parasite that is most often picked up from handling **cat feces** or **undercooked meat**. Infection by toxoplasmosis is common, with up to half of the world's population carrying this parasite around. Almost all carriers of toxoplasmosis are completely asymptomatic. However, two groups in particular are at high risk for a major toxoplasmosis infection: **newborns** and **immunocompromised adults**.

An infected mother can pass this parasite across the placenta onto her fetus, whose immune system is not able to fight it off as effectively. Babies with **congenital toxoplasmosis** are often born with the classic triad of **chorioretinitis** (inflammation of the eyes), **hydrocephalus**, and **intracranial atherosclerosis**, though they are also at risk of developing additional problems such as deafness, cognitive delays, and seizures. For this reason, pregnant women should not change cat litter!

In adults, the majority of people with active toxoplasmosis are those with compromised immune systems, with **HIV/AIDS** being the most common cause. Neuroimaging will reveal abscesses in a particular pattern known as **ring-enhancing lesions** as seen in the image below. This combination (multiple ring-enhancing lesions in a patient with HIV/AIDS) is so highly suggestive of toxoplasmosis that treatment is often started even before the diagnosis can be confirmed! Treatment generally consists of an **antiparasitic** and multiple **antibiotics**. You can remember the link between multiple ring-enhancing lesions and t**OXO**plasmosis by focusing on the **OXO**. Imagine the two **O**'s as the multiple ring-enhancing lesions surrounding an X superimposed on top of a brain to suggest that its function has been wiped out!

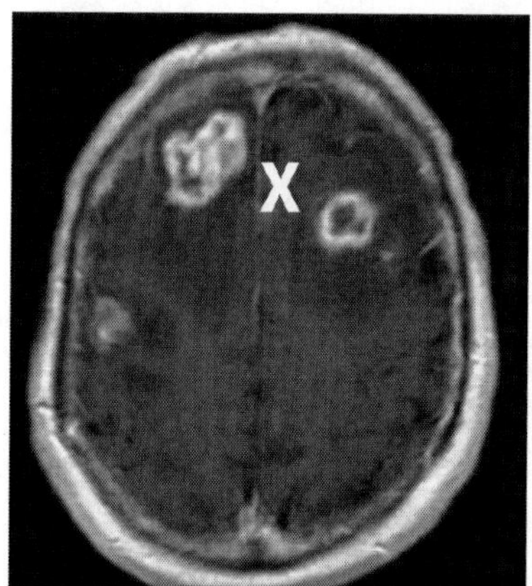

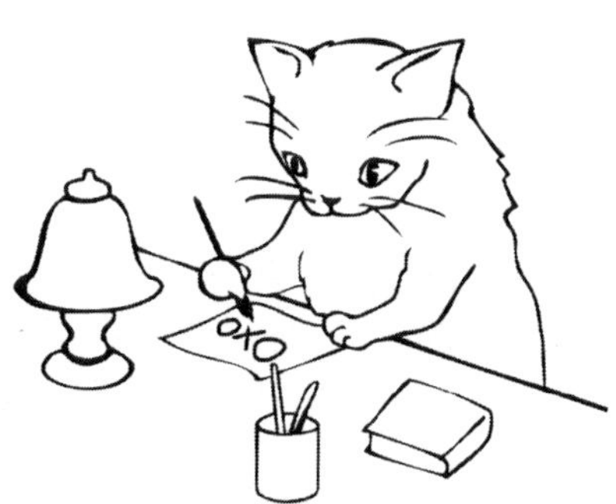

*MRI showing **ring-enhancing lesions** in a patient with **toxoplasmosis**.*

> ***Toxoplasma gondii*** is a **protozoal parasite** that can lead to **encephalitis** in **newborns** and **immunocompromised adults** (particularly those with **HIV/AIDS**).
>
> *Think of the **OXO** in t**OXO**plamosis as multiple **ring-enhancing lesions** in the brain.*

PRIMARY CNS LYMPHOMA

Wait a minute, isn't a lymphoma a type of *neoplasm*? Then why are we studying it in this chapter and not in Chapter 21? The reason is that cases of primary CNS lymphoma are almost always associated with infection by the **Epstein-Barr virus**, making it one of the few kinds of cancer that have a direct relationship to a viral infection. There is a great deal of overlap between central nervous system toxoplasmosis and primary CNS lymphoma, as both occur almost exclusively in **immunosuppressed** patients and can present with **ring-enhancing lesions**. While this combination should always make you think of toxoplasmosis *first*, in cases where a patient is not getting better after adequate treatment of toxoplasmosis, consider primary CNS lymphoma! Treatment consists of **chemotherapy**.

PRION DISEASE

Finally, we will talk about a very unusual (but also very deadly) form of encephalitis known as **prion disease**. Prions are an odd type of central nervous system infection in which the causative "organisms" are not organisms at all. Instead, prion diseases are characterized by the presence of **misfolded proteins** that are toxic to neurons (the word prion itself being short for "**pr**otein **i**nfecti**on**"). These proteins cause other nearby proteins to misfold as well, setting off a cascade of neurotoxicity that punches microscopic holes into nervous tissue, giving it a "spongy" appearance as seen in the following image:

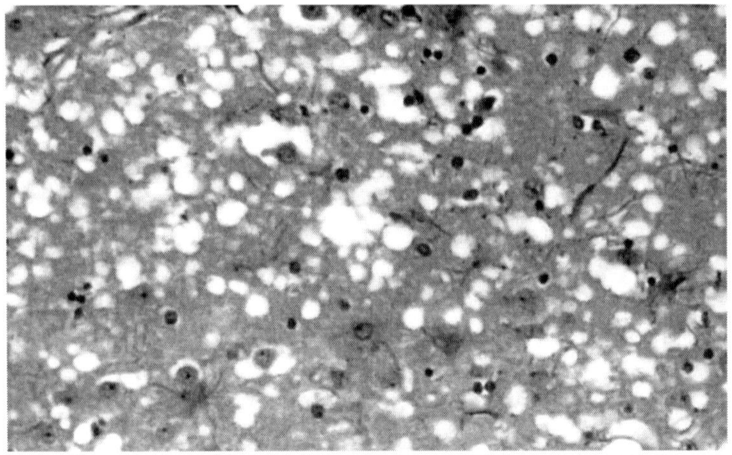

*Microscope image of the **prion disease** showing multiple holes in the gray matter.*

In humans, there are a few specific prion diseases that have been recognized, including **Creutzfeldt-Jakob disease**, **kuru**, and **fatal familial insomnia**. The misfolded protein that sets off the whole deadly cascade can be picked up from the environment (often through eating infected animal products), inherited, or acquired sporadically. The presenting signs and symptoms are highly variable but tend to include memory problems, changes in behavior, and poor coordination. One thing that is a big red flag for prion diseases is the **rapid speed** at which it progresses, as most people die within one year of diagnosis. Unfortunately, there are currently no treatments that have been shown to stop or reverse the disease.

Prions are **misfolded proteins** that are **toxic to neurons** and induce nearby proteins to misfold, resulting in **rapidly progressive neurodegenerative diseases**.

__Prion__s are __pr__otein __i__nfecti__on__s.

PUTTING IT ALL TOGETHER

The number of infectious diseases that can affect the nervous system is vast, and there is no way to cover them all in just a couple chapters. Instead, we have focused on those diseases that are the most **common** (the ones most likely to appear in patients and on tests), the most **devastating** (the ones that must be recognized and treated promptly to avoid a poor outcome), or the most **educational** (the ones that reinforce what we have learned about the anatomy and physiology of the nervous system by illustrating what happens when one aspect of it becomes dysfunctional).

Ultimately a lot of what we've covered can feel like trivia ("Which one is cat feces and which is bird droppings again?"). However, in high-stress clinical situations, this sort of information suddenly becomes relevant for helping to figure out what might be the cause of the patient's disease. Use the mnemonics here to try and remember as much information as you can. You never know when one of them will pop back into your head! Use the table below to identify the unique features of each disease that has been discussed in this chapter:

Disease	Cause	Treatment	Features
Herpes	Viral	Acyclovir	Temporal lobe seizures
Rabies	Viral	Immunization	Hydrophobia
SSPE	Post-viral	None	Long latent period (years)
Arboviruses	Viral	None	Mosquito-borne
Brain abscess	Bacterial	Antibiotics, surgery	Focal symptoms through mass effect
Neurosyphilis	Bacterial	Penicillin	General paresis, tabes dorsalis
Neurocysticercosis	Parasitic	Antiparasitics, anticonvulsants	Cavitary cysts
Toxoplasmosis	Parasitic	Antiparasitics, antibiotics	Multiple ring-enhancing lesions in immunocompromised adult (HIV/AIDS)
Primary CNS lymphoma	Viral	Chemotherapy	Presents similarly to toxoplasmosis
Prion disease	Prions	None	Rapid progression of cognitive decline

REVIEW QUESTIONS

1. A 44 y/o F who recently returned from travel overseas several months ago comes to see her primary care doctor for pain and tingling in her arm that she first noticed while cooking. The doctor diagnoses her with carpal tunnel syndrome and prescribes ibuprofen (a nonsteroidal anti-inflammatory drug) for pain. Several days later, she comes to the emergency department of a local hospital reporting shortness of breath and difficulty swallowing. During the initial interview, she seems confused and in distress. Vital signs are unremarkable. She is admitted for further work-up. Overnight, the nurse notices that she is becoming increasingly agitated. She is unable to drink the water that the nurse brings to her and is seen violently gasping for air while attempting to hold the cup to her mouth. Despite various interventions, she continues to decline over the next few days and soon requires mechanical ventilation for respiratory failure. She passes away one week later. Which of the following is most likely to be observed on post-mortem autopsy?
   A. Spongy appearance of brain tissue
   B. Multiple cysts within the brain
   C. Demyelination of the dorsal columns
   D. Intracellular neuronal inclusion bodies
   E. Localized collections of pus within the brain

2. A 15 y/o M is brought to the hospital by his parents who report that he has been "acting crazy." Starting a few days ago, he began talking constantly about "things that make no sense" and at times appears to be having conversations with people who are not there. When asked, he reports hearing voices but is unable to clarify further. A complete examination is unremarkable except for a low-grade fever of 100.9°F. His attention, concentration, and memory are all poor on mental status examination. He has no psychiatric history prior to this episode. A urine drug screen is negative. He is admitted to the psychiatric hospital for further evaluation. The next day, he becomes lethargic and develops swelling of his lips. He is then observed having a tonic-clonic seizure lasting about one minute. Brain imaging shows localized inflammation of the temporal lobes. Which of the following is the best next step for definitive treatment of this condition?
   A. Supportive care
   B. Ceftriaxone (a cephalosporin antibiotic)
   C. Penicillin (a β-lactam antibiotic)
   D. Acyclovir (an antiviral)
   E. Amphotericin (an antifungal)
   F. Valproic acid (an anticonvulsant)

3. A 41 y/o M is admitted to the hospital for confusion and disorientation. He is HIV positive but has a long history of non-compliance with antiretroviral medications. A review of his chart reveals a 20 lb. weight loss in the past 3 months. On exam, he is oriented to person and place only. His temperature is elevated to 102.0°F. Neurological exam reveals left-sided hemiparesis with hyperreflexia and an upgoing plantar reflex. An MRI is obtained which shows multiple ring-enhancing lesions in the brain, so a presumptive diagnosis of toxoplasmosis is made and empiric treatment with antitoxoplasmosis medications is started. Despite treatment, he shows no improvement over the next several days. He experiences two tonic-clonic seizures on hospital day 5 and does not recover, remaining unresponsive afterwards. Which of the following would most likely explain his lack of response to treatment?
    A. Failure to use antiparasitic medication
    B. Failure to surgically drain the abscess
    C. Failure to vaccinate
    D. Missed diagnosis of prion disease
    E. Missed diagnosis of viral infection

1. **The best answer is D.** This vignette describes a case of rabies as evidenced by the presence of hydrophobia and a fatal outcome. Negri bodies, or intracellular inclusion bodies, are pathognomonic for rabies and can be seen on autopsy. A spongy appearance of brain tissue is more consistent with prion disease (answer A), multiple cysts would be seen in neurocysticercosis (answer B), dorsal column demyelination is seen in syphilis (answer C), and localized collections of pus are seen in brain abscesses related to bacterial infection (answer E).

2. **The best answer is D.** This vignette describes a case of herpesviral encephalitis which has a tendency to localize to the temporal lobe. The involvement of the temporal lobe explains some features of this case including impaired memory (from the hippocampus) and auditory hallucinations (from the auditory cortex). Definitive treatment of herpesviral encephalitis involves high-dose acyclovir, although supportive care and an anticonvulsant (answers A and F) could play a supporting role as well. Ceftriaxone is used in cases of bacterial meningitis (answer B), while penicillin would be used in cases of syphilis (answer C). Amphotericin would be used in cases of fungal meningitis (answer E).

3. **The best answer is E.** While an immunocompromised patient presenting with multiple ring-enhancing lesions in the brain is highly suggestive of toxoplasmosis, it is not the only possible explanation. This presentation can also be seen in cases of primary CNS lymphoma which are almost always associated with the Epstein-Barr virus. Use of an antiparasitic medication would not be helpful in cases of primary CNS lymphoma (answer A). Surgical drainage is primarily helpful in cases of brain abscesses (answer B). There is no vaccine yet available for Epstein-Barr virus (answer C). While prion disease can similarly present with a rapid decline in cognitive function, it does not present with ring-enhancing lesions (answer D).

24 PERIPHERAL NEUROPATHY

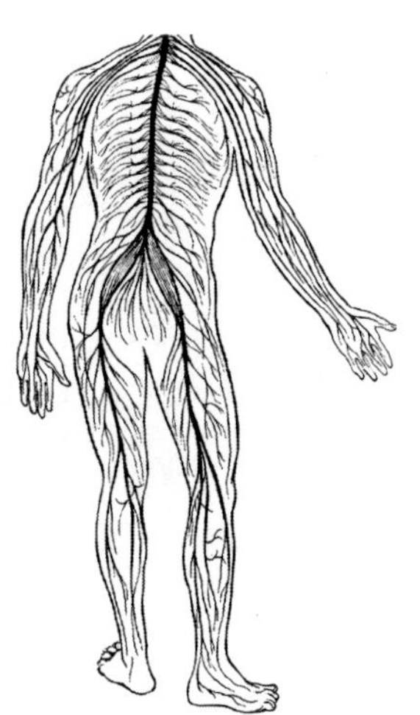

We learned in Chapter 9 that there are 12 pairs of cranial nerves and 31 pairs of spinal nerves in the human body. However, each of these nerves splits into many smaller subdivisions, creating the seemingly infinite number of unique nerves that make up the peripheral nervous system. When dysfunction arises in any of these nerves, it is known as a **peripheral neuropathy**. In some cases, only one nerve is affected a time, creating a focal neurologic deficit (for example, when compression of the sciatic nerve running through the pelvis leads to pain and weakness in the leg). In other cases, multiple nerves can be affected at once (such as a cervical plexus injury leading to symptoms in the arm and hand). In still other cases, a systemic disease can affect *all* nerves in the body, leading to widespread dysfunction (for example, when exposure to a neurotoxin causes death of nerves throughout the body). Dysfunction of a single nerve is known as a **mononeuropathy**, while a generalized dysfunction of multiple nerves is known as **polyneuropathy**.

Because of the wide variability in which nerves are affected from patient to patient, the presenting signs and symptoms of peripheral neuropathy can be totally different from one case to the next. Nevertheless, some general themes do emerge! In this chapter, we'll explore some key patterns when it comes to diagnosing peripheral neuropathies before talking about some of the most common causes. We'll wrap up by talking about a few high-yield diseases involving peripheral neuropathy that are most likely to pop up on boards and wards!

SIGNS AND SYMPTOMS OF PERIPHERAL NEUROPATHY

Because most nerves have both motor and sensory aspects, peripheral neuropathies often present as a combination of **sensory abnormalities** (such as numbness and/or pain) and **motor deficits** (like weakness or paralysis). If a nerve makes up part of the sympathetic or parasympathetic nervous system, signs and symptoms of **autonomic dysfunction** (like hypotension or constipation) can be present as well. We'll talk about each of these one by one.

Sensory disturbances related to peripheral neuropathy can involve not only the *absence* of *normal* sensations but also the *presence* of *abnormal* sensations. These sensations can range from the merely uncomfortable (such as a "pins and needles" tingling sensation known as **paresthesia**) to the outright painful (including "burning," "stabbing," or "electrical" sensations known as **neuropathic pain**). On the other hand, **sensory loss** can occur in some modalities but not others (such as someone who is unable to sense vibration or proprioception in their toes but can still feel pain and temperature) or can be complete (with a total absence of *all* sensory signals coming from a particular part of the body). In some cases, this lack of sensation can lead to injury if the patient is unable to sense that they are damaging a part of their body.

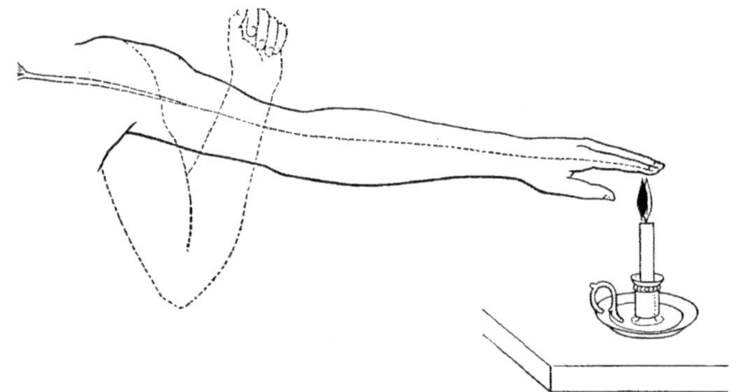

***Numbness** related to **peripheral neuropathy** can lead to a lack of protective reflexes.*

Motor deficits are generally associated with **lower motor neuron** signs, which makes sense as it is the peripheral nerve (and not a higher-up part of the chain like the motor cortex or basal ganglia) that is involved. Lower motor neuron signs should be familiar to you by now, but as a reminder they tend to involve flaccid paralysis, poor reflexes, low muscle tone, diminished power, and decreased bulk.

Autonomic dysfunction can involve basically any part of the sympathetic or parasympathetic nervous systems, including the ability to regulate vascular tone (producing an inability to constrict the blood vessels in response to postural changes known as **orthostatic hypotension**), bowel and bladder functions (which can lead to constipation or incontinence), and sexual function (which can result in impotence).

The specific nerves affected also have implications for the presenting signs and symptoms. In a *mono*neuropathy, the specific nerve that is damaged will determine what parts of the body are affected. We discussed a few common mononeuropathies back in Chapter 9 (such as wrist drop related to radial neuropathy or winged scapula resulting from long thoracic neuropathy). In contrast, in cases of a *poly*neuropathy, the most common pattern is for the most *distal* parts of the nerves to be affected first, while more proximal areas are spared. This results in a characteristic "**stocking glove**" pattern in which the ends of the extremities are most severely affected, as seen below:

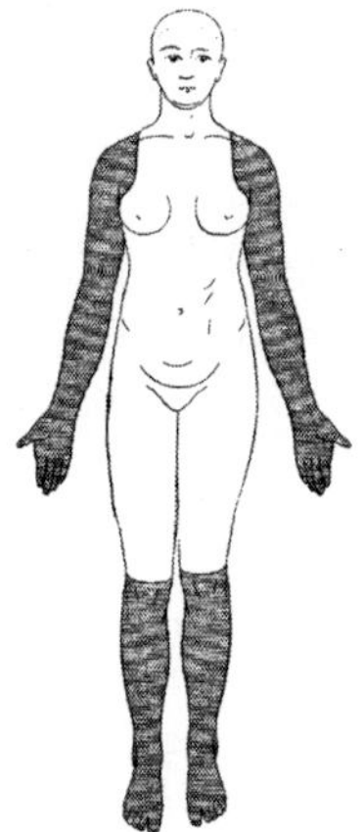

*A **"stocking glove" distribution** of **peripheral neuropathy**.*

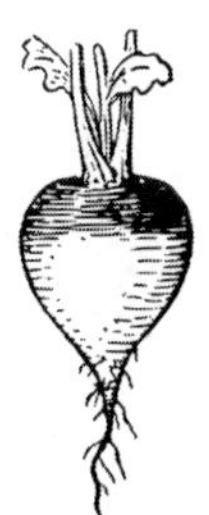

A specific form of localized neuropathy known as a **radiculopathy** occurs when a spinal nerve is affected at its **root** just after exiting from the spinal cord. This often occurs due to an injury or degeneration of the spinal bones, resulting in a narrowing of the space through which the nerve travels on its way out of the spinal cord (radiculopathies are often called a "pinched nerve" for this reason). This has a tendency to cause pain, sensory loss, and weakness in a **strict dermatomal and myotomal distribution**. You can remember the association of **radi**culopathy with compression of the nerve **root** by thinking of a **radish**-ulopathy to link it to a common **root** vegetable.

A **radiculopathy** involves dysfunction of a **nerve root**, leading to pain, numbness, and weakness in a **strict dermatomal and myotomal distribution.**

*A **radish**-culopathy involves the nerve **root** (just like a **radish** is a **root** vegetable).*

In some cases, dysfunction can affect areas that are not close together enough to be considered part of the same group of nerves but are not dispersed enough to be considered a generalized polyneuropathy. Instead, the affected nerves are almost randomly distributed throughout the body (as in a case of someone who develops simultaneous neuropathies in both the left wrist and right thigh). These cases are referred to as **mononeuritis multiplex** (with the "mono-" prefix referring to the fact that it seems to hit individual nerves and the "multi-" prefix suggesting that it is hitting multiple nerves at once). In many cases, mononeuritis multiplex represents a kind of "pre-polyneuropathy" in that it progresses and becomes more widespread to the point that it is mostly indistinguishable from a generalized polyneuropathy.

CAUSES OF PERIPHERAL NEUROPATHY

While peripheral neuropathies can occur "out of the blue," in most cases they are a *symptom* of an underlying disease rather than the disease itself. For this reason, any patient presenting with peripheral neuropathy should undergo a thorough work-up to determine where the damage is coming from! To remember all of the potential causes of peripheral neuropathy, use the mnemonic **GOSH DARNED PAIN**:

G is for Genetic. Several **genetic disorders** can damage peripheral nerves, including some that we will talk about later in this chapter like Charcot-Marie-Tooth disease.

O is for Oncologic. Several forms of **cancer** can cause peripheral neuropathies, especially those that are based in the blood rather than in a solid organ (such as lymphoma or multiple myeloma). Many forms of **chemotherapy** used to treat cancer can themselves damage peripheral nerves as well.

S is for Sugars. Diabetes mellitus is the single **most common cause** of peripheral neuropathy, as high levels of **sugar** in the bloodstream can injure the small blood vessels that supply nerves with oxygen and lead to ischemic damage.

H is for Hematologic. Various diseases of the blood can affect peripheral nerves. One example is **amyloidosis**, a disease in which amyloid proteins deposit into tissues throughout the body. When these proteins deposit into peripheral nerves, they can produce a sensory neuropathy that begins distally and moves in proximally.

D is for Drugs. We've made mention of the fact that chemotherapy can result in peripheral neuropathy, but this is just the tip of the iceberg! All sorts of **medications** have the nasty side effect of damaging peripheral nerves, including those used for infections (like metronidazole, nitrofurantoin, and isoniazid), seizures (phenytoin), heart conditions (amiodarone and digoxin), high blood pressure (hydralazine), hyperlipidemia (statins), and psychiatric conditions (lithium), just to name a few.

A is for Alcohol. By far the most common toxin that causes a peripheral neuropathy is **alcohol**. Alcoholic neuropathy involves degeneration of both motor and sensory nerves throughout the body. It's unclear whether alcohol itself is directly responsible for the nerve damage or whether it results from the nutritional deficiencies that frequently accompany cases of chronic alcoholism. Nevertheless, abstinence from alcohol does appear to reduce the severity of alcoholic neuropathy, suggesting that there is some direct effect.

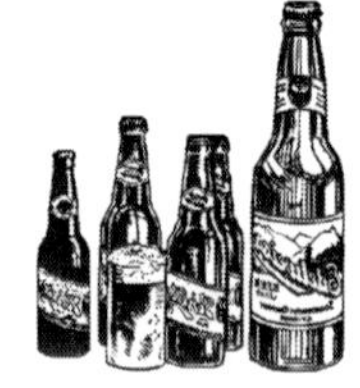

R is for Rheumatologic. Several diseases of the joints and connective tissue can be associated with peripheral neuropathy. An example is **sarcoidosis**, a disease in which immune cells collect into discrete lumps known as granulomas. These granulomas can grow and cause problems in almost any area of the body, with the nervous system being no exception. Sarcoidosis has a tendency to affect the central nervous system and cranial nerves, although spinal nerves can be affected as well.

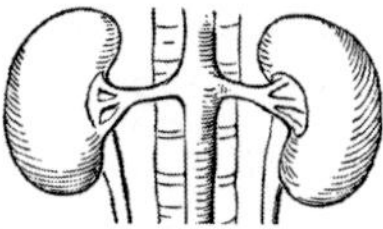

N is for Nephrogenic. Failure of the **kidneys** to properly clear out waste products from the body can lead to peripheral neuropathy if these toxins build up to excessive amounts, a condition known as **uremic neuropathy**.

E is for Environmental. A variety of chemicals can be neurotoxic, making it essential to screen for **environmental exposures** in patients presenting with a peripheral neuropathy. In particular, **heavy metals** such as lead, arsenic, mercury, and gold are often associated with various forms of nerve damage.

D is for Diet. Various nutritional deficiencies can lead to damage in peripheral nerves, with **vitamins B_{12} and B_6** being the two you should be most aware of!

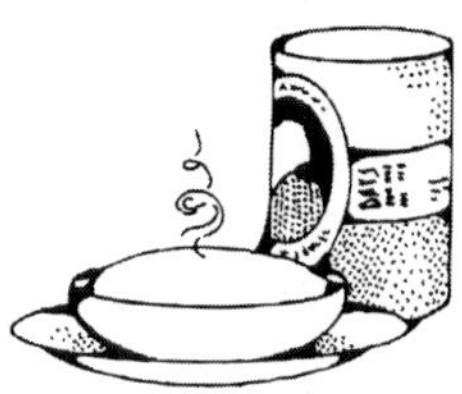

Recall from Chapter 8 that a deficiency of vitamin B_{12} can lead to "not 1 but 2" forms of nerve damage, with both epicritic numbness (from damage to the dorsal columns) as well as motor weakness (from damage to the corticospinal tract) being seen. Vitamin B_{12} deficiency can result from an inability to absorb this nutrient through the gut, or it can come from a heavily restricted diet (with a "**tea and toast**" diet being the classic buzzwords on a boards question!).

A deficiency in vitamin B_6 (also known as **pyridoxine**) can also lead to peripheral neuropathy, as this vitamin is needed to synthesize a molecule that forms a part of nerve cell membranes.

P is for Physical injury. Direct physical trauma to a nerve is a very common cause of peripheral neuropathy, especially in cases involving a focal mononeuropathy. While major injuries like stab wounds are obvious causes, even more subtle damage can lead to dysfunction, especially if it is chronic. A common example of this is **carpal tunnel syndrome** in which the median nerve becomes compressed as it travels through the wrist, leading to pain and weakness in the hand.

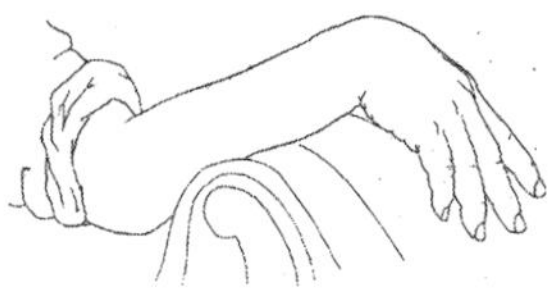

A is for Autoimmune. A few **autoimmune diseases** (such as Guillain–Barré syndrome, which we will talk about in the next chapter) can use the body's own immune system to attack peripheral nerves.

I is for Infections. As we covered in the last few chapters, several **infectious diseases** have a tendency to affect the nervous system, and peripheral nerves are no exception! We'll cover a few more (like shingles and Lyme disease) later in this chapter. Another common culprit is **HIV/AIDS** which can cause a distal symmetric polyneuropathy in some patients with the disease (although this may partly be attributable to the drugs used to treat HIV, many of which can themselves cause peripheral neuropathy!).

N is for No known cause. Unfortunately, it's not always possible to find an underlying cause in all patients presenting with a peripheral neuropathy! These are known as **idiopathic** cases, and they can be just as painful and debilitating to the patient as those related to an underlying condition. Idiopathic cases of peripheral neuropathy can affect a single nerve or can involve multiple nerves across the body.

Peripheral neuropathies are a symptom of an **underlying disease** in most cases, although **idiopathic neuropathies** can occur as well.

GOSH DARNED PAIN:

***G**enetic*	***D**rugs*	***P**hysical injury*
***O**ncologic*	***A**lcohol*	***A**utoimmune*
***S**ugars*	***R**heumatologic*	***I**nfectious*
***H**ematologic*	***N**ephrogenic*	***N**o known cause*
	***E**nvironmental*	
	***D**iet*	

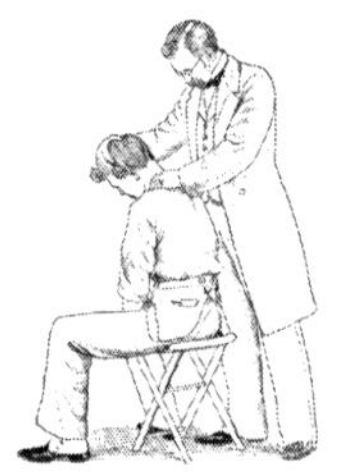

In cases where a peripheral neuropathy is related to an underlying condition, treatment involves identifying the upstream cause and addressing it (like helping a patient cut down on alcohol or better control their blood sugar levels). In some cases, additional testing is warranted, such as **nerve conduction studies** (to assess for abnormalities in the ability of peripheral nerves to conduct an impulse) and/or **electromyography** (to detect problems with both the muscle itself as well as the nerve supplying it).

When peripheral neuropathy cannot be addressed through these measures (or when there is no known cause), additional treatments aimed specifically at reducing symptoms and improving quality of life can be helpful. For cases with motor involvement, **physical and occupational therapy** can help to restore function. For cases involving neuropathic pain, specific medications like **anticonvulsants** (such as gabapentin and topiramate), **antidepressants** (amitriptyline and duloxetine), and **anesthetics** (lidocaine and capsaicin) can relieve suffering. Non-pharmacologic treatments such as a **transcutaneous electrical nerve stimulator** (TENS) device can also improve neuropathic pain by using electric signals to block transmission of pain signals on peripheral nerves. All in all, make sure to consider **both drugs and non-pharmacologic strategies** for managing painful peripheral neuropathies!

DISEASES ASSOCIATED WITH PERIPHERAL NEUROPATHY

While the **GOSH DARNED PAIN** mnemonic will remind you of the broad categories of diseases that can cause peripheral neuropathies, it's worth discussing a few specific conditions that include peripheral neuropathy as a core aspect of the pathology. The diseases featured here are all high-yield, either because they are common in clinical settings or because they help to illustrate the structure and function of various aspects of the nervous system. Many of these will be infectious diseases, but we'll also cover a few genetic conditions as well. Let's dive in!

LYME DISEASE

Lyme disease is a tick-borne illness caused by the bacterium ***Borrelia burgdorferi***. The hallmark sign of early infection is a characteristic "bull's eye" rash known as **erythema migrans** (as seen in the image below) which is often accompanied by flu-like symptoms. Following this initial localized infection, *Borrelia* can travel through the bloodstream and cause problems in other areas of the body, causing pain in various joints (arthritis) as well as abnormal heart rhythms (cardiac conduction abnormalities).

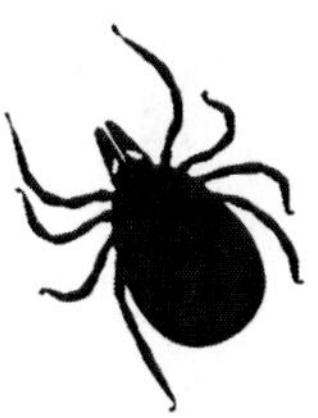

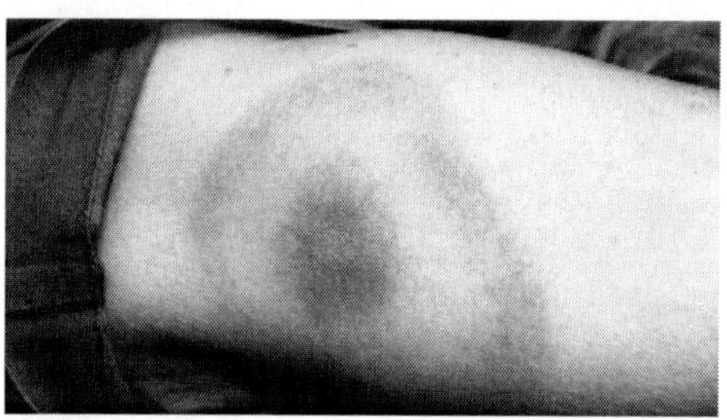

Erythema migrans *in a patient infected with* ***Lyme disease****.*

When *Borrelia* infects the nervous system, it causes a syndrome known as **neuroborreliosis** which can damage both the central and peripheral nervous system. Central nervous system involvement can present as **encephalitis** (with confusion, mood changes, and cognitive deficits) as well as the possibility of developing **meningitis**. However, Lyme disease is perhaps best known for its peripheral nerve manifestations, including a generalized **peripheral neuropathy** as well as **Bell's palsy** or a paralysis of the facial nerve as seen below:

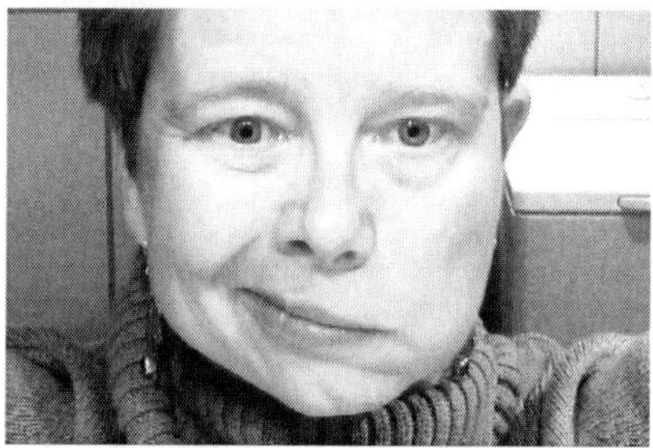

Bell's palsy *related to* ***Lyme disease****.*

Treatment of Lyme disease involves **antibiotics** such as doxycycline to target the *Borrelia* bacteria. However, as with other infections, the most important step is prevention, which in this case involves **avoidance of ticks** (such as by wearing long-sleeve clothing, using insect repellent, or even staying out of areas that are known to have ticks altogether!).

To remember the key associations with **Lyme** disease, use the word "**B-lime**y!" to add a B to this disease. The B should help you remember **B**ell's palsy and the "**B**ull's eye" rash which are the two most distinctive findings related to Lyme disease!

Lyme disease is a **tick-borne disease** that causes a **"bull's eye" rash** in its initial stages, followed by **Bell's palsy** and other peripheral neuropathies.

***B-lime**y will help you remember the two most distinctive findings in **Lyme** disease: **B**ell's palsy and a "**B**ull's eye" rash.*

SHINGLES

Shingles is a **painful blistering rash** that occurs as the result of an infection by the **varicella zoster virus** (the same virus that causes chickenpox). After an infection with chickenpox, the virus is not cleared from the body but instead lays dormant in the **dorsal root ganglion** of specific spinal nerves. The virus can then reactivate years or even decades later, at which point it travels down the axons of the spinal nerve to the skin where it causes inflammation, including the characteristic rash (as seen below). Notably, this rash occurs in a **dermatomal distribution** depending on the specific spinal nerve involved, so make sure to know your dermatomal landmarks!

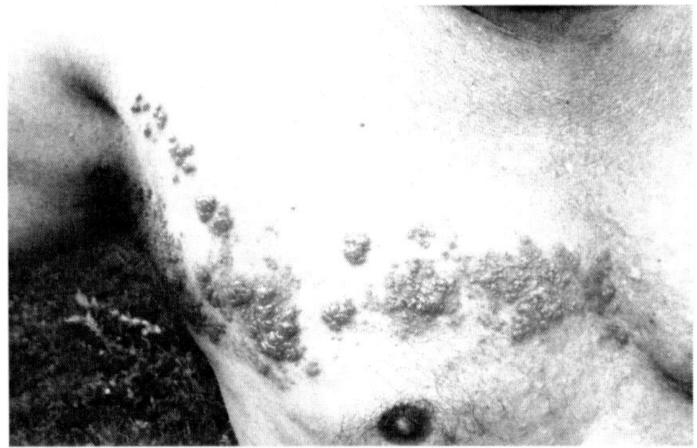

***Shingles** infection in the T3 dermatome.*

This rash typically lasts several weeks before the virus returns to a latent state. However, in some people the nerve damage caused by shingles can lead to lasting pain even after the infection has gone back to being dormant (known as **postherpetic neuralgia**). Treatment with acyclovir can help to shorten the duration of the rash, though the best strategy is to prevent shingles from occurring through **vaccination**.

LEPROSY

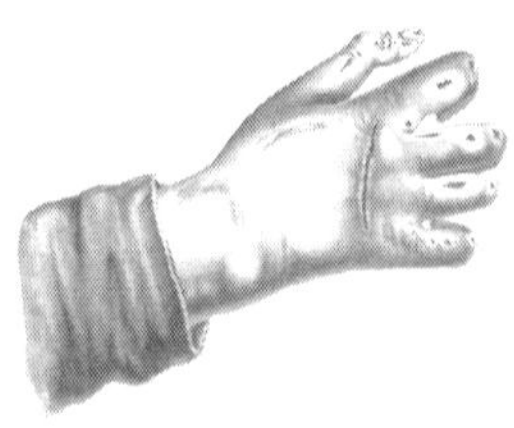

Leprosy (or Hansen's disease) occurs when infection with the *Mycobacterium* bacteria leads to nerve damage. **Loss of pain and temperature sensation** is often the most pronounced finding, although muscle weakness can occur as well. Due to the lack of pain sensation, people with leprosy are at high risk of injuring themselves, particularly their hands and feet. Leprosy is rare in the modern world, although it is not unheard of! Treatment involves a combination of multiple antibiotics for maximum efficacy.

TRIGEMINAL NEURALGIA

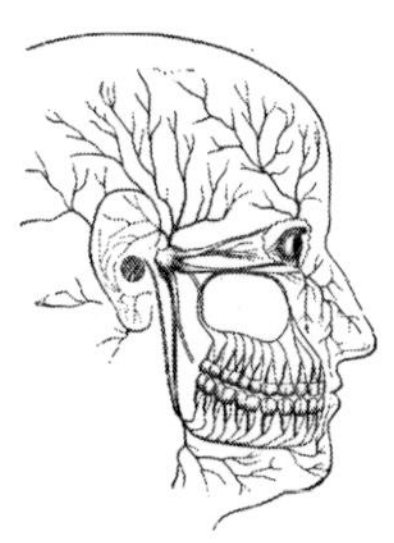

One particularly high-yield idiopathic mononeuropathy to know is **trigeminal neuralgia** which presents as severe pain in regions supplied by the trigeminal nerve, including all parts of the face. These can either occur in sudden "attacks" lasting a few minutes or may be present in a more chronic form. Trigeminal neuralgia is one of the most painful conditions known. The exact cause is unclear, although it may be related to demyelination as higher rates of trigeminal neuralgia can be seen in patients with demyelinating diseases like multiple sclerosis.

CHARCOT–MARIE–TOOTH DISEASE

We will round out this chapter by talking about a few genetic diseases in which peripheral neuropathy plays a major role. The first is **Charcot–Marie–Tooth disease**, a condition involving a mutation in one or more of the genes that directly contribute to the **myelin sheath**. This leads to both **motor weakness and epicritic numbness** that begins during childhood and progressively gets worse with age. While pain *sensation* is generally preserved (as those nerves are unmyelinated), many patients with this disease often experience **neuropathic pain** as well.

Charcot–Marie–Tooth disease is associated with various physical abnormalities, including prominent **foot deformities** like the high arch seen in the following image. You can remember the shape of the foot in this disease by thinking of its name as "**Shark**-o"–Marie–Tooth disease (as that is how the first part of the name is pronounced), as the high arch looks like a shark took a bite out of it!

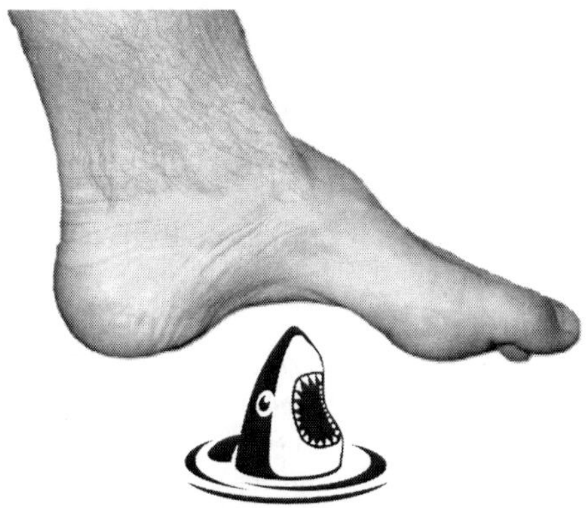

***Foot deformity** related to **Charcot–Marie–Tooth disease**.*

Charcot–Marie–Tooth disease is a genetic disorder involving defects in the **myelin sheath**, leading to a **motor and sensory neuropathy**.
Physical deformities like an **arched foot** are common.

*It looks like a **shark** took a **bite** out of a foot in "**Shark**-o"–Marie–Tooth disease!*

FRIEDREICH'S ATAXIA

Another form of inherited peripheral neuropathy is **Friedreich's ataxia** which, like Charcot-Marie-Tooth disease, involves damage to **myelinated nerves**. For unclear reasons, **epicritic nerves** are affected to a greater extent than motor nerves (as opposed to Charcot-Marie-Tooth disease where both are affected about equally).

As you might guess from the word "ataxia" in its name, this disease also features widespread atrophy of the **spinocerebellar pathways** connecting the cerebellum to the spinal cord, leading to a variety of cerebellar signs like those captured in the "dizzy AUNT with 3 dishes" mnemonic. Furthermore, many patients have abnormalities in other organ systems as well, including **hypertrophic cardiomyopathy** (an enlarged heart), **diabetes mellitus**, and various skeletal abnormalities such as **scoliosis** (an abnormal curvature of the spine) and **arched feet** (another similarity with Charcot-Marie-Tooth disease!). You can link together these seemingly random findings using the mnemonic "**fried rich CANDI**" which will remind you of **C**ardiomyopathy, **A**taxia, **N**europathy, **D**iabetes, and **I**rregular anatomy.

Friedreich's ataxia is an **autosomal recessive disorder** resulting in atrophy of **spinocerebellar pathways.** It is associated with **hypertrophic cardiomyopathy**, **diabetes mellitus**, and **skeletal deformities** like scoliosis.

Friedreich's ataxia *should make you think of* ***fried rich CANDI****:*
__C__ardiomyopathy
__A__taxia
__N__europathy
__D__iabetes
__I__rregular anatomy

Friedreich's ataxia is an **autosomal recessive** disease in which mutations in the **frataxin gene** are passed down to one's offspring. However, affected individuals often don't show signs of the disease until later childhood (usually around the age of 10). A suspected diagnosis can be confirmed by genetic testing which will show a **trinucleotide repeat sequence GAA** on **chromosome 9**. You can connect the trinucleotide sequence GAA to this disease by thinking of a child going **GAA GAA** over **fried rich CANDI**.

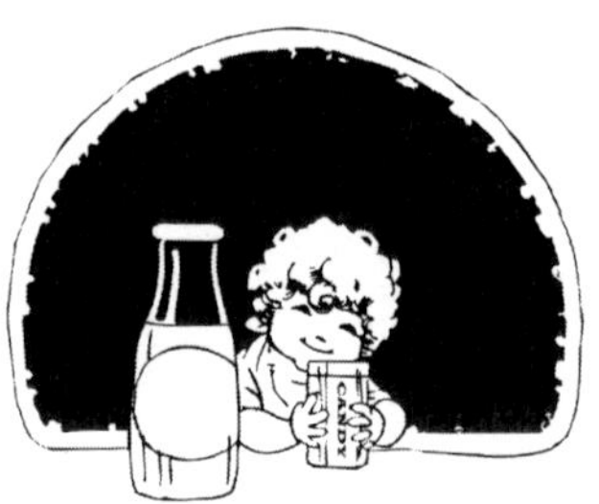

Friedreich's ataxia results from an expansion of the **trinucleotide sequence GAA** on **chromosome 9**.

Think of a child going ***GAA GAA*** *over* ***fried rich CANDI****.*

PORPHYRIAS

Finally, we will talk about one last genetic disorder that is associated with peripheral neuropathy. The **porphyrias** are a group of diseases in which enzyme deficiencies lead to excessive levels of substances called porphyrins in the body. When porphyrins build up, they can lead to a syndrome involving a triad of **abdominal pain**, **psychiatric symptoms** such as anxiety and hallucinations, and a generalized **polyneuropathy**. The neuropathy in porphyria tends to preferentially affect motor neurons (in contrast to Friedreich's ataxia which more often targets epicritic sensory neurons). Changes in vital signs, such as tachycardia or hypertension, are often seen as well. Of note, porphyrins are excreted in the urine where they can add a **dark purple coloration** which can be diagnostic in some cases. You can remember these core signs and symptoms of **P**orphyrias by thinking of them as the **4 Ps**: **P**olyneuropathy, **P**ain in the abdomen, **P**sychiatric symptoms, and **P**urple urine.

While most causes of peripheral neuropathy come on slowly over months or years, in porphyria these episodes tend to happen acutely over a period of just a day or two. This **rapid onset** is the key to accurately recognizing porphyrias when they occur! For this reason, consider porphyria in cases of **acute onset polyneuropathy**, especially when accompanied by the other signs and symptoms in the 4 Ps.

Porphyrias are a potential cause of **acute onset polyneuropathy**. Episodes will be accompanied by **abdominal pain**, **psychiatric symptoms**, and/or **purple urine**.

__P__orphyrias should make you think of the __4 Ps__:
__P__olyneuropathy
__P__ain in the abdomen
__P__sychiatric symptoms
__P__urple urine

PUTTING IT ALL TOGETHER

Peripheral neuropathy can be a diagnosis in and of itself, although more often it is a result of an underlying condition. The most important thing to remember from this chapter is the **GOSH DARNED PAIN** mnemonic which will help you to identify some of the most common culprits (and thus open the door to treatment!). In idiopathic cases of peripheral neuropathy, don't give up! There is often still something that you can do to help, including both medications and other forms of intervention. Finally, take a moment to review some of the high-yield diseases that are associated with peripheral neuropathy!

REVIEW QUESTIONS

1. A 57 y/o M living in rural Canada sees a primary care doctor for the first time in several decades with a chief complaint of a slow but steady onset of pain in his feet and calves bilaterally. He describes the pain as "burning," saying, "It's like when you try to walk on hot concrete during the summer." He also describes a "pins and needles" sensation in his feet. The pain is particularly severe at night, resulting in poor sleep for several months. He denies any other symptoms of depression. His exam is notable for decreased plantar flexion of both feet, reduced ankle jerk reflexes, and diminished sensation for pain, temperature, vibration, and proprioception in both feet. Dry crusty skin with mild bruising in both sets of toes is apparent, as seen below:

   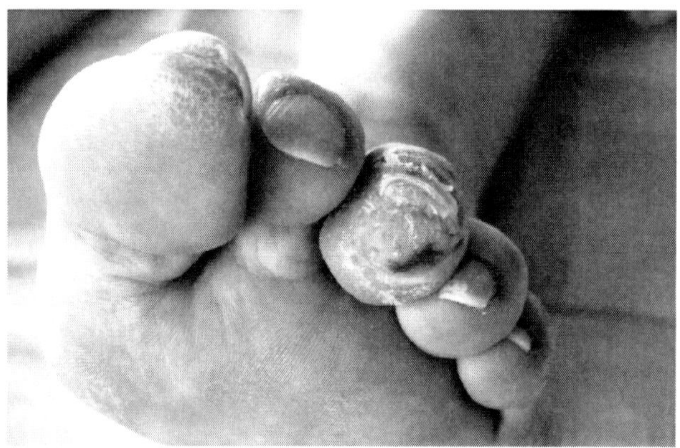

   Which of the following is the most likely explanation for his symptoms?
   A. Compression of a nerve root in the spinal cord
   B. Resistance to insulin
   C. Antibodies directed against his own nerves
   D. Damage to the anterior horn of the spinal cord
   E. Undiagnosed malignancy
   F. Idiopathic peripheral neuropathy

2. (Continued from previous question.) All of the following are likely to result in improvement in the patient's symptoms and quality of life *except*:
   A. Treatment of the underlying disorder
   B. Gabapentin, an anticonvulsant
   C. Capsaicin, a topical anesthetic
   D. Duloxetine, an antidepressant
   E. Physical therapy
   F. All of the above are likely to improve the patient's symptoms

3. A 71 y/o M experiences the loss of his wife due to cancer. For 6 months following her death, he becomes severely depressed and has little appetite, restricting his food intake to old crackers and other items he finds in the pantry. He drinks several bottles of beer per day and will sometimes drink vodka and other distilled drinks when he thinks of his wife. Several months later, he presents to his primary care nurse practitioner reporting difficulty walking without a cane. He has never had need of a cane previously and has no significant past medical history. He is not on any medications. On interview, he reports a feeling of "sharp" pain on the back of his left calf which worsens when he stands up from a chair. His vital signs are within normal limits. His exam is notable for left foot drop, though all other muscles of the left leg are at full motor strength. There is diminished sensation to proprioception and vibration in the left foot. Which of the following is most likely to result in improvement of his symptoms?
    A. Treatment of his depression
    B. Expanded food selection
    C. Reduction in alcohol intake
    D. Improved glycemic control
    E. Spinal surgery

4. A 12 y/o F comes to see her pediatrician. She has been having difficulty walking over the past year and experiences frequent falls if she does not steady herself using a nearby wall or banister. She has particular difficulty walking down stairs. Her speech is slurred, with difficulty enunciating words clearly. Family history is positive for an uncle with a similar condition. On exam, there is wasting of lower leg muscles bilaterally, with an inability to stand on her tip toes. She is scheduled to undergo surgery for scoliosis. An x-ray of the spine is below:

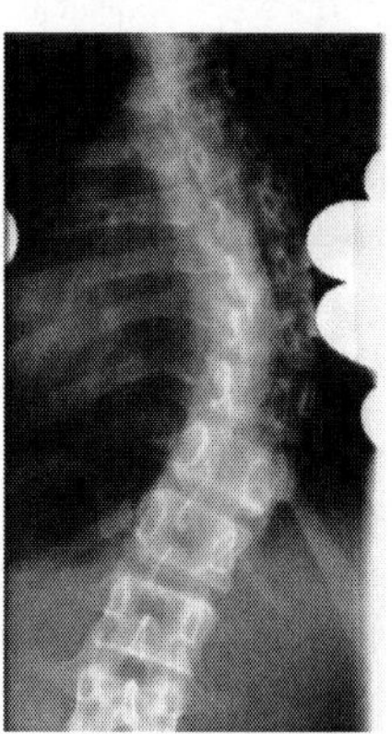

Which of the following features is *least* likely to be found on further exam?
    A. Arched feet
    B. Impaired proprioception in the toes
    C. Loss of pain and temperature sensation in the hands
    D. Impaired glucose tolerance
    E. Progressive systolic dysfunction of the heart
    F. Trinucleotide repeats on chromosome 9 on genetic testing

1. **The best answer is B.** The most common cause of peripheral neuropathy in developed countries is diabetes mellitus, as high levels of sugar in the blood are damaging to neurons, especially those in the most distal parts of the extremities. Autoimmune disorders (answer C) and malignancies (answer E) are both causes that should be considered as well, as should an idiopathic onset (answer F); however, statistically speaking none of these are the most likely explanation. A radiculopathy would be unlikely to cause bilateral findings (answer A), while damage to the anterior horn of the spinal cord would not present with sensory loss (answer D).

2. **The best answer is F.** Treatment of diabetic peripheral neuropathy should be comprehensive, involving not only medications but also physical therapy as well (answer E). A variety of medications have been shown to be effective in treating peripheral neuropathy including anticonvulsants (answer B) and topical anesthetics (answer C). Certain antidepressants, particularly those that interact with norepinephrine, are effective at reducing symptoms, even in patients who are not suffering from depression (answer D).

3. **The best answer is E.** This case describes an L5 radiculopathy as evidenced by pain in a dermatomal distribution with weakness in the corresponding myotome. An L5 radiculopathy is often related to a herniated disc for which a surgical discectomy may be performed. As there appears to be only a single nerve root involved, treatment of systemic causes of peripheral neuropathy such as vitamin B_{12} deficiency (answer B), excess alcohol intake (answer C), and diabetes mellitus (answer D) are unlikely to result in significant improvements. While some antidepressants can be used for symptomatic treatment of neuropathic pain, they would not address the nerve root compression that is the current cause of his symptoms (answer A).

4. **The best answer is C.** This vignette describes a case of Friedreich's ataxia, an autosomal genetic disease involving a GAA repeat on chromosome 9 (answer F). Aside from various cerebellar signs resulting from damage to the spinocerebellar pathways, Friedreich's ataxia involves a variety of other signs and symptoms encompassing various organ systems, including musculoskeletal deformities such as scoliosis and arched feet (answer A), difficulties in glycemic regulation (answer D), and cardiomyopathy (answer E). Epicritic sensation is affected, resulting in impaired vibration, proprioception, and fine touch (answer B). In contrast, protopathic sensation is generally spared.

25 DEMYELINATING DISEASES

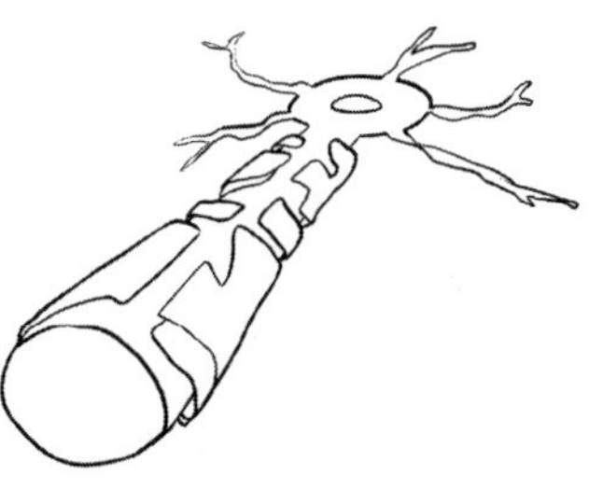

The **myelin sheath** that covers many neurons in both the central and peripheral nervous system is essential for rapid transmission of signals, particularly in neurons carrying motor impulses and proprioceptive information where lightning-fast communication is key. Because the body relies on this speed, any disease that strips the myelin sheath off neurons can result in noticeable deficits, including decreased motor strength, impaired coordination, and loss of sensation.

These **demyelinating diseases** come in a variety of forms, including environmental exposures, nutrient deficiencies, infectious diseases (like tabes dorsalis in syphilis), and even some genetic diseases. However, a surprisingly large proportion of demyelinating diseases are **autoimmune diseases** or those in which the patient's immune system becomes confused and attacks its own body in the same way it would attack an invading pathogen. As we talk about these diseases, keep in mind which neurons are myelinated and which are not, as this will help to identify when a demyelinating disease is present (for example, if someone presents with loss of motor strength and numbness of fine touch, vibration, and proprioception but has intact crude touch, pain, and temperature sensation).

In addition, try to focus on whether demyelination is occurring in the central nervous system, the peripheral nervous system, or both, as this forms a line of separation between **central** and **peripheral demyelinating diseases**. We'll start this chapter with a discussion of several central demyelinating diseases before wrapping up with a couple of peripheral demyelinating diseases.

CENTRAL DEMYELINATING DISEASES

The prototypical central demyelinating autoimmune disease is **multiple sclerosis**, so that is where we will spend the most time. However, there are a few others to know as well, including **neuromyelitis optica**, **acute disseminated encephalomyelitis**, and **progressive multifocal leukoencephalopathy** which each have their own features.

MULTIPLE SCLEROSIS

The name **multiple sclerosis** means "many scars," and this helps to illustrate that the autoimmune attack on myelin is occurring in numerous locations across the central nervous system. For this reason, the presenting signs and symptoms can be quite variable from person to person. In fact, patients with multiple sclerosis can present with **virtually any neurologic sign or symptom**, including muscle weakness, sensory changes, autonomic instability, cerebellar dysfunction, and even neuropsychiatric phenomena including mood and cognitive changes. Visual deficits are particularly common in multiple sclerosis, including a sudden **loss of vision** due to inflammation of the optic nerve. **Internuclear ophthalmoplegia** is common as well, as the medial longitudinal fasciculus is quite heavily myelinated.

Because of this inconsistency, multiple sclerosis is not diagnosed on the basis of any one neurologic sign or symptom. Instead, attacks in multiple sclerosis must be both **disseminated in *space*** (affecting multiple areas of the central nervous system) and **disseminated in *time*** (occurring over weeks or months). Dissemination in space can often be demonstrated on repeat neuroimaging which will show migration of the characteristic scars as seen below:

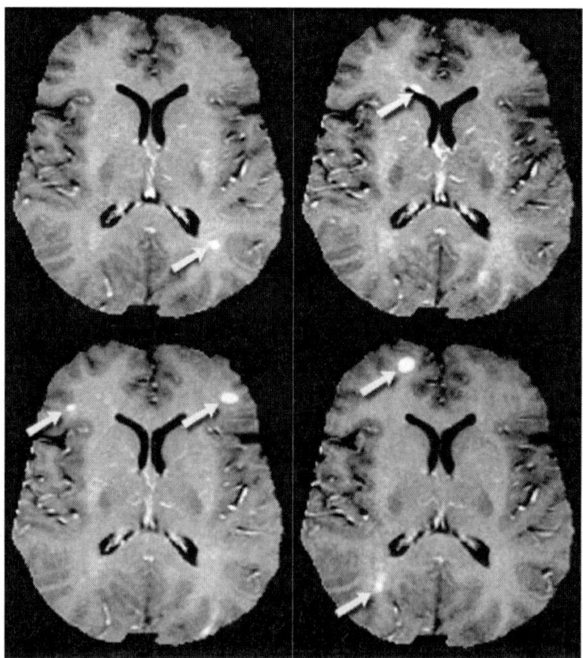

*Serial MRIs in a patient with **multiple sclerosis** showing dissemination of lesions in both **time and space**.*

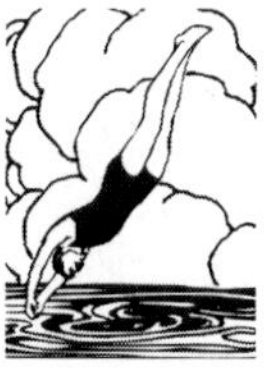

To remember the importance of both dissemination in time and dissemination in space, it can be helpful to think of multiple sclerosis as **multi-pool sclerosis**, with each "pool" being a different neurologic deficit. People with this disease may be in one pool for a time, then be outside the pool symptom-free for a few months, then find themselves in a different pool!

Multiple sclerosis is an **autoimmune disease** involving **demyelination in the central nervous system**. Attacks must be **disseminated in both time and space**.

__Multi-pool sclerosis__ involves getting in and out of different "__pools.__"

For the most patients with the disease, multiple sclerosis follows a **relapsing-remitting course** in which the deficits wax and wane seemingly at random. In between exacerbations, function is often restored due to remyelination of affected neurons. Because of its "here today, gone tomorrow" nature, misdiagnosis of multiple sclerosis is quite common, especially in the initial stages of the illness. (In places where there is a wait time for medical care, someone with multiple sclerosis may find that their neurologic problems have all resolved by the time they actually get an appointment and end up canceling the visit, only to find that their symptoms have returned a few weeks later.) However, it's worth noting that while many cases *begin* with a relapsing-remitting course, over time the disease often shifts to a progressive course, with slowly accumulating deficits even between episodes (this is known as "**secondary progressive multiple sclerosis**").

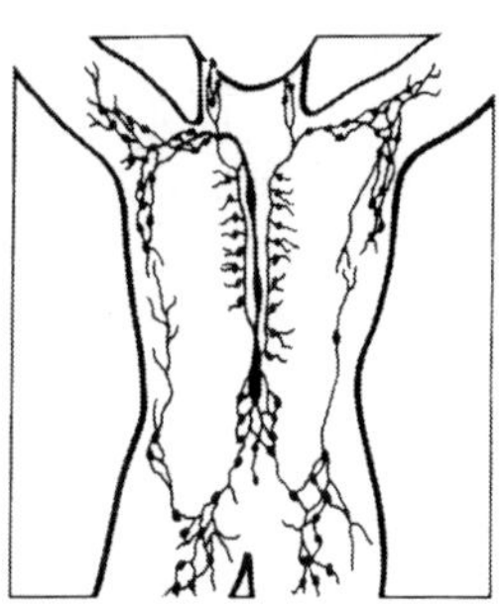

A diagnosis of multiple sclerosis is based on the characteristic clinical history, neurological exam findings, and imaging results demonstrating demyelinating attacks that are disseminated in both time and space. Lumbar puncture can also reveal the presence of **oligoclonal bands** which is a sign that a wider-than-normal range of antibodies are present in the cerebrospinal fluid. In fact, the *absence* of oligoclonal bands strongly argues *against* a diagnosis of multiple sclerosis, as almost all patients with multiple sclerosis will have oligoclonal bands. You can remember this association by thinking of multiple sclerosis as a disease of **oligo**clonal bands attacking the **oligo**dendrocytes that make myelin in the central nervous system.

Oligoclonal bands in cerebrospinal fluid are diagnostic for **multiple sclerosis**.

__Oligo__clonal bands destroy __oligo__dendrocytes in the central nervous system.

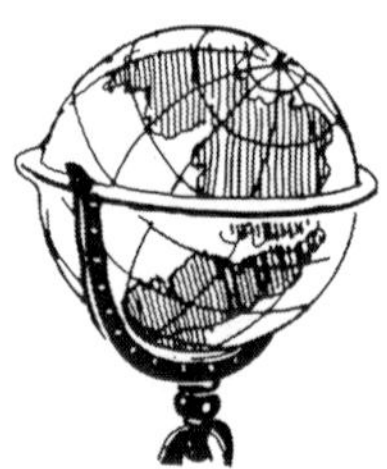

Multiple sclerosis is more common in **women** than men. It tends to begin in one's 20s or 30s. (For this reason, you should think of multiple sclerosis in **any young person presenting with upper motor neuron signs or sudden visual changes**, as these are findings that are typically seen in older adults!) For unclear reasons, the incidence of multiple sclerosis seems to go up the farther away you go from the equator, with a low incidence in tropical areas like Central America and Southeast Asia and a higher incidence in cooler climates like Europe and North America. To remember this, think of how much worse it is to get into multiple **pool**s in **frigid climates** (as opposed to a hot tropical climate near the equator where getting into a pool is fun).

The **incidence of multiple sclerosis** is higher in people living in **temperate climates** compared to **tropical areas.**

*Being in **multi**ple **pool**s is worse the farther away from the equator you go.*

There is **no definitive cure** for multiple sclerosis. Instead, treatment is aimed at managing acute attacks as well as preventing future episodes. Acute treatment involves **steroids** to quickly calm an overactive immune system. However, steroids cannot be used for long-term treatment due to their side effects, so chronic treatment instead involves **disease-modifying drugs** aimed at *preventing* attacks. The first-line treatment is either **glatiramer acetate** or a class of drugs known as **interferons**. Glatiramer acetate is a mixture of proteins that resembles **myelin basic protein** (the antigen found in myelin) which can serve as a "decoy" of sorts for the body's immune system. (To remember the association of g-**ladder**-amer acetate with multi-**pool** sclerosis, think of someone needing a **ladder** to get out of a **pool**.) In contrast, interferons are **cytokines** (or compounds that are involved in signaling between different cells of the immune system) which help to regulate the immune response. Both glatiramer acetate and interferons have been shown to reduce the rate of relapses in multiple sclerosis by about 30%. Other drugs such as **natalizumab** (an antibody targeting a specific protein on white blood cells) are even more effective at preventing relapses, but due to their harsher side effects they are generally not the first drugs used.

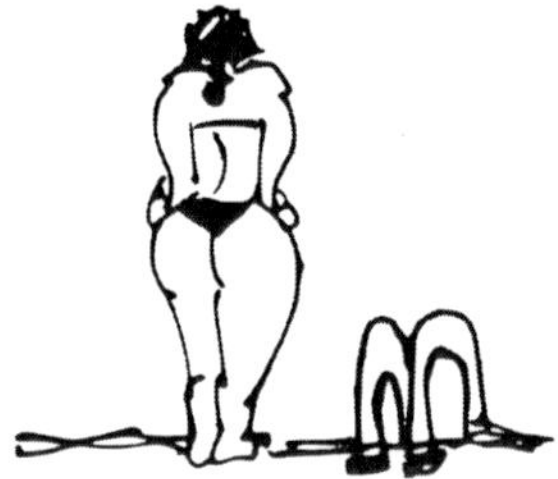

Glatiramer acetate and **interferons** can both be used as a **first-line treatment** for **multiple sclerosis.**

*Use g-**ladder**-amer acetate to get out of multi-**pool** sclerosis.*

Despite the availability of treatment, most people with multiple sclerosis will develop increasing levels of disability with time. Life expectancy is reduced by around 5 or 10 years, with most patients passing away in their 60s or 70s.

NEUROMYELITIS OPTICA

Neuromyelitis optica (also known as NMO or **Devic's disease**) is an autoimmune central demyelinating disease involving inflammation of both the spinal cord (known as **transverse myelitis**) and the optic nerve (**optic neuritis**). Specifically, antibodies are generated that target the **astrocytes** supporting neurons in both of these regions. Because neuromyelitis optica targets these two areas of the central nervous system preferentially, the signs and symptoms can often be traced to both of these structures, with optic neuritis leading to **visual loss** and transverse myelitis leading to **weakness and numbness** of the extremities as well as **bowel and bladder dysfunction**.

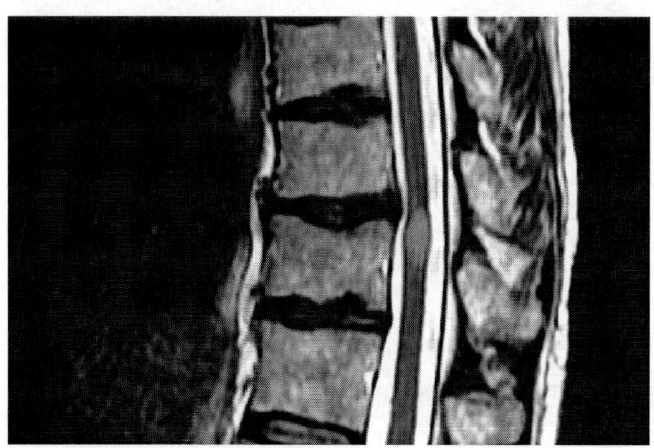

*MRI showing **transverse myelitis** in the lower thoracic spinal cord.*

There is ongoing debate as to whether neuromyelitis optica is simply a variant of multiple sclerosis or an entirely different disease. Like multiple sclerosis, the majority of cases are characterized by a **relapsing-remitting course**. Unlike multiple sclerosis, however, the regions affected are pretty narrow (the optic nerve and spinal cord only), and in some cases the presence of **antibodies against aquaporin-4** (which are not present in multiple sclerosis) can be demonstrated on specialized lab testing. Further, treatment for neuromyelitis optica involves **steroids** and/or **plasmapheresis** (rather than the immune-modulating drugs used in multiple sclerosis).

Whether it ends up ultimately being classified as a different disease or not, on a clinical level it can help to differentiate between them so you know when to use the correct treatment! To differentiate between the widespread destruction seen in multiple sclerosis and the more **narrow** focus of neuromyelitis optica (which targets just the spinal cord and optic nerve), think of it as **narrow**-myelitis optica.

Neuromyelitis optica is a **demyelinating autoimmune disease** involving both **optic neuritis** and **transverse myelitis**.

__Narrow__-myelitis optica is like multiple sclerosis but more __narrow__ in its scope.

ACUTE DISSEMINATED ENCEPHALOMYELITIS

Acute disseminated encephalomyelitis (or ADEM) is a rare but notable central demyelinating disease. Let's use the mnemonic **APPLE** (as in ADEM's APPLE) to learn about the distinguishing features of this disease:

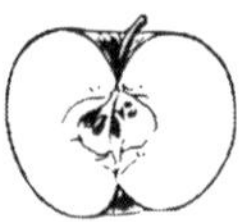

A is for Autoimmune. ADEM is an autoimmune disease involving widespread inflammatory demyelination throughout the central nervous system. Due to the broad distribution of targets, ADEM can present with many different signs and symptoms, including headache, vision loss, weakness, and sensory changes. The extent of the damage can also be visualized in neuroimaging as seen below:

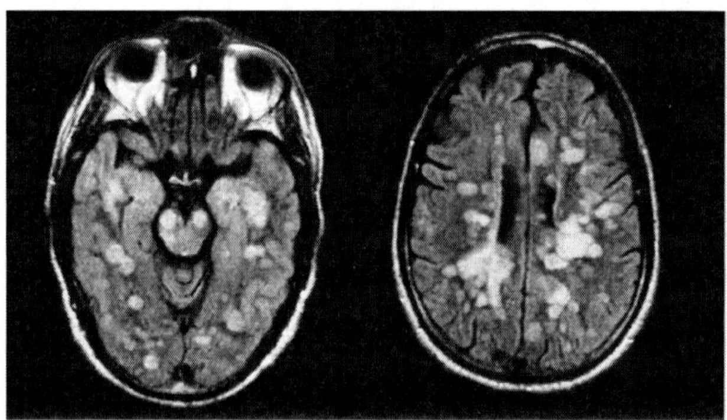

*MRI showing the **widespread lesions** characteristic of **acute disseminated encephalomyelitis**.*

P is for Post-infectious. ADEM most often occurs following exposure to an antibody-generating infection. The **measles virus** is a common culprit, although other viruses like influenza, mumps, and rubella have been implicated as well.

P is for Pediatric. ADEM tends to hit **children**, with an average age of 5 to 8 years.

L is for Life-threatening. ADEM has a relatively high mortality rate, with up to 5% of children with the disease dying as a result. Treatment involves high-dose **steroids** and other measures aimed at reducing immune system activity. Survivors often take many months to recover, though the majority will go on to have no lasting deficits.

E is for Event. ADEM is generally a **one-time event** rather than a chronic condition.

Acute disseminated encephalomyelitis is an **autoimmune disease** leading to **central nervous system demyelination** after exposure to an **infection**.

*Think of ADEM's **APPLE**:*
***A**utoimmune*
***P**ost-infectious*
***P**ediatric*
***L**ife-threatening*
***E**vent*

When learning about these diseases, it's easy to confuse ADEM for multiple sclerosis, as both are central demyelinating diseases with widespread inflammation. To help differentiate, focus on the key features as captured in the **APPLE** mnemonic, including the **P**ost-infectious onset (which isn't seen in multiple sclerosis), the **P**ediatric age group (versus multiple sclerosis which generally begins in middle-aged adults), the **L**ife-threatening nature (compared to multiple sclerosis which shortens lifespan only a little, if at all), and the fact that it is a one-time **E**vent (as opposed to the relapsing-remitting course of multiple sclerosis).

Another disease that is easily confused with ADEM is subacute sclerosing panencephalitis (which we learned about in Chapter 23), as both occur following exposure to an antibody-generating infection like the measles virus. Despite having the connection to measles in common, these diseases are otherwise quite different, with a different presentation (central nervous system *demyelination* in ADEM versus *inflammation* in SSPE) and time of onset (occurring *weeks* after the measles infection in ADEM versus *years* in SSPE). The prognosis is also better in ADEM, with survival and recovery occurring in the majority of cases (versus SSPE which is fatal in the majority of cases).

PROGRESSIVE MULTIFOCAL LEUKOENCEPHALOPATHY

The final central demyelinating disease we will talk about is **progressive multifocal leukoencephalopathy** (or PML) which is characterized by widespread **destruction of oligodendrocytes** in the brain. The key features are all packed into the name itself, with "progressive" capturing the persistent course, "multifocal" reminding you that multiple areas of the brain are hit at once, "leuko" linking to the white matter of the brain, and "encephalopathy" showing that brain-related symptoms such as confusion, clumsiness, and personality changes are all common.

Progressive multifocal leukoencephalopathy is related to **JC virus** (short for **J**ohn **C**unningham virus, after a patient who contracted the disease). Most people who are infected with JC virus are healthy and asymptomatic. However, in cases where someone is **immunocompromised** (such as with **HIV/AIDS**), the virus can overwhelm their defenses and wreak havoc. There is no treatment available for the virus *itself*, so management consists of trying to bolster the patient's immune system (such as by treating the HIV or by stopping any immunosuppressant medications). Even with treatment, the disease has a **poor prognosis**, with up to half of all patients dying within several months due to its rapidly progressive nature. You can remember the aggressive nature of **P**rogressive **M**ultifocal **L**eukoencephalopathy by linking it to the word **P**u**M**me**L** (meaning "to beat with fists").

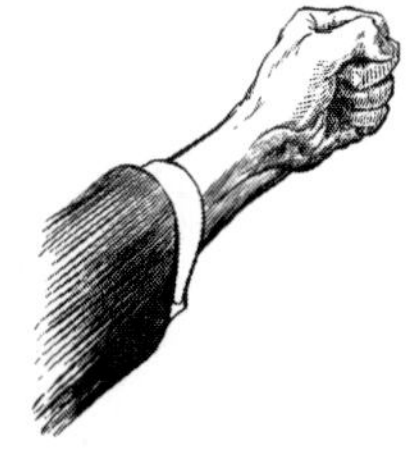

Progressive multifocal leukoencephalopathy is a **central demyelinating disease** related to infection with **JC virus** in an **immunocompromised patient**.

*Progressive **M**ultifocal **L**eukoencephalopathy will **P**u**M**me**L** you (poor prognosis).*

PERIPHERAL DEMYELINATING DISEASES

While central demyelinating diseases strip the myelin sheath off of neurons in the *central* nervous system, peripheral demyelinating diseases do the same for *peripheral* nerves. Here, the prototype disease is **Guillain–Barré syndrome** along with its longer-lasting cousin known as **chronic inflammatory demyelinating polyneuropathy**.

GUILLAIN–BARRÉ SYNDROME

Guillain–Barré syndrome is the peripheral nervous system's counterpart to multiple sclerosis. Both are **autoimmune** diseases in which the myelin sheath is attacked by the immune system, leading to motor deficits (like weakness) as well as changes in sensation (such as numbness and tingling). You can remember the demyelinating nature of this disease by thinking of it as Guillain–**Bare**-é.

Guillain–Barré syndrome is a **demyelinating disease** involving **autoimmune destruction** of **peripheral nerves.**

*Guillain–**Bare**-é leaves your peripheral nerves **bare**.*

The motor deficits in Guillain–Barré syndrome tend to present in a **symmetric** fashion, beginning in the limbs and then **ascending** towards the trunk and face over several weeks. (Of note, the neurological exam will reveal only *lower* motor neuron signs as opposed to the upper motor neuron signs that are seen in multiple sclerosis!). Worryingly, this paralysis will end up hitting the diaphragm in around 25% of patients, leading to **respiratory failure** and death without medical treatment. The autonomic nervous system is also affected in most patients with this condition, leading to an irregular heart beat, unstable blood pressure, and/or absent pupillary responses.

Interestingly, many cases of Guillain–Barré syndrome are preceded by exposure to an infectious disease, with ***Campylobacter jejuni*** being the culprit in around a third of all cases. It is believed that this infection induces the immune system to make antibodies against these pathogens. However, on a molecular level these bugs bear a striking resemblance to **gangliosides** or the fatty molecules found in the myelin of peripheral nerves. Because of this **molecular mimicry**, these newly created antibodies attack not only the pathogens but also the gangliosides present on peripheral nerve cells, leading to demyelination. You can remember the association of Guillain–**Berry** syndrome with ***Camp**ylobacter je**juni*** by thinking of going **camp**ing in **Jun**e which is when **berries** are most ripe.

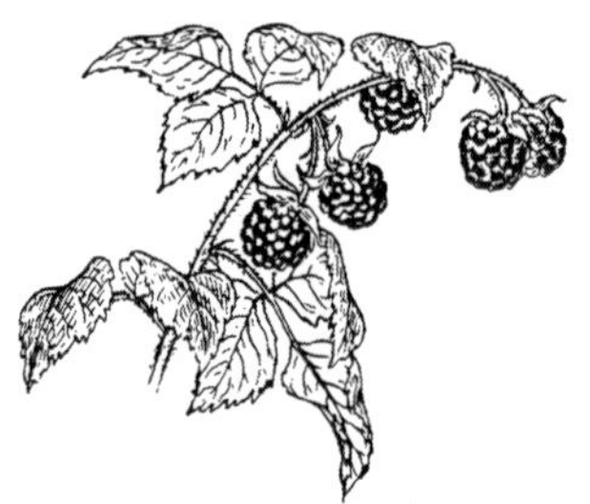

Guillain–Barré syndrome is often preceded by a ***Campylobacter jejuni*** infection.

*You go **camp**ing in **Jun**e (**Camp**ylobacter je**jun**i) when the **berries** (Guillain-**Berry** syndrome) are most ripe.*

Diagnosis is based on the patient's history, physical findings, and lab test results. Lumbar puncture will often show **albuminocytologic dissociation** or an increased protein level combined with a normal cell count in the cerebrospinal fluid. Imaging can help to rule *out* other conditions that may resemble the findings in Guillain–Barré syndrome (such as compression of the spinal cord by a tumor) but is not necessarily helpful for ruling this *in*. Other findings include slowed conduction on EMG (which makes sense, as the main function of myelin is to speed up neuronal transmission).

Treatment is aimed at removing the autoantibodies out of the bloodstream. This is done by either **plasmapheresis** or by administering **intravenous immunoglobulins** (both of which we discussed back in Chapter 17 in the context of autoimmune neuromuscular junction diseases). These treatments are equally effective, with neither being superior to the other. With treatment, there is usually a **good prognosis**, with most patients recovering lost functions within a few weeks and surviving without long-term complications.

CHRONIC INFLAMMATORY DEMYELINATING POLYNEUROPATHY

Chronic inflammatory demyelinating polyneuropathy (or CIDP) is best thought of as the **chronic counterpart** to Guillain–Barré syndrome, as it involves many of the same signs and symptoms with a similar pathophysiology. This time, however, the disease does not simply go away on its own but instead lingers for months or even years. Some people with CIDP have persistent deficits, while others experience a relapsing-remitting course similar to multiple sclerosis. Treatment is the same as for Guillain–Barré syndrome.

PUTTING IT ALL TOGETHER

Demyelination is a pathologic feature of many neurologic diseases, and you will see the characteristic pattern (impaired motor strength and epicritic sensation with intact protopathic sensation) pop up again and again. In this chapter, we have primarily focused on those diseases that feature demyelination as the *core* pathology. Use the table below to identify key patterns that will help you to tease apart the different demyelinating diseases on boards and wards!

Disease	Type	Distribution	Course	Features
MS	Central	Widespread	Relapsing-remitting	Oligoclonal bands
NMO	Central	Optic nerve, spinal cord	Relapsing-remitting	Aquaporin-4 antibodies
ADEM	Central	Widespread	Single episode	Post-infectious
PML	Central	Widespread	Rapidly progressive	HIV/AIDS, immunocompromised
GBS	Peripheral	Ascending, symmetric	Single episode	Albuminocytologic dissociation
CIDP	Peripheral	Ascending, symmetric	Persistent or relapsing-remitting	Albuminocytologic dissociation

REVIEW QUESTIONS

1. A 42 y/o M who has lived in Nicaragua all his life immigrates to the United States. He makes an appointment to see a primary care doctor. At his first appointment, he reports difficulty walking for the past 2 years. He initially noticed weakness in his left lower limb while working as a construction worker. He said that this weakness would "come and go," with weeks where he had trouble walking interspersed with months where his strength was intact. However, he was always able to compensate for his weakness and never sought medical care. He denies sensory loss, visual abnormalities, or any flu-like symptoms. A lumbar puncture shows oligoclonal bands in his cerebrospinal fluid. Which of the following argues most strongly *against* a diagnosis of multiple sclerosis at this time?
    A. Recurrent nature of neurologic deficits
    B. Neurologic deficits in only the left lower leg
    C. Male gender
    D. Upbringing in a tropical region
    E. Ability to work even after disease onset
    F. Presence of oligoclonal bands in cerebrospinal fluid

2. (Continued from previous question.) At his follow-up appointment one month later, the patient reports a tremor of his right hand along with an "hormigueo" (tingling) sensation in his right arm. He also reports difficulty swallowing which causes occasional coughing while eating. An MRI of his brain shows multiple plaques around the ventricles bilaterally as seen below:

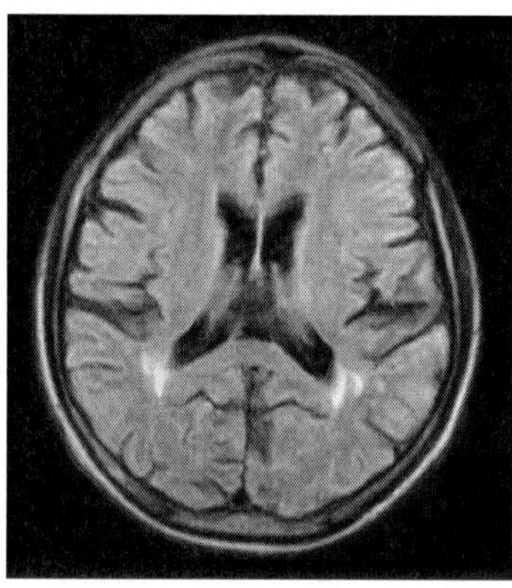

Which of the following is the best next step in management?
    A. Prescribing corticosteroids
    B. Prescribing glatiramer acetate
    C. Prescribing an interferon
    D. Prescribing natalizumab
    E. Arranging for plasmapheresis
    F. Administering intravenous immunoglobulins
    G. Referring to physical therapy

3. A 51 y/o M with a history of HIV infection presents to his infectious disease specialist reporting recent onset of difficulty walking and speaking. He has been treated for HIV for the past 15 years, although his particular strain of the virus is resistant to multiple types of antiviral medications, leading to recurrent treatment failures. His current $CD4^+$ count is less than 10 cells/µl. On exam, his speech is dysarthric, with difficulty enunciating words. His gait is ataxic. He has difficulty with finger-to-nose testing, and his Romberg sign is positive. At a follow-up visit two weeks later, he is in a wheelchair due to extreme difficulty walking. His speech is weak to the point of being unable to communicate. He is admitted to the hospital for supportive care. An MRI of the brain shows multiple areas of widespread demyelination as seen below:

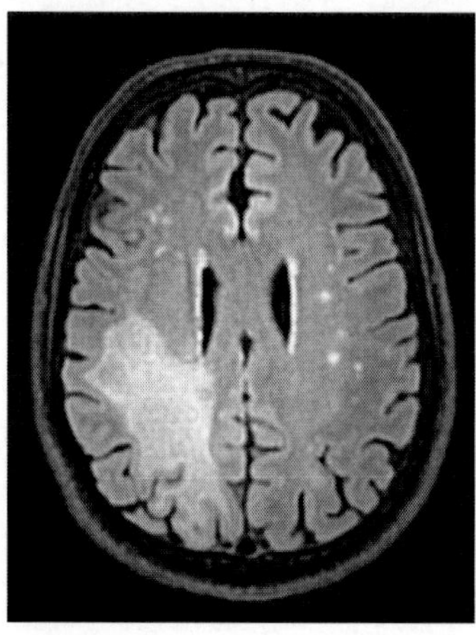

Which of the following is the most likely explanation for his condition?

A. Autoimmune demyelination
B. Direct neurotoxicity of HIV
C. Concurrent infection by more than one virus
D. Post-infectious reactivation of the measles virus
E. Inflammation of the spinal cord

4. A 15 y/o F is brought to the emergency department after 2 days of progressively worsening motor weakness in all 4 limbs. She had a case of "food poisoning" involving diarrhea and vomiting 2 weeks ago that had resolved without medical treatment. On exam, there is 1/5 motor function in each of her limbs. A nerve conduction study is performed which shows a predominantly demyelinating pattern. Which of the following additional findings is most likely to be seen on further examination?

A. Active bloodstream bacterial infection
B. Muscle spasticity to palpation
C. Upgoing plantar responses
D. Loss of pain and temperature sensation over both arms
E. Areflexia in the biceps, patellar, and ankle jerk reflexes
F. None of the above are likely to be found

1. **The best answer is B.** A diagnosis of multiple sclerosis requires that any neurologic signs or symptoms are disseminated in both time and space. This patient's relapsing and remitting course shows a pattern of dissemination in time (answer A), but the fact that his neurologic deficits are localized to a single area does not demonstrate dissemination in space. His sex (answer C) and upbringing in a tropical region (answer D) are both less common in multiple sclerosis, but they are not incompatible with the diagnosis. While some people with multiple sclerosis become functionally impaired by this disease, others are not (answer E). Finally, the presence of oligoclonal bands in cerebrospinal fluid is evidence in favor of a diagnosis of multiple sclerosis, not against it (answer F).

2. **The best answer is A.** Now that dissemination in space has been demonstrated for this patient's neurologic deficits, a diagnosis of multiple sclerosis can be confirmed. In the setting of an acute attack, steroids should be used as the first-line treatment. Glatiramer acetate and interferons are both effective treatments for multiple sclerosis, but they are generally used for long-term prevention of attacks rather than acute management (answers B and C). Natalizumab is a second-line treatment for multiple sclerosis and should generally not be used until other drugs have failed (answer D). Neither plasmapheresis nor intravenous immunoglobulins are first-line treatments for acute attacks of multiple sclerosis (answers E and F). Physical therapy is a key part of long-term management but is not the immediate priority (answer G).

3. **The best answer is C.** This vignette describes a case of progressive multifocal leukoencephalopathy, a potentially fatal demyelinating disease caused by the JC virus. While the JC virus is typically harmless, in people with a compromised immune system (such as this patient with HIV/AIDS) it can lead to severe neurologic dysfunction. Unlike multiple sclerosis and Guillain–Barré syndrome, an autoimmune mechanism is not thought to account for progressive multifocal leukoencephalopathy (answer A). While HIV itself can cause neuronal damage, on its own it would not lead to the rapidly progressive disease seen in this case (answer B). Post-infectious reactivation of the measles virus is related to acute disseminated encephalomyelitis (answer D), while inflammation of the spinal cord is seen in neuromyelitis optica (answer E).

4. **The best answer is E.** Guillain–Barré syndrome is a demyelinating disease that primarily affects the peripheral nervous system, including both motor and sensory neurons. Notably, unmyelinated neurons such as those carrying pain and temperature sensation are not affected (answer D). As Guillain–Barré syndrome affects the peripheral nervous system, lower motor neuron signs including areflexia should be seen, while upper motor neuron signs such as spasticity and a positive Babinski signs should be absent (answers B and C). Guillain–Barré syndrome is thought to be mediated by autoantibodies whose production is induced by exposure to the *Campylobacter jejuni* bacteria rather than being associated with an active bacterial infection (answer A).

26 HEADACHE

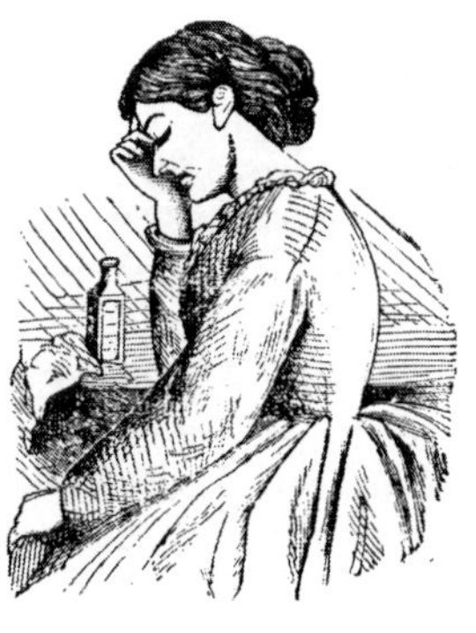

On the surface, a **headache** seems like a simple thing that requires little explanation. Most people have experienced a headache (and if they haven't yet, they probably will in the future!). However, just because headaches are so common doesn't make them any less distressing or disabling, and any health care provider will need to have a systematic way of assessing and treating headaches.

When learning about headaches, it's worth knowing that the *brain itself* does not feel pain! Instead, the sensation of pain during a headache tends to come from structures *in and around* the brain, including the skin of the scalp, the meninges, and the periosteum of the skull.

Headaches can either be a symptom of another disease or a disease in their own right. Headaches that occur on their own are called **primary headaches**, while those that are related to another condition are known as **secondary headaches**. While secondary headaches tend to get the most attention (as they are associated with some pretty scary diseases including cancer, infections, and bleeding), that does not make primary headaches any less deserving of diligent medical care!

For the rest of this chapter, we will focus first on the various ways that primary headaches can present, including **tension headaches**, **migraine headaches**, and **cluster headaches**. We will then look at some of the most common causes of secondary headaches. Some of these causes we have talked about already in previous chapters (such as a subarachnoid hemorrhage), but for the sake of completeness we will make reference to them again here.

PRIMARY HEADACHES

The vast majority of headaches (around 90%) are **primary headaches**. There are a number of different forms of primary headaches, but we will limit our discussion to the three most high-yield forms: tension headaches, migraine headaches, and cluster headaches. Of these, tension and migraine headaches are by far the most common, while cluster headaches are so severe that they have a tendency to show up frequently on standardized tests even if they are relatively rare in real life.

TENSION HEADACHES

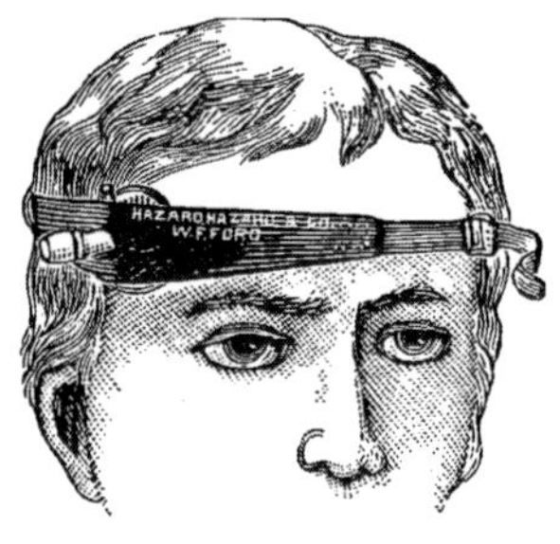

A **tension headache** is the single most common form of headache, with around 20% of people experiencing them on a regular basis. As their name implies, they are experienced as a sense of "tension" or "pressure," almost as if the head were being squeezed. Notably, tension headaches are felt **bilaterally** and tend to be located in a **band-like** pattern around the forehead, the sides of the heads, or the back of the head near the neck. Tension headaches usually last for a **few hours** at a time. They are often precipitated by situational factors, including high stress and poor sleep. While tension headaches can be uncomfortable or even painful, they are usually not incapacitating.

Treatment involves over-the-counter drugs including acetaminophen or NSAIDs like aspirin, ibuprofen, and naproxen. However, these must be taken with caution, as excessive use may actually make headaches *worse* in the long-term (a condition known as a **medication overuse headache** or **rebound headache**). Because of the potential downsides of pharmacologic treatment of tension headaches, **prevention** should be the cornerstone of management. Lifestyle modifications such as stress management, sleep hygiene, and adequate hydration may be helpful. In some cases, antidepressants can be used to reduce the frequency of tension headaches.

MIGRAINE HEADACHES

A **migraine headache** is the second most common form of headache, with around 15% of people being affected by them. They are often described as **paroxysmal**, meaning that they tend to come on episodically and are quite severe when they occur.

To understand migraines, it can be helpful to examine how they differ from tension headaches. The word **POUND** can help you to do this:

P is for Pulsatile. Migraine headaches generally have a "throbbing" or "pounding" quality, almost as if the brain is beating like a heart or a drum (which should help you to remember the mnemonic "POUND" itself).

O is for hOurs. The painful phase of a migraine often lasts around **4 hours**, although some people have intractable headaches that can last up to a few days at a time.

U is for Unilateral. Unlike the bilateral pain caused by tension headaches, migraines tend to be felt much more strongly on one side of the head or the other.

N is for Nausea. Nausea and vomiting frequently accompany migraine headaches, with over 90% of patients reporting this symptom during an attack. Vomiting is less common but still affects around a third of migraine sufferers.

D is for Disabling. Finally, migraine headaches are often disabling, and the patient is often unable to work or interact with others during an attack. Partly this is due to pain, although many people with migraines also report an intense sensitivity to lights and sounds (known as **photophobia** and **phonophobia**, respectively) that prevent them from functioning as well. For this reason, it is not uncommon for someone with a migraine to retreat to a dark, quiet room during an attack.

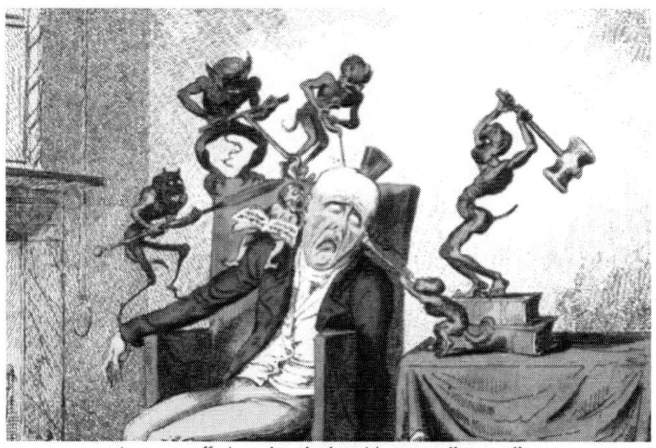

*A person suffering a **headache** with a **pounding quality**.*

Migraines are a **disabling form** of **paroxysmal headache** that presents with **pulsatile unilateral pain** lasting **several hours**.

POUND:
***P**ulsatile*
*h**O**urs*
***U**nilateral*
***N**ausea*
***D**isabling*

A migraine does not involve only the headache itself but also presents with distinct symptoms occurring before and after the attack. Many people experience a **prodrome** for several hours or even days prior to the onset of a migraine which alerts them to the coming episode. The specific symptoms of a prodrome differ from person to person, but they commonly consist of changes in mood, energy levels, toileting habits, and sensitivity to light and noise.

Some people also experience an **aura** that occurs either before or during the headache. An aura is distinct from a prodrome in that it is usually more transient (only a few minutes) and involves distinct **visual abnormalities**. Most often this takes the form of "blurry" or "flickering lights" sensations known as **scintillating scotomas**, as seen in the following picture. However, in some cases these visual abnormalities may even extend to vision loss, as in a hemianopsia. Non-visual sensory abnormalities are less common but can occur as well, including "pins-and-needles" **paresthesias** in the arms and face. In rare cases, **motor weakness** may be observed as part of an aura.

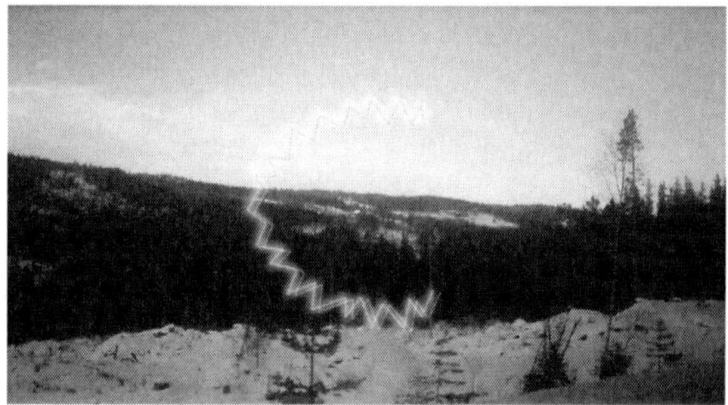

*Depiction of a **scintillating scotoma** during a **migraine**.*

Following a migraine, a **postdromal state** may occur. This is often described as being "not unlike a hangover," with patients reporting fatigue, malaise, cognitive dulling, depressed mood, and soreness in the part of the head where they felt the pain most acutely. A migraine postdrome can last for several days.

Most people who experience one migraine will go on to have more attacks in the future. For this reason, treatment of migraines involves not only acute management of a headache (known as **abortive treatment**) but also **preventive treatment** aimed at reducing the likelihood of future episodes. In mild cases, the same over-the-counter medications that are used in tension headaches can be tried. In more severe cases, drugs known as **triptans** (so-named because many of their names end in -triptan, as in sumatriptan, rizatriptan, and zolmitriptan) can be used. Triptans are effective at reducing both pain and nausea in the majority of patients who take them. Like with over-the-counter pain medicines, however, care must be taken to avoid overuse which can lead to rebound headaches. For this reason, alternative strategies to prevent migraines should be used in people who experience frequent attacks. While the mechanism underlying their use in migraine prophylaxis is unclear, the two best-supported medication classes are **anticonvulsants** like topiramate and valproate and **beta-blockers** like propranolol and metoprolol. Lifestyle modifications and various forms of therapy may help to reduce migraine frequency and severity as well.

CLUSTER HEADACHES

Cluster headaches are an incredibly painful form of headache (so painful, in fact, that they are also known as "**suicide headaches**" because patients who experience them have been known to contemplate killing themselves rather than continuing to live with the unbearable agony of a cluster headache!). The pain is often located around or above the eye on one side and is described as someone "sticking a hot poker" behind the eye. More than just being painful, cluster headaches are associated with several other features that the word **CLUSTER** will help you to remember:

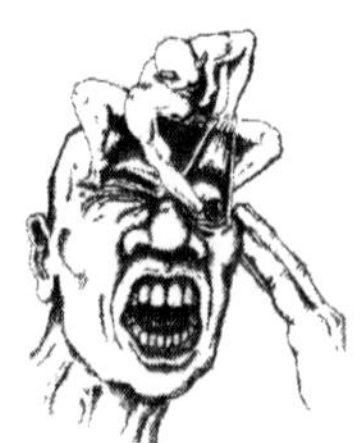

C is for Conjunctival injection. Patients often present with eye redness during a cluster headache.

L is for Lacrimation. Cluster headaches are associated with excessive crying and nasal discharge, typically on the same side as the pain.

U is for Unilateral. Like a migraine (and *unlike* a tension headache), a cluster headache tends to be felt only on one side or the other.

S is for Speedy. Cluster headaches tend to come on quickly and without warning, with no prodrome or aura like in a migraine. They also dissipate just as quickly, with most attacks lasting less than an hour.

T is for Treatable. Cluster headaches are often treatable. **High-flow oxygen** seems to reduce pain within 15 minutes in the majority of patients. **Triptans** also appear to help stop an episode quickly. Preventive treatments include **verapamil**, a calcium channel blocker that is used as an antihypertensive. The mechanism by which these seemingly random treatments work in cluster headaches is not known.

E is for Eyelid drooping. Ptosis is commonly seen on the affected side during a cluster headache.

R is for Recurrent. Finally, cluster headaches are highly recurrent, occurring at the same time each day for most patients. Some patients have even given them the nickname "alarm clock headaches" because of how precisely regular they are.

Cluster headaches are **highly recurrent headaches** that are experienced as **retro-orbital pain**. Autonomic signs such as **lacrimation** and **ptosis** are often seen.

CLUSTER:
***C**onjunctival injection*
***L**acrimation*
***U**nilateral*
***S**peedy*
***T**reatable*
***E**yelid drooping*
***R**ecurrent*

Cluster headaches tend to begin in one's 20s and 30s. For unclear reasons, **men** are affected four times as often as women. The cause of cluster headaches is not known, although there appears to be a genetic component. The majority of people who experience cluster headaches have a history of **smoking**, although unfortunately smoking cessation does not lead to improvement in the headaches, making it unlikely that this is a direct cause.

SECONDARY HEADACHES

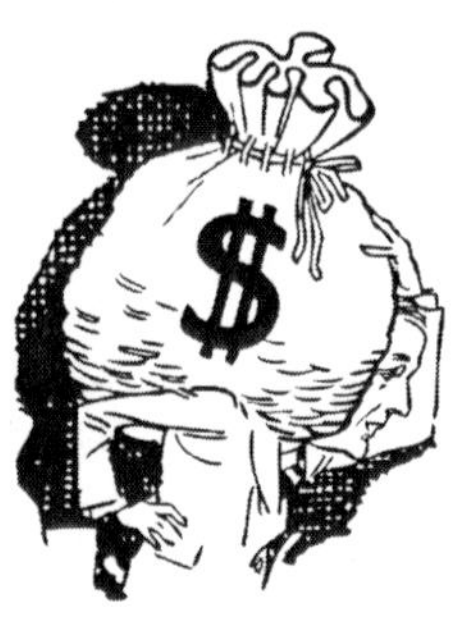

Secondary headaches, or those caused by another medical condition, represent a minority of all headaches seen in clinical practice, with only around 10% of headaches having an underlying cause. However, because of the potential seriousness of some of these causes, secondary headaches must always be on your differential! The key to picking up secondary headaches is to look for **red flags** that signal the need for a more thorough work-up. You can remember these red flags with the mnemonic **PAID 40 TAXMEN** (a situation that would give just about anyone a headache!):

P is for Papilledema. The presence of papilledema or any other signs of increased intracranial pressure could be suggestive of a brain tumor, an infection, or other potentially serious diseases.

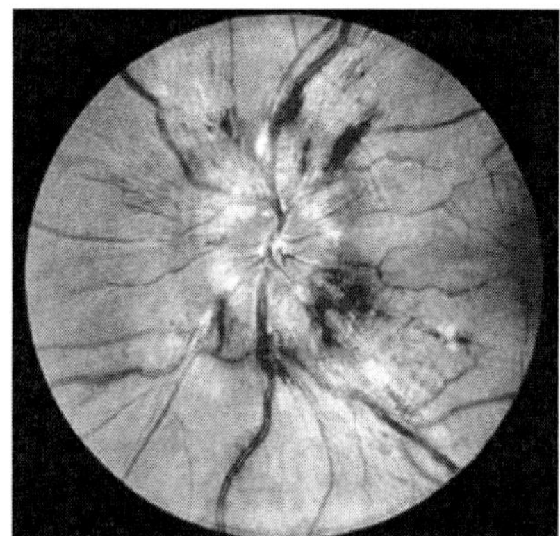

Papilledema *in a patient who initially presented with a headache.*

A is for Abrupt onset. A headache that arrives with an abrupt and sudden onset may be a sign of an intracranial bleed, with the "thunderclap" headache that we talked about in Chapter 15 as a sign of subarachnoid hemorrhages being a notable example.

I is for Immunosuppressed. Cancer, HIV, steroid use, and other situations that result in an immunocompromised state increase the risk of central nervous system infections significantly, so a headache in these patients should be investigated as a potential sign of a dangerous disease.

D is for Different than before. Someone who suddenly presents with a headache that feels completely different than anything they have experienced previously in their life should receive an additional work-up.

40 is for 40 years or older. It is unusual for someone above the age of 40 who has never experienced headaches before to suddenly start having them, so this may warrant further investigation.

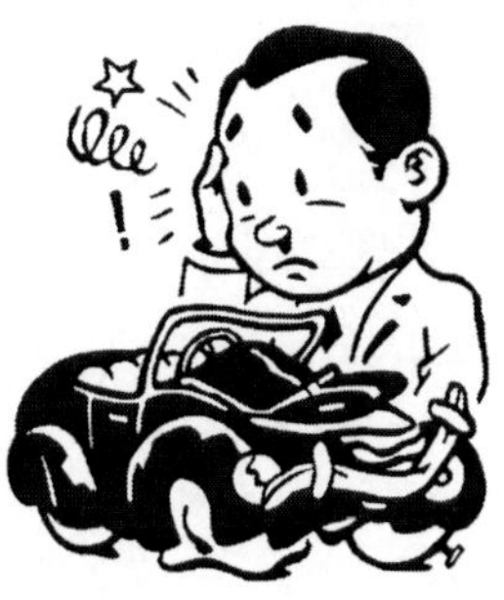

T is for Trauma. While some degree of headache following a mechanical trauma (such as a car crash or fall) may be completely normal, it is still wise to order imaging to rule out an intracranial bleed.

A is for Altered mental status. A headache in the context of accompanying changes in one's mental status (including confusion, cognitive impairment, or unusual behavior) can be concerning for an infection, an inflammatory disease, or a tumor.

X is for eXertional. Heavy exertion, frequent coughing, or other activities that tend to increase intracranial pressure may lead to bursting of a blood vessel with subsequent bleeding. Any headache that is triggered by this kind of exertion should prompt a work-up for a possible bleed.

M is for Morbid. Signs of morbid illness, including systemic findings such as a fever, rash, or abnormal vital signs, could indicate an infection or tumor.

E is for Escalating. Any recurrent headache that is steadily increasing in frequency and/or severity is worrying for a progressive disease process such as a brain tumor or a subdural hematoma.

N is for Neurologic signs or symptoms. With some exceptions (primarily migraines), most primary headaches do not present with accompanying neurologic changes, so a headache with neurologic findings (including weakness, sensory changes, visual loss, or seizures) should prompt clinical concern for a secondary headache.

While **secondary headaches** are the **exception rather than the rule**, be on the lookout for any **red flags** that might signal the presence of an underlying cause.

PAID 40 TAXMEN:
***P**apilledema*
***A**brupt onset*
***I**mmunosuppressed*
***D**ifferent than before*
***40** years or older*
***T**rauma*
***A**ltered mental status*
*e**X**ertional*
***M**orbid*
***E**scalating*
***N**eurologic signs or symptoms*

DISEASES ASSOCIATED WITH HEADACHES

Now that we have an understanding of when to look for upstream causes of headache, let's look at a couple causes of secondary headache that we haven't already addressed elsewhere.

GIANT-CELL ARTERITIS

Giant-cell arteritis (formerly known as **temporal arteritis**) is a rheumatologic disease involving inflammation of the temporal artery. It often presents as a **unilateral headache** overlying the temporal region, although there are often other signs and symptoms as well including fever. This inflammation causes narrowing of nearby blood vessels which manifests as **claudication** (soreness and pain related to tissue ischemia) in the jaw and tongue when chewing. If the ischemia extends to the ophthalmic artery, **vision loss and blindness** can occur. For this reason, giant-cell arteritis is considered to be a **medical emergency**, as permanent damage can occur if it is not diagnosed and treated quickly!

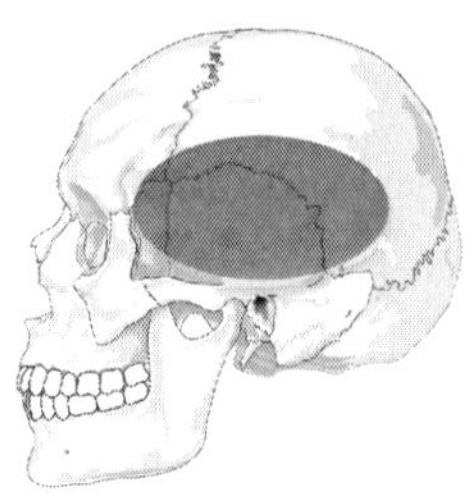

You can use the acronym **TEMPL3** to assist you in identifying the signs and symptoms of giant-cell arteritis:

T is for Temporal artery signs and symptoms. Any symptoms in the region of the temporal artery, including tenderness or reduced arterial pulse strength, should put giant-cell arteritis on your differential. On exam, the skin over the temporal region may be tender to palpation, and there may be signs of poor perfusion (including decreased pulses and ischemic changes on ophthalmologic exam).

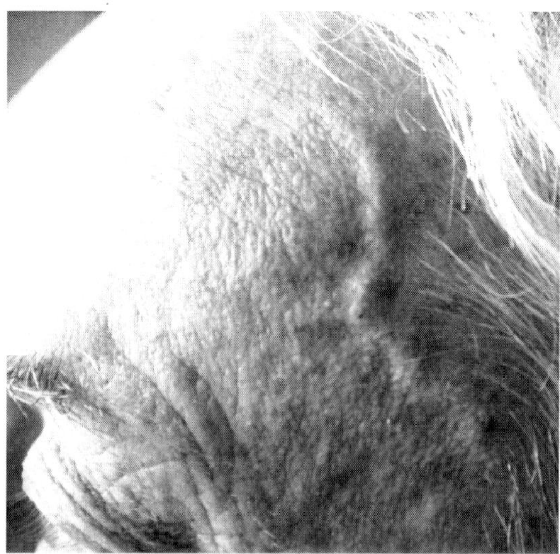

*Inflamed **temporal artery** in a patient with **giant-cell arteritis**.*

E is for ESR elevated. Lab testing often shows elevations in inflammatory markers, with a high **erythrocyte sedimentation rate** (ESR) being common.

M is for Mononuclear cell infiltrates or Multinucleate giant cells on biopsy. The gold standard for diagnosing giant-cell arteritis is a **temporal artery biopsy** which will show mononuclear cell infiltrates or multinucleate giant cells invading the tissues as seen below:

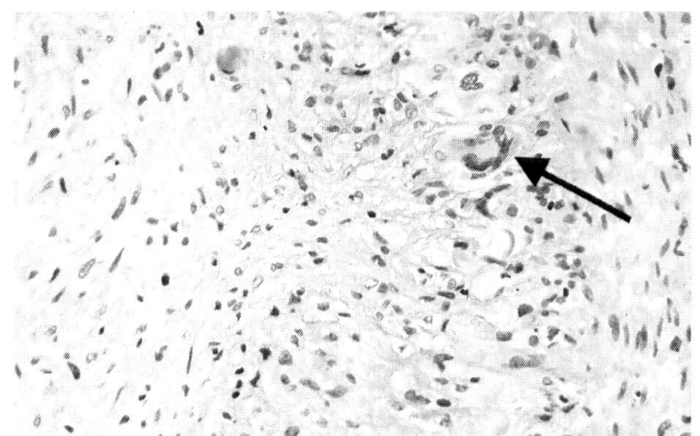

*Microscope image of a **multinucleate giant cell** in a biopsy of the **temporal artery**.*

P is for Painful new-onset localized headache. As noted above, giant-cell arteritis most often presents as pain localized to the temporal region.

L is for Late onset. Giant-cell arteritis almost exclusively begins in **older adults** above the age of 50. For unclear reasons, **men** are affected more often than women.

3 is for 3 or more of these features. If at least 3 of these features are present, giant-cell arteritis should be high on your differential (and if less than 3 are present, then you can feel more comfortable that the diagnosis has been ruled out).

Giant-cell arteritis is an **inflammatory disease** that results in a **unilateral headache**, **jaw and tongue claudication**, and **vision loss** if left untreated.

TEMPL3:

__T__emporal artery tenderness or reduced pulse strength
__E__SR elevated
__M__ononuclear cell infiltrates or __M__ultinucleate giant cells on biopsy
__P__ainful new-onset localized headache
__L__ate in life onset (over 50 years)
__3__ or more of these features

Once giant-cell arteritis is suspected, treatment with **corticosteroids** should be administered promptly to reduce inflammation. Given the risk of permanent damage, you don't need to wait for diagnostic testing results before administering treatment!

IDIOPATHIC INTRACRANIAL HYPERTENSION

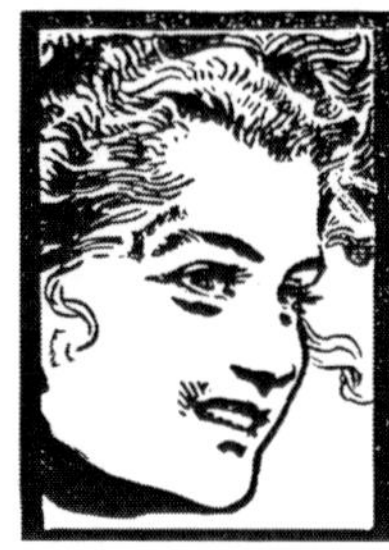

Another cause of secondary headache that we will talk about in this chapter is **idiopathic intracranial hypertension**. This involves increased pressure within the skull ("intracranial hypertension") with no known cause ("idiopathic"). Idiopathic intracranial hypertension tends to present similarly to the other causes of intracranial hypertension that we talked about in Chapter 15, with **headaches** and **papilledema** often being major findings on exam. (As a matter of fact, the clinical presentation of this disease so strongly resembles a brain tumor that it used to be called "**pseudotumor cerebri**"!) Notably, however, there should be **no other focal neurologic findings**, with the only exception to this being that the increased pressure can sometimes lead to dysfunction of specific **cranial nerves** (most often those involved in extraocular muscles but occasionally the facial nerve as well).

By definition, idiopathic intracranial hypertension is a **diagnosis of exclusion** because it assumes that all other causes have been ruled out (it wouldn't be "idiopathic" otherwise!). Imaging of the brain typically should be ordered to rule out any intracranial lesions (like an *actual* tumor).

Idiopathic intracranial hypertension tends to be diagnosed primarily in three groups: the **young** (typically patients in their 20s and 30s), the **overweight** (with the incidence going up drastically as the patient's weight increases), and **women** (who are diagnosed more than 5 times as often as men). Use of certain drugs, including hormonal contraceptives and vitamin A derivatives (like those used to treat acne), increase the risk as well.

Immediate treatment of idiopathic intracranial hypertension involves a **lumbar puncture** to drain cerebrospinal fluid and relieve some of the pressure. This helps to reduce the risk of developing long-term complications of uncontrolled intracranial hypertension, including permanent visual loss and cranial nerve damage. A medication known as **acetazolamide** can be used to reduce cerebrospinal fluid production as well. Over the long-term, weight loss can help to reduce the severity of the condition. In severe cases where other efforts have failed, **venous sinus stenting** and other neurosurgical techniques can help to reduce intracranial pressure.

In summary, you can remember the typical case presentation for idiopathic intracranial hypertension using the mnemonic **HAPY NOW** which stands for **H**eadaches **A**nd **P**apilledema in a **Y**oung, **N**ormal, **O**bese **W**oman (with normal referring to the negative neurological exam, imaging, and lab findings seen in patients with this condition). You can connect this mnemonic to this condition by thinking that someone will be relieved when they are told that their recurrent headaches are *not* in fact a sign of brain cancer!

Idiopathic intracranial hypertension presents as **headaches** and **papilledema**, typically in **young obese women**.

HAPY NOW*: **H**eadaches **A**nd **P**apilledema in a **Y**oung, **N**ormal, **O**bese **W**oman.*

PUTTING IT ALL TOGETHER

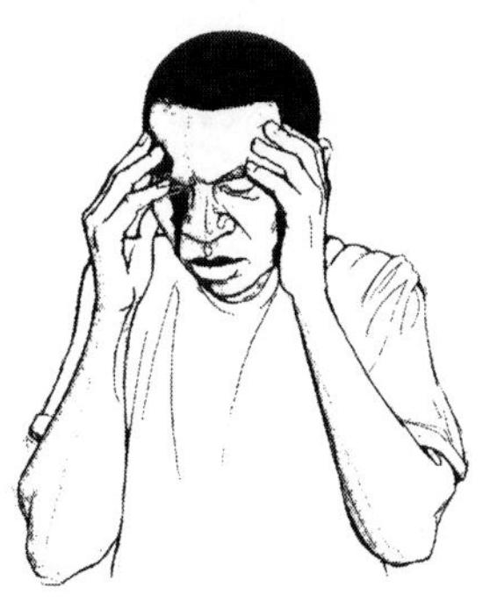

Any patient presenting with a headache should always receive additional questioning to get more information about what is going on. Even in cases of primary headaches where no cause has been identified, knowing about the type of headache can help to identify the best treatments (such as triptans in migraine headaches or high-flow oxygen in cluster headaches). In cases where any of the red flags in the **PAID 40 TAXMEN** mnemonic are present, you should go beyond just a history and physical by considering lab testing and/or neuroimaging to rule out other more serious (and potentially even deadly) causes. Take some time to review conditions from previous chapters that can present as headaches including **strokes** (Chapter 14), **intracranial bleeds** (Chapter 15), **hydrocephalus** (Chapter 15), **post-ictal headaches** (Chapter 20), **brain tumors** (Chapter 21), and infections such as **meningitis** (Chapter 22) and **encephalitis** (Chapter 23)! From there, integrate that information with the new diseases you've learned about in this chapter as summarized in the table below:

Disease	Description	Distribution	Course	Features
Tension	"Tension," "pressure"	Bilateral	Few hours	Band-like pattern
Migraines	"Pounding," "throbbing"	Unilateral	Few hours	Nausea, photo/phonophobia, prodrome, aura, postdromal state
Cluster	"Hot poker behind my eye"	Unilateral	Few hours	Red eyes, ptosis, lacrimation
Giant-cell arteritis	Soreness, tender to palpation	Unilateral	Persistent	ESR ↑, older men, giant cells on biopsy
IIH	Generalized, throbbing	Bilateral	Persistent	Papilledema, otherwise healthy young woman

REVIEW QUESTIONS

1. A 23 y/o F is seeing a neurologist for management of recurrent headaches. Several times per month, she experiences a severe headache on the left side of her head which she describes as "someone sticking my head in a bag and hitting it with a sledgehammer." These headaches generally last around 4 hours during which time she tries to lay down in a quiet dark room, as "seeing any light is like staring into the sun." She often experiences nausea during these episodes and occasionally vomits as a result. During the appointment, she tells her neurologist that in the past week she has had 2 attacks. For half an hour prior to each attack, she noticed small "dots that change color" appearing in her field of view that were "kind of like looking through a kaleidoscope." These dots were then followed by complete loss of vision in one eye, although she notes that it was a different eye each time (left the first time, right the second time). Which of the following is the best explanation for her visual symptoms?
    A. Transient ischemic attacks
    B. Migraine headaches
    C. Mononeuritis multiplex
    D. Occipital lobe seizures
    E. Optic neuritis related to multiple sclerosis

2. A 71 y/o M presents to the emergency department with sudden vision loss accompanied by "the worst headache of my life." He reports that for the past month he has had recurrent headaches of an "agonizing" quality on the right side of his head. Over this same time period, he has had a few episodes of blurry vision in his right eye that have resolved on their own. Review of symptoms is positive for reduced food intake related to pain in his jaw while chewing. Vital signs are HR 102, BP 136/88, RR 14, and T 101.4°F. On exam, there is extreme tenderness to palpation of his right scalp with diminished pulse strength. Which of the following in the best next step?
    A. Ordering a CT scan of the head
    B. Ordering an MRI scan of the head
    C. Obtaining a tissue sample for biopsy
    D. Obtaining a blood sample to test the erythrocyte sedimentation rate
    E. Administering corticosteroids
    F. Administering tissue plasminogen activator
    G. Administering high flow oxygen

3. A 24 y/o M is brought to the emergency department by ambulance around 11:00 at night after telling his girlfriend he wanted to die. This is his third time coming to the hospital in the past month. On interview, he reports a desire to die related to severe retro-orbital pain on his right side "like someone is jabbing a knife directly into my eyeball over and over and over." He denies any plans to actively harm himself but says, "I can't keep living like this!" The pain began around 25 minutes ago and awakened him shortly after falling asleep. He is having trouble sitting still during the interview which he attributes to the pain. All of the following features are likely to be seen in this case *except*:
    A. Unilateral eyelid drooping
    B. Impaired pupillary light reflex
    C. Progression to both eyes
    D. Spontaneous termination of symptoms
    E. Good response to treatment
    F. History of tobacco use

4. A 44 y/o F sees her primary care doctor for management of headaches. She has been having headaches "off and on" for over 10 years. Since changing jobs 4 months ago, however, her headaches have been "almost constant." The pain is located over her forehead and feels like "pressure." If she massages her forehead, it brings a small degree of relief but only temporarily. She also describes pain on her back between her neck and left shoulder. Over the past few months, she has taken various medications in an effort to relieve her pain, including caffeine, over-the-counter medications (ibuprofen, naproxen, acetaminophen, and some herbal supplements), antidepressants (amitriptyline), and anticonvulsants (gabapentin). Each drug brought partial relief at the time it was started but then slowly lost efficacy over time. In the past week, she has had episodes of nausea and vomiting which she has not experienced before. She also had an episode where she fell while walking up stairs at work, though she says, "It's probably because I was wearing high heels." Examination reveals increased muscle tone in her trapezius muscles bilaterally, though she is able to reduce this tone when asked. Motor strength is intact throughout exam for 4/5 strength in her right leg and 3/5 in her right ankle. Which of the following is the best next step?
    A. Starting lorazepam, a benzodiazepine
    B. Starting tramadol, an opioid
    C. Stopping her existing medications
    D. Referring for psychotherapy
    E. Ordering head imaging
    F. None of the above

1. **The best answer is B.** While headaches are the hallmark symptom of migraines, they are not the only manifestation of this condition. Many people with migraines experience visual symptoms either before or during an attack, with scintillations, scotomas, and even blindness occurring. The patient's description of her headache matches the presentation of a migraine closely, with a pulsatile quality, nausea, vomiting, and photophobia. For this reason, it is unlikely that another condition is needed to explain her visual symptoms (answers A, C, D, and E).

2. **The best answer is E.** This case describes a classic presentation of giant-cell arteritis, an inflammatory disease affecting large blood vessels including the temporal artery. It often presents as a unilateral headache in an elderly patient along with jaw claudication, visual abnormalities, and constitutional symptoms such as fever. Giant-cell arteritis is a medical emergency, as delays in treatment can lead to permanent vision loss. For this reason, treatment should not be delayed for diagnostic tests if there is a reasonably high degree of certainty about the diagnosis (answers A—D). Corticosteroids are the treatment of choice for giant-cell arteritis as they are effective at rapidly reducing the inflammatory state brought on by this disease. High flow oxygen is effective at treating cluster headaches (answer G). Given the gradual onset of the patient's symptoms, a stroke is less likely (answer F).

3. **The best answer is C.** Cluster headaches are also known as "suicide headaches," as their excruciatingly painful nature has been said to make death sound like an attractive option compared to experiencing them. Cluster headaches are associated with autonomic signs including ptosis (answer A) and constriction of the pupils (answer B). Most cluster headaches will end on their own in around 30 minutes (answer D), although during a cluster of attacks the recurrence rate is high. Cluster headaches are treatable using high flow oxygen or triptans (answer E). There is an association between smoking and cluster headaches, although the exact mechanism linking the two is not clear (answer F). Most cluster headaches are unilateral, so progression to both eyes is unlikely to be seen.

4. **The best answer is E.** This vignette describes what initially appears to be a tension headache with a possible contribution from medication overuse. However, there are several features of this case that are concerning for a secondary headache, including a distinct change in how her headaches present beginning 4 months ago, atypical symptoms such as nausea and vomiting, and focal neurologic deficits on exam. For this reason, other causes of headaches, such as a brain tumor, must be ruled out. If no primary cause is found, then stopping her existing medications would be an appropriate treatment for a medication overuse headache (answer C). Starting a new medication is not likely to provide lasting relief, and both benzodiazepines and opioids are prone to dependence (answers A and B). Psychotherapy can be a helpful adjunct for helping to cope with headaches but is not the highest priority compared to working up a potential brain tumor (answer D).

27 NEUROCUTANEOUS DISORDERS

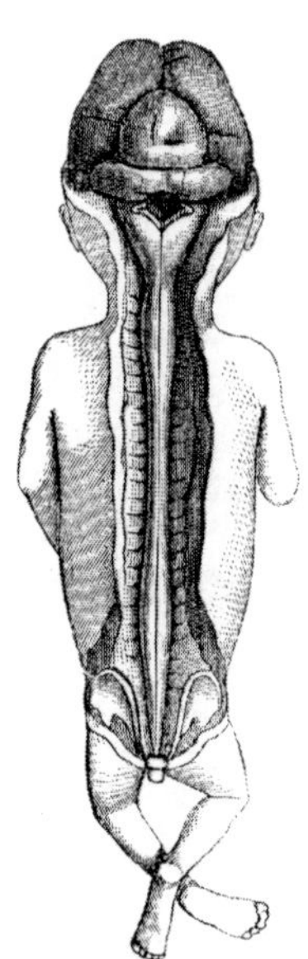

Okay, we're almost done! In our next-to-final chapter, we will talk about a class of genetic diseases known as **neurocutaneous disorders** that have effects on both the **nervous system** ("neuro-") and the **skin** ("-cutaneous"). The link between these two organ systems isn't immediately obvious. However, if you consider that nerves and skin both derive from the **ectoderm**, or one of the three germ layers that form during early embryonic development, it starts to make more sense. In particular for our study of neurology, these diseases tend to increase one's risk of developing **nervous system tumors**, as we will discover here.

Because genes contribute in some way to just about everything in the body, it makes sense that genetic diseases can have deleterious effects on multiple organ systems. For that reason, the disorders we will be studying in this chapter do not always make intuitive or logical sense and will instead require a lot of memorization. (Like, *a lot.*) But that's just the sort of situation that mnemonics were made for! So buckle up and strap in for the final ride of this book as we explore the wild world of neurocutaneous disorders.

NEUROFIBROMATOSIS

The term **neurofibromatosis** doesn't refer to only a single disease but rather to a collection of diseases that are all characterized by rampant growth of tumors in the nervous system. Of note, these tumors arise not in the neurons themselves but rather in the supporting cast members (the **glial cells** we talked about back in Chapter 2). These tumors are known as **neurofibromas** and are generally made up of *non-myelinating* Schwann cells (or those that provide other forms of support to neurons in the peripheral nervous system). We will talk about the two most highest-yield forms of this disease here! (The third, known as schwannomatosis, is so incredibly rare that it is unlikely to show up clinically or on tests.)

NEUROFIBROMATOSIS TYPE I

Neurofibromatosis type I (NF1, or previously **von Recklinghausen disease**) is an **autosomal dominant disorder** caused by a mutation in the neurofibromin 1 gene on chromosome **17.** (Conveniently, "von Recklinghausen" is made up of 17 letters, which should help you remember this association.)

Neurofibromatosis type I (previously known as **von Recklinghausen disease**) is an **autosomal dominant disease** caused by a mutation on **chromosome 17.**

*"Von Recklinghausen" has **17** letters which should help you remember chromosome **17**.*

Neurofibromatosis type I is characterized by a triad of **neurofibromas** (tumors of Schwann cells), **café-au-lait spots** (hyperpigmented birthmarks named after the French term for "coffee with milk," referencing their light brown color), and **Lisch nodules** (tumor-like aggregations known as **hamartomas** consisting of melanocytes, or pigment-producing cells, found in the iris of the eye).

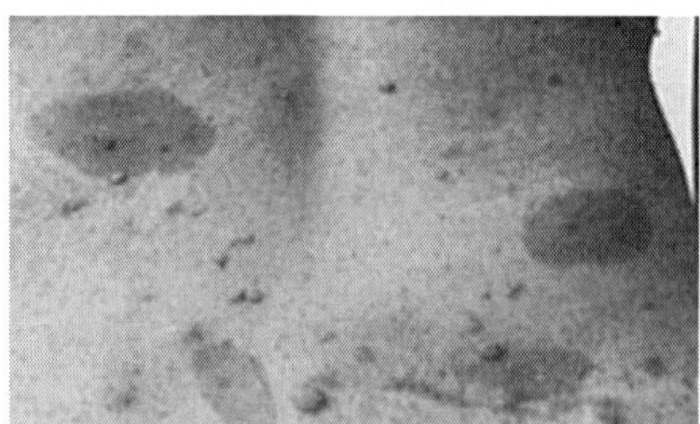
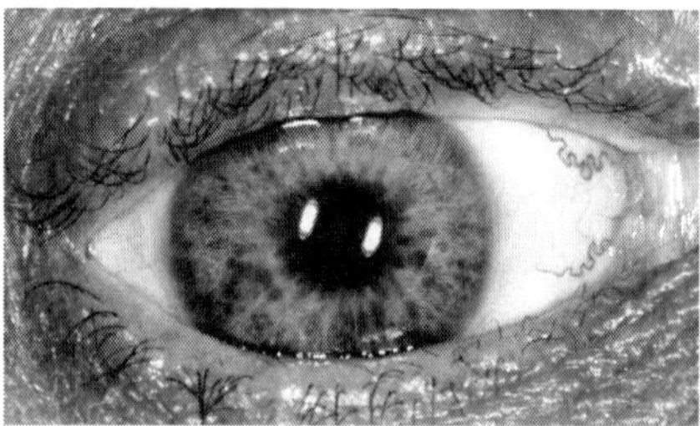

*Left: **Neurofibromas** and **café-au-lait spots** on the skin of the back.*
*Right: Hyperpigmented **Lisch nodules** in the iris.*

Other signs of neurofibromatosis type I include freckling of the skin around the armpit and groin, skeletal deformities, and gliomas (or more tumors of glial cells) in the optic nerve. You can put all of these presenting signs and symptoms together into the mnemonic **CAFÉ SPOT** which stands for **C**afé-au-lait spots, **A**xillary/inguinal freckling, **F**ibromas, **E**ye hamartomas (Lisch nodules), **S**keletal deformities, **P**assed down from parents, and an **O**ptic nerve **T**umor.

Neurofibromatosis type I is quite variable in its severity, as many patients are only mildly affected while others are completely disabled. There is **no cure**, but care can still be provided to minimize symptoms and maximize functional ability.

Neurofibromatosis type I is characterized by a triad of **neurofibromas**, **café-au-lait spots**, and **Lisch nodules** as well as other associated signs.

CAFÉ SPOT:
C*afé-au-lait spots*
A*xillary/inguinal freckling*
F*ibromas*
E*ye hamartomas (Lisch nodules)*
S*keletal deformities*
P*assed down from parents*
O*ptic nerve* ***T****umor*

NEUROFIBROMATOSIS TYPE II

Neurofibromatosis type II goes by the name **MISME syndrome** which, conveniently, is also a mnemonic for what this disease involves! **MISME** stands for **M**ultiple **I**nherited **S**chwannomas, **M**eningiomas, and **E**pendymomas which actually sums up the clinical presentation of patients with this disease quite nicely. The schwannomas are often found in the sheath around the **vesticulocochlear nerve** and tend to be **bilateral** (in contrast to sporadic schwannomas which are generally unilateral). Treatment often involves **surgical removal** of the schwannomas as well as **hearing aids** and other assistive devices if needed.

Neurofibromatosis type II involves **bilateral benign brain tumors**, particularly **bilateral schwannomas** as well as **meningiomas** and **ependymomas**.

MISME: ***M****ultiple* ***I****nherited* ***S****chwannomas,* ***M****eningiomas, and* ***E****pendymomas.*

Like type I, neurofibromatosis type II is inherited in an **autosomal dominant** fashion, with the defect having been localized to the NF2 gene on chromosome **22**. In contrast to type I, however, it often presents a little later in life (usually around one's teenage years or early 20s). You can remember these distinctions using the **2** in its name to remind you of the **bi**lateral occurrence of vestibular schwannomas, the location on chromosome **22**, and the onset around the age of **2**0.

Neurofibromatosis type II is inherited in an **autosomal dominant** fashion and is localized to the **NF2 gene** on **chromosome 22**.

Neurofibromatosis type ***II*** *involves* ***bi****lateral vestibular schwannomas, is located on chromosome* ***22****, and begins around the age of* ***2****0.*

OTHER NEUROCUTANEOUS DISORDERS

Aside from neurofibromatosis types I and II, there are a few other particularly high-yield neurocutaneous disorders to know! These are all **complex syndromes** involving many organ systems, meaning that treatment often involves a multidisciplinary team to address the various biological, psychological, and social aspects of the disease.

TUBEROUS SCLEROSIS

Tuberous sclerosis is an **autosomal dominant** genetic disorder in which mutations of two **tumor suppressor genes** (TSC1 and TSC2, both named after this disease) lead to the development of **multiple benign tumors** in various organs of the body. The main clinical features of tuberous sclerosis can be captured in the mnemonic **I ♥ TUBERS**:

I is for Intellectual disability. Cognitive deficits are seen in about half of all cases.

♥ is for Heart. One type of tumor seen commonly in tuberous sclerosis is a **cardiac rhabdomyoma** or a tumor of the muscles cells of the heart.

TU is for TUmors. Lots of tumors.

B is for Brain. Tuberous sclerosis is associated with three types of brain tumors in particular: **giant cell astrocytomas**, **cortical tubers**, and **subependymal nodules**.

E is for Epilepsy. Most patients with tuberous sclerosis suffer from recurrent **seizures** and generally require treatment with anticonvulsants.

R is for Renal. The majority of tuberous sclerosis cases involve benign tumors in the kidney known as **angiomyolipomas**, named for the combination of vascular ("angio"), muscular ("myo"), and fatty ("lipo") tissues seen in these tumors.

S is for Skin. Skin involvement in seen in basically all cases of tuberous sclerosis. Hypopigmented areas known as **ash leaf spots** are incredibly common (compare this to the *hyper*pigmented lesions seen in neurofibromatosis type I!). Another finding is **facial angiofibromas** or small flesh-colored papules as seen in the image below:

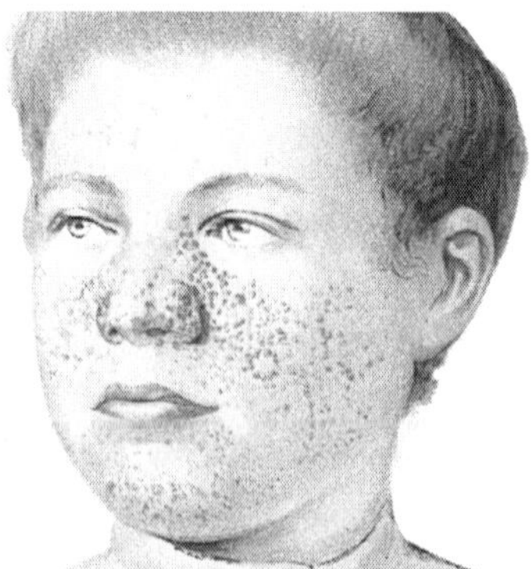

***Facial angiofibromas** in a patient with **tuberous sclerosis**.*

Tuberous sclerosis is an **autosomal dominant neurocutaneous disorder** that involves the growth of **multiple benign tumors** in various organs of the body.

I ♥ TUBERS:
__I__ntellectual disability
♥ (cardiac rhabdomyomas)
Multiple benign __TU__mors
__B__rain tumors
__E__pilepsy
__R__enal angiomyolipomas
__S__kin findings (ash leaf spots and facial angiofibromas)

STURGE-WEBER SYNDROME

Sturge-Weber syndrome (also known as **encephalotrigeminal angiomatosis**—quite the mouthful!) is a neurocutaneous disorder whose most notable feature is dark red cutaneous hemangiomas known as **port-wine stains** that are found on the patient's face at birth. If this were the only anomaly associated with this condition, it wouldn't be quite so bad! However, patients with Sturge-Weber syndrome also present with other deficits as well. You can remember these by making an acronym out of **STURGE** to associate the port-wine **S**tains with **T**umors (specifically **angiomas** or tumors of vascular tissues), **U**nilateral muscle weakness (generally on the side *opposite* of the port-wine stain!), mental **R**etardation (now called intellectual disability), **G**laucoma (increased intraocular pressure that can lead to vision loss), and **E**pilepsy (recurrent seizures). Unlike most other neurocutaneous diseases, Sturge-Weber syndrome does not have a clear genetic cause, with most cases being **sporadic**.

Sturge-Weber syndrome is a **sporadic neurocutaneous disease** seen at the time of birth. **Port-wine stains** are a notable feature.

***STURGE**-Weber syndrome:*
Port-wine __S__tains
__T__umors (angiomas)
__U__nilateral muscle weakness
Mental __R__etardation (intellectual disability)
__G__laucoma
__E__pilepsy

VON HIPPEL-LINDAU DISEASE

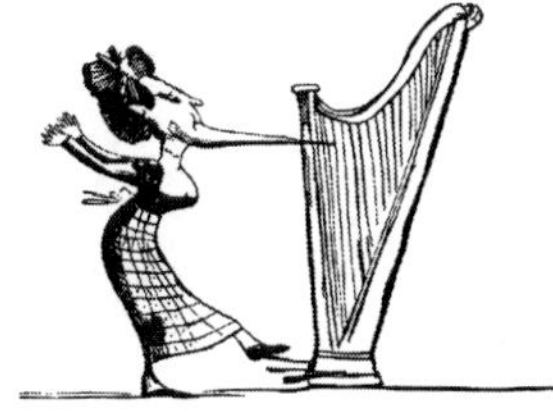

Von Hippel–Lindau disease is an **autosomal dominant** genetic disorder involving a mutation in a tumor suppressor gene on **chromosome 3**, leading to tumors popping up in multiple areas of the body. You can remember the four most common manifestations of this condition by thinking of it as von **HARP**el—Lindau disease to stand for **H**emangioblastomas (generally in the cerebellum and spine), **A**ngiomas (the same vascular tumors as are seen in Sturge-Weber syndrome), **R**enal cell carcinomas (often bilateral), and **P**heochromocytomas (tumors of the adrenal glands producing excessive amounts of norepinephrine which can cause a state of sympathetic nervous system overactivation). These tumors can all occur on their own, but when they appear in children or as more than one tumor at a time, this is strongly suggestive of von Hippel-Lindau disease!

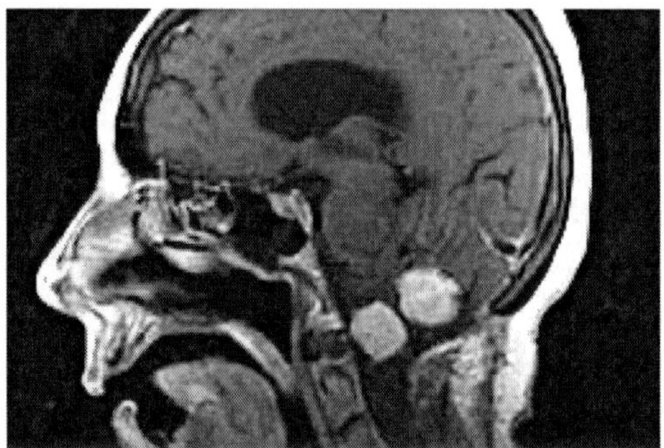

Von Hippel-Lindau disease *manifesting as multiple* ***hemangioblastomas****.*

Von Hippel-Lindau disease is an **autosomal dominant genetic disorder** resulting in **multiple tumors** across the body.

*von **HARP**el—Lindau disease:*
***H**emangioblastomas*
***A**ngiomatosis*
***R**enal cell carcinomas*
***P**heochromocytomas*

ATAXIA TELANGIECTASIA

The last neurocutaneous disorder we will talk about is **ataxia telangiectasia**. Luckily, the two biggest manifestations of the disease (ataxia and multiple telangiectasias) are both written right into the name! We've talked about **ataxia** and its associated "**dizzy AUNT with 3 dishes**" signs already so you should be able to recognize those. In contrast, **telangiectasia** might be a new word for you, but it refers to **small dilated blood vessels** located right under the surface of the skin that make small points of redness, as seen in the following image:

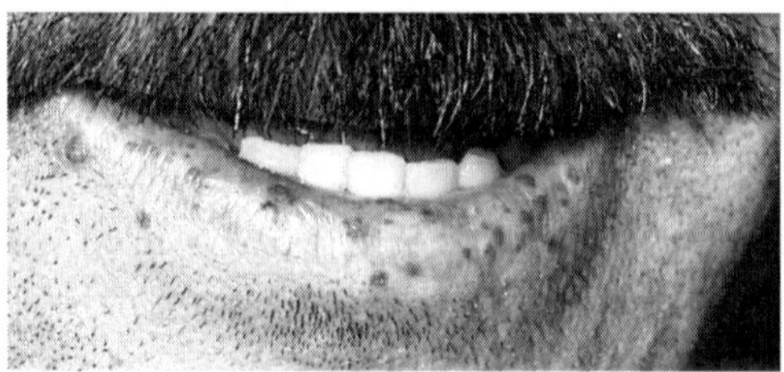

Telangiectasias *on the lip.*

While ataxia and telangiectasias are the core features of this disease, most people with ataxia telangiectasia also suffer from **immunodeficiency** and are at an increased risk for infections (particularly in the lungs). There is also an increased risk of various types of **cancer**, with lymphomas and leukemia being the most common.

Ataxia telangiectasia is an **autosomal recessive** genetic disease caused by a mutation in the **ATM gene** on **chromosome 11**. The ATM gene is involved in repairing broken DNA, which explains why people with ataxia telangiectasia are at an increased risk of cancer (due to their inability to repair DNA damage) and dysfunction of the immune system (as creation of antibodies requires rearranging DNA sequences that are normally put back together by ATM). You can remember the mechanism of this disease by thinking of a situation in which someone **attacks ya tel**evision set. What do you do? **Repair IT**! This will help you associate "**ataxia tel**angiectasia" with DNA **repair** as well as the risk of both **I**mmunodeficiency and **T**umors.

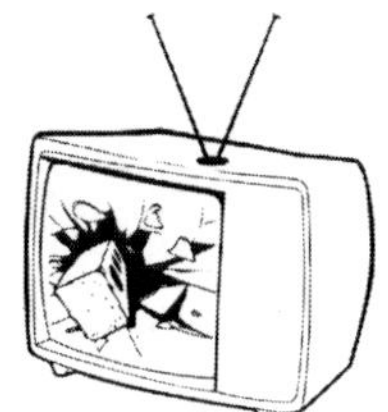

Ataxia telagiectasia is an **autosomal recessive** disorder involving **malfunctioning DNA repair** that leads to **ataxia**, **telangiectasias**, **immunodeficiency**, and an increased risk of **cancer**.

*What do you do when someone **attacks ya tel**evision set? **Repair IT**!*
*Defect of DNA **repair***
***I**mmunodeficiency*
***T**umors*

PUTTING IT ALL TOGETHER

The diseases found in this chapter can admittedly come across as a hodgepodge of different conditions that have few, if any, unifying themes between them. However, try to remember the core pattern of both **nervous system** and **skin involvement** due to the origin of both of these organs in the **ectoderm**! From there, use the mnemonics provided to look for patterns that will help you to identify the specific diagnosis.

Disease	Inheritance	Chromosome	Features
NF1	AD	17	Neurofibromas, café-au-lait spots, Lisch nodules
NF2	AD	22	Schwannomas, meningiomas, ependymomas
Tuberous sclerosis	AD	9, 16	Multiple benign tumors (heart, brain, kidneys, skin)
Sturge-Weber	Sporadic	n/a	Port-wine stains, tumors, hemiparesis, intellectual disability, glaucoma, epilepsy
Von Hippel-Lindau	AD	3	Hemangioblastomas, angiomatosis, renal cell carcinomas, pheochromocytomas
Ataxia telangiectasia	AR	11	Ataxia, telangiectasias, immunodeficiency, tumors

REVIEW QUESTIONS

1. A 27 y/o F has seen a primary care doctor for the past decade. She comes in today for a check-up. Her medical history is notable for blindness in her right eye due to radiation treatment of an optic nerve tumor as a child. She also underwent corrective surgery for scoliosis at the age of 12. Her physical exam is notable for several hyperpigmented areas on her back with small soft skin nodules dispersed across her body as seen below:

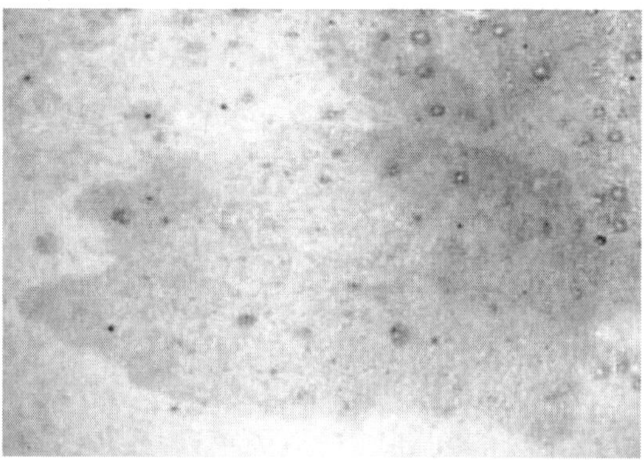

These findings have all been noted by the doctor since the time he first saw her, and he does not believe there has been any change in their pattern or distribution. On interview, she reports increasing fatigue for the past 2 weeks, with nausea yesterday and today. She also reports occasional abdominal pain over the same time period. A urine pregnancy test is positive. Her partner has no significant personal or family history of disease. Which of the following is the most appropriate statement for the doctor to make at this time?

    A. "The likelihood of your child inheriting this condition from you depends on whether it is a boy or a girl."
    B. "It is almost certain that your child will be affected by your condition."
    C. "There is a 50% chance that you will pass your condition to your child."
    D. "It is highly unlikely that your child will be affected."
    E. "There is no chance that your child will develop your condition."

2. A 3 y/o M is brought to the hospital for fever and lethargy over the past 2 days. He has a history of recurrent ear infections, and his exam today is consistent with a repeat infection. His medical history is notable for developmental delays in both motor and speech milestones as well as a prior hospitalization for aspiration pneumonia. His pediatrician documented in his chart for the past several visits that his gait was unsteady, with a tendency to fall when walking more than a few feet at a time. His height and weight are appropriate for his age. Small dilated blood vessels are seen over his ears and nose but are particularly prominent on his sclerae as seen in the following image:

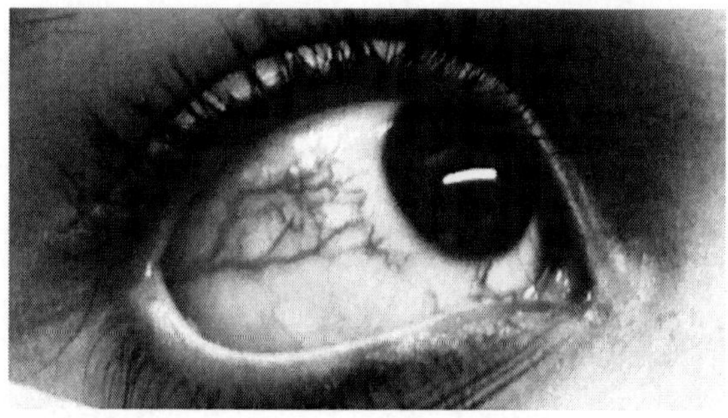

Which of the following should most be *avoided* in this patient?

A. CT scans of the chest to diagnose pulmonary infections
B. MRI scans of the head to evaluate cerebellar volume
C. Prophylactic antibiotics to prevent future infections
D. Mechanical bracing of the legs to improve leg stability
E. Feeding tubes to prevent aspiration

3. A 3 m/o M is brought to the emergency department after he is seen having several tonic-clonic seizures involving the right half of his body. On exam, a deep purple patch of skin is noticeable on the left side of the patient's face as seen below:

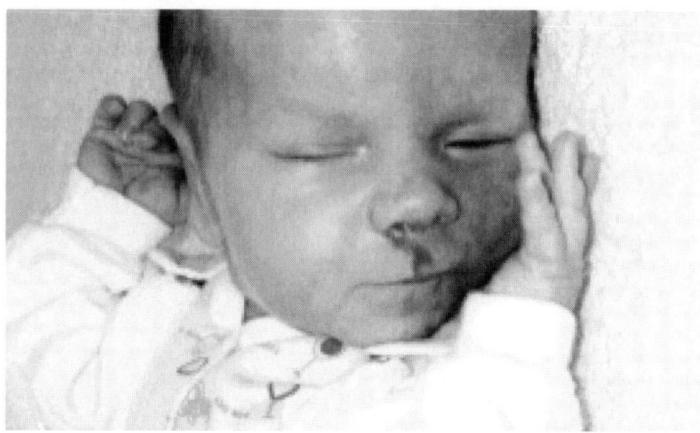

Which of the following conditions is this patient at risk for later in life?

A. Recurrent seizures
B. Increased intraocular pressure leading to damage of the optic nerve
C. Delayed attainment of motor and speech milestones
D. Weakness of right-sided muscles
E. All of the above
F. None of the above

1. **The best answer is C.** This patient likely has neurofibromatosis type I given the presence of café-au-lait spots, neurofibromas, and several associated conditions including scoliosis and optic nerve tumors. Neurofibromatosis type I is an autosomal dominant disorder, so this patient has about a 50% chance of passing the disease to her offspring, not lower or higher (answers B, D, and E). Neurofibromatosis type I is not an X-linked condition (answer A).

2. **The best answer is A.** Patients with ataxia–telangiectasia have a mutation in the ATM gene which normally produces a protein that is involved in repairing DNA damage. For this reason, exposure to radiation and other potential sources of DNA damage should be avoided to reduce the risk of developing cancer as much as possible (although in some cases the benefits of doing an x-ray or CT scan will outweigh this risk). MRI scans do not involve radiation and will not increase the risk of cancer (answer B). While overuse of antibiotics is a concern, for a patient who is at high risk of recurrent infections, prophylactic use may be appropriate (answer C). A feeding tube is an invasive procedure, although it may be appropriate if the patient is unable to eat by mouth without aspirating food (answer E). Mechanical bracing of the legs is an appropriate measure to improve mobility (answer D).

3. **The best answer is E.** The combination of infantile seizures with a port-wine stain is characteristic of Sturge–Weber syndrome, a neurocutaneous disorder that affects multiple organ systems. Patients with Sturge–Weber syndrome are at risk for recurrent seizures (answer A), glaucoma (answer B), intellectual disability (answer C), and unilateral hemiparesis (answer D), the latter of which notably tends to occur on the opposite side of the body as the port-wine stain.

28 FINAL REVIEW

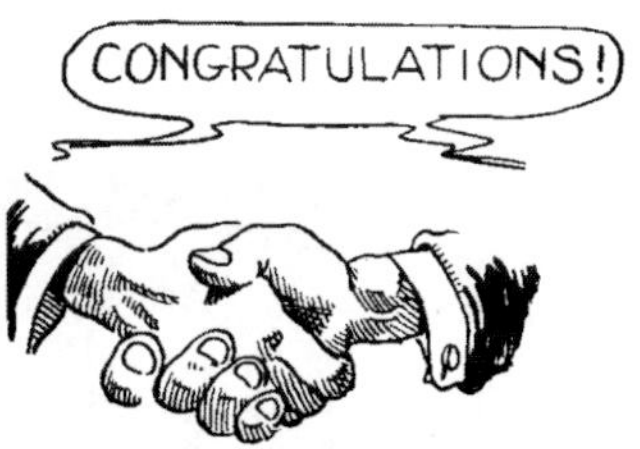

Okay, that's a wrap! At this point, we have covered many of the most common **neurologic diseases** found on exams and in the real world. We have also covered the **foundational neuroanatomy** that allows us to explain what we are seeing on a clinical level. This is not to say that we have gone over every possible detail of neurologic pathology, as such a feat would require volumes of books and a lifetime of learning. Because of this, it is possible that as you continue on in your clinical career, you will encounter neurologic diseases that we haven't explicitly covered here. Don't be put off by this! By keeping our neuroanatomical framework in mind, learning about new diseases doesn't have to be scary or confusing. Try to use everything you have learned so far about neuroanatomy to make predictions about what kinds of signs and symptoms you might observe with any new disease you come across—because you'll probably be right! This is because the nervous system is an understandable and predictable structure, and those that take the time to learn it will find themselves rewarded.

We will close out this book with a final set of review questions that will hopefully bring together much of what you have learned into a cohesive whole. After all, when practicing in the real world, patients will not come to you with their diseases neatly organized into discrete chapters. Instead, you will need to be prepared to see whatever pathology may come through the door at any given moment. Use this opportunity to make connections and comparisons between the various signs, symptoms, and clinical findings that are shared across different types of diseases so that you can come to the right diagnosis and treatment.

Good luck!

FINAL REVIEW QUESTIONS

1. A 10 y/o F is adopted from an orphanage in Laos and brought to live in the United States. Her medical history is unknown. At the age of 12, she is brought to a pediatrician for an evaluation after she develops intermittent jerking movements of her arms and legs. Her adopted mother says that over the same period of time her personality began to change and that the "bright sunny girl" she used to be has gone away. The pediatrician diagnoses her as having a tic disorder, says that her personality changes are a normal part of pre-adolescent development, and prescribes her a medication to treat her tics. Over the next several months, the jerky movements begin to happen more frequently and more violently. She begins to struggle in school, and she is much more irritable and withdrawn. She is brought to the hospital after she drops "like a rag doll" several times at school. She does not lose consciousness during these episodes. In the emergency department, her exam is notable for difficulty following simple commands such as being asked to raise her hand or hop on one leg. There is mild cogwheel rigidity in her upper extremities bilaterally. Her vital signs are within normal limits for her age. A lumbar puncture is performed which shows no abnormalities in cell counts, glucose, or protein. An MRI of the brain reveals abnormal signals in the white matter of the left frontal lobe as below:

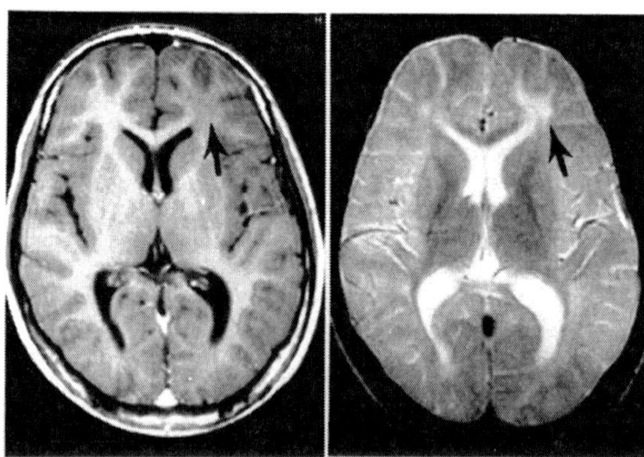

The patient is admitted to the hospital. Which of the following is the most likely explanation for her presentation?

A. Bacterial meningitis
B. Viral encephalitis
C. Fungal meningoencephalitis
D. Childhood absence epilepsy
E. Juvenile myoclonic epilepsy
F. Lennox-Gastaut syndrome
G. Pilocytic astrocytoma
H. Acute disseminated encephalomyelitis
I. Subacute sclerosing panencephalitis
J. None of the above

2. An 18 y/o M plays football on his high school team. During a championship game, he sustains two hard hits to the head but does not lose consciousness. Worried about being ejected from the game, he does not tell his coach about this. Over the next 5 days, he begins to experience a progressive headache and increasing nausea with three episodes of vomiting. One week after the game, he tells his parents to take him to the hospital. In the emergency department, he is initially fully alert and oriented. However, as time passes he begins to look increasingly sedated and is unable to understand the questions being asked of him. Concerned, the emergency medicine team orders a head CT. Which of the following images is most likely to be seen?

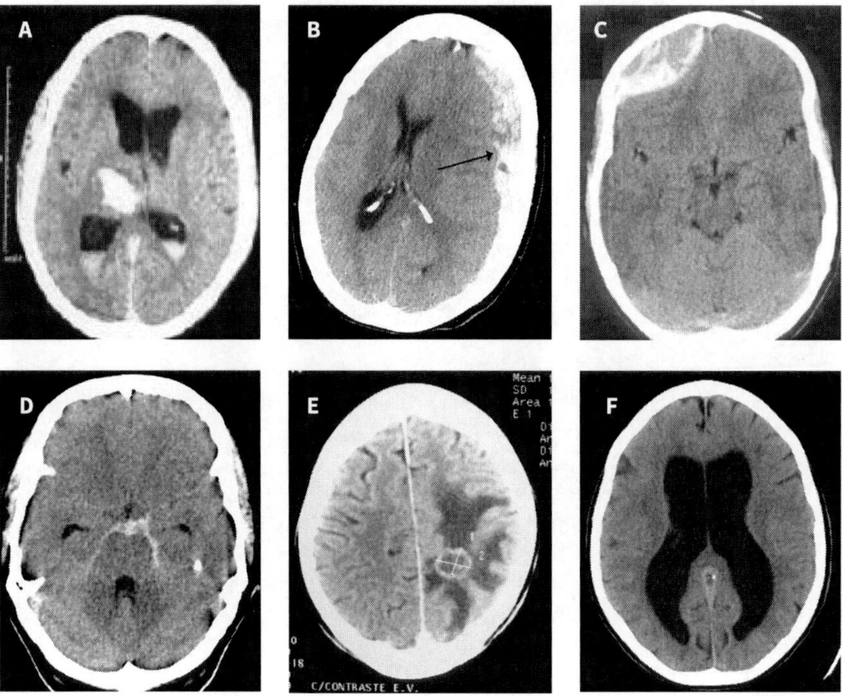

3. A 28 y/o F is training to be a neurologist. She is reading the results of a genetic test that she recently ordered for one of her patients. The report says that her patient has an expansion of the trinucleotide repeat sequence GAA on chromosome 9. Which of the following is most likely to describe her patient?
    A. A 2 m/o F with new onset of a complete loss of motor tone
    B. A 10 y/o F with unsteady gait, no proprioception, and an enlarged heart
    C. A 42 y/o M with involuntary swinging movements of the arms and legs
    D. A 15 y/o F with epilepsy, hyperpigmented spots, and skin nodules
    E. A 28 y/o M with bilateral hand weakness and slowed muscle relaxation
    F. A 50 y/o F with diffuse muscle weakness, spasticity, and atrophy
    G. None of the above

4. A 58 y/o F with a history of hypertension and diabetes mellitus presents to the emergency department with left-sided weakness. When she awoke this morning, she noticed that her left arm was weak and that she was having difficulty speaking. Left leg weakness developed several hours later. She denies any loss of consciousness or changes in vision. Vital signs are HR 92, BP 182/114, RR 16, and T 99.1°F. Neurological exam is notable for an absent gag reflex, weakness of the left upper and lower extremities, loss of vibration and proprioception on the left, and deviation of the tongue to the right as seen in the following image:

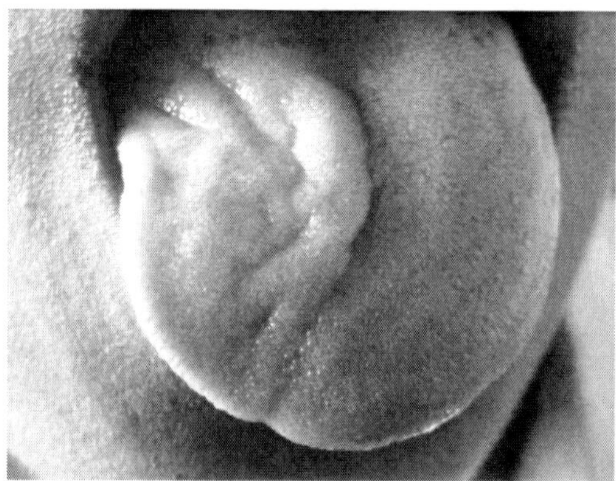

No facial weakness or asymmetry is seen. Extraocular movements are intact for both eyes. Pain and temperature sensation are intact throughout. Which of the following arteries is most likely to reveal an occlusion?

A. Left anterior cerebral artery
B. Right anterior cerebral artery
C. Left middle cerebral artery
D. Right middle cerebral artery
E. Left posterior cerebral artery
F. Right posterior cerebral artery
G. Basilar artery
H. Left anterior inferior cerebellar artery
I. Right anterior inferior cerebellar artery
J. Left posterior inferior cerebellar artery
K. Right posterior inferior cerebellar artery
L. Left vertebral artery
M. Right vertebral artery
N. Anterior spinal artery

5. A 19 y/o F with no past medical history presents to the emergency department complaining of severe headaches for the past 3 weeks along with blurry vision for the past 5 days. She describes her headaches as "throbbing" and continuous. She denies fever, chills, or muscle weakness but does note that she has felt more tired recently. Vital signs are HR 92, BP 130/84, RR 16, and T 99.1°F. Exam reveals a moderately obese young woman who is alert and oriented to person, place, time,

and situation. Motor strength and sensation is intact in all four extremities. Gait is steady and balanced. Her Romberg test is negative. Cranial nerve exam reveals limited ability to look laterally in both eyes. Visual acuity is decreased with an enlarged blind spot bilaterally. Fundoscopic examination reveals blurring of the optic discs bilaterally as seen in the following image:

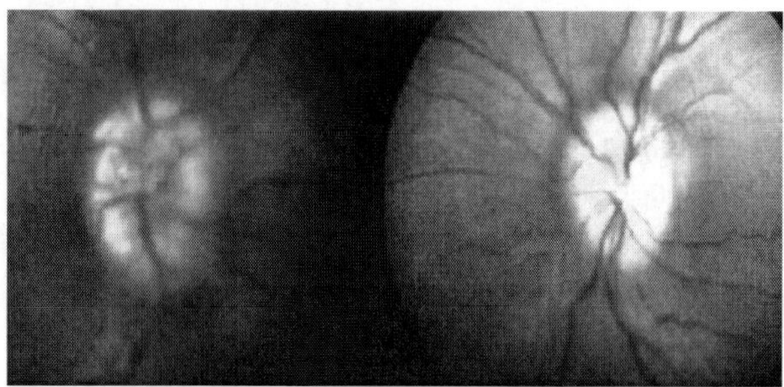

An MRI of the brain is ordered which shows no abnormalities. Which of the following is most likely to relieve her symptoms?

A. Short course of corticosteroids
B. Lumbar puncture
C. Ibuprofen
D. Neurosurgical tumor resection
E. Sumatriptan
F. Broad-spectrum antibiotics
G. High flow oxygen by nasal cannula
H. Full recovery is expected without treatment

6. A 25 y/o right-handed M who is a graduate student in archaeology comes to the student health clinic reporting shaking of his right hand for the past several months. This shaking is most noticeable when he is writing and recently has resulted in him being unable to take written tests for his coursework. The shaking seems to "come and go," though at times it is so pronounced that his friends will ask him about it. He denies a history of excessive alcohol intake but says, "Now that you mention it, the shaking does seem to get better when I drink." A full neurological exam is unremarkable, with intact cranial nerves, full motor strength, no sensory deficits, and a steady gait. There is no resting tremor in his arms, but when asked to hold his arms out a tremor is seen in both hands, greater on the right than the left. The tremor increases in amplitude when asked to write his name and the date using a pencil, as seen below:

Which of the following is the best next step in management?

A. Genetic testing
B. MRI of the brain
C. PET scan of the brain
D. Prescribing a blood pressure medication
E. Injecting botulinum toxin
F. Electromyography of both upper extremities

7. A 23 y/o M goes to the urgent care clinic reporting severe pain and a rash on his left chest. He has never had a rash like this before. He denies recent sick contacts or unsafe sexual practices. He is otherwise healthy and takes no medications. Vital signs are HR 74, BP 126/84, RR 14, and T 98.8°F. Exam reveals a linear grouping of red vesicles as seen below:

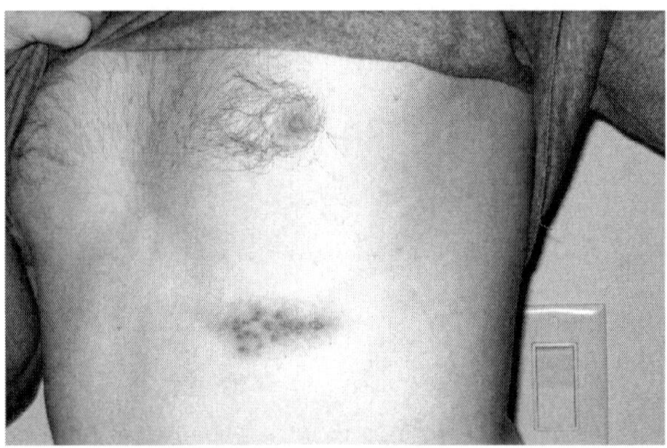

The remainder of the physical and neurological exam is completely normal. Viral particles are most likely to be found in which of the following spinal nerve roots?

A. C5
B. C7
C. T1
D. T4
E. T7
F. T10
G. L2
H. L4
I. S1

8. An 18 y/o F with a history of epilepsy is brought to the emergency department after a generalized tonic-clonic seizure lasting 2 minutes. She regularly sees a neurologist in clinic and has been taking lamotrigine for the past several years. On interview, she appears tired but is alert and oriented to person, place, time, and situation. Neurological exam reveals 2/5 motor strength in the left arm and leg. Her voice is soft and faint, though she is able to both speak and understand instructions. Vital signs are HR 114, BP 136/78, RR 18, and T 99.5°F. Which of the following is most likely to be seen on neuroimaging?

A. Hemorrhage in the region of the right anterior cerebral artery
B. Hemorrhage in the region of the left anterior cerebral artery
C. Hemorrhage in the region of the right middle cerebral artery
D. Hemorrhage in the region of the left middle cerebral artery
E. Hemorrhage in the region of the right posterior cerebral artery
F. Hemorrhage in the region of the left posterior cerebral artery
G. Ischemia in the region of the right anterior cerebral artery
H. Ischemia in the region of the left anterior cerebral artery
I. Ischemia in the region of the right middle cerebral artery
J. Ischemia in the region of the left middle cerebral artery
K. Ischemia in the region of the right posterior cerebral artery
L. Ischemia in the region of the left posterior cerebral artery
M. None of the above

9. A 79 y/o F is brought to the hospital after being found on the floor by her daughter. It is unclear whether she had lost consciousness or how long she had been on the floor. Neurologic exam reveals intact motor strength and preservation of all sensory modalities throughout her extremities. The most notable finding is profoundly impaired visual acuity, as the patient is observed to walk directly into objects, ignore a plate of food that is placed directly in front of her, and ask for lights to be turned on during the daytime. On more thorough testing, visual acuity is lost in all four quadrants of both eyes. When asked about her vision, she adamantly denies visual loss. When the doctor asks her to name various objects that are being held in front of her, she gives seemingly random responses, calling a watch "a pen" and a clipboard "a bottle." Her pupillary light reflexes are intact bilaterally. There is no evidence of other neurologic deficits. Where is the most likely location of the injury accounting for her deficits?
   A. Eye
   B. Optic nerve
   C. Optic chiasm
   D. Optic tract
   E. Lateral geniculate nucleus
   F. Optic radiations
   G. Occipital lobe
   H. Medial longitudinal fasciculus
   I. Paramedian pontine reticular formation
   J. Edinger-Westphal nuclei

10. A 71 y/o right-handed F is brought to the hospital from a local pier after a passerby found her sitting on a bench looking confused. When asked questions, she did not respond but looked very frustrated and upset about her situation. She was able to follow commands such as "Hold up your right hand" or "Shake your head." She was unable to write when given a paper and pencil. No other deficits are noted during a full neurological exam. Magnetic resonance angiography is most likely to reveal severe narrowing of which of the following arteries?

A. Right anterior cerebral artery
B. Left anterior cerebral artery
C. Right middle cerebral artery
D. Left middle cerebral artery
E. Right posterior cerebral artery
F. Left posterior cerebral artery
G. None of the above

11. A 19 y/o M is brought to the hospital after not eating for the past 3 weeks related to a belief that all food has been poisoned. He calls his family members "deceivers" and claims that he cannot trust them as they have "all been replaced by demons." For the past 6 months, he has stopped bathing or going to work. He is given a diagnosis of schizophrenia and started on a medication that blocks dopamine receptors in the brain. Which of the following effects is *least* likely to be seen as a side effect of this medication?
    A. Difficulty initiating movements
    B. Increased muscular rigidity
    C. Decreased production of prolactin
    D. Decreased goal-directed behavior
    E. All of the above are likely to be observed

12. An 11 y/o F is brought to see an optometrist after she tells her parents she is having trouble reading. She has been increasingly accident prone over the past few months and has been hit in the side of the head by a ball during recess on two separate occasions. In both instances, she says that she did not see the ball coming before it hit her. Visual acuity testing reveals no refractive errors. However, there are significant deficits in her field of vision as seen below:

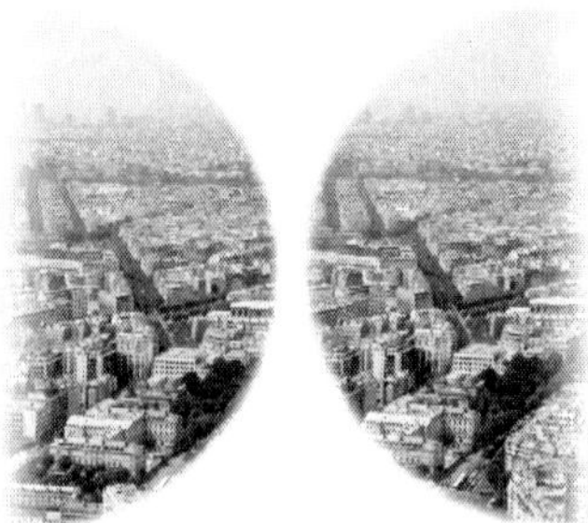

She is referred to an ophthalmologist for further evaluation. Her review of systems is positive for headache and increased thirst. Her weight is in the 12th percentile, though she was in the 64th percentile one year ago. An MRI is ordered which shows the following:

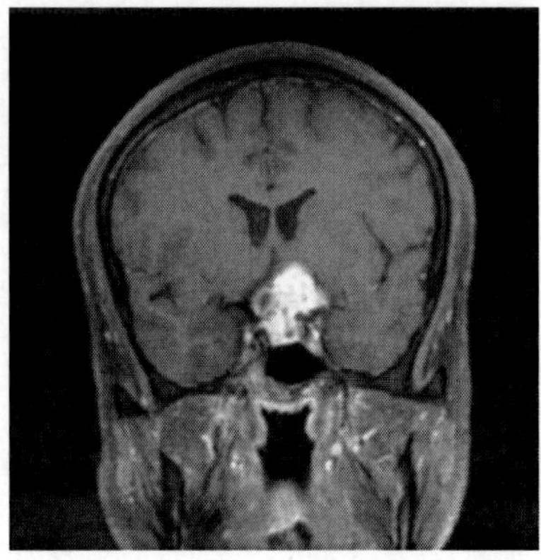

Which of the following best explains the patient's presentation?

A. Clonal expansion of glial cells in the central nervous system
B. Tumor of cerebellar stem cells
C. Growth of cerebrospinal fluid-producing cells in the ventricular system
D. Neoplastic growth of the vascular system supplying the brain
E. Growth of embryonic cell remnants in the pituitary gland
F. None of the above

13. (Continued from previous question.) The patient is scheduled for surgical resection followed by radiation therapy. Both of these are successful, and the patient is deemed to be in remission. Over the next year, however, she is noted to have an increased appetite resulting in excessive weight gain. Within two years, her BMI is in the morbidly obese range, and she is diagnosed as having insulin resistance. Her change in appetite is most likely attributable to damage in which of the following areas?

A. Ventral posterolateral nucleus of the thalamus
B. Ventral posteromedial nucleus of the thalamus
C. Lateral geniculate nucleus of the thalamus
D. Medial geniculate nucleus of the thalamus
E. Anterior nucleus of the hypothalamus
F. Lateral nucleus of the hypothalamus
G. Ventromedial nucleus of the hypothalamus
H. Suprachiasmatic nucleus of the hypothalamus
I. Supraoptic nucleus of the hypothalamus
J. Paraventricular nucleus of the hypothalamus

14. A 53 y/o F with a history of poorly controlled diabetes mellitus type 2 presents to the emergency department complaining of new-onset double vision. She says that over the past week she has had blurriness of vision, with difficulty focusing on objects beginning yesterday. On exam, there are no focal motor or sensory deficits in her extremities. Her eyes are deviated in separate directions as seen in the following image:

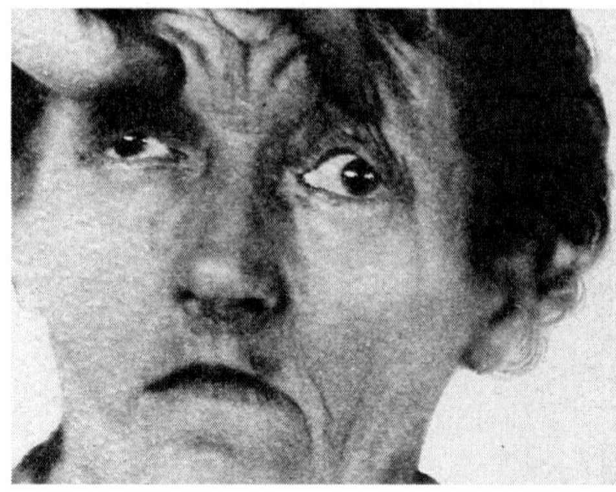

Her pupils are equal and reactive bilaterally. Vital signs are within normal limits. Her blood glucose is elevated at 280 mg/dL. A CT scan of the brain shows no evidence of ischemic changes. Which of the following cranial nerves is most likely affected?

A. Oculomotor nerve
B. Trochlear nerve
C. Abducens nerve
D. Oculomotor and trochlear nerves
E. Oculomotor and abducens nerves
F. Trochlear and abducens nerves
G. Oculomotor, trochlear, and abducens nerves
H. None of the cranial nerves

15. A 4 y/o F is brought to the hospital by her parents after she begins repeatedly falling to one side while walking "like she's drunk." Her medical history is unremarkable except for an episode of vomiting and diarrhea that occurred 5 days prior to this episode. Her parents do not believe she has ingested any alcohol, poisons, or other substances. She is up to date on her immunizations. Her vital signs are entirely within normal limits with no fever. There are no deficits in either motor strength or any sensory modality noted on neurological exam. There is no facial asymmetry or nystagmus. Her mental status appears to be grossly intact, and her parents deny any episodes of lost consciousness. CT and MRI scans of the head are ordered, and both show no focal abnormalities. Urine toxicology testing is negative for all substances including alcohol. Within 2 weeks, her gait has returned to normal. What is the most likely etiology?

A. Acute cerebellar ataxia
B. Acute disseminated encephalomyelitis
C. Subacute sclerosing panencephalitis
D. Encephalitis
E. Meningitis
F. Guillain-Barré syndrome
G. Multiple sclerosis
H. Hydrocephalus
I. Atonic seizures

16. A 24 y/o F gives birth to a healthy baby boy after a 39-week gestation. The mother lives in a rural area and objects to medical care, so she gives birth at home. One week after birth, the infant begins crying inconsolably and refuses to nurse. After several hours, the mother is sufficiently concerned and takes him to the emergency department. On exam, the patient is noted to have increased muscle tone throughout his body leading to an arched position as seen below:

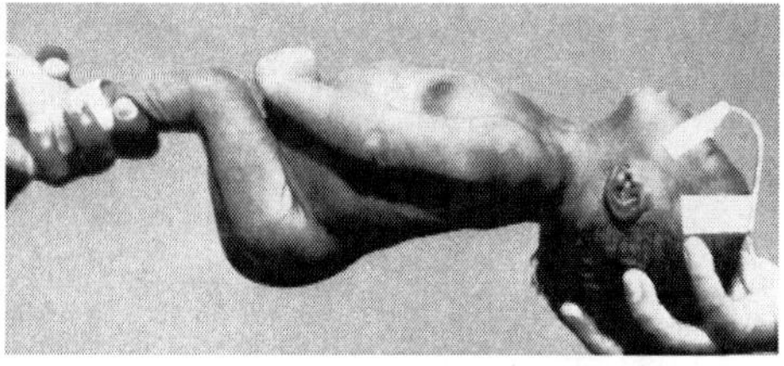

The exam is also notable for a malodorous purulent discharge from his umbilicus. No abnormalities in the fontanelles are observed. The patient is afebrile. Which of the following is the most likely cause of the patient's presentation?

A. Group B *Streptococci*
B. *Escherichia coli*
C. *Clostridium tetani*
D. *Clostridium botulinum*
E. Genetic defect in the SMN1 gene
F. None of the above

17. A 30 y/o F clutches her head and cries out suddenly while at work. She appears to be in a state of panic, so a nearby coworker calls 911. Upon initial evaluation in the hospital, she is completely unresponsive. Her body shows decerebrate extensor posturing. A CT is ordered which shows an acute left subdural hematoma. A follow-up MRI shows transtentorial herniation as below:

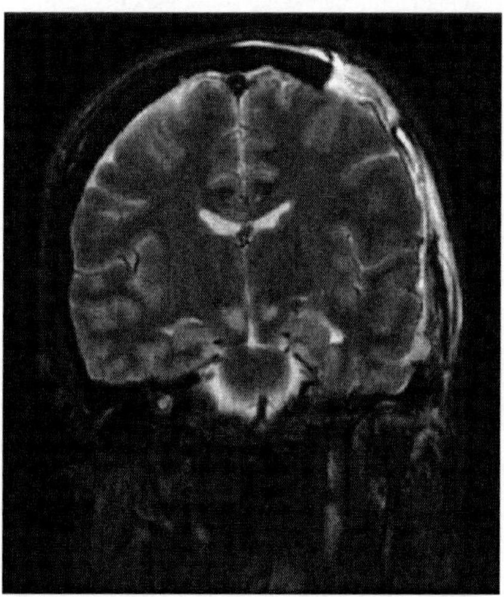

Which of the following is most likely to be seen on examination?

A. Fixed constricted pupils bilaterally
B. Downward and outward positioning of right eye
C. Upward and inward drift of the left eye
D. Outward drift of both eyes
E. None of the above

18. A 70 y/o F is referred to a neurologist after she develops slurring of her speech gradually over a period of one year. Her past medical history is significant for hypertension and diabetes both of which are well controlled with medications and lifestyle changes. While speaking with the patient, the neurologist notes that the patient's emotions will vacillate wildly from one moment to the next, and she switches between laughing and crying several times. Her emotional expression does not appear to correlate with the topic of the conversation. After additional evaluation, the patient is diagnosed with primary lateral sclerosis. Which of the following is most likely to be found on further examination?

    A. Absent gag reflex
    B. Tongue atrophy
    C. Urinary incontinence
    D. Rapid functional decline and death within several months
    E. Difficulty swallowing
    F. None of the above

19. A 72 y/o M with a history of poorly controlled hypertension and hyperlipidemia presents to the hospital after a sudden onset of headache with a "spinning" sensation. When he tried to walk around after this, he felt that he was perpetually falling to the left. On the way to the hospital, he developed severe nausea with several episodes of vomiting. On initial evaluation, his vital signs are within normal limits. Neurological exam is normal except for a slow unsteady gait, rapid darting eye movements when looking to the left, and inability to flip his hands over repeatedly when asked. While his visual acuity is intact, during the exam he notes that his vision is "not keeping up" with his eyes. He is unable to elaborate further when asked about this. The cranial nerve exam is otherwise intact. There is full motor strength and sensation in all four extremities. His memory and cognition are grossly normal. Which of the following is the most likely explanation for his symptoms?

    A. Thromboembolic occlusion of the anterior cerebral circulation
    B. Tearing of the inner lining of the vertebral artery
    C. Acute blockage of the ventricular system
    D. Buildup of fluid in the endolymphatic compartment of the inner ear
    E. Viral infection of the vestibular nerve
    F. None of the above

20. A 37 y/o M sees his primary care doctor after he awoke with severe low back pain and numbness in both legs. When he tried to get out of bed, his legs could not support his weight, and he collapsed onto the floor. On interview, he reports that several days ago he developed shooting pains in his back while lifting weights at the gym, but these resolved on their own. On exam, the patient is alert and oriented. His vital signs are within normal limits. Motor strength is intact in both upper extremities but is significantly decreased in the left lower extremity, with mild weakness in the thigh, moderate weakness in the calf, and complete paralysis in the foot. The left patellar reflex and bilateral Achilles reflexes are all absent. Sensory numbness is noted in the scrotum and perianal area. Urine is seen soaking his pants. When asked about this, the patient reports that he has had dribbling of urine since this morning. Magnetic resonance imaging of the back is most likely to reveal a herniated disk in which region of the spine?
    A. Cervical
    B. Thoracic
    C. Lumbar
    D. Sacral
    E. Coccygeal

21. A 18 y/o F college student is spending a semester abroad. On her first day, she goes to dinner with her host family at a local restaurant. She is offered a dish that she does not recognize. Not wanting to be rude, she takes a bite and tries to swallow it. However, she is repulsed by the taste and gags on the food, spitting it back out. She feels nauseous and about to vomit for the next several minutes. Which of the following neural structures is *least* involved in these processes?
    A. Facial nerve
    B. Glossopharyngeal nerve
    C. Vagus nerve
    D. Hypoglossal nerve
    E. Edinger-Westphal nuclei
    F. Nucleus solitarius
    G. Nucleus ambiguus
    H. Area postrema

22. A 21 y/o M comes to the hospital reporting a 4-day history of increasing nausea. His initial exam is unremarkable, with normal vital signs and no focal neurologic deficits. He is given fluid hydration and an outpatient follow-up appointment. When the nurse tries to give him his discharge paperwork, she notices that he appears somnolent and confused. Repeat vital signs are HR 38, BP 168/90, RR 18, and T 98.8°F. A new exam is notable for an unsteady gait and a positive Romberg sign. A third set of vital signs show HR 36, BP 190/100, RR 8, and T 99.0°F. Which of the following is the most likely explanation for his rapidly changing condition?
    A. Thromboembolism leading to ischemic brain damage
    B. Ruptured artery leading to increased intracranial pressure
    C. Viral infection leading to widespread inflammation of the brain
    D. Epileptic activity leading to alteration of consciousness
    E. Autoimmune attack leading to central nervous system demyelination

23. A 70 y/o M with no past medical history presents to his primary care doctor after he was told by a friend that his walking was "abnormal" while golfing. On exam, his cranial nerves are all intact. There are no signs of weakness or sensory deficits in any of his extremities. No tremor or rigidity is seen. He is able to perform finger-to-nose, heel-to-shin, and rapid alternating movement testing. The patient's gait is slowed, and he finds himself needing to place his hand on the wall to steady himself. His performance on the MoCA, a cognitive screening test, shows no signs of mental decline. Labs are all within normal limits, and an MRI of the head shows no significant findings outside of some mild cerebral atrophy which is considered normal for his age. His primary care doctor is unable to arrive at a diagnosis and suggests monitoring his symptoms without treatment for now. Over the next 6 months, the patient's gait progressively worsens to the point where he cannot walk without a cane. He begins to have frequent urination including several episodes where he soils himself. He stops playing games with friends at his senior center as he finds himself confused and unable to remember the rules. He returns for his follow-up visit with his primary medical doctor with the results of a new MRI which shows only "enlargement of the ventricles consistent with cerebral volume loss." He asks his doctor, "What's happening to me? Am I dying?" Which of the following is the most appropriate response at this time?
    A. "This is a treatable condition. Let me prescribe you a new medication."
    B. "This is a treatable condition. Let me refer you to a neurosurgeon."
    C. "The disease you have is related to loss of neurons in the substantia nigra. It is slowly progressive, with no known cure."
    D. "You likely have a form of dementia. Medications may be able to help, although they cannot reverse the deficits you have already suffered."
    E. "You may have suffered a stroke in your cerebellum. The important thing now is to focus on preventing future strokes."

24. A 71 y/o F is brought to the hospital following an unwitnessed fall at her nursing home. On arrival to the emergency department, she appears lethargic but is able to follow commands. A CT scan is obtained showing an intracerebral bleed with subfalcine herniation as seen below:

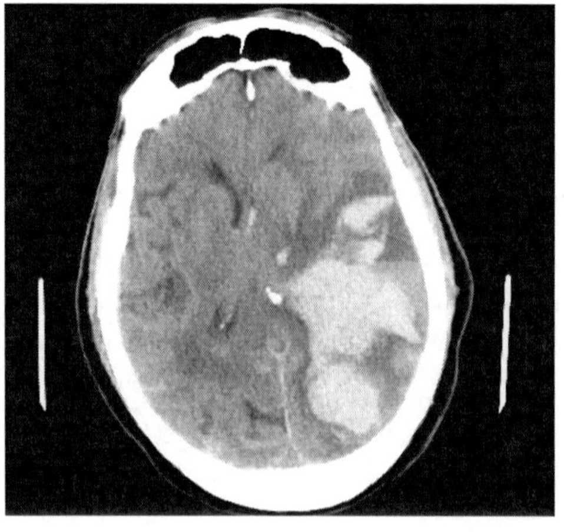

Which of the following is most likely to be seen secondary to arterial compression by herniation of the brain across the falx cerebri?

A. Weakness of the legs and urinary incontinence
B. Weakness of the arms and expressive aphasia
C. Contralateral homonymous hemianopsia with macular sparing
D. Unsteady wide-based gait
E. Full body weakness without sensory disturbance
F. Absent sensation in all extremities with full motor strength

25. A 42 y/o M is involved in a motor vehicle accident in which he was the driver. The right side of his head hit the steering wheel, resulting in a large bruise above his right ear. He did not lose consciousness but did report a headache and "dizzy" feelings for several minutes following the crash. In the emergency department, his pupils are equal and reactive. His right eye shows full range of movement, but his left eye is divergent as seen below:

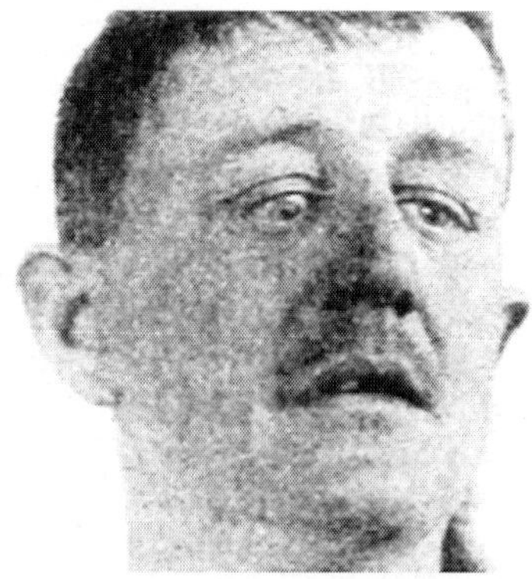

The affected cranial nerve exits from which part of the central nervous system?

A. Brain
B. Midbrain
C. Pons
D. Medulla oblongata
E. Cervical spine
F. None of the above

26. A 34 y/o M working in healthcare decides to become trained in administering injections of botulinum toxin. Which of the following patients is *not* likely to benefit from his training?

A. A 68 y/o F retiree with muscle spasticity following a stroke
B. A 19 y/o M college student with excessive underarm sweating
C. A 38 y/o F cartoonist with recurrent cramping of her right hand
D. A 55 y/o M lawyer with overactive bladder and occasional incontinence
E. A 13 y/o F student with inward misalignment of the eyes
F. All of these patients are likely to benefit from botulinum toxin injections

27. A 60 y/o F wakes up in the morning and notices "stiffness" on her right side. When she gets up to go to the bathroom, she feels that her gait is slow, and she finds that she needs to steady herself on the wall and nearby objects to avoid falling. Concerned, she calls an ambulance. On evaluation in the emergency department, she is fully alert and oriented. She reports no significant past medical history outside of hypertension. Vital signs are HR 90, BP 160/88, RR 16, and T 99.5°F. Her neurological exam is notable for limb rigidity on the right, cogwheeling in the right elbow, and a slow shuffling gait with forward leaning of her upper body. There are no motor or sensory deficits in the head or any of her extremities. Finger-to-nose testing and rapid alternating movements are both intact. Her MoCA cognitive screen is 30/30, although her writing is noticeably small. An MRI is ordered. An ischemic lesion is most likely to be seen in which of the following structures?

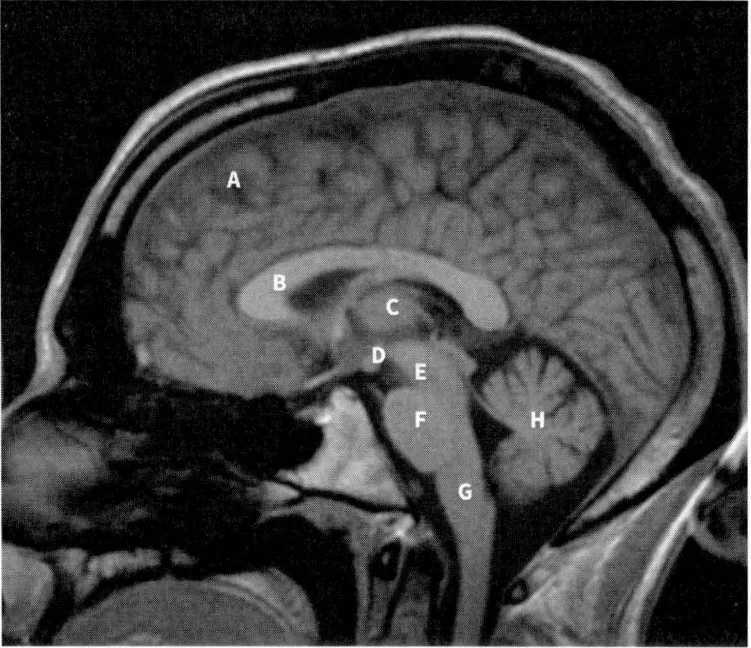

28. A 12 y/o M is brought to the emergency department after a witnessed generalized tonic-clonic seizure. His mother reports that he has been complaining of daily headaches and a tingling sensation in his hands for the past 2 weeks. On exam, there is limited abduction of the right eye and impaired hearing on the left. There is full motor strength throughout his body, with no sensory deficits. Finger-to-nose testing is impaired, though his gait is intact. Fundoscopic exam reveals bilateral swelling of the optic discs, prompting the doctor to order an MRI which is seen in the following image:

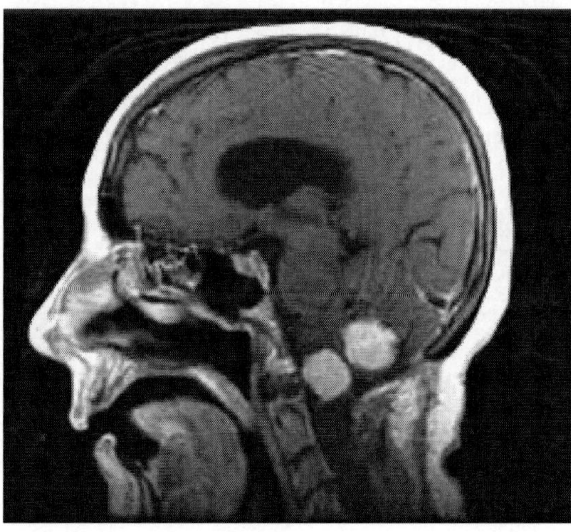

He is diagnosed with two tumors arising from the vascular system within the cerebellum and brainstem. Which of the following laboratory abnormalities is most likely to be seen on testing?

A. Elevated red blood cell count
B. Decreased white blood cell count
C. Elevated platelets
D. Decreased sodium
E. Elevated glucose
F. None of the above

29. (Continued from previous question.) He is sent for genetic testing which reveals an autosomal dominant genetic disorder involving a mutation in a tumor suppressor gene on chromosome 3. Based on these findings, he is at risk for developing all of the following *except*:

    A. Proliferation of capillaries in the retinas
    B. Neoplastic growth of cells lining the renal tubules
    C. Episodes of excess release of epinephrine and norepinephrine from the adrenal medulla
    D. Benign tumor of striated muscle in the heart
    E. All of the above are likely to be seen

30. A 64 y/o F presents to her primary care doctor complaining of weakness. She first noticed this 4 months ago when she began having difficulty getting up from her chair at night to go to bed. However, her weakness has progressed to the point where she has extreme difficulty climbing stairs or reaching for high objects in her kitchen cupboards. On exam, there is decreased motor strength in her shoulders, hips, and knees bilaterally, with preservation of the muscles of the hands and feet. Her exam is also notable for skin atrophy with punctate red dots over her joints on the backs of her fingers as seen in the following image:

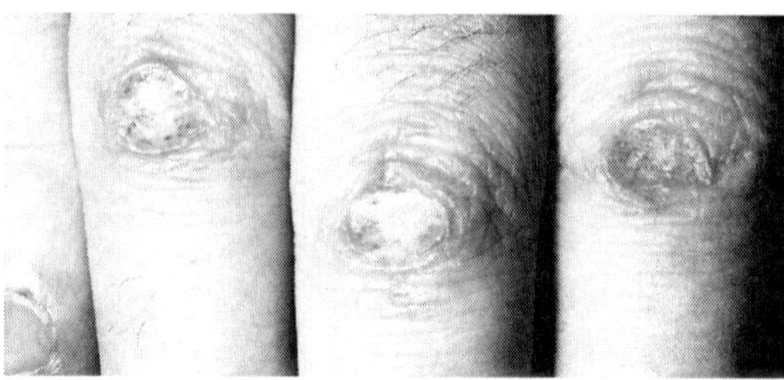

Which of the following is most likely to be seen on further investigation?

A. Fatiguing pattern on repetitive nerve stimulation testing
B. Mononuclear white blood cells between muscle cells on biopsy
C. Oligoclonal bands in cerebrospinal fluid on lumbar puncture
D. Decreased creatine kinase concentration on laboratory testing
E. Scarring of the internal capsule on magnetic resonance imaging
F. None of the above

31. A 38 y/o F presents to the emergency department complaining of headache and chills for the past several months. Around 6 months ago she had "the flu" for several weeks which resolved on its own. She has a history of opioid dependence and has scars on her arm suggestive of intravenous drug use. Vital signs are HR 78, BP 140/92, RR 16, and T 101.3°F. Her exam is notable for drooping of her right eyelid as well as weakness of her left arm and leg. An MRI with contrast is ordered which reveals a ring-enhancing lesion as seen below:

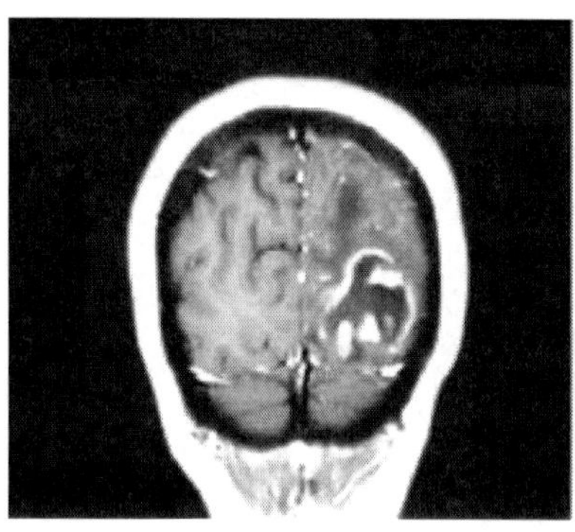

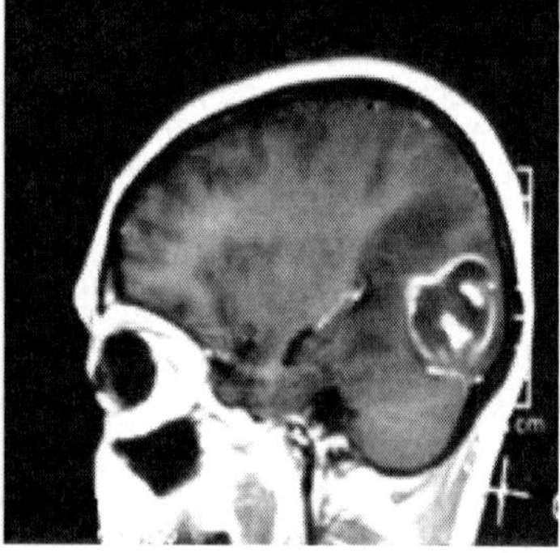

Serological testing is positive for antibodies against *Toxoplasma gondii*. Which of the following most likely accounts for the patient's presentation?

A. Recent change in immune system function
B. Exposure to cat feces
C. Handling of undercooked meat
D. Undetected pregnancy
E. Transmission through intravenous injection
F. None of the above

32. A 70 y/o M is brought to the emergency department by his wife after he was found looking confused while at the bank. His wife was waiting in the car while the patient went to withdraw money from the ATM. However, when the patient did not return for 15 minutes, his wife went to go see what was taking so long. When his wife found him, he was staring at the computer screen on the ATM and appeared frustrated and confused about what was happening. The patient denies other symptoms. He has a past medical history of hypertension, hyperlipidemia, and atrial fibrillation. His neurological exam is notable for right homonymous hemianopsia. There are no deficits in either motor or sensory function. His gait is steady. Testing of his speech reveals intact expression, comprehension, and repetition. While undergoing brief cognitive testing, the patient is unable to follow instructions that are handed to him on a piece of paper. He is able to write a sentence when asked, although he is then unable to read that same sentence aloud. An MR angiogram is most likely to reveal ischemic damage in the territory of which artery?

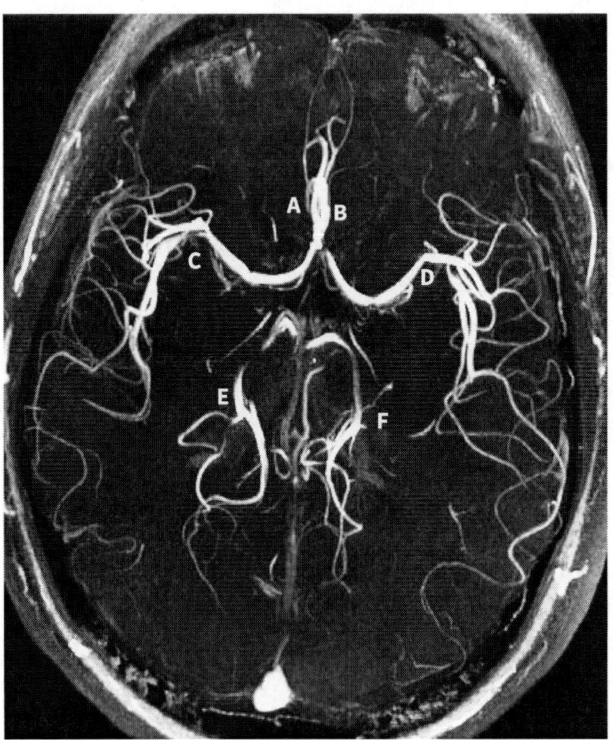

33. A 71 y/o F with a history of osteoporosis falls during a game of tennis and is brought to an urgent care clinic. She undergoes a full examination which reveals no neurologic deficits. She is diagnosed with a compression fracture and discharged home. At a follow-up appointment 2 weeks later, she complains of severe pain in her neck and upper back. Examination continues to reveal no focal neurologic deficits. She is scheduled for vertebral augmentation surgery to relieve her pain. After the operation, she awakens to find that she is unable to move the muscles in her lower limbs, though motor strength in her upper limbs is preserved. Further testing reveals a loss of pain and temperature sensation in the lower limbs, though both vibration and proprioception are intact. Her deep tendon reflexes are intact in the upper extremities, with hyporeflexia in the patellar joints and areflexia in the ankle joints bilaterally. Which of the following best explains the patient's post-operative findings?
    A. Hypotensive ischemia in the basal ganglia
    B. Surgical injury of the posterior spinal cord
    C. Ischemia of the anterior spinal artery
    D. Unilateral hemorrhage in the lateral spinal cord
    E. Compression of spinal nerve roots
    F. None of the above

34. A 55 y/o M presents to the hospital with weakness of his right arm and leg. He first noticed this one month ago but did not seek care until today. He notes that the weakness has worsened over time to the point where he has difficulty raising his right arm and leg against gravity. A CT scan in the emergency department reveals the following:

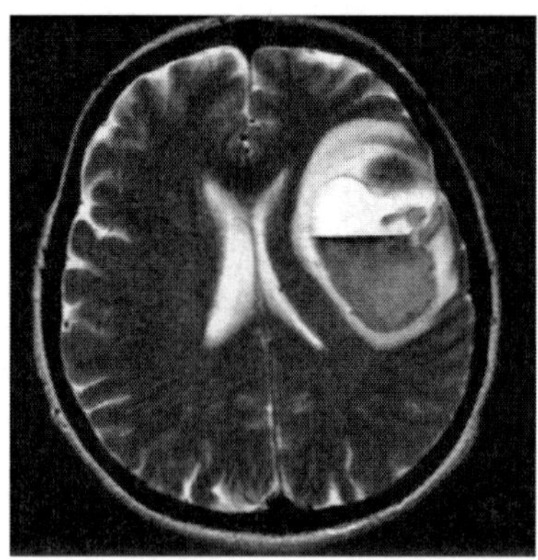

A diagnosis of a brain metastasis is made. Which of the following is *least* likely to be the source organ in this case?
    A. Breast
    B. Colon
    C. Kidney
    D. Lung
    E. Skin
    F. Stomach

35. (Continued from previous question.) The patient is admitted to the hospital. When the doctor informs him of the poor prognosis for his diagnosis, he does not react with any emotion. Later, when his nurse asks him, "How are you holding up with the news?" he responds by saying, "What news?" He is later seen attempting to eat the remote control to his television. The next morning, the nurse comes in the room and finds him masturbating. She shrieks and runs out, but he continues his behavior as though nothing had happened. His current presentation is most consistent with damage to which of the following structures?
    A. Anterior cingulate cortex
    B. Thalamus
    C. Amygdala
    D. Paraventricular hypothalamic nucleus
    E. Subthalamic nucleus
    F. Mammillary bodies
    G. Hippocampus

36. A 25 y/o F is brought to the hospital after becoming non-responsive following a chiropractic treatment earlier in the day. She presented for her treatment in the morning and then went to work immediately after. Upon arriving to work, she appeared confused and dizzy. An ambulance was called after she stumbled and passed out on her way to the bathroom. In the emergency department, she is alert but appears puzzled. She remains unsteady in her gait. Cerebellar testing reveals an inability to perform finger-to-nose, heel-to-shin, and rapid alternating movement testing on the left side. MRI reveals an acute infarction in the territory of the left posterior inferior cerebellar artery. Which of the following findings is *least* likely to be seen in this patient?
    A. Deficits in pain and temperature sensation in the right limbs
    B. Deficits in pain and temperature sensation in the left face
    C. Absent gag reflex
    D. Difficulty swallowing
    E. Drooping eyelid on the left
    F. All of the above are likely to be seen

37. A 16 y/o F is brought to see her pediatrician for a recent change in her personality. Previously she was a bright and engaged student, but for the past several months she has appeared very tired and has been failing her schoolwork. She is a talented softball player, but over the past month she has been benched due to poor performance. On exam, there is a mild but noticeable tremor in both hands that increases in intensity during active motion. Her gait is slowed but steady. Her facial expression appears "frozen" to the doctor, and her speech is monotone. Examination of her eyes reveals decreased visual acuity and bilateral cataracts as seen in the following image:

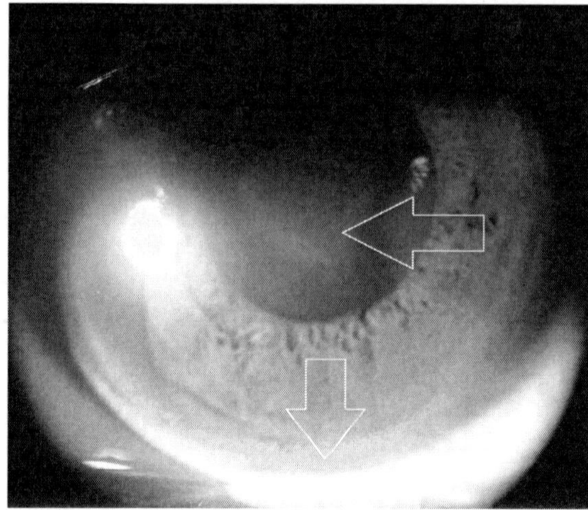

Which of the following statements is most appropriate to make to her parents at this time?

A. "This is normal behavior for her age. Don't worry about it too much."
B. "This is a treatable condition. Let me give you a prescription and a referral for a dietician."
C. "This is a treatable condition. Let me give you a prescription and a referral for a psychiatrist."
D. "This is a treatable condition. Let me give you a prescription and a referral for a transplant surgeon."
E. "This is an untreatable condition, but we can do our best to manage it with physical and occupational therapy."
F. "This is an untreatable condition, and it will likely only get worse from now on."

38. A 40 y/o F comes to her nurse practitioner complaining of right arm weakness and pain for the past month. The pain is localized primarily in the right forearm on the radial side but radiates into her hand as well. There is also a "tingling" sensation in the same distribution. She reports difficulty with movements in her right hand, saying, "I can't open jars anymore." On exam, there is diffuse numbness in the right thumb, index finger, and middle finger. Grip strength is reduced in the right hand compared to the left, with flaccid paralysis of the involved muscles. Hyporeflexia of the biceps reflex is appreciated on the right. On further exam, there is hyperreflexia in the patellar and ankle jerk reflexes on the right, with spasticity in the calf and ankle flexors. Which of the following explanations best accounts for these findings?

A. Demyelinated plaques in the left primary motor cortex
B. Ischemic damage to the posterior limb of the internal capsule
C. Whiplash injury at the level of the pyramidal decussation
D. Compressive arthritis in the cervical spine
E. Infectious damage to the anterior horn of the spinal cord
F. None of the above

39. A 45 y/o M is brought to a publicly funded hospital after he was found wandering on a hot desert road. On initial evaluation in the emergency department, he appears confused and does not know his name, though he is able to follow simple commands. His physical exam is notable for enlarged cervical and inguinal lymph nodes as well as a healed ulcer on his penis. The venereal disease research laboratory (VDRL) and rapid plasma reagin (RPR) tests, which evaluate for the presence of syphilis, are both positive. Which of the following findings is *least* likely be found on exam?
    A. Pupil constriction in response to light
    B. Pupil constriction in response to a nearby object
    C. Impaired vibration and proprioceptive sensation
    D. Poor performance on cognitive testing
    E. None of the above are likely to be found

40. A 47 y/o F presents for follow-up with her neurologist. She was diagnosed with amyotrophic lateral sclerosis a year ago after she began having weakness in her legs. The diagnosis was frustrating to her, but it did not come as a surprise as she had two immediate family members who were also diagnosed with the disease. She is now reliant on a wheelchair for mobility. Since her last appointment one month ago, she has developed new swinging movements of her arms that occur constantly. She maintains that these movements are involuntary, saying through a weak voice, "Sometimes I feel like one of those flailing tube men they have outside of car dealerships." Cognitive testing is performed and is within normal limits. What is the most likely explanation for her new movements?
    A. Neuronal loss in the subthalamus
    B. Upper motor neuron degeneration in the anterior horns
    C. Epileptiform activity in the primary motor cortex
    D. Exposure to dopamine-blocking medications
    E. Physician misdiagnosis of amyotrophic lateral sclerosis
    F. Patient misrepresentation of voluntary movements
    G. None of the above

41. A 16 y/o F is brought to the hospital by her caregiver after she was seen having a generalized tonic-clonic seizure. She was born to parents belonging to a religious group that forbid contact with the government or health care providers, so her medical history is unknown. When her parents died 2 weeks ago, she became a ward of the state. She is currently living in a group home and was there when the seizure occurred. On interview, the patient appears to have difficulty producing verbal responses to questions asked. The caregiver provides results of recent testing showing her IQ to be in the range of severe intellectual disability. Her exam is notable for small growths on her cheeks extending onto her nose and her forehead as seen in the following image:

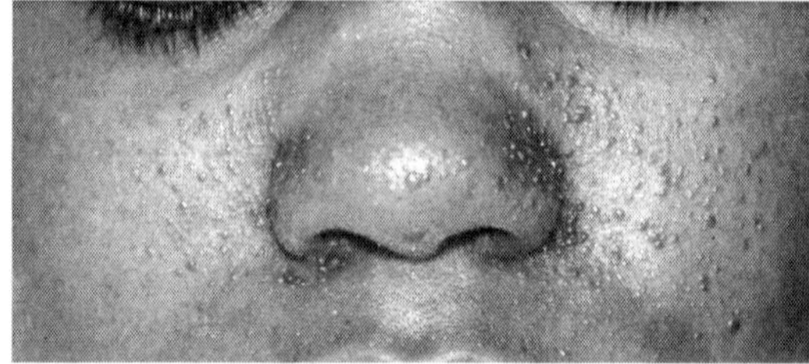

Which of the following is *least* likely to be of value in this patient's care?

A. Starting an anticonvulsant
B. Obtaining an MRI of the brain
C. Drawing blood to evaluate renal function
D. Arranging for electroencephalography
E. Ordering an echocardiogram
F. All of the above are likely to be of value

42. A 25 y/o M with no prior medical history presents to a primary care doctor with a 6 month history of a "ringing" sound in his ears and a sense that he cannot hear things as well as he used to. He works as a DJ and has played several parties each week for the past few years without ear protection. A Weber test reveals equal sound intensity in both ears, while a Rinne test reveals air conduction greater than bone conduction in both ears. His gait is unsteady. A Romberg test is positive. The remainder of his neurological exam is normal, with no motor or sensory deficits. An MRI is ordered which reveals the following:

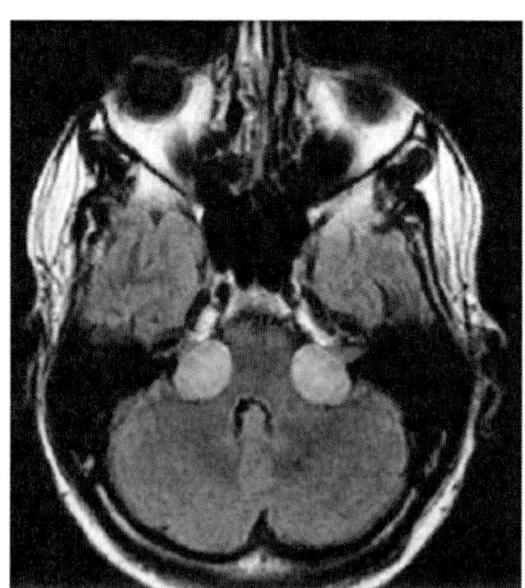

Which of the following is the most likely cause of this patient's presentation?

A. Physiological hearing loss due to aging
B. Sensorineural hearing loss due to latent infection
C. Conductive hearing loss due to ear canal occlusion
D. Progressive hearing loss due to a genetic mutation
E. Environmental hearing loss due to loud noise exposure
F. None of the above

43. A 7 y/o F is brought to the hospital following a "fit." The patient was sleeping in her bed when her mother heard "choking noises" from outside the door. Upon entering the room, the mother saw the patient's face twisting and contorting repeatedly. The patient's entire body then became stiff for several seconds followed by a period of shaking lasting approximately 2 minutes. The episode had ended by the time the patient arrived in the emergency department. Her neurological exam shows no focal abnormalities. Vital signs are entirely within normal limits. A 24-hour EEG reveals centrotemporal spikes during sleep. The mother is worried about her daughter and wants to know what will happen next. Which of the following is the most appropriate statement to make?
    A. "This seizure occurred as the result of neuronal damage in the brain. As long as the damage is there, she will be at risk of further seizures."
    B. "This seizure is the result of a brain tumor. The prognosis is good, but we need to operate right away."
    C. "There's nothing to be worried about. This condition tends to get better even without treatment. This may be the last seizure she'll ever have."
    D. "Unfortunately this condition does not just involve seizures. She is at high risk of developing an intellectual disability."
    E. "This was not a seizure. I think your daughter may be trying to get your attention."
    F. None of the above

44. A 77 y/o F comes to the emergency department complaining of repeated attacks of sharp pain in her head behind her right eye. She denies a history of any recent head trauma. On exam, there is noticeable drooping of her right upper eyelid, with a downward and outward displacement of her right eye. Her right pupil is dilated compared to the left. The rest of her neurological exam is normal, with intact motor strength, sensation, and coordination throughout. CT angiography is ordered which shows the following:

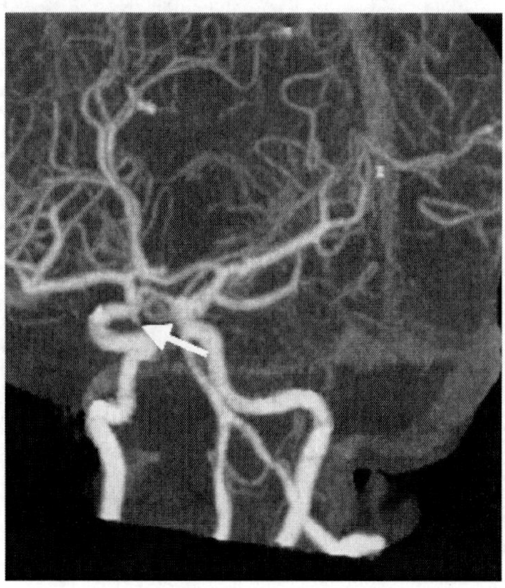

A focal outpouching in which of the following blood vessels is most likely responsible for her presenting signs and symptoms?

A. Anterior communicating artery
B. Left anterior cerebral artery
C. Right anterior cerebral artery
D. Left middle cerebral artery
E. Right middle cerebral artery
F. Left posterior cerebral artery
G. Right posterior cerebral artery
H. Left posterior communicating artery
I. Right posterior communicating artery
J. None of the above

45. (Continued from previous question.) While in the emergency department, the patient suddenly cries out. She reports the onset of a "10 out of 10" headache located "all over my head." She develops nausea and vomiting several minutes later. Her mental status is unchanged, as she remains fully oriented and able to follow verbal commands. A repeat CT scan is most likely to show which of the following images?

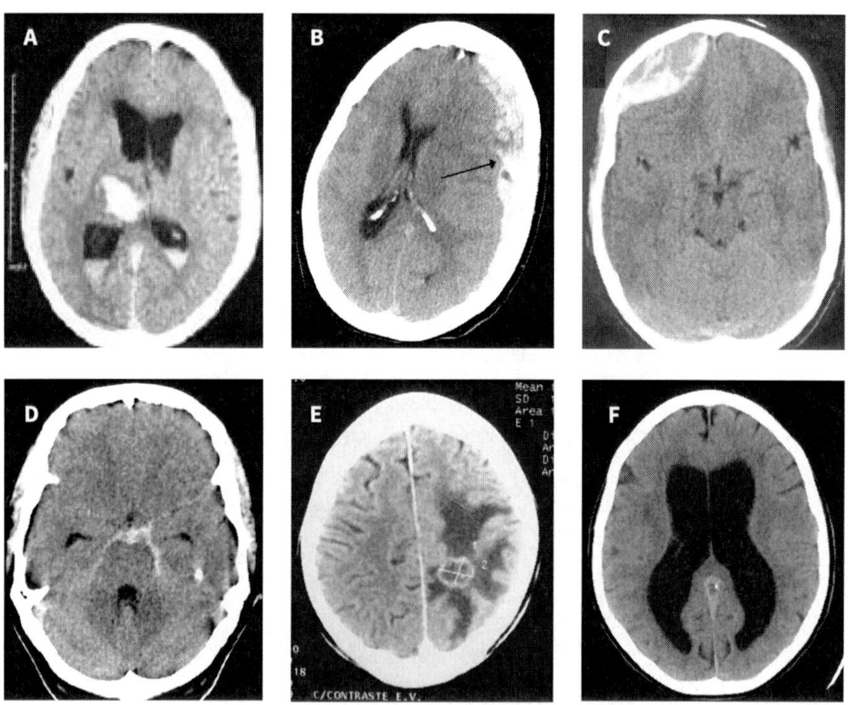

46. A 22 y/o F comes to the student health clinic reporting headaches of increasing intensity, duration, and frequency over the past 3 months to the point where they are near constant. She has also had difficulty sleeping over the past month and feels that she is not tired at night but then "super tired during the day." The nurse at the clinic is concerned and refers her for urgent neurological evaluation. At her appointment with the neurologist one week later, she reports a recent onset of blurry vision and severe nausea. She is not certain whether the blurry vision and nausea are related to her headaches. Neurological exam is notable for downward trending eyes with weakness of upward gaze. A CT scan reveals asymmetric expansion of the ventricles and a well-circumscribed lesion as seen in the following image:

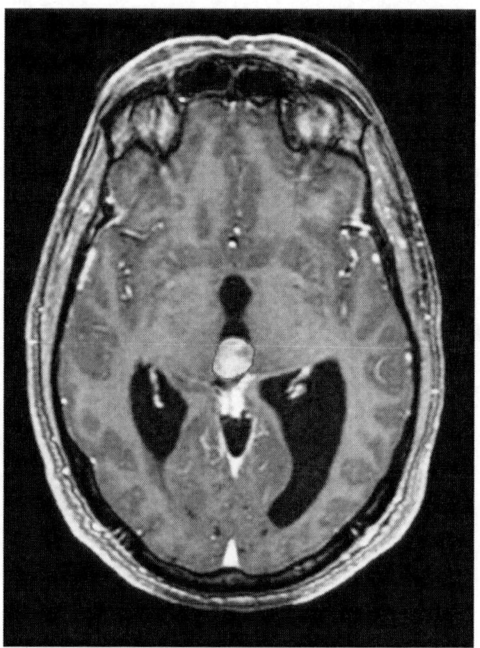

Which of the following best explains her presentation?

A. Autoimmune-mediated inflammation of the optic nerve
B. Toxin-related dysfunction of the oculomotor nerves bilaterally
C. Abducens nerve palsy due to compression at the level of the pons
D. Trochlear nerve ischemia due to arterial narrowing
E. Central herniation of the cerebrum through the tentorium cerebelli
F. Dysfunction of the epithalamus due to unregulated cell growth
G. Focal plaques of demyelination in the central nervous system
H. Atrophy of the suprachiasmatic nucleus in the hypothalamus
I. None of the above

47. A 57 y/o right-handed F with a history of diabetes and hyperlipidemia experiences a sudden sensation of coldness in the left half of her body "almost like someone turned me on my side and dipped me into the ocean." She notes that her left side is numb as well, as she is unable to feel her clothes. She is able to perceive some sensation with vigorous rubbing of her hand against her left arm and leg, but even then the sensation feels "distant." After several hours without a change in status, she calls 911. In the emergency department, she is alert and fully oriented. Her vital signs are HR 102, BP 176/98, RR 18, and T 98.9°F. She reports that the feeling of coldness now feels like "burning." Her neurological exam is notable for absent touch and pinprick sensation in the left face, arm, and leg. Her motor strength, reflexes, and gait are all normal. Which of the following mechanisms best accounts for this patient's presentation?
    A. Occlusion of the right middle cerebral artery
    B. Ischemic stroke in the right thalamus
    C. Infarction of the spinothalamic tract at the level of the medulla
    D. Damage to the right cervical spinal cord
    E. Narrowing of the posterior spinal artery
    F. None of the above

48. A 43 y/o F goes to the emergency department for evaluation of double vision. She reports that for the past 9 months she has had intermittent episodes of her vision losing focus which seem to happen most often when reading, saying, "It's like there's a ghost of each letter lurking just behind it." She previously had perfect vision. Attempts at using corrective eyeglasses to fix the problem have not been helpful. A head CT in the emergency department shows no focal abnormalities. After further workup is unrevealing, she is discharged with an outpatient referral to see a neurologist. By the time of her appointment 2 weeks later, her vision has improved. On interview, she notes that this is the general pattern, saying, "My visual stuff comes and goes like it has a mind of its own." However, she does report fatigue over the same time period that is persistent rather than episodic. Her fatigue increases throughout the day to the point where even sitting upright to work on her computer in the evening is a struggle. Which of the following is *least* likely to be helpful at finding the cause of this patient's symptoms?
    A. Laboratory testing of blood
    B. Lumbar puncture
    C. Computed tomography
    D. Magnetic resonance imaging
    E. Electromyography
    F. Full neurological exam

49. (Continued from previous question.) The patient is sent for various tests, with a plan to return in 2 weeks. However, 5 days later she is admitted to the hospital for difficulty breathing. Vital signs are HR 102, BP 138/84, RR 24, T 99.6°F, and decreased oxygen saturation at 85%. She is intubated and put on ventilation. Meanwhile, the treatment team reviews her chart. A recent MRI showed no focal abnormalities, while repetitive nerve stimulation showed a fatiguing pattern. Which of the following treatments should be administered at this time?

A. A short course of oral corticosteroids
B. An inhibitor of the enzyme responsible for metabolizing acetylcholine
C. A drug with a molecular resemblance to myelin basic protein
D. An antidote against the offending bacterial toxin
E. A mixture of donated antibodies from healthy volunteers
F. None of the above

50. A 10 y/o is brought to the hospital with signs and symptoms of meningitis. An emergent lumbar puncture is performed. Fifteen minutes after the procedure, the patient's mental status suddenly deteriorates, and he becomes comatose. Repeat vital signs are HR 44, BP 160/90, RR 14, and T 102.3°F. Exam reveals fixed dilated pupils bilaterally and decerebrate posturing in his extremities. Corneal and gag reflexes are absent. The patient is quickly intubated. Imaging reveals bilateral downward displacement of the cerebellar tonsils. Which of the following is most likely to have prevented this outcome?
    A. Proper sterile technique prior to needle insertion
    B. Earlier radiographic imaging of the head
    C. Rapid administration of tissue plasminogen activator
    D. Surgical removal of the blood clot under the dura mater
    E. Strict blood pressure control
    F. None of the above could have prevented this outcome

51. A 38 y/o F who is 39-weeks pregnant desires to give birth at home. During her delivery, she is seen losing large amounts of blood. Concerned, her husband drives her to the hospital where she receives several liters of transfused blood. She is discharged home the next day after her vital signs stabilize. One week later, while caring for her infant, she suddenly feels faint and collapses. She is brought back to the hospital and resuscitated. Magnetic resonance imaging of her brain reveals an abnormal signal in the pituitary gland suggestive of ischemic damage. Which of the following findings is *least* likely to be seen in this patient?
    A. Lack of milk production
    B. Low blood sugar
    C. Lack of urination
    D. Hypothyroidism
    E. Lack of a feeling of bonding with her child

52. A 45 y/o F is out walking in the woods with her dog when she notices a tick on her leg. She quickly brushes it off of her leg. Three weeks later, she presents to an urgent care clinic reporting a severe headache, fevers, and excessive thirst. Vital signs are normal except for a temperature of 102.7°F. During the exam, a rash is discovered on her leg as seen below:

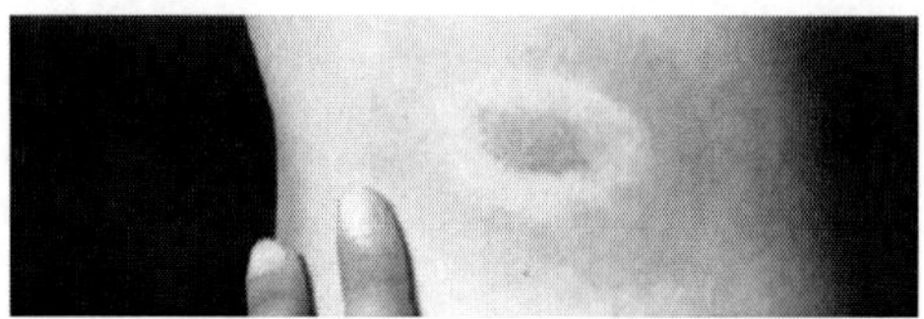

Which of the following is *least* likely to be found in patients with this condition?

A. Severe joint pain in multiple joints
B. Cardiac conduction abnormalities on EKG
C. Pain with neck flexion
D. "Electrical" pain running down her legs
E. Lopsided weakness of the muscles of facial expression
F. All of the above are likely to be found

53. A 42 y/o M sees his nurse practitioner after developing right ear pain, headache, and fever over the past 2 days. He is diagnosed as having an infection of the middle ear and is prescribed antibiotics. Within several hours of taking the medication, he feels better. However, 3 days later, he begins feeling feverish and confused. His husband rushes him to the hospital after he is unable to say his own name. Vital signs in the emergency department are HR 108, BP 142/84, RR 20, and T 102.9°F. His exam is notable for a bulging left eye as seen below:

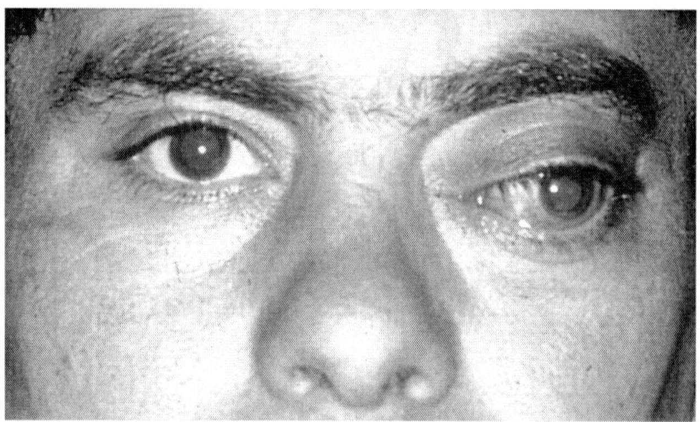

There are unilateral deficits in visual acuity and pupillary response on the left. A CT scan with contrast reveals irregular vascular filling within the cavernous sinus with engorgement of several nearby veins. Which of the following findings is *least* likely to be seen on exam?

A. Inability to move the left eye towards the nose
B. Inability to move the left eye towards the ear
C. Inability to move the left eye towards the forehead
D. Inability to move the left eye towards the chin
E. Sensory loss over the forehead
F. Sensory loss over the cheeks
G. Sensory loss over the jaw
H. All of the above are likely to be seen

1. **The best answer is I.** This vignette describes a case of subacute sclerosing panencephalitis, a devastating condition that affects some people who were infected by measles earlier in life. The patient's earlier medical history is unknown, though earlier in life she lived in an area where the prevalence of measles was significantly higher than in the United States. Subacute sclerosing panencephalitis often presents as changes in cognition and personality, with subsequent development of focal neurologic signs including myoclonic jerks and atonic seizures. The diagnosis could likely be confirmed by testing for the presence of anti-measles antibodies. Meningitis and/or encephalitis are unlikely given the patient's normal vital signs and lack of cerebrospinal fluid findings (answers A—C). While the patient is presenting with myoclonic and atonic seizures, an epilepsy syndrome is unlikely as seizures alone cannot explain the presence of personality changes, cognitive decline, and lesions on neuroimaging (answers D—F). A brain tumor would likely be seen on MRI and is more likely to be found in an infratentorial location in a child (answer G). Acute disseminated encephalomyelitis tends to occur weeks after an infection, not years as in subacute sclerosing panencephalitis, and would present with central nervous system demyelination (answer H). *(Chapter 23—Viral Encephalitis and Chapter 25—Central Demyelinating Diseases)*

2. **The best answer is B.** This vignette describes a case of a subdural hematoma which is consistent with the history of head trauma, subacute onset of symptoms, and progressive nature of symptoms including headache and nausea. A subdural hematoma often presents as a crescent-shaped strip of blood between the brain and the skull on CT. Epidural hematomas can present similarly but are often much faster in their progression and tend to involve an immediate loss of consciousness (answer C). Subarachnoid hemorrhages tend to involve a sudden "thunderclap" headache and neck irritation (answer D). Signs and symptoms of an intracerebral hemorrhage tend to come on much more quickly as well (answer A). The clinical history here is not suggestive of either a brain tumor (answer E) or hydrocephalus (answer F). *(Chapter 15—Intracranial Bleeds)*

3. **The best answer is B.** An expansion of the trinucleotide repeat sequence GAA on chromosome 9 is associated with Friedreich's ataxia. Huntington's disease is associated with the repeat sequence CAG (answer C), while myotonic dystrophy is instead associated with the repeat sequence CTG (answer E). Spinal muscular atrophy (answer A), neurofibromatosis type 1 (answer D), and amyotrophic lateral sclerosis (answer F) are all genetic diseases, but none of them are associated with trinucleotide repeat sequences. *(Chapter 24—Diseases Associated with Peripheral Neuropathy, Chapter 19—Huntington's Disease, Chapter 16—Muscular Dystrophies, Chapter 18—Motor Neuron Diseases, and Chapter 27—Neurocutaneous Disorders)*

4. **The best answer is N.** This vignette describes a case of right medial medullary syndrome which is most often related to a stroke in the anterior spinal artery. We can determine the location of this stroke in the medulla by looking at what cranial nerves are involved. The presence of tongue deviation implicates the 12th cranial nerve which exits the brainstem at the level of the medulla, while the presence of intact extraocular movements argues against either midbrain or pons involvement as the 3rd, 4th, and 6th cranial nerves exit from these two regions. To determine whether the lesion is medial or lateral, consider the presence of both motor weakness and loss of epicritic sensation. This shows that the corticospinal tract and medial lemniscus, both of which travel medially in the medulla, are involved. Notably, protopathic sensation is intact, arguing against a lateral medullary syndrome which tends to be involved in a stroke in the posterior inferior cerebellar artery (answers J and K). The presence of cranial nerve involvement localizes the lesion to the brainstem, arguing against a stroke in the anterior, middle, or posterior cerebral arteries (answers A—F). Strokes in the region of the vertebral and basilar arteries more often present with cerebellar signs (answers G, L, and M). Anterior inferior cerebellar artery strokes are more associated with lateral pontine syndrome which would present with facial weakness and/or asymmetry (answers H and I). *(Chapter 14—Brainstem Strokes)*

5. **The best answer is B.** Idiopathic intracranial hypertension often presents with headache and visual abnormalities in an obese but otherwise healthy young woman. Papilledema is classically seen on fundoscopic exam. The first step in management is often a lumbar puncture which not only helps to confirm the diagnosis but also provides immediate relief of symptoms by rapidly reducing the intracranial pressure. This case is unlikely to be a primary headache such as a tension headache, cluster headache, or migraine given the presence of papilledema and focal neurologic deficits, so treatments like nonsteroidal anti-inflammatory drugs, oxygen, or triptans will likely not be effective (answers C, E, and G). The MRI showed no evidence of a tumor, so neurosurgical resection is not necessary (answer D). The patient is afebrile and shows no other signs of bacterial infection (answer F). Steroids would help if this were a case of giant-cell arteritis, but the patient's presenting symptoms and demographics make this unlikely (answer A). *(Chapter 26—Diseases Associated with Headaches)*

6. **The best answer is D.** This vignette describes a prototypical case of essential tremor as evidenced by the presence of an intention tremor that improves with alcohol with onset in a young person. Essential tremor is often a clinical diagnosis, and in the absence of any other neurologic signs, neuroimaging is not required to rule out other potential causes of tremor such as Parkinson's disease (answers B and C). Essential tremor does appear to run in families with an autosomal dominant pattern, but a specific gene has not been identified (answer A). Initial management of essential tremor often involves prescribing a beta-blocker. Botulinum toxin is generally used for focal dystonias and is rarely used for treatment of essential tremor unless if multiple other treatments have been ineffective (answer E). Electromyography is unlikely to reveal any abnormalities in the absence of motor or sensory deficits (answer F). *(Chapter 19—Tremor)*

7. **The best answer is E.** A vesicular rash in a dermatomal distribution is classic for shingles, an infectious disease caused by the varicella zoster virus. Knowing your dermatomal landmarks is essential for localizing the infection to a specific spinal nerve root. Two important landmarks on the torso are the nipples at T4 and the belly button at T10. As this patient's infection is between these two, T7 is the best answer. *(Chapter 9—Spinal Nerves and Chapter 24—Diseases Associated with Peripheral Neuropathy)*

8. **The best answer is M.** Postictal paralysis, also known as Todd's paralysis, is known to affect around 10% of all patients following a generalized tonic-clonic seizure. In a young patient with no significant medical history presenting with focal neurologic deficits immediately after a seizure, there is little reason to suspect a concurrent stroke, as no additional pathology is necessary to explain these findings (answers A—L). *(Chapter 20—Generalized Seizures)*

9. **The best answer is G.** This vignette describes a case of Anton's syndrome, a condition in which someone experiences blindness but does not admit to this and will even confabulate to fill in for the missing sensory input. Anton's syndrome is associated with injury to the primary visual cortex in the occipital lobe. The presence of an intact pupillary light reflex bilaterally rules out any injury to more anterior portions of the visual pathway, as does the loss of visual acuity in all quadrants rather than a hemianopsia or quadrantanopsia (answers A–F). The medial longitudinal fasciculus, paramedian pontine reticular formation, and Edinger-Westphal nuclei are all involved in control over extraocular muscles, not visual acuity (answers H–J). *(Chapter 3—The Four Lobes of the Brain and Chapter 10—The Visual Pathway)*

10. **The best answer is D.** This patient is suffering from an expressive aphasia, also known as Broca's aphasia, as evidenced by her inability to speak or write despite intact language comprehension. Expressive aphasias are most often related to damage in Broca's area which lies in the frontal lobe of the dominant hemisphere in an area supplied by the middle cerebral artery. As the patient is right-handed, it is most likely that her dominant lobe is on the left, not the right (answer C). The anterior and posterior cerebral arteries do not supply Broca's area (answers A, B, E, and F). *(Chapter 3—Language Centers and Chapter 14—Cortical Strokes)*

11. **The best answer is C.** Dopamine is a neurotransmitter that is involved in a variety of processes in the brain. It is highly involved in modulating movements in the basal ganglia, so someone taking a dopamine-blocking medication is likely to experience increased muscular rigidity and difficulty initiating movements as a result of its effects here (answers A and B). Dopamine is involved in goal-directed behavior through its action in the ventral tegmental area (answer D). Finally, dopamine is involved in prolactin production, but its effect here is to *decrease* the release of prolactin, so someone taking a dopamine-blocking medication would instead see *increased* production of prolactin as a result. *(Chapter 4—The Pituitary Gland, Chapter 5—The Basal Ganglia, Chapter 7—The Midbrain, and Chapter 19—Parkinsonism)*

12. **The best answer is E.** Craniopharyngiomas often present with bitemporal hemianopsia due to their typical location above the optic chiasm. Other features of this patient's presentation are related to dysfunction of the pituitary gland itself, as decreased levels of growth hormone and vasopressin can lead to growth restriction and diabetes insipidus, respectively. The MRI shows the characteristic location of the tumor in the brain. Craniopharyngiomas represent neoplastic growth of Rathke's pouch, which is the embryonic precursor of the anterior pituitary gland. Pilocytic astrocytomas (answer A), medulloblastomas (answer B), ependymomas (answer C), and hemangioblastomas (answer D) all have different presentations. *(Chapter 21—Pediatric Brain Tumors and Chapter 4—The Pituitary Gland)*

13. **The best answer is G.** Cases of severe obesity have been documented following treatment for a craniopharyngioma, as surgery and radiation can damage nearby structures such as the hypothalamus. In particular, damage to the ventromedial hypothalamic nucleus, which normally responds to the presence of leptin by inducing a state of satiety and reducing food intake, can lead to dramatic increases in food intake. In contrast, the lateral hypothalamic nucleus produces feelings of hunger, so damage here would likely *decrease* food intake, not increase it (answer F). The thalamus is involved in processing sensory information and does not play a large role in appetite (answers A—D). The anterior hypothalamic nucleus is involved in thermoregulation and autonomic regulation (answer E), the suprachiasmatic nucleus is involved in the circadian rhythm (answer H), the supraoptic nucleus produces vasopressin (answer I), and finally the paraventricular nucleus produces oxytocin (answer J). *(Chapter 4—The Hypothalamus)*

14. **The best answer is A.** Hyperglycemia related to diabetes mellitus is the most common cause of oculomotor nerve palsy in adults. This classically presents as an acute onset of diplopia and unilateral ptosis. Because the oculomotor nerve controls 4 of the 6 extraocular muscles, the actions of the unopposed lateral rectus and superior oblique muscles lead to a characteristic "down and out" deviation of the affected eye as seen in this image. While muscles controlling pupil size travel on the oculomotor nerve, these are typically spared in cases of oculomotor nerve palsy related to diabetes mellitus. There is no evidence in this vignette suggestive of either trochlear or abducens nerve involvement (answers B—G). *(Chapter 10—Organization of the Oculomotor Nerve)*

15. **The best answer is A.** We have not talked about acute cerebellar ataxia directly, so this question is more about ruling out the other causes than your knowledge of this condition in particular. Acute cerebellar ataxia is an inflammatory central nervous system disease involving a rapid onset of ataxia with subsequent recovery. It is most often seen in young children following a viral illness. Most patients recover within several weeks without long-lasting deficits, so the goal here is to rule out any other explanations that would require more intensive treatment. Acute cerebellar ataxia is frequently confused for acute disseminated encephalomyelitis, as both are post-infectious inflammatory diseases. However,

acute disseminated encephalomyelitis tends to present with focal neurologic findings as well as abnormalities on brain imaging (answer B). Subacute sclerosing panencephalitis is also post-infectious and may involve ataxia, but it is generally characterized by a much more dramatic presentation, including behavioral abnormalities, changes in mental status, seizures, loss of vision, and progressive cognitive decline (answer C). Encephalitis and meningitis are both less likely given the patient's normal vital signs, lack of focal neurologic findings, and stable mental status (answers D and E). Guillain–Barré syndrome is tempting as it is also post-infectious, but this would specifically involve findings in the peripheral nervous system such as motor weakness or sensory abnormalities (answer F). Multiple sclerosis is highly unlikely in a young child and should not be diagnosed based on a single episode given the requirement for dissemination in both space and time (answer G). Hydrocephalus would be observable on brain imaging (answer H). Finally, atonic seizures would present with loss of consciousness which was not present in this patient (answer I). *(Chapter 6—Cerebellar Signs, Chapter 15—Hydrocephalus, Chapter 20—Generalized Seizures, Chapter 23—Viral Encephalitis, and Chapter 25—Multiple Sections)*

16. **The best answer is C.** A neonate presenting with generalized muscle rigidity and an opisthotonus position is concerning for either tetanus or meningitis. In this case, the lack of fever or bulging fontanelles makes meningitis less likely (answers A and B). The tetanus toxin blocks the release of inhibitory neurotransmitters in the neuromuscular junction, leading to widespread excitation of muscles. It is normally preventable through vaccination of the mother, though in this case the mother's objections to medical care have made it so that she was not immunized. Botulism (answer D) and spinal muscular atrophy (answer E) would both be expected to produce generalized muscle *weakness*, not rigidity. *(Chapter 17—Neuromuscular Junction Diseases, Chapter 22—Diagnosis of Meningitis, and Chapter 18—Motor Neuron Diseases)*

17. **The best answer is E.** Transtentorial herniation can be caused by a variety of conditions that increase intracranial pressure. In this case, a spontaneous rupture of an artery led to a subdural hematoma with subsequent herniation. Transtentorial herniation most often compresses the oculomotor nerve, leading to fixed *dilated* pupils (answer A) and a "down and out" positioning of the ipsilateral eye. In this case, the subdural hematoma was on the left, so the oculomotor nerve palsy would be on the left, not the right (answer B). Palsies of either the trochlear nerve (answer C) or abducens nerve (answer D) are not commonly seen in a transtentorial herniation. *(Chapter 15—Brain Herniation)*

18. **The best answer is E.** Primary lateral sclerosis is a motor neuron disease that affects upper motor neurons exclusively, leaving lower motor neurons intact. For this reason, lower motor neuron signs such as absent reflexes (answer A) and muscle atrophy (answer B) are absent, replaced by an exaggerated gag reflex and tongue spasticity, respectively. Dysphagia is common due to involvement of the brainstem. In contrast to amyotrophic lateral sclerosis, primary lateral sclerosis has a much better prognosis, and most people die from unrelated causes (answer

D). Urinary incontinence is uncommon, though a state of *emotional* incontinence known as pseudobulbar affect is seen in this case (answer C). *(Chapter 18—Motor Neuron Diseases)*

19. **The best answer is B.** Vertigo has a wide variety of possible causes that are often categorized into central causes (those involving a lesion in the cerebellum or brainstem) and peripheral causes (those involving the vestibular system of the inner ear). In this case, the patient presented with an acute onset of vertigo along with several cerebellar signs including dysdiadochokinesia, nystagmus, and ataxia. These all make a central cause of vertigo more likely than a peripheral cause, as patients with peripheral vertigo tend to perform well on finger-to-nose, heel-to-shin, rapid-alternating movements, and other tests of cerebellar function (answer E). In this case, the patient is experiencing vertebral artery dissection. Ménière's disease is unlikely given the absence of hearing loss or ringing in the ears (answer D). An acute blockage of the ventricular system leading to obstructive hydrocephalus could cause symptoms of cerebellar dysfunction, although most cases of hydrocephalus tend to have a slower onset and would present with changes in mental status and other signs of increased intracranial pressure (answer C). There are no cortical signs such as motor deficits, sensory loss, or impaired cognition to suggest a stroke in the anterior cerebral circulation (answer A). *(Chapter 6—Cerebellar Signs, Chapter 11—Balance, and Chapter 14—Cerebellar Strokes)*

20. **The best answer is C.** This patient has cauda equina syndrome as evidenced by the presence of low back pain, saddle anesthesia, weakness and numbness in the legs, and urinary incontinence. The cauda equina represents the bundle of spinal nerves that continues even after the spinal cord ends in the lumbar region. Recall that, although nerves from the cauda equina *exit* in the lumbar, sacral, and coccygeal regions, the cauda equina itself is located in lumbar spine (answers D and E). Cervical nerves innervate the neck and arms which are not involved in this case (answer A), while thoracic nerves innervate the arms and chest (answer B). *(Chapter 8—Spinal Cord Pathology and Chapter 9—Spinal Nerves)*

21. **The best answer is E.** Several neuroanatomical structures are involved in tasting and reacting to food. The hypoglossal nerve is used to move the food inside the mouth (answer D), while the nucleus ambiguus contains the cell bodies of neurons involved in swallowing (answer G). The facial and glossopharyngeal nerves (answers A and B) carry taste sensations from the anterior and posterior aspects of the tongue, respectively, to the nucleus solitarius (answer F). When it senses food that it wants to reject, the nucleus solitarius sends signals to the area postrema to induce nausea and vomiting (answer H). In addition, the vagus nerve activates the pharyngeal muscles responsible for gagging (answer C). Of the listed options, only the Edinger-Westphal nuclei are not directly involved in these processes. Instead, the Edinger-Westphal nuclei play a role in the pupillary light reflex. *(Chapter 7—The Medulla Oblongata, Chapter 9—Cranial Nerves, and Chapter 11—Taste)*

22. **The best answer is B.** This patient is demonstrating Cushing's triad of irregular breathing, a slow heart rate, and elevated blood pressure. Cushing's triad is classically associated with a sudden increase in intracranial pressure as would occur due to a ruptured artery. Viral encephalitis could lead to similar alterations in consciousness but would likely present with fever as well (answer C). Neither an ischemic stroke nor a seizure would produce the sudden changes in vital signs seen here (answers A and D). Finally, autoimmune demyelination tends to move at a much slower pace, causing changes in presentation over weeks or months rather than hours (answer E). *(Chapter 15—Signs and Symptoms of Intracranial Hypertension)*

23. **The best answer is B.** This vignette describes a case of normal pressure hydrocephalus, a disease characterized by a triad of gait instability, incontinence, and cognitive deficits. Of these, gait instability is the most common sign and is typically the first presentation of the illness, with incontinence and cognitive deficits occurring later. Normal pressure hydrocephalus is a treatable condition, with surgical placement of a shunt resulting in rapid improvements for the majority of patients. Medication does not play a large role in management of this disease (answer A). Normal pressure hydrocephalus is often misdiagnosed. It can be diagnosed as dementia, especially as the enlargement of the ventricular spaces seen on imaging can resemble the hydrocephalus *ex vacuo* caused by cerebral atrophy; however, in dementia gait disturbance is typically a late finding, not the initial presenting complaint (answer D). The presence of gait disturbance puts Parkinson's disease on the differential, although a lack of tremor or rigidity is not characteristic (answer C). Finally, a cerebellar stroke may impact gait but would not be expected to lead to cognitive deficits or urinary incontinence (answer E). *(Chapter 14—Cerebellar Strokes, Chapter 15—Hydrocephalus, and Chapter 19—Parkinsonism)*

24. **The best answer is A.** Subfalcine herniation occurs when the brain is displaced under the anterior edge of the falx cerebri due to increased intracranial pressure. For this reason, frontal structures in the brain including the anterior cerebral artery are at risk of compressive injury in a subfalcine herniation. Compression of the anterior cerebral artery leads to weakness of the lower limbs as well as urinary incontinence. Compression of the middle cerebral artery would lead to arm weakness and expressive aphasia (answer B), while compression of the posterior cerebral artery would lead to contralateral homonymous hemianopsia with macular sparing (answer C). Ataxia is more likely to be related to compression of the arteries supplying the cerebellum (answer D). Pure motor or pure sensory strokes are more often seen in lacunar than cortical strokes (answers E and F). *(Chapter 15—Brain Herniation and Chapter 14—Cortical Strokes)*

25. **The best answer is B.** This image shows an upward and inward drift of the left eye which is consistent with a trochlear nerve palsy. The trochlear nerve exits from the midbrain along with the oculomotor nerve, while the abducens nerve exits from the pons (answer C). The cranial nerves exit in groups of four, with the first four exiting from the brain (answer A) and midbrain, the middle four exiting

from the pons, and the final four exiting from the medulla oblongata (answer D). Cranial nerves by definition do not exit from the spinal cord (answer E). *(Chapter 10—Extraocular Movements and Chapter 7—The Midbrain)*

26. **The best answer is F.** Botulinum toxin works by preventing the release of acetylcholine into synapses, and it is effective at reducing activation of acetylcholine receptors wherever they are found. Injection of botulinum toxin can be an effective treatment for a variety of disorders characterized by overactive muscles, including muscle spasticity (answer A) and focal dystonia (answer C). It can be an effective treatment for some cases of strabismus, or misalignment of the eyes, by relaxing specific extraocular muscles to allow for the gaze to become aligned again (answer E). Botulinum toxin can also be effective for non-skeletal muscles such as those in the bladder, as acetylcholine is the neurotransmitter used here (answer D). Finally, while sweating is a function of the sympathetic nervous system, it uses acetylcholine as its neurotransmitter, so botulinum toxin injections can be effective at addressing this as well (answer B). *(Chapter 2—The Autonomic Nervous System and Chapter 17—Neuromuscular Junction Diseases)*

27. **The best answer is E.** This patient is presenting with clear signs of Parkinsonism including rigidity, cogwheeling, and a forward-flexed shuffling gait. While most cases of idiopathic Parkinson's disease have a slow insidious onset, there are reports of vascular Parkinsonism related to ischemic injury that can be much more sudden in their onset. Imaging in vascular Parkinsonism often shows damage to the substantia nigra which is located in the midbrain. The other labeled structures are the frontal cortex (answer A), corpus callosum (answer B), thalamus (answer C), hypothalamus (answer D), pons (answer F), medulla (answer G), and cerebellum (answer H). *(Chapter 19—Parkinsonism and Chapter 7—The Midbrain)*

28. **The best answer is A.** This patient has tumors in the brainstem and cerebellum that have been diagnosed as hemangioblastomas, which are tumors not of the nervous tissue itself but of the vasculature supplying it. Hemangioblastomas have an association with polycythemia, or increased red blood cell count, due to excess production of the hormone erythropoietin. Leukopenia (answer B), thrombocythemia (answer C), hyponatremia (answer D), and hyperglycemia (answer E) do not have known associations with hemangioblastomas. *(Chapter 21—Pediatric Brain Tumors)*

29. **The best answer is D.** This patient has von Hippel–Lindau disease, a genetic disorder with manifestations in various organs throughout the body, including hemangioblastomas, angiomatosis (answer A), renal cell carcinomas (answer B), and pheochromocytomas (answer C). In contrast, there is no association with cardiac rhabdomyomas which are instead seen more commonly in tuberous sclerosis. *(Chapter 27—Neurocutaneous Disorders)*

30. **The best answer is B.** The presence of proximal muscle weakness combined with skin rashes is highly suggestive of dermatomyositis. Diagnosing dermatomyositis often involves laboratory testing, electromyography, and a muscle biopsy, the latter of which will show white blood cells invading the space *between* muscle fibers, which is in contrast to the cells being *within* muscle fibers as occurs in polymyositis. Creatine kinase concentrations are generally *increased*, not decreased (answer D). A fatiguing pattern on repetitive nerve stimulation is more suggestive of myasthenia gravis (answer A), while oligoclonal bands suggest a diagnosis of multiple sclerosis (answer C). Damage to the internal capsule can lead to motor weakness, though this would be unlikely to show a pattern of exclusively proximal weakness as seen in this case (answer E). *(Chapter 16—Inflammatory Myopathies)*

31. **The best answer is A.** It is estimated that up to half of the world's population is infected by *Toxoplasma gondii*. However, toxoplasmosis generally produces symptoms only in patients with compromised immune systems. In this case, the patient's intravenous drug use provides a mechanism for contracting HIV. While exposure to cat feces (answer B) and handling of undercooked meat (answer C) are common means of transmission of toxoplasmosis, they would not lead to a symptomatic state in and of themselves without the change in immune status. While pregnancy is a concern for someone with toxoplasmosis, this is due to the effect it would have on the infant, as pregnancy itself does not predispose the mother to developing active toxoplasmosis (answer D). Transmission of toxoplasmosis is generally oral or congenital rather than intravenous (answer E). *(Chapter 23—Parasitic Encephalitis)*

32. **The best answer is F.** A homonymous hemianopsia in combination with alexia without agraphia is highly suggestive of a stroke in the left posterior cerebral artery. Keep in mind that head imaging is displayed as though you are looking at the patient's brain from their feet, so the *left* posterior cerebral artery is found on the *right* side of the page, not the left (answer E). A stroke in the anterior cerebral arteries (answers A and B) would result in motor weakness in the lower extremities while a stroke in the middle cerebral arteries would result in motor weakness in the upper extremities (answers C and D). *(Chapter 12—Cerebral Blood Supply and Chapter 14—Cortical Strokes)*

33. **The best answer is C.** An anterior spinal artery syndrome is a rare complication of spinal surgery. Paraplegia in the lower extremities with loss of protopathic sensation should immediately bring to mind the anterior spinal cord, as the structures containing these neurons both travel in the front parts of the cord. In contrast, epicritic sensation travels posteriorly in the spinal cord and would not be affected (answer B). Unilateral damage to the lateral spinal cord would produce Brown-Séquard syndrome (answer D). A radiculopathy would be unilateral and would likely only produce deficits in the distribution of a single nerve (answer E). Finally, damage to the basal ganglia would produce a movement disorder rather than sudden onset of weakness (answer A). *(Chapter 8—Spinal Cord Pathology and Chapter 14—Spinal Cord Strokes)*

34. **The best answer is F.** The most common sources of brain metastases include the lungs, breasts, skin, kidneys, and colon. In contrast, brain metastases from a primary malignancy of the stomach are rarely seen clinically. *(Chapter 21—Brain Metastases)*

35. **The best answer is C.** This vignette describes a case of Klüver–Bucy syndrome which is characterized by docility, amnesia, hypersexuality, and hyperorality. Docility and amnesia are the key features localizing this disorder to the amygdala, as the amygdala is responsible both for activating the fear response (such as the fear most people would feel about engaging in sexual behavior in a public place) and for assigning emotional meaning to experiences (such as learning about a devastating diagnosis). Damage to the other areas involved in memory including the hippocampus and mammillary bodies would also produce these memory failures but would not likely lead to these types of behavior (answers F and G). In contrast, damage to the anterior cingulate cortex may lead to socially unacceptable behavior but would not produce the memory failures (answer A). The thalamus (answer B) and subthalamic nucleus (answer E) are involved in sensory and motor processes, respectively, and would not produce the syndrome described here when damaged. The paraventricular nucleus of the hypothalamus produces oxytocin which tends to promote prosocial, rather than antisocial, behavior (answer D). *(Chapter 3—The Limbic System)*

36. **The best answer is F.** Lateral medullary syndrome, also known as Wallenberg's syndrome, can occur following a stroke in the posterior inferior cerebellar artery or vertebral artery. It affects structures that are found to the side of the medulla, resulting in contralateral loss of protopathic sensation from involvement of the spinothalamic tract (answer A), an absent gag reflex from involvement of the glossopharyngeal and vagus nerves (answer C), and dysphagia from involvement of the nucleus ambiguus (answer D). Protopathic sensation from the face is carried on the trigeminal nerve which exits out of the pons; however, the nucleus of the trigeminal nerve lies within the medulla, so a stroke here can produce ipsilateral loss of protopathic sensation as well (answer B). Loss of facial muscles is more typically associated with a stroke in the *anterior* inferior cerebellar artery and lateral pontine syndrome; however, recall that nerve fibers belonging to the sympathetic nervous system travel through the lateral medulla as well, so it is possible to see ptosis in lateral medullary syndrome (answer E), although other muscles of facial expression should be intact. *(Chapter 14—Brainstem Strokes)*

37. **The best answer is B.** This patient is showing signs of a movement disorder including a slowed gait, tremor, and a mask-like face. Any young person presenting with a movement disorder should have Wilson's disease high on the differential, as in general movement disorders are primarily found in older individuals. Kayser-Fleischer rings, as seen in the image, are caused by the accumulation of copper in the cornea and are considered to be diagnostic for Wilson's disease. Wilson's disease is associated with a poor prognosis if untreated (answer A), but fortunately there are effective treatments available (answers E and F). Treatment involves use of penicillamine, a drug that helps to clear excess

copper from the system. Dietary avoidance of high copper foods can also be effective. While Wilson's disease can present with psychiatric manifestations, psychiatric medications are not the first line of treatment (answer C). In rare cases, liver transplantation may be considered; however, this is reserved for patients with fulminant liver failure who have not responded to conventional treatments (answer D). *(Chapter 19—Wilson's Disease)*

38. **The best answer is D.** The presence of both upper motor neuron and lower motor neuron findings at the same time is highly suggestive of a lesion at the level of the spine, as the spine is the only area in which both upper and lower motor neuron signs can be produced by the same lesion. In this case, arthritis of the spine is compressing not only the C5 spinal nerve root but also the spinal cord itself. The radiculopathy causes sensory loss and lower motor neuron signs in the C5 distribution, while the spinal cord compression leads to upper motor neuron signs in the legs. Damage to motor neurons in the cerebral cortex (answer A), internal capsule (answer B), medulla (answer C), or anterior horn (answer E) would all produce exclusively upper *or* lower motor neuron signs. *(Chapter 24—Signs and Symptoms of Peripheral Neuropathy, Chapter 18—Motor Neuron Disease, and Chapter 8—Spinal Cord Anatomy)*

39. **The best answer is A.** If left untreated, syphilis can wreak havoc on the nervous system, with several conditions resulting from with this. General paresis refers to the psychiatric manifestations of neurosyphilis which often include cognitive deficits (answer D). Tabes dorsalis refers to demyelination of the dorsal columns of the spinal cord leading to impaired vibration and proprioceptive sensation (answer C). Argyll Robertson pupils will constrict when the patient focuses on a nearby object (answer B) but notably will not constrict when exposed to a bright light. *(Chapter 8—Spinal Cord Pathology, Chapter 10—Pupillary Reflexes, and Chapter 23—Bacterial Encephalitis)*

40. **The best answer is A.** Involuntary flailing movements of the limbs are known as hemiballismus. Hemiballismus is most often caused by a stroke in the area of the subthalamic nucleus, but any disease that causes neuronal damage in this area can lead to hemiballismus, including amyotrophic lateral sclerosis. While upper motor neuron damage can lead to muscle spasticity, it would not lead to the dramatic ballistic movements described here (answer B). The constant nature of these movements argues against a seizure (answer C). Dopamine-blocking medications can cause extrapyramidal symptoms, but hemiballismus is not one of them (answer D). While hemiballismus is a rare outcome of amyotrophic lateral sclerosis, there is no reason to suspect that the diagnosis is incorrect (answer E) or that the patient is feigning illness (answer F). *(Chapter 5—The Basal Ganglia and Chapter 18—Motor Neuron Diseases)*

41. **The best answer is F.** This patient likely has tuberous sclerosis as evidenced by the characteristic triad of epilepsy, intellectual disability, and cutaneous findings. Tuberous sclerosis is a multi-system disorder that requires an interdisciplinary medical team for appropriate management. For this patient, ordering an EEG and starting an anticonvulsant are appropriate given her recent seizure (answers A and D). The patient is at high risk of brain tumors, so an MRI of the brain can help to rule those out (answer B). Tuberous sclerosis is associated with both renal angiomyolipomas and cysts, so evaluating renal function is essential (answer C). Finally, patients with this condition are at high risk of cardiac rhabdomyomas, so an echocardiogram should be obtained (answer E). *(Chapter 27—Neurocutaneous Disorders)*

42. **The best answer is D.** Hearing loss has a wide variety of causes. Some degree of hearing loss with age is expected, especially if the patient has been chronically exposed to loud noises. However, the presence of ataxia and an unsteady gait are strongly suggestive of a more pathological process (answers A and E). A sensorineural or conductive hearing loss would not account for these findings (answers B and C). In this case, the largest clue comes from the MRI which reveals bilateral schwannomas in the nerve sheath of the vestibulocochlear nerve. Because they are symmetrical, an observer may assume they are normal, but don't make this mistake: those two tumors should not be there! Bilateral vestibular schwannomas are diagnostic for neurofibromatosis type II, a genetic disorder that can either be inherited in an autosomal dominant fashion or develop through *de novo* mutations. *(Chapter 27—Neurocutaneous Disorders, Chapter 21—Adult-Onset Brain Tumors, and Chapter 11—Hearing)*

43. **The best answer is C.** This vignette describes a case of benign Rolandic epilepsy as evidenced by the focal onset of the seizure during sleep and the characteristic centrotemporal spikes on EEG. Benign Rolandic epilepsy has a good prognosis, and many patients with this condition will not need treatment. There is no association between structural damage in the brain and this condition like there is with temporal lobe epilepsy and mesial temporal sclerosis (answer A). There is no evidence of a brain tumor at this time, with the presence of centrotemporal spikes and absence of neurologic deficits making this a remote possibility (answer B). Benign Rolandic epilepsy does not involve intellectual disability as other forms of epilepsy such as Lennox-Gastaut syndrome do (answer D). Finally, positive findings on EEG argue strongly against psychogenic non-epileptic seizures in this patient (answer E). *(Chapter 20—Epilepsy Syndromes)*

44. **The best answer is I.** The oculomotor nerve and the posterior communicating artery are right next to each other, so an aneurysm of this artery can lead to compressive dysfunction in that nerve. In fact, posterior communicating artery aneurysms are so common that an acute painful oculomotor nerve palsy with pupil dilation is often assumed to be a posterior communicating artery aneurysm unless proven otherwise. The oculomotor nerve palsy is ipsilateral to the side of the aneurysm, so the aneurysm is on the right, not the left (answer H). The anterior communicating artery is a common site for aneurysms, but it is not

located near the oculomotor nerve (answer A). The anterior, middle, and posterior cerebral arteries are not located near the oculomotor nerve, nor do they supply oxygen to the nerve (answers B—G). *(Chapter 15—Intracranial Bleeds and Chapter 10—Organization of the Oculomotor Nerve)*

45. **The best answer is D.** When aneurysms become large enough to compress nearby structures and produce neurologic symptoms, it suggests a high degree of instability in the arterial wall. Unstable aneurysms are prone to rupturing and causing a subarachnoid hemorrhage which often presents as the sudden "thunderclap" onset of a severe headache (answer A). While an intracerebral hemorrhage can present similarly, it is less likely given the presence of a known unstable aneurysm and a lack of recent head trauma. A lack of recent head trauma also argues against either a subdural hematoma (answer B) or an epidural hematoma (answer C). A brain tumor (answer E) or hydrocephalus (answer F) both tend to come on more slowly compared to the acute onset described here. *(Chapter 15—Intracranial Bleeds)*

46. **The best answer is F.** This vignette describes a tumor of the pineal gland in the epithalamus leading to an obstructive hydrocephalus, melatonin insufficiency, and Parinaud's syndrome (or a weakness of upward gaze related to compression of the vertical gaze center in the medial longitudinal fasciculus). Upward gaze is mediated by the superior rectus muscle which is controlled by the oculomotor nerve; however, the oculomotor nerve also controls several other extraocular muscles, so dysfunction of the nerve itself would not lead to an isolated upward gaze palsy (answer B). The trochlear and abducens nerves do not control upward gaze (answers C and D). Central herniation can produce "sunset eyes" as well, but this would likely present with a sudden onset of coma due to compression of vital structures in the brainstem (answer E). The suprachiasmatic nucleus does regulate sleep, but a lesion here would not account for Parinaud's syndrome and would likely present with other signs of hypothalamic dysfunction as well (answer H). Optic neuritis would result in impaired vision rather than weakness in extraocular movements (answer A). Finally, multiple sclerosis is an unlikely cause of hydrocephalus (answer G). *(Chapter 4—The Epithalamus, Chapter 10—Extraocular Movements, and Chapter 15—Hydrocephalus)*

47. **The best answer is B.** This case describes a pure sensory stroke which is most often related to a lacunar infarct in the thalamus on the side contralateral to the observed deficits. A pure sensory stroke can present not only with numbness but also paresthesias and pain as well. A stroke in the territory of the middle cerebral artery would tend to produce motor deficits in addition to sensory loss (answer A). A lesion in the spinothalamic tract at the level of the medulla would not produce the facial numbness seen in this case (answer C). Damage to the right spinal cord would produce Brown-Séquard syndrome and would not involve the face (answer D). Finally, occlusion of the posterior spinal artery would primarily affect the dorsal columns leading to deficits in vibration and proprioceptive sensation, not pain and temperature as seen here (answer E). *(Chapter 14—Lacunar Strokes)*

48. **The best answer is C.** For a patient presenting with neurologic symptoms in a relapsing-remitting pattern, consideration should be given to a diagnosis of multiple sclerosis. However, a patient with diplopia and fatigue that worsens in the evening is also suggestive of myasthenia gravis. This patient's history is not immediately diagnostic of one or the other, so steps should be taken to evaluate further. A diagnosis of multiple sclerosis would be supported by the presence of oligoclonal bands on lumbar puncture (answer B) or the characteristic plaques on MRI (answer D), while a diagnosis of myasthenia gravis would be supported by identifying antibodies against the acetylcholine receptor in the blood (answer A) or abnormal action potential patterns on electromyography (answer E). Only a CT scan would not have diagnostic value in either multiple sclerosis or myasthenia gravis, as it is primarily used for identifying infarctions, bleeds, tumors, and bone abnormalities. A neurological exam is always of diagnostic value in working up a neurologic complaint (answer F). *(Chapter 25—Central Demyelinating Diseases and Chapter 17—Neuromuscular Junction Diseases)*

49. **The best answer is E.** This patient's MRI and fatiguing pattern on repetitive nerve stimulation are both suggestive of myasthenia gravis. She has now developed weakness of her respiratory muscles known as a myasthenic crisis, which is a medical emergency requiring immediate treatment. While acetylcholinesterase inhibitors are effective treatments for myasthenia gravis, they do not work quickly enough in a potentially life-threatening situation (answer B). Instead, either plasmapheresis or intravenous immunoglobulins (IVIGs) should be administered to rapidly clear the offending antibodies from the system. Steroids (answer A) and glatiramer acetate (answer C) are both treatments used for multiple sclerosis, not myasthenia gravis. Myasthenia gravis is an autoimmune disease and is not related to toxins as with botulism or tetanus (answer D). *(Chapter 17—Neuromuscular Junction Diseases)*

50. **The best answer is B.** Cerebral herniation following a lumbar puncture is a rare event, but given the morbidity and mortality associated with it, it is important to keep in mind. As a rule, it is not necessary to order a CT scan prior to performing a lumbar puncture. However, in certain cases, such as a young patient presenting with seizures, it may have helped to identify a source of increased intracranial pressure that would make herniation more likely if a lumbar puncture is performed. As this was not a stroke, administration of either tissue plasminogen activator or antihypertensives is unlikely to have been of benefit (answers C and E). The patient had signs of meningeal infection prior to the lumbar puncture, so the quality of sterile technique is unlikely to account for this outcome (answer A). While a subdural hematoma can lead to brain herniation in some cases, the lack of focal head trauma and a clear alternative explanation in meningitis makes this a much less likely source (answer D). *(Chapter 13—Lumbar Puncture and Chapter 15—Brain Herniation)*

51. **The best answer is C.** This vignette describes a case of postpartum pituitary gland necrosis, also known as Sheehan's syndrome. The pituitary gland is sensitive to ischemic damage, so in cases of severe blood loss the pituitary gland can stop functioning, leading to deficits in many of its endocrine functions. These include milk production from prolactin (answer A), release of glucose in the bloodstream from adrenocorticotropic hormone (answer B), proper thyroid function from thyroid-stimulating hormone (answer D), and a feeling of bonding with the child from oxytocin (answer E). Damage to the posterior pituitary can result in lack of vasopressin release, which would make the frequency of urination likely to *increase*, not decrease. *(Chapter 4—The Pituitary Gland)*

52. **The best answer is F.** Lyme disease is a tick-borne infectious disease involving the bacterium *Borrelia burgdorferi*. A characteristic "bull's eye" rash known as erythema migrans is highly suggestive of the disease. Lyme disease affects both the central and peripheral nervous systems and is a potential cause of peripheral neuropathy (answer D), Bell's palsy (answer E), and meningitis (answer C). However, it can affect other organs as well, including the heart (answer B) and joints (answer A). *(Chapter 24—Diseases Associated with Peripheral Neuropathy)*

53. **The best answer is G.** The cavernous sinuses contain veins that drain blood from the eyes and other anterior parts of the head. However, they also contain several important structures including the internal carotid artery and all three of the cranial nerves responsible for extraocular movements. When the cavernous sinus becomes thrombosed, these structures can be injured, leading to loss of extraocular movements in all directions (answers A—D). The ophthalmic and maxillary divisions of the trigeminal nerve, which supply the upper and middle face respectively, also pass through the cavernous sinus (answers E and F). Notably, the mandibular division of the trigeminal nerve does not, so sensation to the jaw and lower face would likely be preserved. *(Chapter 12—Venous Drainage)*

ATTRIBUTIONS

The fonts **Oswald** and Source Sans Pro were used for the cover and inside text, respectively. They were accessed from Google Fonts under an open-source license.

With the following exceptions, all images displayed in this book are in the public domain and/or are not associated with any known copyright restrictions. Most images have been modified for formatting. Use of this content does not suggest that the content's original creator(s) endorse this book or its author in any way.

COVER AND BACK

- Cover and back design by Stephen Sauer (SingleFinDesign.com).
- Images and icons designed by Iconfinder.

CHAPTER 2 | THE NERVOUS SYSTEM

- "Dissection of the head and neck, cranial, spinal and sympathetic nerves." Credit: Thomas Fisher Rare Book Library, UofT (Creative Commons Attribution 2.0 Generic license).
- "HE stain of brain autopsy specimen (formalin-fixated, paraffin embedded) showing oligodendrocytes with fried-egg appearance." Credit: Jensflorian (Creative Commons Attribution-Share Alike 4.0 International license).
- "Typing consciousness." Credit: Akiyao and LucasVB; modified by Cangjie6 (Creative Commons Attribution-Share Alike 3.0 Unported license).
- "Shows termination of nerve in muscle." Credit: Wellcome Images (Creative Commons Attribution 4.0 International license).
- "Anatomy and Physiology of the Neuromuscular Junction." Credit: Open Learning Initiative, provided by Carnegie Mellon University (Creative Commons Attribution 3.0 United States license).
- "Comment utiliser cette latrines." Credit: SuSanA Secretariat (Creative Commons Attribution 2.0 Generic license).
- "Divisions of the nervous system." Credit: Fuzzform at English Wikipedia (Creative Commons Attribution-Share Alike 3.0 Unported license).

CHAPTER 3 | THE CEREBRAL CORTEX

- "Motor homunculus." Credit: ralf@ark.in-berlin.de (Creative Commons Attribution-Share Alike 4.0 International license).
- "Sensory homunculus." Credit: btarski (Creative Commons Attribution-Share Alike 4.0 International license).
- "The classical Wernicke-Lichtheim-Geschwind model of the neurobiology of language." Credit: Peter Hagoort (Creative Commons Attribution 3.0 Unported license).
- "Optic tract and optic nerve." Credit: Anatomist90 (Creative Commons Attribution-Share Alike 3.0 Unported license).

CHAPTER 4 | THE THALAMUS, EPITHALAMUS , AND HYPOTHALAMUS

- "12 Line Field Telephone Switchboard." Credit: Sam Stokes (Creative Commons Attribution-ShareAlike 2.0 Generic license).

- "Parinaud syndrome." Credit: Luciobgomes (Creative Commons Attribution-Share Alike 4.0 International license).
- "The Hypothalamus-Pituitary Complex." Credit: OpenStax College (Creative Commons Attribution 3.0 Unported license).
- "A giant and a dwarf, London, 1927." Credit: Wellcome Images (Creative Commons Attribution 4.0 International license).
- "Pituitary tumor." Credit: Elgee (Creative Commons Attribution 3.0 Unported license).

CHAPTER 5 | THE BASAL GANGLIA AND INTERNAL CAPSULE

- "Basal Nuclei Connections." Credit: OpenStax (Creative Commons Attribution 4.0 International license).
- "Back End of a Bus." Credit: Andrew Bone from Weymouth, England (Creative Commons Attribution 2.0 Generic license).
- "DBS simulation of subthalamic nucleus." Credit: Hartmann CJ, Chaturvedi A, and Lujan JL (Creative Commons Attribution 4.0 International license).

CHAPTER 6 | THE CEREBELLUM

- "Push-up-with-feet-on-an-exercise-ball." Credit: Everkinetic (Creative Commons Attribution-Share Alike 3.0 Unported license).
- "Cerebellar Peduncles." Credit: OpenStax College (Creative Commons Attribution 3.0 Unported license).
- "Major Regions of the Cerebellum." Credit: OpenStax College (Creative Commons Attribution 3.0 Unported license).
- "Left sided cerebellar stroke due to occlusion of a vertebral artery." Credit: James Heilman, MD (Creative Commons Attribution-Share Alike 3.0 Unported license).

CHAPTER 7 | THE BRAINSTEM

- None.

CHAPTER 8 | THE SPINAL CORD

- "The human body in anatomical position." Credit: Osteomyoamare (Creative Commons Attribution 3.0 Unported license).
- "Apparatus for the treatment of paralysis." Credit: Wellcome Images (Creative Commons Attribution 4.0 International license).
- "T2-weighted MRI of a syrinx located at C6–C7 in the cervical spine." Credit: Cyborg Ninja at English Wikipedia (Creative Commons Attribution 4.0 International license).

CHAPTER 9 | THE PERIPHERAL NERVOUS SYSTEM

- "2nd nerve-figure, by Vesalius." Credit: Wellcome Images (Creative Commons Attribution 4.0 International license).
- "Trigeminal nerve." Credit: Harrygouvas (Creative Commons Attribution-Share Alike 3.0 Unported license).
- "Automatic Innervation." Credit: OpenStax College (Creative Commons Attribution 3.0 Unported license).
- "Bells palsy diagram." Credit: Patrick J. Lynch, medical illustrator (Creative

Commons Attribution 2.5 Generic license).
- "Ear Schema." Credit: Didier Descouens (Creative Commons Attribution-Share Alike 3.0 Unported, 2.5 Generic, 2.0 Generic and 1.0 Generic license).
- "Reflexo da tosse." Credit: Ericneuro (Creative Commons Attribution-Share Alike 4.0 International license).
- "Autonomic Nervous System." Credit: Paul Walker (Creative Commons Attribution-ShareAlike 2.0 Generic license).
- "Down Curved Arrow." Credit: Star and Anchor Design, US (Creative Commons CCBY license).
- "spinalstudy." Credit: James. P Well on Flickr (Creative Commons Attribution-NoDerivs 2.0 Generic license).
- "Pancoast Tumor." Credit: Jmarchn (Creative Commons Attribution-Share Alike 1.0 Generic license).

CHAPTER 10 | VISION

- "Optical Fields." Credit: OpenStax College (Creative Commons Attribution 3.0 Unported license).
- "Cranial nerve III visceral." Credit: Patrick J. Lynch, medical illustrator (Creative Commons Attribution 2.5 Generic license).
- "Dilated and Undilated Pupil." Credit: National Eye Institute Creative Commons Attribution 2.0 Generic license).
- "Argyll Robertson pupil." Credit: Chainwit (Creative Commons Attribution-Share Alike 4.0 International license).
- "Nerve Structure." Credit: OpenStax College (Creative Commons Attribution 3.0 Unported license).
- "An example of eye divergence." Credit: Scumbag at English Wikipedia (Creative Commons Attribution-Share Alike 3.0 Unported license).

CHAPTER 11 | HEARING, BALANCE, TASTE, AND SMELL

- "Weber test being performed on a volunteer." Credit: DrSaltMD (Creative Commons Attribution-Share Alike 4.0 International license).
- "Rinneversuch." Credit: FOX 52 (Creative Commons Attribution-Share Alike 4.0 International license).
- "falling." Credit: Lovelorn Poets (Creative Commons Attribution 2.0 Generic license).
- "Anatomy and physiology of animals Olfactory organ the sense of smell." Credit: Sunshineconnelly at English Wikibooks (Creative Commons Attribution 3.0 Unported license).

CHAPTER 12 | THE MENINGES, VENTRICLES, AND BLOOD SUPPLY

- "Carotidian pulse." Credit: Rama (Creative Commons Attribution-ShareAlike 3.0 license).
- "Vesalius, figure of the brain." Credit: Wellcome Images (Creative Commons Attribution 4.0 International license).
- "Arteries, from Diderot's Encyclopedie." Credit: Science Museum Group, in the United Kingdom (Creative Commons Attribution 4.0 International license).
- "MRA Circle of Willis." Credit: © Nevit Dilmen (Creative Commons Attribution-

Share Alike 3.0 Unported license).

- "Oedema." Credit: Klaus D. Peter (Creative Commons Attribution-Share Alike 1.0 Generic license).

CHAPTER 13 | THE NEUROLOGICAL EXAM

- "A doctor skating past a group of people whilst inspecting their tongues and running down a street throwing pills to patients in houses." Credit: Wellcome Images (Creative Commons Attribution 4.0 International license).
- "Moro Reflex." Credit: Ashley Arbuckle (Creative Commons Attribution 2.0 Generic license).
- "Rooting Reflex." Credit: Ashley Arbuckle (Creative Commons Attribution 2.0 Generic license).
- "Palmar Grasp Reflex." Credit: Ashley Arbuckle (Creative Commons Attribution 2.0 Generic license).
- "Romberg." Credit: Gonad (Creative Commons Attribution-Share Alike 1.0 Generic license).
- "Trendelenburg's sign." Credit: Foto H.-P.Haack (Creative Commons Attribution-Share Alike 3.0 Unported license).
- "CT and MRI of cerebral hemorrhages and effective T2 MRI of subsequent hemosiderosis." Credit: Hongwei Zhao, Jin Wang, Zhonglie Lu, Qingjie Wu, Haijuan Lv, Hu Liu, Xiangyang Gong (Creative Commons Attribution 4.0 International license).

CHAPTER 14 | STROKE

- "Ischemic Stroke." Credit: ElinorHunt (Creative Commons Attribution-Share Alike 4.0 International license).
- "A patient paying a dentist after having a tooth removed with gas." Credit: Wellcome Images (Creative Commons Attribution 4.0 International license).
- "FLAIR MRI of cerebral infarction." Credit: Shazia Mirza and Sankalp Gokhale (Creative Commons Attribution 4.0 International license).
- "CT of lacunar strokes." Credit: Prashanthsaddala (Creative Commons Attribution-Share Alike 3.0 Unported license).
- "Cerebellum arteries." Credit: Petit B (Creative Commons Attribution-Share Alike 4.0 International license).
- "Arteries entering spinal canal." Credit: Wellcome Images (Creative Commons Attribution 4.0 International license).
- "Arteries at base of brain and anterior spinal arteries." Credit: Wellcome Images (Creative Commons Attribution 4.0 International license).
- "Neuroimaging in Acute Stroke." Credit: Shazia Mirza and Sankalp Gokhale (Creative Commons Attribution 4.0 International license).
- "TOF MRI angiography of right middle cerebral artery stenosis." Credit: Shazia Mirza and Sankalp Gokhale (Creative Commons Attribution 4.0 International license).
- "Oculomotor nerve palsy." Credit: Wang Y, Wang XH, Tian MM, Xie CJ, Liu Y, Pan QQ, Lu YN (Creative Commons Attribution 4.0 International license).
- "Palatine Uvula." Credit: Luigithemetal64 (Creative Commons Attribution-Share Alike 3.0 Unported license).

CHAPTER 15 | INTRACRANIAL HYPERTENSION

- "An illustration of the different types of brain hemorrhage." Credit: https://www.myupchar.com/en (Creative Commons Attribution-Share Alike 4.0 International license).
- "Epidurale Blutung in der Computertomographie rechts." Credit: Hellerhoff (Creative Commons Attribution-Share Alike 3.0 Unported license).
- "Large left sided frontal parietal subdural hematoma with associated midline shift." Credit: James Heilman, MD (Creative Commons Attribution-Share Alike 3.0 Unported license).
- "A subarachnoid hemorrhage." Credit: James Heilman, MD (Creative Commons Attribution-Share Alike 3.0 Unported license).
- "An intra parenchymal bleed with surrounding edema." Credit: James Heilman, MD (Creative Commons Attribution-Share Alike 4.0 International license).
- "Ruptured 7mm left vertebral artery aneurysm." Credit: James Heilman, MD (Creative Commons Attribution-Share Alike 4.0 International license).
- "Skull and brain human normal." Credit: Patrick J. Lynch, medical illustrator (Creative Commons Attribution 2.5 Generic license).
- "Stress ball." Credit: Eptihal alghamdi - 171 psy (Creative Commons Attribution-Share Alike 4.0 International license).
- "Brain herniation types." Credit: Delldot, with derivative work by RupertMillard (Creative Commons Attribution-Share Alike 3.0 Unported license).
- "Schematic representation of Kernohan's notch." Credit: Ragesh Panikkath, Deepa Panikkath, Sian Lim, and Kenneth Nugent (Creative Commons Attribution 3.0 Unported license).
- "Anisocoria." Credit: Tair1978 (Creative Commons Attribution-Share Alike 4.0 International license).
- "Hydrocephalus with sunset eyes." Credit: شهاب (Creative Commons Attribution-Share Alike 4.0 International license).
- "Papilledema Stages." Credit: Ambika S., Arjundas D., Noronha V. (Creative Commons Attribution-Share Alike 2.0 Generic license).
- "Anterior communicating artery aneurysm before and after GDC coil embolization." Credit: J Neal Rutledge (Creative Commons Attribution-ShareAlike 3.0 license).
- "Brain atrophy from vascular dementia." Credit: James Heilman, MD (Creative Commons Attribution-Share Alike 4.0 International license).

CHAPTER 16 | MYOPATHY

- "Polymyositis HE." Credit: Jensflorian (Creative Commons Attribution-Share Alike 3.0 Unported license).
- "High magnification micrograph of dermatomyositis, a type of inflammatory myopathy. H&E stain." Credit: Nephron (Creative Commons Attribution-Share Alike 3.0 Unported license).
- "Dermatomyositis." Credit: Elizabeth M. Dugan, Adam M. Huber, Frederick W. Miller, Lisa G. Rider (Creative Commons Attribution-Share Alike 3.0 Unported license).
- "Patient with DMD enlarged calf muscles." Credit: Sohail A, et al. (Creative Commons Attribution license).

CHAPTER 17 | NEUROMUSCULAR JUNCTION DISEASES

- "Shows termination of nerve in muscle." Wellcome Images (Creative Commons Attribution 4.0 International license).
- "Botulism." Credit: Herbert L. Fred, MD and Hendrik A. van Dijk (Creative Commons Attribution 2.0 Generic license).
- "Botox Injections from Dr Braun." Credit: Dr. Braun (Creative Commons Attribution-ShareAlike 2.0 Generic license).
- "Myasthenia gravis ptosis reversal." Credit: Mohankumar Kurukumbi, Roger L Weir, Janaki Kalyanam, Mansoor Nasim, Annapurni Jayam-Trouth (Creative Commons Attribution 2.0 Generic license).

CHAPTER 18 | MOTOR NEURON DISEASES

- "A boy affected by konzo, causing a spastic paraparesis with walking difficulties. It also shows the upper motor neuron, the suspected site of the neurodamage." Credit: Thorkild Tylleskar (Creative Commons Attribution-Share Alike 3.0 Unported license).
- "Chin-ups-1." Credit: Everkinetic (Creative Commons Attribution-Share Alike 3.0 Unported license).
- "Amyotrophic lateral sclerosis." Credit: Frank Gaillard (Creative Commons Attribution-Share Alike 3.0 Unported license).

CHAPTER 19 | MOVEMENT DISORDERS

- "Spiral drawing - essential tremor." Credit: Undescribed/Pharexia (Creative Commons Attribution-Share Alike 4.0 International license).
- "Kayser-Fleischer ring." Credit: Herbert L. Fred, MD, Hendrik A. van Dijk (Creative Commons Attribution 3.0 Unported license).
- "Face of the giant panda sign in Wilson's disease." Credit: S Chakraborty,1 MB BS, MD (Radiodiagnosis); S Mondal,2 MB BS, DMRD; D Sinha,2 MB BS; A Nag,2 MB BS. Corresponding author: S Mondal (drmsumantro@gmail.com) (Creative Commons Attribution 4.0 International license).

CHAPTER 20 | SEIZURES

- "A group of people standing around a man having an epileptic fit." Credit: Wellcome Images (Creative Commons Attribution 4.0 International license).
- "Attaque: Periode Epileptoide. Planche XVII." Credit: Wellcome Images (Creative Commons Attribution 4.0 International license).
- "Human EEG with prominent alpha-rhythm." Credit: Andrii Cherninskyi (Creative Commons Attribution-Share Alike 4.0 International license).
- "Frontal lobe tumor." Credit: Roland Schmitt et al (Creative Commons Attribution 2.0 Generic license).
- "A figure with four arms and four legs." Credit: Wellcome Images (Creative Commons Attribution 4.0 International license).
- "Generalized 3 Hz spike and wave discharges in a child with childhood absence epilepsy." Credit: Der Lange (Creative Commons Attribution-Share Alike 2.0 Generic license).
- "Normal axial T2-weighted MR image of the brain." Credit: Novaksean (Creative Commons Attribution-Share Alike 4.0 International license).

CHAPTER 21 | NEOPLASMS

- "Brain MRI of 39YO man with lung cancer metastasis." Credit: Nevit Dilmen (Creative Commons Attribution-Share Alike 3.0 Unported license).
- "A posterior fossa tumor causing mass effect." Credit: James Heilman, MD (Creative Commons Attribution-Share Alike 3.0 Unported license).
- "Glioblastoma multiforme - MRT T2 ax." Credit: Hellerhoff (Creative Commons Attribution-Share Alike 3.0 Unported license).
- "MRI, coronal image, of a meningioma with contrast." Credit: James Heilman, MD (Creative Commons Attribution-Share Alike 4.0 International license).
- "Meningioma high mag." Credit: Nephron (Creative Commons Attribution-Share Alike 3.0 Unported license).
- "Oligodendroglioma high mag." Credit: Nephron (Creative Commons Attribution-Share Alike 3.0 Unported license).
- "Medulloblastoma with rosettes." Credit: Jensflorian (Creative Commons Attribution-Share Alike 3.0 Unported license).
- "Rose window on the front of the cathedral of Saint Vigilius." Credit: Matteo Ianeselli (Creative Commons Attribution-Share Alike 3.0 Unported license).
- "Ependymoma: MRI T1." Credit: User Hellerhoff (Creative Commons Attribution-Share Alike 3.0 Unported license).
- "Ependymoma pseudorosette." Credit: Jensflorian (Creative Commons Attribution-Share Alike 3.0 Unported license).
- "Hemangioblastoma of cerebellum." Credit: Public Library of Science (Creative Commons Attribution-Share Alike 2.5 Generic license).
- "Craniopharyngioma." Credit: Hellerhoff (Creative Commons Attribution 3.0 Unported license).
- "Large Acoustic Neuroma coronal MRI." Credit: Student30 (Creative Commons Attribution-Share Alike 4.0 International license).
- "Brain Metastasis From Breast Cancer." Credit: Jmarchn (Creative Commons Attribution-Share Alike 3.0 Unported license).
- "Glioblastoma showing areas of pseudopalisading necrosis." Credit: Jensflorian (Creative Commons Attribution-Share Alike 3.0 Unported license).
- "Pituitary Tumor." Credit: OpenStax College (Creative Commons Attribution 3.0 Unported license).

CHAPTER 22 | MENINGITIS

- "Petechial rash." Credit: DrFO.Jr.Tn (Creative Commons Attribution-Share Alike 3.0 Unported license).
- "HSV1 encephalitis CSF specimen." Credit: Jensflorian (Creative Commons Attribution-Share Alike 4.0 International license).
- "Purpura." Credit: Hektor (Creative Commons Attribution-Share Alike 3.0 Unported license).

CHAPTER 23 | ENCEPHALITIS

- "HSV encephalitis." Credit: Dr Laughlin Dawes (Creative Commons Attribution 3.0 Unported license).
- "Brain abscess - MRI T1 KM axial." Credit: Hellerhoff (Creative Commons Attribution-Share Alike 3.0 Unported license).

CHAPTER 24 | PERIPHERAL NEUROPATHY

- "Diabetic foot syndrome." Credit: Pflegewiki-User ApoPfleger (Creative Commons Attribution-Share Alike 3.0 Unported license).
- "Herpes zoster chest." Credit: Fisle (Creative Commons Attribution-Share Alike 1.0 Generic license).
- "Bullseye Lyme Disease Rash." Credit: Hannah Garrison (Creative Commons Attribution-Share Alike 2.5 Generic license).
- "Bell's palsy." Credit: Andrea Kamphuis (Creative Commons Attribution-Share Alike 4.0 International license).
- "Hand showing leprosy." Credit: Wellcome Library, London (Creative Commons Attribution 4.0 International license).
- "The foot of a person with Charcot-Marie-Tooth." Credit: Benefros at English Wikipedia (Creative Commons Attribution-Share Alike 3.0 Unported license).
- "Surgical result after ventral fusion of scoliosis." Credit: Weiss HR, Goodall D (Creative Commons Attribution 2.0 Generic license).

CHAPTER 25 | DEMYELINATING DISEASES

- "The demyelination of the Central Nervous System." Credit: Gonz2019 (Creative Commons Attribution-Share Alike 4.0 International license).
- "Fulminating ADEM showing many lesions." Credit: Rodríguez-Porcel F, Hornik A, Rosenblum J, Borys E, Biller J (Creative Commons Attribution 4.0 International license).
- "Multiple Sclerosis in a Nigerian Alcoholic Male: A Case Report from Enugu, South East Nigeria." Credit: IO Onwuekwe and O. Ekenze, © Annals of Medical and Health Sciences Research (Creative Commons Attribution-Noncommercial-Share Alike 3.0 Unported license).

CHAPTER 26 | HEADACHE

- "The Cluster Headache." Credit: JD Fletcher (Creative Commons Attribution-Share Alike 3.0 Unported license).
- "Papilledema." Credit: Jonathan Trobe, M.D. - University of Michigan Kellogg Eye Center (Creative Commons Attribution 3.0 Unported license).
- "Superficial temporal artery." Credit: Opzwartbeek (Creative Commons Attribution-Share Alike 4.0 International license).
- "Micrograph of giant cell arteritis." Credit: Nephron (Creative Commons Attribution-Share Alike 3.0 Unported license).

CHAPTER 27 | NEUROCUTANEOUS DISORDERS

- "Embryo at three months. Brain and spinal cord exposed." Credit: Wellcome Images (Creative Commons Attribution 4.0 International license).
- "Back of a person with neurofibromas." Credit: Seiradcruz at English Wikipedia (Creative Commons Attribution-Share Alike 3.0 Unported license).
- "Lisch nodules." Credit: Dimitrios Malamos (Creative Commons Attribution 4.0 International license).
- "Lip telangiectases in hereditary hemorrhagic telangiectasia." Credit: Herbert L. Fred, MD and Hendrik A. van Dijk (Creative Commons Attribution 2.0 Generic license).

- "Photo personnelle d'une 'tache café au lait.'" Credit: Accrochoc at fr.wikipedia (Creative Commons Attribution-Share Alike 3.0 Unported license).
- "Ocular telangiectasia in a person with A-T." Credit: Thomas O. Crawford (Creative Commons Attribution-Share Alike 3.0 Unported license).
- "A new born child with M-CM syndrome." Credit: ArturroD (Creative Commons Attribution-Share Alike 3.0 Unported license).

CHAPTER 28 | FINAL REVIEW

- "Intracerebral hemorrhage." Credit: Yadav YR, Mukerji G, Shenoy R, Basoor A, Jain G, Nelson A (Creative Commons Attribution 2.0 Generic license).
- "Large left sided frontal parietal subdural hematoma with associated midline shift." Credit: James Heilman, MD (Creative Commons Attribution-Share Alike 3.0 Unported license).
- "Traumatic acute epidual hematoma." Credit: Jpogi (Creative Commons Attribution-Share Alike 3.0 Unported license).
- "Subarachnoid haemorrhage." Credit: Lipothymia (Creative Commons Attribution-Share Alike 1.0 Generic license).
- "CT brain tumor." Credit: Bobjgalindo (Creative Commons Attribution-Share Alike 1.0 Generic license).
- "Hydrocephalus." Credit: Lucien Monfils (Creative Commons Attribution-Share Alike 1.0 Generic license).
- "Shingles on the chest." Credit: Preston Hunt (me@prestonhunt.com) (Creative Commons Attribution 3.0 Unported license.
- "Unilateral hypoglossal nerve injury." Credit: Mukherjee SK, Gowshami CB, Salam A, Kuddus R, Farazi MA, Baksh J (Creative Commons Attribution 2.0 Generic license).
- "Brain herniation MRI." Credit: Rocque BG, Başkaya MK (Creative Commons Attribution 2.0 Generic license).
- "Saggital transection through the human brain." Credit: Christian R. Linder (Creative Commons Attribution-Share Alike 3.0 Unported license).
- "Papilledema Stages." Credit: Ambika S., Arjundas D., Noronha V. (Creative Commons Attribution-Share Alike 2.0 Generic license).
- "Craniopharyngioma." Credit: Hellerhoff (Creative Commons Attribution 3.0 Unported license).
- "Paris as seen with bitemporal hemianopsia." Credit: Nunh-huh at English Wikipedia (Creative Commons Attribution-Share Alike 3.0 Unported license).
- "Subfalcine herniation." Credit: RadsWiki (Creative Commons Attribution-Share Alike 3.0 Unported license).
- "MRA shows the circle of Willis." Credit: SBarnes (Creative Commons Attribution-Share Alike 3.0 Unported license).
- "Dermatomyositis." Credit: Elizabeth M. Dugan, Adam M. Huber, Frederick W. Miller, Lisa G. Rider (Creative Commons Attribution-Share Alike 3.0 Unported license).
- "Cerebral melanoma metastasis in the left frontal lobe." Credit: Dr Laughlin Dawes (Creative Commons Attribution 3.0 Unported license).
- "KF ring and Sunflower cataract." Credit: Imrankabirhossain (Creative Commons Attribution-Share Alike 4.0 International license).

- "Toxoplasmic Encephalitis in an AIDS Patient with Normal CD4 Count: A Case Report" Credit: Eissa Soleymani et al © Iranian Society of Parasitology & Tehran University of Medical Sciences (Creative Commons Attribution license).
- "Volume rendered CT angiography of posterior communicating artery aneurysm." Credit: Shazia Mirza and Sankalp Gokhale (Creative Commons Attribution 4.0 International license).
- "Pineocytoma, MRI T1 with contrast, axial." Credit: Tdvorak (Creative Commons Attribution-Share Alike 1.0 Generic license).
- "Patient with facial angiofibromas caused by tuberous sclerosis." Credit: Herbert L. Fred, MD and Hendrik A. van Dijk (Creative Commons Attribution-Share Alike 3.0 Unported license).

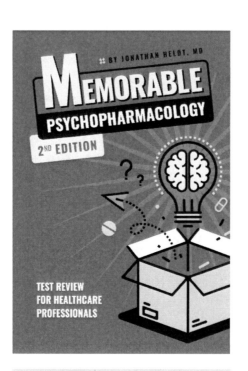
BY JONATHAN HELDT, MD
MEMORABLE
PSYCHOPHARMACOLOGY
2ND EDITION
TEST REVIEW
FOR HEALTHCARE
PROFESSIONALS

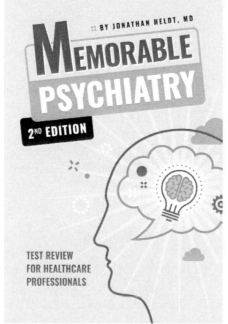
BY JONATHAN HELDT, MD
MEMORABLE
PSYCHIATRY
2ND EDITION
TEST REVIEW
FOR HEALTHCARE
PROFESSIONALS

INTERESTED IN LEARNING MORE?

Get ***Memorable Psychopharmacology*** and ***Memorable Neurology***, both available now from the same author!

Memorable Psychopharmacology

Now that you have the information needed to approach psychiatric diagnosis, take your learning to the next step by understanding the evidence behind the treatment of these disorders! ***Memorable Psychopharmacology*** uses a conversational tone, catchy mnemonics, visual aids, and practice questions to ensure that you not only learn the material but retain it far into the future. For anyone preparing to meet the mental health needs of their patients, ***Memorable Psychopharmacology*** is an indispensable review.

Memorable Psychiatry

The best and most effective way to learn about psychiatry! ***Memorable Psychiatry*** breaks down the complex but fascinating world of mental health using simple explanations, frequent mnemonics, visual aids, and a focus on mechanisms over memorization to catch you up to speed and put you ahead of the curve on the art and science of psychiatric diagnosis.

BOTH AVAILABLE NOW ON AMAZON.COM!

ABOUT THE AUTHOR

Jonathan Heldt is currently on faculty at the UCLA Semel Institute for Neuroscience & Human Behavior. He completed his Bachelor's degree in Biochemistry at Pacific Union College, his medical degree at the Loma Linda University School of Medicine, and his residency at the UCLA Psychiatry Residency Training Program. He is interested in both mental health and medical education and hopes that this book will inspire these interests in others. He has no conflicts of interest to disclose.

For questions, comments, and updates, please visit ***memorablepsych.com*** *or email* ***memorablepsych@gmail.com***.

Memorable Neurology by Jonathan Heldt

The Nervous System

Organization

Brain = Capital city
Brainstem = Bridge
Spinal cord = Highway
Peripheral nerves = Side streets

Neuron Types

Afferent =
Ascend to **A**lert the brain (sensory)
e**F**ferent =
Flow down to e**F**fect change (motor)

Sensory Neurons

Protopathic ("primitive")
Non-discriminative touch, **P**ain, **T**emperature

Epicritic ("snobby")
Fine touch, **V**ibration, **P**roprioception

Glial Cells

Ol-**egg**-odendrocytes.myelinate in CNS
Sch-wann cells myelinate in PNS
(wann cell at a time)
Astro-cytes & **satellite** cells in **space** between neurons
E-**pen**-dyma dipped in (cerebrospinal) **fluid**

Autonomic Nervous System

Sympathetic
"Fight or flight"

Parasympathetic
"Feed and breed, then rest and digest"

Muscarinic effects = SLUDG-E BM:
Salivation
Lacrimation
Urination
Diaphoresis
Gastrointestinal hypermotility
Emesis
Bradycardia
Miosis

Nicotinic receptors = **Nic's muscle memory**

Cerebral Cortex

Lobes of the Brain

FPOT:
Frontal = Executive function, Motor (in the front like a **car**)
Parietal = Sensory (**pariah**-tal)
Occipital = Vision (bin**oc**ulars)
Temporal = Sound (hear music's **tempo**)

Language Centers

Broca's = expressive (**broken** pull string doll **won't talk**)
Wernicke's = receptive (can't listen but can still be quite **Wer**-dy)
Arcuate fasciculus = conduction (need **accurate** fasciculus to **accurately** repeat)

Limbic System

Emo-gdala involved in **emo**-tions
You would **remember** a "**hippo** on **campus**"
Mammillary bodies for **mam**ory formation
Anterior **c**ingulate **c**ortex = error recognition ("**Acc**!")
Nucleus **accum**bens = **accum**ulate money and other rewards

Cerebral Subcortex

Thalamus

Thalamus = **th**en**th**ory
Ventral **P**ostero**L**ateral nucleus = **V**ery **P**ainful **L**imbs
Ventral **P**ostero**M**edial nucleus = **V**ery **P**ainful **M**outh
Lateral **G**eniculate **N**ucleus = **L**ooking **G**ood **N**aked (visual)
Medial **G**eniculate **N**ucleus = **M**aking **G**reat **N**oise (auditory)

Epithalamus

Epi**thalamus** contains **pi**neal gland
Parinaud's = **peerin' odd**

Hypothalamus

6 H's of the **H**ypothalamus
Hot (temperature regulation)
Hungry (food intake)
Hourly (circadian rhythm)
Hydrated (water balance)
Horny (reproduction)
Hormonal (hormone release)

Anterior Pituitary Hormones = FLAT PiG:
Follicle-stimulating hormone (FSH)
Luteinizing hormone (LH)
Adrenocorticotropic hormone (ACTH)
Thyroid-stimulating hormone (TSH)
Prolactin
Growth hormone (GH)

Hypothalamic Nuclei

Anterior = **C**ooling (**A/C** = **A**ir **C**onditioning)
Posterior = **H**eating ("Got a **hot posterior**!")

Lateral = hunger (make you **fatter**-al)
Ventro-**meal** = satiety (make you feel **full**)

Supra-**chiasmatic** = sleep (need sleep to be **charismatic**).

Supra-optic = fluid balance (**look above** at clouds to see if it's going to rain)

Para**V**entricular **N**ucleus = reproduction (**Par**ental **V**iewing is **N**eeded)

The Basal Ganglia and Internal Capsule

Basal Ganglia

Basal **gangli**a prevent **gangly** movement

Direct pathway **C**omes **S**traight **I**nto the **T**halamus = **C**ortex → **S**triatum → **I**nternal GP → **T**halamus

Indirect pathway **C**omes **S**traight, **E**xits, then **S**idesteps **I**nto the **T**halamus = **C**ortex → **S**triatum → **E**xternal GP → **S**TN → **I**nternal GP → **T**halamus

Components of the Basal Ganglia

Caudate nucleus = most **cau**gnitive part
Put-am-en = exclusively **motor** ("**put-an-M**" for Motor)
"**Slow bus**" pallidus = inhibitory (**slows**)
Subthalamic **N**ucleus = hemi**ball**ismus (**S**unday **N**ight football)
Nigro**S**triatal **P**athway = i**N**voluntary movement like **S**tuttering and **P**arkinson's

Internal Capsule

Posterior **L**imb of the **I**nternal **C**apsul**e** (**PoLICe**) = corticospinal tract (bypasses the basal ganglia)

Genu contains corticobulbar tract (**geni**us with an idea in their **cranium** = light **bulb!**)

The Cerebellum

Lobes of the Cerebellum

Anterior & posterior = body
Vermis = middle (trunk)
Lateral = sides (limbs)

Flocculonodular = eyes (**flock** of **see**-gulls)

Cerebellar Peduncles

Superior **C**erebellar **P**eduncle = **S**ends **C**rossed **P**athways

Middle = receives from pons

Inferior = receives from spinal cord

Ipsilateral deficits (cerebellum is a **dirty double crosser**!)

Cerebellar Signs (Ataxia)

Dizzy AUNT with **3 dishes**:
Dizziness
Ambulation
Unsteadiness
Nystagmus
Tremor
Dysdiadochokinesia, **D**ysarthria, and **D**ysmetria

Memorable Neurology by Jonathan Heldt

Brainstem

General Functions

Brainstem Can Do It All:
Bridge between brain and spinal cord
Cranial nerves
Distinct functions
Integral functions
Arousal (re-**tickler** formation)

Rule of 4 for Cranial Nerves

First 4 (1-4) exit from **brain & midbrain**
Middle 4 (5-8) exit from **pons**
Last 4 (9-12) exit from **medulla**

Midbrain & Pons

IMPRESSV:
Inferior colliculi
Medial longitudinal fasciculus
Periaqueductal grey
Red nuclei
Eye movement cranial nerves
Substantia nigra
Superior colliculi
Ventral tegmental area

PONS:
Pneumotaxic and apneustic centers
Ocular movements
Neurotransmitter production
Sound (superior olivary nuclei & lateral lemniscus)

Medulla

SCARPH:
Nucleus Solitarius (**sole-lick**-tarius = taste makes you gag, HR & BP increase)
Crossing of motor and epicritic pathways
Nucleus Ambiguus (ambig-**uh**-**uh**'s = speech)
Respiratory center
Area Postrema ("p.o. streamer")
Heart (cardiovascular) center (gold **medul** placed over heart and lungs)

The Spinal Cord

Corticospinal Tract

Flexing Involves Pyramids, Cords, & Horns:
Frontal lobe
Internal capsule
Pyramidal decussation
Corticospinal tract
Anterior Horn

All 3 tracts have legs lateral and arms medial *except* dorsal column—**medial leg**-niscus pathway!

Dorsal Column—Medial Lemniscus Pathway

Discover New Directions for Moving Vibration & Proprioception:
Dorsal columns
Nucleus gracilis & nucleus cuneatus ("**walk gracefully** and **eat** with your **hands**")
Decussation
Medial lemniscus
Ventral posterolateral nucleus (thalamus)
Parietal lobe

Fine touch, Vibration, Proprioception = Feeling Very Patient (wait to cross)

Spinothalamic Tract

List Some Proper Avenues for Sending Temperature & Pain:
Lissauer's (posterolateral) tract
Substantia gelatinosa and nucleus Proprius
Anterior white commissure
Spinothalamic tract
Thalamus
Parietal lobe

Non-discriminative touch, Temperature, Pain = Not That Patient (cross immediately)

Spinal Cord Pathology

Anterior cord = motor ×, protopathic ×, epicritic ✓

Posterior cord = motor ✓, protopathic ✓, epicritic ×

Brown-Séquard = ipsilateral motor & epicritic, contralateral protopathic (BackStabs but only **halfway**)

Central cord = motor × (arms affected > legs)
Ex: **syringomyelia** = "see-him-go-fly"-lia (superhero = **cape-like** distribution)

Subacute combined degeneration = dorsal columns × & corticospinal tract × (lack of B**12** → not **1** but **2** forms of injury!)

Cauda equina syndrome = **horse**'s tail (**saddle** distribution)

The Peripheral Nervous System

Cranial Nerves

Ooh, Ooh, Ooh, To Touch And Feel Very Green Vegetables, **AH!**:
Olfactory
Optic
Oculomotor
Trochlear
Trigeminal
Abducens
Facial
Vestibulocochlear
Glossopharyngeal
Vagus
Accessory
Hypoglossal

Cranial Nerve Types

Some Say Marry Money But My Brother Says Big Brains Matter More:
Sensory (olfactory)
Sensory (optic)
Motor (oculomotor)
Motor (trochlear)
Both (trigeminal)
Motor (abducens)
Both (facial)
Sensory (vestibulocochlear)
Both (glossopharyngeal)
Both (vagus)
Motor (accessory)
Motor

Specific Cranial and Spinal Nerves

LR_6SO_4 = Lateral Rectus 6th, Superior Oblique 4th cranial nerve (everything else is 3rd!)

Bell's palsy = **Bell**-lateral face symmetry lost

VEGAS = Vital signs, Entire body, Gag reflex, Autonomics, Speaking and swallowing

"**C3, 4, and 5** keep the **diaphragm** alive."

Dermatomal Landmarks

T4 = **Teat pore**
T10 = Belly but-**ten**
L1 = **1**nguinal **L**igament
L4 = down on **all fours** (L4s) = knee

Vision

Visual Pathway

2 Charismatic Travelers Looking Good Naked at the **Radia**nt **Oc**ean:
Optic nerve (Cranial nerve **2**)
Optic **Chiasm**
Optic **Tract**
Lateral **G**eniculate **N**ucleus (thalamus)
Optic **Radia**tions
Occipital cortex (damage to the **back** leads to sparing of the **mac**!)

Extraocular Movements

Oculomotor palsy = "**down and out**"
OOMMPP: OculOmotor = Motor Middle, Pupils Periphery
Trochlear palsy = "**up and in**"
Abducens palsy = can't look to the side

Medial Longitudinal Fasciculus + InterNuclear Ophthalmoplegia = Midline Look Fails Ipsilaterally, Nystagmus Opposite

Pupillary Reflexes

2 priests educated 3 cili (silly) **pupils**:
Optic nerve (cranial nerve **2**)
Pretectal nucleus
Edinger-Westphal nuclei ("**EW!** I don't want to look at that...")
Oculomotor nerve (cranial nerve **3**)
Ciliary sphincter → **pupil**lary constriction

Argyll Robertson = Accommodate, not Reac

Memorable Neurology by Jonathan Heldt

Hearing, Balance, Taste, and Smell

Auditory Pathway

8 Cocky SONs Laughing **'N M**aking **G**reat **N**oise in the **Te**nt:
Vestibulocochlear nerve (CN **8**)
Cochlear nucleus
Superior **O**livary **N**uclei
Lateral lemniscus
i**N**ferior colliculus
Medial **G**eniculate **N**ucleus (thalamus)
Temporal cortex

Tests of Hearing

Weber = symmetry (**W** is a symmetric letter)
Rinne = damage is on the **R**ight or left

MAN BBC GAS:
Midline + **A**ir>Bone = **N**ormal
Bad ear + **B**one>Air = **C**onductive
Good ear + **A**ir>Bone = **S**ensorineural

Balance

3 semicircular canals & 2 otoliths
Utricle = horizontal
Saccule = vertical (drop it like a **sack** of potatoes)

Taste

Anterior 2/3 = facial nerve (make a face)
Posterior 1/3 = glossopharyngeal nerve (gag)

The Meninges, Ventricles, and Blood Supply

Ventricular System

CSF is **LIT AF**:
Choroid plexuses
Lateral ventricle
Interventricular foramina
Third ventricle
Cerebral **A**queduct
Fourth ventricle

Anterior Circulation

Draw **circle** from bottom using word **WILLI** w/
W = **Posterior** cerebral arteries
I = **Middle** cerebral arteries
L = **Anterior** cerebral arteries

Meninges

PAD:
Pia → **A**rachnoid → **D**ura (in to out)

Posterior Circulation

Draw **stick figure** w/
Head = **Circle of Willis**
Neck = **Basilar** artery
Arms = **Ant. inferior cerebellar** arteries
Legs = **Vertebral** arteries
Endowment = **Anterior spinal** artery

Venous Drainage

Draw **VEIN**, then fill w/ "**S**uper **I**cy **S**hower **O**f **C**a**TS** & **C**anine **Pet**s":
(1) **S**uperior sagittal, (2) **I**nferior sagittal → **S**traight, (3) **O**ccipital
Confluence → **T**ransverse → **S**igmoid
Cavernous → **Pet**rosal
i**N**ternal jugular vein

N

Cavernous Sinus

Tom COAT:
Trigeminal nerve (**o**phthalmic & **m**axillary)
Internal **C**arotid artery
Oculomotor, **A**bducens, & **T**rochlear nerves

The Neurological Exam

Exam Elements

"Head and hammer, feet like tots
Bulk and tone, pretend we fought
Stroking, poking, shaking, hot
Touch my finger, stand and walk!"

Head = **cranial nerves**, **mental status**
Hammer = **reflexes**
Feet like tots = **primitive reflexes**
Bulk & tone, pretend we fought = **motor**
Stroking, poking, shaking, hot = **sensory**
Touch my finger = **coordination**
Stand & walk = **Romberg**, **gait**

Reflexes

Draw **stick figures** w/
6s for arms = **biceps** (C5-C**6**)
7s for arms = **triceps** (C6-C**7**)
2 Ls for legs = kneeling or on **L4**s (L2-L4)
Ach-**I**-**II**-e**S** reflex (S**1**-S**2**)

Babinski sign = only normal in **Babi**s

Neuroimaging

CT = like a **C**a**T** (quick but harmful)

MRIs = **M**ake **R**ealistic **I**mages, but the patient **M**ust **R**emain **I**dle

Lumbar Puncture

LP in **L3**!

C (see) **FIRST**:
Central nervous system disease
Focal neurologic deficits
Immunocompromised
Raised intracranial pressure
Seizures (new-onset or unexplained)
Thinking unclear

Strokes

Diagnosis

BE FAST:
Balance
Eyes/vision
Face droop
Arm/leg weakness
Speech
Timing (sudden)

Treatment

Hemorrhagic:
No treatment available

Ischemic:
tPA within 3h ("Where's -teplase tPA?!")

Risk Factors

DASHCAM:
Diabetes
Atrial fibrillation
Smoking
Hypertension
Cholesterol
Age
Male

Cortical Strokes

Anterior vs Middle vs Posterior:
Draw a **stick** figure w/
A = **legs** (lower body)
M = **arms** (upper body)
P = glasses (**eyes**)

Left PCA = **alexia w/o agraphia** (can't read letters if **post** office workers have **left** for the day!)

Lacunar Strokes

Pure **motor** = post. limb internal capsule
Pure **sensory** = thalamus
Sensorimotor = internal capsule + thalamus

Brainstem Strokes

Crossed findings = **B**rain**S**tem stroke!
(Crossed fingers = **BS** promise)

4 Medial structures:
Motor pathway
Medial lemniscus
Medial longitudinal fasciculus
Motor component of cranial nerves

4 Side structures:
Spinocerebellar pathway
Spinothalamic tract
Sympathetic pathway
Sensory nuclei of trigeminal nerve

Brainstem Strokes

Medial **M**edullary = **M**cDonald's (eating w/ **tongue**, **arch**-shaped **ant. spinal artery**)

Lateral medullary = **PICA-chew** (**P**osterior **I**nf. **C**erebellar **A**rtery stroke → can't **chew**)

Lateral pontine = **A**nterior **I**nferior **C**erebellar **A**rtery stroke → ↓ f**AICA**l sensation

Medial pontine = facial asymmetry, INO (branches off **base** → problems in **face**)

Midbrain = Weber syndrome (spider **web** in **eye** = eyelid shut, move ipsilat. arm but leave contra. arm still)

Locked in = entire basilar artery

Memorable Neurology by Jonathan Heldt

Intracranial Hypertension

Signs and Symptoms

General: HA, N/V, confusion, papilledema
Cushing's triad: **I**ntra**C**ranial **P**ressure → **I**rregular **I**nspirations, **C**rawling **C**ardiac, & **P**ushed up blood **P**ressure

Hydrocephalus

Obstructive (upstream, use "CSF LIT AF")
Communicating (all ventricles)
NPH = **DIG** (**D**ementia, **I**ncontinence, **G**ait)
Ex vacuo = Alzheimer's (not real hydro)

Intracranial Bleeds

Epidural = **epic M**ixed **M**artial **A**rts (**M**iddle **M**eningeal **A**rtery) match (head trauma)
Subdural = **Sub** under **bridge** (bridging veins) w/ **crescent** moon (shape on CT) to **slowly sneak up** on its target (slow onset)
SAH = **CT HEAD**: **C**onsciousness, **T**hunderclap headache, **H**urt neck, **E**xertional, **A**ge 40+, **D**ecreased neck flexion
Intracerebral = based on location
Pontine hemorrhages = **pin**point **pup**ils

Brain Herniation

Sub-**falcon**: **CAN**-ary in a coal mine = **C**ingulate cortex & **AN**terior cerebral a.
Transtentorial: **Uncle CHIP**, the **Third** = **Uncal** herniation → **C**ontralateral **H**emianopsia, **I**psilateral **P**aralysis (2/2 Kernohan's notch), CN**3** palsy
Thentral = all **three** **th**alami involved
Upward = basically same as central
Tonsillar = thru foramen magnum
Transcalvarial = thru skull (injury, surgery

Motor Diseases

Muscular Dystrophy

Duchenne's = **do shins** (calf hypertrophy)
Becker's = like Duchenne's w/ ↑ prognosis
Myotonic = "It's **my otonic dystrophy**!" (trouble **letting go**)

Inflammatory Myopathies

Polly-myositis = **Polly** wants cracker but **can't get up** so is stuck **inside**
Derm-**out**-omyositis = **out**side (skin) & **out**side muscle fibers (on biopsy)
Inclusion **B**ody **M**yositis = **older man** typing on **IBM** using **finger flexors**

Neuromuscular Junction Diseases

Myasthenia gravi-**T**: nico-**T**-inic, **T**op down, fa-**T**-iguing, **T**ensilon test, **T**hymoma, **T**reatable
ROBOT-ulism = **R**apid onset, **O**xygen, **B**abies, **O**pen wounds, **T**op down,
Legbert eatin' **small**, **dry pre**tzels (**leg** paralysis, **small**-cell lung cancer, **dry** mouth, **pre**-synaptic antibodies)
Bea**T** (**B**otulism, **T**etanus) on **SNARE** drum
Tetanus = **on** beat
Botulism = **off** beat

Motor Neuron Diseases

Amyotrophic **L**atera**L** sclerosis = **ALL** over the place (both UMN & LMN)
Primary **L**atera**L** sclerosis = **P**u**LL-up** (**up**per MN, moves **up** the body)
PRogr**ESS**ive musc. atrophy = **PRESS-dow** (**lower** motor neuron)
Ps**EU**dobulbar = **E**motional incontinence & **U**pper motor neurons
Pole-io = can't **pole** vault
SMALL = **S**pinal **M**uscular **A**trophy affects **L**ower MN in **L**ittle babies
Werdnig-H**offman**n = baby looks **off man**

Movement Disorders

Parkinson's Disease

Parkinson's **D**isease = do**Pa**mine **D**epleted

TRAPped inside of a statue:
Tremor
Rigidity
Akinesia/bradykinesia
Postural instability

Tx: **Car**bidopa is the **car** that drives levodopa to its destination (the brain)

Parkinson-Plus Syndromes

Multi**S**ystem **A**trophy = **M**issing **S**table **A**utonomics
Progressive **S**upranuclear **P**alsy = **P**lease **S**top **P**eering (**looks down**)
Cortico**B**asilar **D**egeneration = **C**ontrolled **B**y **D**eep space (alien hand)

Tremor

PAIR of tremulous hands = **P**hysiologic, **A**ction, **I**ntention, **R**esting

Hyperkinetic Movement Disorders

"You **caun't date** (caudate) **Huntington's daughter**! Her **father** is very (autosoma **dominant**. He'll hunt **4** you and put you in a **CAGe** (CAG repeat, chromosome 4).

WILSON's disease = **I**nherited, **L**iver disea **S**erum (↑ copper, ↓ ceruloplasmin), **O**cular (Kayser-Fleischer rings), **N**eurologic (movement disorders)

Seizures

Generalized Seizures

General McTATA:
Myo**c**lonic (my-old-clinic = bunch of jerks)
Tonic-clonic (town-ic = stiff, clown-ic = shaking)
Atonic (**ate**-onic, like someone "ate it")
Tonic
Absence (of mind, motor, postictal period)

Focal Seizures

Impaired-awareness (complex partial)
Aware seizures (simple partial)

Epilepsy Syndromes

Temporal lobe = memory, mood, halluc.
Frontal lobe = abnormal movements
Benign Rolandic = **FAST ROLL**: **F**ocal **A**ware **S**eizures **T**hat **R**arely **O**utlast **L**ater **L**ife
Roll-andic = centrotempo-**Roll** spikes
Juvenile myoclonic = bunch of jerks
Absence = **absent** from school (beach day) to play volleyball ("**Spike**!") & surf the **waves**
Tx: etho-**sucks-the-mind**
Lennox-**G**astaut **S**yndrome = **L**e**G**S & **ARMS**: **A**ll seizure types, **R**esistant to treatment, **M**ental disabilities, **S**low spike-and-wave

Psychogenic Non-epileptic Seizures

2 minute RAGES:
2+ minutes
Recall
Asynchronous movement
Gradual onset
Eyes (closed or crying)
Side-to-side head shaking

Structured Evaluation of Seizures

CAPPELLA = **C**onsciousness, **A**ctivity, **P**ostictal state, **P**rovoked, **E**EG, **L**ocalizi sx, **L**abs and imaging, **A**ge of onset

Neoplasms

Adult Neoplasms (Supratentorial)

Glio**Blast**oma **M**ultiforme = **blasting off** (fast), **G**FAP+, **B**utterfly glioma, **M**en
Meningioma = (**psam**moma bodies, **Ben**ign prognosis, prefers women)
Schw-one-omas = **Schw-100** (S-100+)
Ol-**egg**-odendroglima = **fried egg** cells, **chicken wire** capillaries, seizures
Pituitary adenoma = **G**o **L**ook **F**or **T**he **A**denoma **P**lease (**G**H > **L**H > **F**SH > **T**SH > **A**CTH > **P**rolactin)

Pediatric Neoplasms (Infratentorial)

Pilocytic astrocytoma = **pile o' roses enthralls** children (**Rosenthal** fibers)
Medusa-blastomas (**stone**-like tumor, "**drop metastasis**," **dangerous**, **cut open** quickly!
Ependymomas = **pretendy-rosas** (**pseudo-rosettes**)
He-Man(glioblastoma) = **red-blooded** male
Craniopharyngioma = child afraid of rat bite (**Rat**hke's pouch, **bite**-temporal hemianopsia, **calcified** teeth, good prognosis)

Brain Tumors

S/Sx: headaches,seizures, papilledema
Tx: surgery, radiation, and/or chemo
Adults = **supra**tentorial
Children = **infra**tentorial
(Adults protect children **under the tent**)

Brain Metastasis

Lotsa **B**ad **S**tuff **C**an **K**ill:
Lung > **B**reast > **S**kin > **C**olon > **K**idney

Memorable Neurology by Jonathan Heldt

Infections

Meningitis

S/Sx: Fever, headache, neck stiffness
Ker**n**ig = pain on **Kn**ee extension
Br**u**dzinski = pain on **B**rain flexion
Bacterial/fungal LP findings = **strong** (high protein), **high pressure** (↑ opening pressure), **not sweet** (low glucose)
Back i**N** the **Fun Limo**: **Bac**terial = **N**eutrophils, **Fun**gal = **Lym**ph**o**cytes

Fungal Meningitis

Crypto-**caca** neoformans (pigeon **poop**)
Coccidioides immitis (SW USA)
O-HIst**O**plasma (Midwest USA)
Blastomyces dermatitidis (Midwest USA)

Viral Meningitis

Enteroviruses, herpes simplex
Better prognosis
Tx: supportive care

Bacterial Meningitis

Infants = **GEL**:
Group **B** **S**trep (**G**iving **B**aby a **S**urprise)
E. coli (K-one heads = K-1 antigen)
Listeria

Children/adults = **HeNS**:
H. influenzae
Neisseria meningitides (**Water**house-Friderichsen = adrenal insufficiency → **fluid** balance)
Streptococcus pneumoniae

Tx: **cephalo**sporins to get into the **head** plus others to cover **LAME** organisms

Parasitic Encephalitis

T**OXO**plamosis (O's ring-enhancing lesions)
Cysticercosis (T. solium, tapeworm in pigs)

Viral Encephalitis

Herpes (**herpe-campus** in temporal lobe)
Rabies = FINISH: **F**atal w/o treatment, **I**ncubation period, **N**egri bodies, Tx=**I**mmunization, **S**alivary glands, **H**ydrophobia
Ar-bo-viruses (**ar**thropod-**bo**rne)
SSPE = years after measles (**SS**ss…**P**p**E**ee!)
Primary CNS lymphoma (Epstein-Barr virus)

Bacterial Encephalitis

Syphilis = **PARESIS**: **P**ersonality Δ, **A**ffect Δ, ↑ **R**eflexes, **E**yes (Argyll-Robertson), **S**ensorium Δ, **I**ntellect ↓, **S**peech slurred

Prion Disease

Prions = **Pro**tein **in**fecti**on**s (e.g. mad cow)

Other Neurologic Diseases

Peripheral Neuropathy

Causes = **GOSH DARNED PAIN**:
Genetic, **O**ncologic, **S**ugars (diabetes), **H**ematologic, **D**rugs, **A**lcohol, **R**heumatologic, **N**ephrogenic, **E**nvironmental, **D**iet, **P**hysical injury, **A**utoimmune, **I**nfectious, **N**o cause

Lyme disease = **B-lime**y (**B**ell's palsy, "**B**ull's eye" rash)
Shingles (**dermatomal** distribution!)
Leprosy (loss of **pain** sensation)
Trigeminal neuralgia (very **painful**)
Shark-o-Marie-Tooth = **arched feet** (like a **shark** bite)
Fried rich ataxia = **GAA GAA** for **CANDI**: **C**ardiomyopathy, **A**taxia, **N**europathy, **D**iabetes, **I**rregular anatomy
GAA repeat on chromosome 9
Porphyrias = **4 Ps**: **P**olyneuropathy, abd **P**ain, **P**sych sx, **P**urple urine

Demyelinating Diseases

Multi-pool sclerosis = in and out of "**pools**" (disseminated in time & space)
Oligoclonal bands = **oligo**dendrocyte damage
Tx: g-**ladder**-amer acetate (get out of pool), interferons, steroids (acute)

Narrow-myelitis optica = **narrow** (eyes & spinal cord only)

ADEM's **APPLE** = **A**utoimmune **P**ost-infectious **P**ediatric **L**ife-threatening **E**vent (one-time)

Progressive **M**ultifocal **L**eukoencephalopathy = **P**u**M**me**L** (HIV+, poor prognosis)

Guillain–**Bare**-é leaves peripheral nerves **bare** **Camp**ing in **Jun**e (**Camp**ylobacter je**jun**i) w/ ripe **berries** (Guillain-**Berry** syndrome)
CIDP = chronic version of Guillain–Barré

Headache

Tension (bilateral, band-like, ~hours, stress)
Migraine = **POUND** (**P**ulsatile, h**O**urs, **U**nilateral, **N**ausea, **D**isabling)
CLUSTER (**C**onjunctival injection, **L**acrimation, **U**nilateral, **S**peedy, **T**reatable, **E**yelid drooping, **R**ecurrent)

Secondary headaches = **PAID 40 TAXMEN**:
Papilledema
Abrupt
Immunosuppressed
Different than before
40 years or older
Trauma
Altered mental status
e**X**ertional
Morbid
Escalating
Neurologic s/sx

Headache Syndromes

Giant-cell arteritis = **TEMPL3**:
Temporal artery tenderness/weak pulse
ESR ↑
Mononuclear infiltrates and/or **M**ultinucleate giant cells on biopsy
Painful new-onset localized headache
Late in life onset (50+)
3 or more of these

Idiopathic intracranial hypertension = **HAPY NOW** (**H**eadaches **A**nd **P**apilledema in a **Y**oung, **N**ormal, **O**bese **W**oman)

Neurocutaneous Disorders

Neurofibromatosis Type I = **CAFÉ SPOT**:
Café-au-lait spots
Axillary/inguinal freckling
Fibromas
Eye hamartomas (Lisch nodules)
Skeletal deformities
Passed down from parents
Optic nerve **T**umor

Neurofibromatosis Type II = **MISME**:
Multiple **I**nherited **S**chwannomas, **M**eningiomas, **E**pendymomas
2 = **bi**lateral schwannomas, chromosome **22**, begins age **20**

Tuberous sclerosis = I ♥ TUBERS:
Intellectual disability
♥ (cardiac rhabdomyomas)
Multiple benign **TU**mors
Brain tumors
Epilepsy
Renal angiomyolipomas
Skin (ash leaf spots, facial angiofibromas)

Neurocutaneous Disorders (cont.))

STURGE-Weber syndrome:
Port-wine **S**tains
Tumors (angiomas)
Unilateral muscle weakness
Mental **R**etardation (intellectual disability)
Glaucoma
Epilepsy

von **HARP**el—Lindau disease:
Hemangioblastomas
Angiomatosis
Renal cell carcinomas
Pheochromocytomas

Attacks-ya-telangiectasia = **Repair IT**:
Defect of DNA **repair**
Immunodeficiency
Tumors

Made in United States
North Haven, CT
22 October 2021

10490073R00251